Manual of Toxicologic Emergencies

Manual of Toxicologic Emergencies

EDITORS

ERIC K. NOJI, M.D., M.P.H., F.A.C.E.P.
Assistant Professor of Emergency Medicine
The Johns Hopkins Hospital and School of
    Medicine
Baltimore, Maryland

GABOR D. KELEN, M.D., F.R.C.P., F.A.C.E.P.
Assistant Professor of Emergency Medicine
Residency Director
Director of Research
Department of Emergency Medicine
The Johns Hopkins Hospital and School of
    Medicine
Baltimore, Maryland

ASSISTANT EDITOR

Tracy K. Goessel, M.D.
Assistant Professor of Emergency Medicine
The Johns Hopkins Hospital
Baltimore, Maryland

YEAR BOOK MEDICAL PUBLISHERS, INC.
Chicago • London • Boca Raton

1   2   3   4   5   6   7   8   9   0   CY   93   92   91   90   89

Library of Congress Cataloging-in-Publication Data

Manual of toxicologic emergencies.
   Includes bibliographies and index.
   1. Toxicologic emergencies—Handbooks, manuals, etc.   I. Noji, Eric K.   II. Kelen, Gabor D.   [DNLM: 1. Emergencies. 2. Poisoning.   QV 600 M294]
RA1224.5.M36   1989   615.9′08   88-33868
ISBN 0-8151-6450-5

Sponsoring Editor: David K. Marshall
Associate Managing Editor, Manuscript Services: Deborah Thorp
Copyeditor: Jan Gardner
Production Project Manager: Max Perez
Proofroom Manager: Shirley E. Taylor

To Pam and Laurie

Contributors

E. JACKSON ALLISON, JR., M.D.,
M.P.H., F.A.C.E.P.
Professor and Chairman
Department of Emergency Medicine
East Carolina University School of
Medicine
Chief-of-Service
Emergency Department
Pitt County Memorial Hospital
Greenville, North Carolina

JAMES L. BAKER, M.D., F.A.C.E.P.
Assistant Professor of Emergency
Medicine
The Johns Hopkins University School
of Medicine
The Johns Hopkins Hospital
Baltimore, Maryland

M. DOUGLAS BAKER, M.D.
Assistant Professor of Pediatrics
The University of Pennsylvania School
of Medicine
Attending Physician
Emergency Department
The Children's Hospital of
Philadelphia
Philadelphia, Pennsylvania

RICHARD M. CANTOR, M.D.
Assistant Professor
Department of Critical Care and
Emergency Medicine
University Hospital SUNY Health
Science Center
Syracuse, New York

JULIE A. P. CASANI, M.D.
Assistant Professor
Emergency Medicine
The Johns Hopkins University
Attending Physician
Francis Scott Key Medical Center
Baltimore, Maryland

DONALD R. CHABOT, M.D.
Instructor in Medicine and Surgery
Harvard Medical School
Assistant Physician
Massachusetts General Hospital
Boston, Massachusetts

RICHARD A. CHRISTOPH, M.D.,
F.A.C.E.P.
Assistant Professor of Internal
Medicine and Surgery
University of Virginia School of
Medicine
University of Virginia Prehospital
Program Director
University of Virginia Medical Center
Charlottesville, Virginia

ROBIN M. CUDDY, M.D.
Assistant Professor
The Johns Hopkins School of Medicine
The Johns Hopkins Hospital
Baltimore, Maryland

J. WARD DONOVAN, M.D.,
F.A.C.E.P.
Assistant Professor of Medicine
Pennsylvania State University College
of Medicine

Director, Capital Area Poison Center
University Hospital
M.S. Hershey Medical Center
Hershey, Pennsylvania

MARY L. DUNNE, M.D.
Attending Emergency Physician
St. Francis Hospital
Poughkeepsie, New York

LUIS F. ELJAIEK JR., M.D.
Attending Emergency Physician
Fairfax Hospital
Falls Church, Virginia

WILLIAM P. FABBRI, M.D.,
F.A.C.E.P.
Assistant Professor of Emergency
  Medicine
The Johns Hopkins University School
  of Medicine
Attending Staff Physician
Francis Scott Key Medical Center
Baltimore, Maryland

DOUGLAS J. FLOCCARE, M.D.
Instructor, Emergency Medicine
The Johns Hopkins University School
  of Medicine
Assistant Chief of Service, Emergency
  Medicine
The Johns Hopkins Medical
  Institutions
Baltimore, Maryland

PATRICIA D. FOSARELLI, M.D.
Assistant Professor of Pediatrics
The Johns Hopkins Medical
  Institutions
Baltimore, Maryland

STUART R. FRITZ, M.D.
Clinical Instructor
Department of Family Practice
University of Minnesota Emergency
  Physicians Professional Association
Minneapolis, Minnesota

TRACEY K. GOESSEL, M.D.
Assistant Professor of Emergency
  Medicine
The Johns Hopkins Hospital
Baltimore, Maryland

THOMAS P. GROSS, M.D.
Attending Physician
Emergency Department
Bartlett Hospital
Juneau, Alaska

J. STEPHEN HUFF, M.D.
Assistant Professor
Division of Emergency Medicine
Eastern Virginia Graduate School of
  Medicine
Staff Physician
Medical Center Hospital
Norfolk, Virginia

MICHAEL S. JASTREMSKI, M.D.
Associate Professor
SUNY Health Science Center
Director, Critical Care and Emergency
  Medicine Departments
University Hospital
Syracuse, New York

JOHN G. KEENE, M.D., F.A.C.E.P.
Director, Department of Emergency
  Medicine
St. Francis Hospital
Poughkeepsie, New York

GABOR D. KELEN, M.D., F.R.C.P.,
F.A.C.E.P.
Assistant Professor of Emergency
  Medicine
Residency Director
Director of Research
Department of Emergency Medicine
The Johns Hopkins Hospital and
  School of Medicine
Baltimore, Maryland

CHRISTOPHER J. KNUTH, M.D.
Clinical Instructor of Emergency
  Medicine
Department of Trauma and
  Emergency Medicine
Medical College of Wisconsin
Milwaukee, Wisconsin
Medical Director
Emergency Department
St. Mary's Hospital
Port Washington, Wisconsin

JORDAN M. LAUB, M.D.
Attending Emergency Physician
Holy Cross Hospital
Silver Spring, Maryland

LOUIS J. LING, M.D., F.A.C.E.P.
Medical Director
Hennepin Regional Poison Center
Assistant Residency Director
Department of Emergency Medicine
Hennepin County Medical Center
Minneapolis, Minnesota

CELESTE M. MADDEN, M.D.
Assistant Professor
Departments of Pediatrics and Critical
* Care and Emergency Medicine*
SUNY Health Science Center
Attending Physician
University Hospital
Syracuse, New York

TERI A. MANOLIO, M.D., M.H.S.
Medical Officer
National Heart, Lung, and Blood
* Institute*
National Institutes of Health
Clinical Assistant Professor
Naval Hospital, Bethesda
Bethesda, Maryland

KEVIN S. MERIGIAN, M.D.
Assistant Professor
Department of Emergency Medicine
University Hospital
University of Cincinnati
Cincinnati, Ohio

DAN K. MORHAIM, M.D., F.A.C.E.P.
Clinical Instructor
Department of Emergency Medicine
Georgetown University
Chairman, Department of Emergency
* Medicine*
Franklin Square Hospital
Baltimore, Maryland

CHRISTOPHER T. MORROW, M.D.,
F.A.C.E.P.
Assistant Professor
Emergency Medicine
The Johns Hopkins University School
* of Medicine*
Attending Physician
Emergency Medicine
Francis Scott Key Medical Center
Baltimore, Maryland

BRUCE MOSKOW, M.D., J.D.
Fellow, American College of
* Emergency Physicians*
Assistant Director
Emergency Department
Seton Medical Center
Austin, Texas

ERIC K. NOJI, M.D., M.P.H.,
F.A.C.E.P.
Assistant Professor of Emergency
* Medicine*
The Johns Hopkins Hospital and
* School of Medicine*
Baltimore, Maryland

GARY M. ODERDA, PHARM.D.,
M.P.H.
Director and Professor
Maryland Poison Center
University of Maryland School of
* Pharmacy*
Baltimore, Maryland

EDWARD J. OTTEN, M.D.
Associate Professor
Department of Emergency Medicine
Director of Prehospital Care
University of Cincinnati Medical
* Center*
Cincinnati, Ohio

V. GAIL RAY, M.D., F.A.C.E.P.
Associate Professor
East Carolina University School of
* Medicine*
Pitt County Memorial Hospital
Greenville, North Carolina

BETTY S. RIGGS, M.D.
Clinical Instructor
Department of Surgery (Trauma and
* Emergency Medicine Section)*
University of Colorado Health Sciences
* Center*
University Hospital
Denver, Colorado

TIMOTHY J. RITTENBERRY, M.D.,
F.A.C.E.P.
Assistant Professor of Clinical
* Emergency Medicine*
University of Illinois
Director of Emergency Medicine
* Education*

Illinois Masonic Medical Center
Chicago, Illinois

DAVID ROBERTS, M.D.
Diplomate of American Board of
*   Medical Toxicology*
Clinical Assistant Professor
North Memorial Medical Center
Staff, Emergency Room Physician
North Memorial Medical Center
Robbinsdale, Minnesota

S. RUTHERFOORD ROSE II,
PHARM.D.
Clinical Toxicology Fellow
Maryland Poison Center
University of Maryland
*   School of Pharmacy*
Baltimore, Maryland

JEANNE C. RUBENSTONE, M.D.
Attending Physician
Emergency Department
Chesterfield General Hospital
Cheraw, South Carolina

PAULA A. RYALS, M.D., F.A.C.E.P.
Instructor in Surgery (Emergency
*   Medicine)*
Thomas Jefferson University College of
*   Medicine*
Associate Physician
Department of Emergency Medicine
Medical Center of Delaware
Wilmington, Delaware

RICARDO L. SANCHEZ, M.D., M.P.H.
Instructor in Medicine
Harvard Medical School
Attending Physician
Emergency Services
Brigham and Women's Hospital
Boston, Massachusetts

DANIEL L. SAVITT, M.D.
Attending Physician
Department of Emergency Medicine
Rhode Island Hospital
Providence, Rhode Island

GERALD R. SCHWARTZ, M.D.,
F.A.C.E.P.
Chief, Department of Emergency
*   Medicine*
Englewood Hospital
Englewood, New Jersey

CAROL JACK SCOTT, M.D.
Clinical Instructor
Director, Continuing Education
Department of Emergency Medicine
The Johns Hopkins University School
*   of Medicine*
Baltimore, Maryland

DONNA L. SEGER, M.D., F.A.C.E.P.,
A.B.M.T.
Assistant Professor of Surgery and
*   Medicine*
Department of Surgery
Division of Trauma
Vanderbilt University Hospital
Nashville, Tennessee

ROBERT F. SHESSER, M.D., M.P.H.,
F.A.C.E.P.
Associate Professor of Emergency
*   Medicine*
George Washington University
Vice Chairman
Department of Emergency Medicine
George Washington University
*   Hospital*
Washington, D.C.

KEITH T. SIVERTSON, M.D.,
F.A.C.E.P.
Assistant Professor
The Johns Hopkins University School
*   of Medicine*
Director, Department of Emergency
*   Medicine*
The Johns Hopkins Hospital
Baltimore, Maryland

MARK S. SMITH, M.D., F.A.C.E.P.
Associate Professor and Chairman
Department of Emergency Medicine
The George Washington University
*   Medical Center*
Washington, D.C.

SAMUEL S. SPICER, M.D.
Clinical Assistant Professor of
*   Emergency Medicine*
East Carolina School of Medicine
Emergency Physician
New Hanover Memorial Hospital
Wilmington, North Carolina

ROBERT J. STINE, M.D., F.A.C.E.P.
Associate Professor of Medicine
University of Massachusetts Medical
  School
Chief, Department of Emergency
  Medicine
Worcester City Hospital
Worcester, Massachusetts

HARLAN A. STUEVEN, M.D.,
F.A.C.E.P.
Associate Professor of Surgery
Medical College of Wisconsin
Staff Physician
Milwaukee County Medical Complex
Milwaukee, Wisconsin

J. ANDREW SUMNER, M.D.,
F.A.C.E.P.
Assistant Professor
Emergency Medicine
The Johns Hopkins School of Medicine
Attending Physician
The Johns Hopkins Hospital
Baltimore, Maryland

JAMES J. WALTER, M.D., F.A.C.E.P.
Assistant Professor
Chief, Section of Emergency Medicine
University of Chicago
Chicago, Illinois

EDWARD S. WANG, M.D.
Attending Physician
Emergency Department
Kaiser Medical Center
San Francisco, California

JOHN M. WOGAN, M.D.
Assistant Professor of Emergency
  Medicine
The Johns Hopkins University School
  of Medicine
Attending Physician
Department of Emergency Medicine
The Johns Hopkins Medical
  Institutions
Baltimore, Maryland

Preface

The purpose of this *Manual of Toxicologic Emergencies* is to aid physicians in the initial assessment and management of such emergencies. The book is intended for use by health care providers who deal with toxic ingestions and overdoses and those who evaluate and manage patients during the period immediately after a toxic ingestion or exposure.

Although there are several acceptable approaches to dealing with toxicologic exposures, we have attempted to delineate an approach based on the latest accepted knowledge and methods from the literature, taking into account the experience of the contributing authors, all of whom manage such emergencies as part of their professional lives.

When we began to explore the toxicologic literature and review standard texts, we found that much of the information was fragmented and that no single source contained all the relevant information required to manage the initial stages of poisoning. We do not intend this book to be an exhaustive, classic reference text; however, material in each section and chapter has been distilled from various authoritative sources to bring together in one format all the pertinent information required to manage toxicologic emergencies.

The book has been designed to allow easy access to detailed information, using a systematic format to be followed during the active management of poisonings. It can also stand as a reference.

The text has been divided into five major sections. In Part I, general considerations such as epidemiology, sources of information, first aid, and prehospital management are discussed. Part II presents general management techniques. In this section we introduce the concept of advanced poisoning treatment and life support (APTLS), which should be invoked as the initial approach with all patients with known or possible toxic ingestions or exposures. APTLS is similar in concept to advanced cardiac life support (ACLS), advanced poisoning life support, and advanced trauma life support (ATLS), well known to emergency practitioners. This section also discusses general management measures, such as prevention of absorption, enhancement of elimination, use of the toxicology laboratory, disposition considerations, staff precautions, and medical-legal issues. Part III details approaches to be taken in specific situations that may complicate the evaluation or

treatment of the poisoned patient. Such complexities as the management of concomitant head injury, pregnancy, intoxication with alcohol, violent patients, and
withdrawal states are covered. In Part IV, systematic information to be acquired
during patient evaluation (history, physical examination) that can aid in identifying
the specific poisonings is detailed. Finally, Part V discusses specific poisonings and
exposures.

Each chapter is organized in the same format to allow easy access to information. Within each chapter, controversial areas are acknowledged and special
considerations that may affect management are noted. At the end of each chapter,
guidelines for admission, consultation, discharge, and patient transfer are given.

Virtually all of the contributors are emergency practitioners with academic
backgrounds, each with expertise in his or her area. We are indebted for their
enthusiastic support of this work.

We have enjoyed developing this text and its conceptual approach to poisoning and toxic exposure. We hope you enjoy using the book and find it helpful in
clinical application.

Eric K. Noji, M.D., M.P.H., F.A.C.E.P.
Gabor D. Kelen, M.D., F.R.C.P., F.A.C.E.P.

Acknowledgments

First and foremost, we would like to thank our wives, Pam (EKN) and Laurie (GDK), who have endured virtual widowhood during the last year of the editing process. Without their unyielding support, this book would not have been possible.

We would also like to thank Dr. Keith Sivertson, director of the Department of Emergency Medicine at The Johns Hopkins Hospital for his support of this project and for his fostering of the growth of academic emergency medicine at this institution for the past several years.

Many thanks to Dr. Scott Altman who helped in the early stages of this endeavor and Dr. Tracey Goessel, our assistant editor.

Much appreciation to Dr. Douglas Floccare for his help in preparing computer generated graphs and nomograms.

Finally, thanks and much appreciation to Mr. David Marshall, Executive Editor, Year Book Medical Publishers, for his patience, constant support, and encouragement. He has shared our excitement and passion for the idea behind the creation of this work.

Eric K. Noji, M.D., M.P.H., F.A.C.E.P.
Gabor D. Kelen, M.D., F.R.C.P., F.A.C.E.P.

Contents

PART ONE

General Considerations in the Poisoned Patient

1

Adult Epidemiology

Julie A. P. Casani, M.D.

I. Introduction. Epidemiologic data are collected from regional medical examiners' offices, hospital discharge diagnoses, poison control center registries, and the Drug Abuse Warning Network (DAWN). DAWN is a National Institute of Drug Abuse (NIDA)–sponsored nationwide voluntary system where data are continuously collected regarding drug-related events from emergency departments and medical examiners' offices.
   A. An estimated 4.8 million poisonings occurred nationwide in 1986 according to the American Association of Poison Control Centers (AAPCC) National Data Collection System.
   B. In 1986, of the 1,980,894 poisonings reported to the AAPCC:
      1. Four hundred six resulted in death.
      2. Ninety percent occurred in the home and were accidental.
      3. Suicide attempts represented only 5.6%.
      4. The majority involved children:
         a. Younger than 6 years of age, 63.4%.
         b. Younger than 2 years, 39.1%.
   C. Approximately 22% of the victims of potentially toxic exposures are evaluated in emergency departments, accounting for more than 1 million visits annually.
   D. Those cases resulting in significant morbidity and mortality comprise less than 1% of all toxic exposures.
      1. Fewer than 1% of these patients required use of specific antidotes such as naloxone or aggressive elimination measures such as hemodialysis.
   E. Nearly 80% of all human poison exposures involve the oral route.

TABLE 1–1.
Drugs Commonly Involved in Adult
Poisonings*

Drug	No. of Reports
Alcohol (in combination)	25,032
Diazepam (Valium)	18,557
Heroin and morphine	6,822
Aspirin	6,682
Phencyclidine (in combination)	6,002
Flurazepam (Dalmane)	4,666
Marijuana	4,555
Propoxyphene	3,585
Amitriptyline	3,297
Acetaminophen	3,296
Methaqualone	3,270
Chlordiazepoxide	2,869
Cocaine	2,846
Phenobarbital	2,799
Secobarbital, amobarbital (Amytal)	2,516
Hydantoins	2,466
Methadone	2,415
Sleep aids (over-the-counter)	2,260
Chlorpromazine	2,170
Amphetamines	1,996

*Reported by emergency personnel to DAWN, 1979.

TABLE 1–2.
Emergency Visits*

	Dependence	Suicide	Other
Sex			
Male	27.8	13.3	58.9
Female	12.5	26.5	61.1
Unknown	15.4	23.1	61.5
Age (yr)			
6–17	3.0	28.0	69.0
18–29	18.5	19.4	62.1
>30	26.9	18.1	55.0
Unknown	10.5	10.5	78.9
Drug(s)			
Single drug	21.9	18.3	59.8
Multidrug	17.4	22.4	60.3
Reason for emergency visit			
Unexpected reaction	12.1	2.3	85.5
Overdose	6.8	34.3	58.9
Chronic effects	73.0	—	26.5

(Continued.)

TABLE 1–2 (cont.).

	Dependence	Suicide	Other
Other	41.5	3.1	55.3
Unknown	3.8	3.8	92.4
Patient disposition			
Admitted	1.6	29.3	54.4
Treated and released	22.2	14.5	63.0
Left against medical advice	26.3	7.5	66.2
Died	21.4	14.3	64.3
Unknown	6.9	20.7	72.4

*Percent distribution of drug abuse episodes in each category as reported to DAWN, 1985.

TABLE 1–3.

Medical Examiner Data*

	Accident	Suicide	Unknown
Sex			
Male	39.6	28.5	31.8
Female	21.7	42.2	36.1
Age (yr)			
6–7	46.9	53.1	—
18–29	40.4	27.5	32.1
30–39	42.0	24.2	33.8
>40	19.3	46.3	34.3
Unknown	9.7	12.9	77.4
Race			
White	25.3	41.1	33.5
Black	53.5	14.3	32.2
Hispanic	58.0	17.4	24.5
Other	16.3	26.5	57.1
Unknown	18.9	35.6	45.6
Drug(s)			
Single drug	26.8	37.3	35.9
Multidrug	36.3	31.5	32.2
Cause of death (directly drug induced)			
Single drug	28.2	35.6	36.2
Multidrug	35.2	29.1	35.7

*Percent distribution of drug abuse deaths in each category as reported to DAWN, 1985.

II. Epidemiologic trends in poisonings. Tables 1–1 through 1–3 show trends in drug-related poisonings in adults.

BIBLIOGRAPHY

Litovitz T, Veltri JC: 1984 Annual report of the American Association of Poison Control Centers National Data Collection System. *Am J Emerg Med* 1985; 3:423–450.

2

Pediatric Epidemiology

Patricia D. Fosarelli, M.D.

I. Epidemiology. It is difficult to document the exact number of pediatric poisonings in the United States each year because of trivial cases that never come to medical attention and hence remain unreported.
  A. It is estimated that two to five million poisonings occur each year in the pediatric age group, with most victims younger than 5 years of age.
  B. Data from the National Hospital Discharge Survey, conducted by the National Center for Health Statistics, show that in each year between 1979 and 1982 an estimated 20,000 children younger than 5 years of age were hospitalized in the United States after ingestion of potentially toxic substances.
    1. Medicinal substances accounted for 45% of hospitalizations.
      a. Aspirin and other analgesics accounted for most (11.8%) hospitalizations.
    2. Of nonmedicinal substances, products containing **lead** accounted for 11.7% of hospitalizations.
  C. In 1983 more than 110,000 children younger than 5 years of age were treated in hospital emergency rooms after ingesting potentially toxic substances. Thus for each child hospitalized after unintentional poisoning an estimated six to eight children are treated in emergency rooms and released.
  D. The American Association of Poison Control Centers estimates that of about 1.4 million childhood poison exposures in 1983:
    1. Ninety-one percent occurred in the home.
    2. For each child treated in an emergency department for poisoning about 13 other poison exposures in children are reported to poison control centers.

3. It is unlikely that even these high figures reflect all poisonings. Many poisonings are not reported to poison control centers because they are either treated in a physician's office or not treated at all.

E. Peak age for poisonings is 18 to 36 months.
   1. At this age children are mobile, interested in their environment, and explore by using mouthing behaviors.
   2. These children do not understand the risks of indiscriminately tasting environmental objects.

F. Statistically, poisoned children are more likely to be:
   1. Male.
   2. Described as "daring" by parents.
   3. Hungry or tired at the time of ingestion.

G. Deaths from unintentional ingestion of potentially poisonous substances among children younger than 5 years of age have decreased from a high of 456 in 1959 to a low of 57 in 1981 (Division of Vital Statistics, National Center for Health Statistics, 1981), related to such measures as:
   1. Safety caps on medicine containers.
   2. Better preparation of emergency department staffs to manage pediatric poisoning.
   3. Development of poison control centers, which can quickly relay information about ingested substances to parents and physicians treating victims.

II. Pediatric risks.

A. Whenever an ingestion occurs, one or more of three factors are involved:
   1. Unsafe environment:
      a. Harmful substances within easy reach of a child.
      b. Child poorly supervised.
   2. Susceptible host.
   3. Harmful substance.

B. Parental negligence may be fostered by ignorance or stress (e.g., marital strife, pregnancy, financial or employment concerns, medical or psychiatric problems, recent move, death).

C. In 1979 the 10 most common ingestions by children younger than 5 years reported to the U.S. Division of Poison Control Centers were:
   1. **Plants.**
   2. **Soaps, detergents, cleaners.**
   3. **Antihistamines, cold preparations.**
   4. **Perfumes, colognes.**
   5. **Vitamins.**
   6. **Aspirin.**
   7. **Analgesics other than aspirin.**
   8. **Household disinfectants.**
   9. **Fingernail preparations.**
   10. **Insecticides.**
   Other important ingestants are:
   1. Petroleum products **(hydrocarbons).**
   2. Oven and drain cleaners **(lye).**
   3. **Iron**-containing preparations.

The most lethal poisons in children younger than 5 years are:
1. Medications (especially **aspirin** and **antidepressants**).
2. Household products (especially **pesticides, fertilizers, hydrocarbons** such as **furniture polish**).
3. **Carbon monoxide** inhalation.

BIBLIOGRAPHY

Centers for Disease Control. Poisoning among young children—US. *MMWR* 1984; 33:129–131.
Litovitz T, Veltri JC. 1983 Annual Report of the American Association of PCC National Data Collection System. *Am J Emerg Med* 1984; 2:420–443.
Rivara FP. Epidemiology of childhood injuries. *Am J Dis Child* 1982; 136:399–404.
Update: Childhood poisonings—United States. Leads from the MMWR. *JAMA* 1985; 13:1857.

3

Toxicologic Dangers by Age and Development

Patricia D. Fosarelli, M.D.

TABLE 3–1.

Toxicologic Dangers by Age and Development

Age/Stage	Poisoning Hazard	Comment
Prenatal	Transplacental passage of substances absorbed by the mother orally, dermally, or by inhalation.	
Newborn	Ingestion of breast milk containing maternal ingestants, inhalants.	
Young infant	Exposure to talcum powder or other baby-care products during diaper changing or given by sibling trying to be helpful.	
4–6 mo (grabbing)	Talcum powder (diaper changing).	Keep products out of baby's reach. Do not let a baby "play" with a container of talc.
6–12 mo (crawling, cruising)	Household products in lower cabinets.	Keep products on upper shelves, preferably in locked cabinets.
12–24 mo (walking, imitating)	Medicines, household products.	Keep tabletops free of such products. Never leave child unsupervised.

(Continued.)

TABLE 3–1 (cont.).

Age/Stage	Poisoning Hazard	Comment
Toddler	NOTE: **At greatest risk for poisoning**	
24–36 mo (climbing, tasting)	Medicines that are flavored.	Store medicines on high shelves (never at bedside).
Older preschool, early school-aged child	Any (ingestions rare in age group).	Properly store harmful items. Maintain good parental-child communication and discipline (to counter risk-taking tendencies).
Older child/adolescent	Glue or solvents, street drugs, medications.	Use anticipatory guidance regarding risk taking and dares; maintain parental-child communication to prevent problems (substance abuse, suicide gestures and attempts) **before** they occur.

4

Sources of Poison Information

Gary M. Oderda, Pharm.D., M.P.H.

Sources of poison information include textbooks, journal articles, microfiche systems, computer databases, and poison centers.

I. Micromedex (660 Bannock St., Suite 350, Englewood, CO 80204) produces a series of databases on poisoning of interest to clinicians:
   A. Poisindex (poisonings).
   B. Drugdex (drugs).
   C. Emergindex (emergency medicine).

II. Poisindex is a listing of poisonous commercial products and plants and animals. Where available, ingredients are listed, with amounts or concentration, manufacturer's name, and appropriate management procedures, for example, for generic agents or categories of drugs, such as salicylates, acetaminophen, or chlorinated hydrocarbons. Each management is updated regularly and reviewed by an editorial board, and includes an overview, case reports, clinical effects, laboratory values, treatment, range of toxicity, kinetics, pharmacology and toxicology, and references. Poisindex is available on microfiche or compact disk for use in a microcomputer system, and is updated quarterly.

III. Poison centers serve as a major source of poison information to practitioners and provide:
   A. Consultation to health professionals treating poisoned patients.
   B. Information and advice by telephone to the general public.
   C. Public education and prevention programs.
   D. Health professional training and continuing education.
   E. Research in clinical toxicology and poison prevention.

    Poison information specialists, specially trained registered nurses and pharmacists, answer calls 24 hours a day and work under the direction of an administrative staff including a physician medical director. They develop specific expertise by handling large numbers of poison-related calls. Most regional poison centers answer 20,000 to 50,000 calls per year.

Health professional callers should be prepared to relate pertinent available information, such as history, symptoms and signs and laboratory values. The caller will then be given information on toxicity, expected clinical effects, and specific treatment recommendation as well as answers to any other questions. Clinicians should expect to receive follow-up calls from poison center staff to check on the status of the patient and to provide additional recommendations if necessary.

IV. The American Association of Poison Control Centers (AAPCC) coordinates a data collection system of poison exposures in the United States. Approximately 1 million cases are included each year. Poison epidemiology data are available from the AAPCC. An annual report is published in the *American Journal of Emergency Medicine.*

The AAPCC certifies regional poison centers, which have met a series of criteria related to staffing, available resources, and public education programs. The following is a list of AAPCC-certified regional poison centers as of June 1987:

Alabama Poison Center
Tuscaloosa, AL 35401
800–462–0800 (Alabama only)

Arizona Poison Control System
Arizona Poison & Drug Information
Tucson, AZ 85724
(602) 626–6016
800–362–0101 (Arizona only)

St. Luke's Poison Management Center
Phoenix, AZ 85006
(602) 253–3334

Blodgett Regional Poison Center
Grand Rapids, MI 49506
800–442–4571 (area code 616 only)
800–632–2727 (Michigan only)

Cardinal Glennon Children's Hospital
Regional Poison Center
St. Louis, MO 63104
(314) 772–5200
800–392–9111 (Missouri only)

Central Ohio Poison Center
Columbus, OH 43205
(614) 228–1323;
800–682–7625 (Ohio only)

Duke University Poison Control Center
Durham, NC 27710
(919) 684–8111
800–672–1697 (North Carolina only)

Georgia Poison Control Center
Atlanta, GA 30335
(404) 589–4400
800–282–5846 (Georgia only)

Hennepin Regional Poison Center
Minneapolis, MN 55415
(612) 347–3141

Intermountain Regional Poison Control Center
Salt Lake City, UT 84132
(801) 581–2151
800–662–0062 (Utah only)

Kentucky Regional Poison Center of Kosair Children's Hospital
Louisville, KY 40232
(502) 589–8222
800–722–5725 (Kentucky only)

Long Island Regional Poison Control Center
East Meadow, NY 11554
(516) 542–2323

Los Angeles County Medical Association
Regional Poison Control Center
Los Angeles, CA 90057
(213) 484–5151

Louisiana Regional Poison Control Center
Shreveport, LA 71130
(318) 425–1524
800–535–0525 (Louisiana only)

Maryland Poison Center
Baltimore, MD 21201
(301) 528–7701
800–492–2414 (Maryland only)

Massachusetts Poison Control System
Boston, MA 02115
(617) 232–2120
800–682–9211 (Massachusetts only)

Mid Plains Poison Center
Omaha, NE 68114
(402) 390–5400
800–642–9999 (Nebraska only)
800–228–9515 (surrounding states)

Minnesota Regional Poison Center
St. Paul, MN 55101
(612) 221–2113
800–222–1222 (Minnesota only)

National Capital Poison Center
Washington, DC 20007
(202) 625–3333

New Jersey Poison Information and Education System
Newark, NJ 07112
(202) 923–0764
(800) 962–1253 (New Jersey only)

New Mexico Poison and Drug Information Center
Albuquerque, NM 87131
(505) 843–2551
800–432–6866 (New Mexico only)

New York City Poison Control Center
New York, NY 10016
(212) 340–4494

North Central Texas Poison Center
Dallas, TX 75235
(214) 920–2400
800–441–0040 (Texas only)

Oregon Poison Control and Drug Information Center
Portland, OR 97201
(503) 225–8968
800–452–7165 (Oregon only)

Pittsburgh Poison Center
Pittsburgh, PA 15213
(412) 681–6669

Poison Control Center
Children's Hospital of Michigan
Detroit, MI 48201
(313) 745–5711
800–462–6642 (area code 313 only)
800–572–1655 (remainder of Michigan)

Rhode Island Poison Center
Providence, RI 02902
(401) 277–5727

Rocky Mountain Poison Center
Denver, CO 80204
(303) 629–1123
800–332–3073 (Colorado only)
800–525–5042 (Montana only)
800–442–2702 (Wyoming only)

San Diego Regional Poison Center
San Diego, CA 92103
(619) 294–6000

San Francisco Bay Area Regional Poison Control Center
San Francisco, CA 94110
(415) 476–6600

Southwest Ohio Regional Poison Control System
Cincinnati, OH 45267
(513) 872–5111
800–872–5111

Tampa Bay Regional Poison Control Center
Tampa, FL 33679
(813) 253–4444
800–282–3171

Texas State Poison Center
Galveston, TX 77550
(409) 765–1420
(713) 654–1701 (Houston)
(516) 478–4490 (Austin)
800–392–8548 (Texas only)

UCDMC Regional Poison Control Center
Sacramento, CA 95817
(916) 453–3692

West Virginia Poison Center
Charleston, WV 25304
(304) 348–4211
800–642–3625 (West Virginia only)

Telephone Advice

Patricia D. Fosarelli, M.D.

WARNING: **Many authorities counsel that medical advice should not be given to patients over the phone (see Chapter 20, p. 79).**

I. Remain calm. A parent calling to report a poisoning frequently is upset.
II. Ask the parent's name, address, and phone number so that you can call back if you're disconnected. However, **make every attempt to keep the parent on the line.**
III. Ask if poisoning was by ingestion, inhalation, or exposure; the name of the product; the amount involved; and the time of the episode. If you are not familiar with the product, ask the parent to bring it to the phone and read the label. Record the details.
IV. If you are still unfamiliar with the product, **keep the parent on the line** while you:
   A. Call the local poison control center.
   B. Look up information on the particular ingestion.
   Do not depend on the parent to call a poison control center.
V. Ask the child's age and approximate weight (very important in pediatrics because calculation of toxicity is made in terms of per kilogram weight). Ask what the child is doing now (Playing? Coughing or choking? Having a seizure? Comatose?). Are there lip or mouth burns? If the child is not breathing, instruct the parent to begin cardiopulmonary resuscitation (CPR); have an associate call an ambulance while you stay on the line with the parent.
VI. If the child has ingested something that requires immediate hospital care, **have an associate call an ambulance.**
VII. If the child has ingested something for which the use of ipecac is warranted (and the parent has it on hand), recommend the proper dose (see Chapter

6, pp. 18–19). Instruct the parent to bring the child to the emergency department as soon as possible and to keep the child as calm as possible.

VIII. If the child has ingested a nontoxic substance (see Chapter 49, p. 237), reassure the parent and give information on signs and symptoms to expect and which of these warrant a visit to the emergency department or the child's physician.

IX. If the child has come into contact with a poisonous substance, instruct the parent to remove adjacent clothing (if possible without doing further damage to the skin) and to flood the affected skin with water. Determine the area and location of skin involved and its appearance. Instruct the parent to call an ambulance or take the child to the closest emergency department immediately.

X. If the child has inhaled a poisonous substance, identify it and determine the duration of exposure. Ask what the child is doing now. Instruct the parent to loosen the child's clothing and move him to fresh air (or open the windows if this is impossible). Instruct the parent to begin CPR if the child is not breathing; have an associate call an ambulance. Regardless of the child's condition, he should not be given anything to eat or drink until examined by medical personnel. If the child appears to be well but the inhalant is worrisome, instruct the parent to take him to the closest emergency department (preferably by ambulance).

XI. Even if the substance is nontoxic, call the parent in 1 to 2 hours to check on the patient (remember to get the phone number and address). If there is no phone or address, always advise to go to the nearest hospital.

XII. If home treatment is required (but not hospital care) make follow-up calls at 1, 4, and 24 hours.

XIII. If in doubt, **always** advise an immediate visit to the closest emergency department.

First Aid/Home Management

Patricia D. Fosarelli, M.D.

In the event of a child's ingestion, inhalation, or contact with a poisonous substance, advise the parent to:

I. Call the regional poison control center or nearest emergency department (these numbers should be posted near the phone).

II. Have the container of poison at hand in case the parent is asked about exact labeling or ingredients.

III. Write down all instructions.

IV. For ingested poisons:

    A. Dilute the ingestant by giving the child a cup of water or milk to drink; do not force a child to drink if he or she is drowsy, unconscious, or having a seizure.

    B. Induce emesis if directed to do so. Emesis is contraindicated if the child is drowsy, unconscious, or having a seizure or if the ingestant is a strong acid, or is a base, petroleum product, or has the ability to induce seizures or alter sensorium.

       1. If ipecac is advisable, give the following doses:

Age	Dose	Comment
<6 mo	Not indicated	
6–12 mo		May be indicated, but do not administer outside medical facility.
1–12 yr	15 ml	May repeat once if no emesis in 20 minutes. Follow dose with water or clear juice (not milk).
≥12 yr	30 ml	As above.

2. Do not stick a finger or other object in the child's mouth to induce vomiting (increased risk of injury). Do not give a salt solution to induce emesis.
3. If the child does not vomit bring him or her to an emergency department as soon as possible. Call 911 or other emergency number for an ambulance if ingestion is potentially serious.
4. If the child vomits after administration of ipecac and is given something to drink, he or she is likely to vomit again.
  C. If an emergency department visit is warranted, have the parent bring both child and container of poison to the emergency department.
V. For inhaled toxins:
  A. Remove the child from the vicinity of the toxic fumes (e.g., take the child outdoors or open all windows).
  B. Loosen the child's clothing.
  C. Begin cardiopulmonary resuscitation if necessary.
  D. Call 911 or other emergency number for an ambulance.
VI. For contact poisons:
  A. Remove clothing adjacent to the affected area.
  B. Flood the skin with water.
  C. Call an ambulance or go to the nearest emergency department.

Prehospital Treatment of the Poisoned Patient

Dan K. Morhaim, M.D., F.A.C.E.P.

I. Duties of paramedical personnel at the scene:
  A. Gather and bring items such as pill bottles, needles, suicide notes to emergency department.
  B. Collect information on type, route, and duration of exposure or ingestion.
  C. Identify witnesses with potentially relevant information (i.e., roommates, family, friends).
II. Field precautions for health care providers:
  A. Avoid mouth-to-mouth breathing if possible (risk in certain poisonings such as organophosphate insecticides, cyanide; risk of transmission of infectious disease); use pocket mask.
  B. Wear gloves (risk of skin contact with poisons such as organophosphates; risk of needle-stick injury).
  C. Wash hands between patient encounters.
  D. Dispose of needles and dressings appropriately.
  E. Clean and disinfect reusable items.
  F. Approach hazardous material accident sites upwind if possible (see Chapter 111).
  G. Avoid direct contamination by materials such as organophosphate pesticides.
  H. See Chapter 16 for staff precautions in toxicologic emergencies.
III. Field Treatment
  A. Ipecac and water to induce emesis; contraindicated in caustic or petroleum distillate ingestions. **Physician advice desirable.** (See Chapter 12, Prevention of Absorption.)

B. Fifty percent dextrose solution, 50 ml IV, all unconscious patients.

C. Naloxone in all unconscious patients, 2 mg IV, SC, IM, SL, or via endotracheal tube. NOTE: Some authorities advise not giving naloxone in the field if the patient has adequate respirations and vital signs, because of the risk of vomiting and aspiration when proper suction and airway control are difficult. Further, many patients after regaining consciousness may leave the scene or even jump out of the ambulance before adequate medical assessment of their condition and mental status can be made.

D. Oxygen in all patients (exception: paraquat poisoning).

E. Eye irrigation if topical exposure (see Chapter 28, p. 116).

F. Draw appropriate blood samples if possible.

G. When possible, save urine and stomach contents for toxicologic screening.

H. Alert receiving hospital if paramedics will be bringing a patient contaminated with hazardous materials to allow setup of decontamination area.

I. As in the emergency department, assess the patient for other medical conditions or resultant complications. (For example, carbon monoxide can precipitate angina or myocardial infarction in a patient with ischemic heart disease.)

J. All patients with altered mental status should be carefully assessed for concomitant trauma. If any doubt, transport with trauma precautions, particularly cervical spine immobilization.

IV. Special case: Hazardous materials

A. See Chapter 111 on hazardous chemicals.

B. Decontamination:

1. a. Establish contaminated or "dirty" area.

   b. Remove clothes of contaminated victims; place in laundry bags with proper identification.

   c. Wash contaminated patients thoroughly with soap, cotton-tipped swabs, nail cleaners.

   d. Exit to clean area.

2. Determine water runoff so as not to spread hazardous materials into the general environment and water supply.

3. Establish accurate system of record-keeping to track personnel and materials.

C. Decontamination must be carried out before initiation of triage and medical care. Attention to basic ABCs (*a*irway, *b*reathing, *c*irculation), however, takes precedence over decontamination (i.e., maintaining airway patency, instituting artificial ventilation, cardiac compression, cervical spine immobilization, pressure dressings for hemorrhage control).

PART TWO

General Management of the Poisoned Patient

8

Advanced Poisoning Treatment and Life Support (APTLS)

Gabor D. Kelen, M.D., F.R.C.P.(C), F.A.C.E.P.
Eric K. Noji, M.D., M.P.H., F.A.C.E.P.

WARNING: **All patients with altered mental status have concomitant *trauma* and/or *underlying illness* until proven otherwise.**
All pediatric patients should be assessed for *child abuse* or neglect.
All overdosed and poisoned patients must be assessed for *suicide risk*.

I. Introduction. The management of poisoning is consistent with the approach that should be taken for all emergency medicine problems and incorporates principles of advanced trauma life support (ATLS) and advanced cardiac life support (ACLS). Inherent in this is the notion that the practitioner is mindful of a differential diagnosis in which *all diagnoses of consequence are considered,* particularly the most life-threatening conditions. It is therefore reasonable for the clinician to "always think the worst" when confronted with a poisoned patient and to rule out potentially life-threatening conditions before accepting a more benign diagnosis. It should never be assumed that the patient's signs and symptoms are related solely to drug overdose or even that drugs are involved at all. All other reasonable diagnoses of consequence that may explain the findings must be considered. For example, look for alternate explanations such as trauma, cerebral hemorrhage, infection, or metabolic disorders in poisoned patients with altered mental status or coma.

II. Advanced poisoning treatment and life support. In any emergency involving a severely poisoned patient logical sequential treatment priorities must be established on the basis of overall patient assessment. The assessment must be performed quickly and efficiently. Management must consist of a rapid *primary evaluation, resuscitation* of vital functions, a more detailed *secondary assessment,* leading to initiation of *definitive care,* and finally *disposition.* The following is a logical approach to advanced poisoning treatment and life support (APTLS).

A. Primary survey: During the primary survey immediate life-threatening problems are identified. Appropriate resuscitative measures are performed as each problem is encountered.

1. A—**Airway** maintenance (with cervical spine control in patients with altered or depressed sensorium or concomitant trauma).

2. B—**Breathing:**
   a. Assess ventilation.
   b. Smell breath.

3. C—**Circulation:**
   a. Estimate rate, rhythm, blood pressure by feeling for pulses:
      (1) Radial pulse implies systolic BP at least 80 mm Hg, femoral at least 70 mm Hg, carotid at least 60 mm Hg.
      (2) Do not waste time obtaining cuff blood pressure at this point if hypotension is evident.

4. D—**Disability:**
   a. Assessment of level of consciousness with AVPU method:
      A—*A*lert.
      V—Responds to *v*ocal stimuli.
      P—Responds to *p*ainful stimuli.
      U—*U*nresponsive.
   b. Check pupil size and reactivity.
   c. Calculate initial Glasgow coma score (see Chapter 37, p. 168).

5. E—**Expose. Always** completely undress the patient. Look for **Med-Alert** bracelet.

B. Resuscitation phase: During the resuscitation phase life-threatening conditions are treated as they are discovered. The primary survey and resuscitation phases are essentially accomplished simultaneously. A few immediately life-threatening poisonings **(cyanide, carbon monoxide,** and **opioids)** are specifically treated during this phase before undertaking a full secondary survey.

1. An ECG monitor is placed and supplemental oxygen administered in patients with altered mental status, all patients with unknown diagnosis, all patients with poisonings associated with cardiac arrhythmias, and patients with cardiac and certain other underlying illness (exception: definite paraquat poisonings, see Chapter 107).

2. Intravenous access should be established in all but the most trivial overdoses. When initiating the intravenous line blood should be drawn for basic laboratory work. At this time all patients with altered mental status should be given 50% dextrose solution, **naloxone,** and **thiamine.** Obtain **arterial blood gas** if appropriate.

3. Initiate **antidote** treatment for certain specific symptomatic toxic exposures, if diagnoses established or highly suspected (see inside back cover or Chapter 14, p. 54).
4. **Wash** or **irrigate** any skin or eye contact with the poison.
C. Secondary survey: During the secondary survey a full history is obtained, a head-to-toe physical examination completed, and radiographic and diagnostic laboratory studies obtained.
   1. History (e.g., specific drug ingested). One or more of the **10 Ps** can usually help to identify, locate, or retrieve the specific poisoning(s) involved (see Chapter 36 for details).
      a. Pockets.
      b. Patient.
      c. Parents, partner, pals.
      d. Prehospital personnel.
      e. Personal physician or psychiatrist.
      f. Pedestrians.
      g. Police.
      h. Pharmacy.
      i. Past history (old chart).
      j. Poison center.
   2. **Full examination** (see Chapter 37, p. 165). Search carefully for evidence of trauma or underlying illness.
   3. Additional **diagnostic tests,** if indicated.
D. Definitive care phase: During this phase of treatment the less immediately life-threatening problems and other medical problems or injuries are managed. Social and psychological status are also specifically addressed.
   1. **Continuous reevaluation and monitoring** should be carried out so that new signs and symptoms are not overlooked. Even though the initial life-threatening problems were managed appropriately or ruled out, other serious problems may develop as toxicity sets in or unrecognized associated ingestions take effect. Airway and mental status evaluation is particularly important in patients undergoing gastric decontamination procedures (e.g., emesis, lavage).
   2. Initiate **general and specific treatment measures.** The definitive care phase encompasses in depth management, such as gastric evacuation (see Chapter 12, p. 36) and enhanced elimination (see Chapter 13, p. 48), and measures specific for the toxic exposure.
   3. **Evaluate suicide potential** in all patients and carefully document assessment. Even if a patient is to be admitted, the suicide risk must be evaluated. Patients with risk for suicide may need constant observation.
E. Disposition: Sometimes during the definitive care period (the earlier the better), disposition of the patient should be considered.
   1. Answer the following:
      a. Is consultation required?
      b. Should the patient be admitted, and if so, does the condition or toxin warrant intensive care?
      c. Under what circumstances can this patient be sent home?
   2. Speak with the family and inform them of the patient's condition and planned disposition.
   NOTE: **All patients must be assessed for suicide risk before disposition.**

III. Pediatric priorities.
   A. Priorities in the pediatric patient are basically the same as for adults. Dosages and fluid volumes required for resuscitation differ.
   B. See Chapter 17 for disposition considerations for pediatric patients.
   C. All pediatric patients should be assessed for **child abuse** or **neglect** (see Chapter 31).

9

Airway Management

Douglas J. Floccare, M.D.

I. Indications for endotracheal intubation in poisoned patients*:
   A. Respiratory arrest/hypoventilation unresponsive to naloxone.
   B. Impaired protective airway reflexes.
   C. Need for gastric lavage in unconscious patient.
   D. Severely impaired oxygen diffusion.
   E. Status epilepticus.
II. Indications for mechanical ventilation*:
   A. Respiratory arrest.
   B. Severe hypoxemia.
   C. Alveolar hypoventilation and respiratory acidosis.
   D. Administration of curariform agents.
   E. Shock.
   F. Vital capacity <15 ml/kg.
   G. Tidal volume <5 ml/kg.
   H. Negative inspiratory force <25 cm H_2O.
   I. Pao_2 <70 mm Hg with Fio_2 >50%.
   J. A-ao_2 gradient on 100% Fio_2 >350 mm Hg.
   K. Calculated shunt >15%.
III. Initial parameters of mechanical ventilation†:
   A. Tidal volume, 10–15 ml/kg ideal body weight.
   B. Rate, 10/min.
   C. Fio_2, 100%.

*Adapted from Haddad LM, Winchester JF: *Clinical Management of Poisoning and Drug Overdose.* Philadelphia, WB Saunders Co., 1983, p 209.

†Arterial blood gases should be assessed 20 minutes after starting ventilator. Attempt to maintain Pao_2 >70 mm Hg with Fio_2 <50%.

10

Shock and Hypotension

Louis J. Ling, M.D., F.A.C.E.P.

I. Cause:
   A. Toxins that cause hypotension (see Chapter 38, p. 170).
   B. Other causes of shock (see Table 10–1).
II. Physical examination:
   A. Assess for pulmonary vascular congestion, jugular venous distension.
   B. Assess degree of vascular perfusion (urine output, mental status, skin color, capillary refill, skin temperature, jugular venous pressure).
   C. See Table 10–1.
III. Treatment:
   A. Follow advanced poisoning treatment and life support (see Chapter 8).
   B. Consider nontoxic causes (see Table 10–1).
   C. Administer specific antidotes if available (see inside back cover or Chapter 14).
   D. Respiratory support:
     1. Administer **oxygen,** 100% initially.
     2. Endotracheal intubation and assisted ventilation as needed (see Chapter 9).
     3. Pulmonary edema is treated with fluid restriction and use of positive end-expiratory pressure (PEEP) as necessary.
   E. Cardiovascular support:
     1. Cardiac arrest:
       a. Implement advanced life support. Follow most recent advanced cardiac life support (ACLS) guidelines from the American Heart Association (Standards and guidelines for cardiopulmonary resuscitation and emergency cardiac care: American Heart Association. *JAMA* 1986; 255:2841–3044).

TABLE 10–1.

Differential Diagnosis of Hypotension in the Poisoned Patient*

Cause	History	Examination	Diagnostic Adjuncts
Hypovolemia	Trauma (bleeding), vomiting, diarrhea, pancreatitis, GI bleeding, pregnant	Low JVP Orthostatic BP Abdominal exam for aneurysm, signs of trauma, vaginal bleeding	Low CVP NG, stool (Heme +), low Hct, improvement with fluid challenge
Cardiogenic shock	History of chest pain, dyspnea	High JVP Peripheral edema	High CVP, chest x-ray: ↑cardiothoracic ratio, CHF, ECG
Tamponade	Trauma, cancer, uremia	Increased JVP Muffled heart sounds, cardiac dullness	High CVP, x-ray: normal cardiac silhouette if acute, echo
Anaphylaxis	Previous history of allergy, anaphylaxis	Respiratory distress, wheezing or stridor, angioedema, urticaria	Response to epinephrine
Arrhythmia	History	Irregular pulse	ECG
Sepsis	Cough, UTI symptoms	Fever	CBC, chest x-ray, urinalysis
Endocrine	Thyroid disease, steroid dependent	Neck scar (thyroid)	Electrolytes
Neurogenic	Trauma	Hypotension with normal or slow pulse, paralysis Check rectal tone	X-ray, CT

*CBC = complete blood cell count; CHF = congestive heart failure; CT = computed tomography; CVP = central venous pressure; Hct = hematocrit; JVP = jugular venous pressure; NG = nasogastric; UTI = urinary tract infection.

   b. Some poisonings may not respond to standard ACLS protocols for cardiopulmonary arrest. Consider:
      (1) Sodium bicarbonate for tricyclic antidepressant–induced cardiac arrhythmias.
      (2) Naloxone, 50% dextrose solution in unconscious patients.
      (3) Propranolol or labetolol for cocaine-induced ventricular tachycardia.
      (4) Large doses of naloxone for suspected propoxyphene overdose.
2. Hypotension:
   a. **Volume expansion** with normal saline or Ringer's lactate solution unless contraindicated:
      (1) Fluid challenge:
         a Adult: 500 ml (or two boluses of 250 ml).
         b Child: 20 ml/kg body weight.
      (2) If persistent, consider monitoring central venous pressure or pulmonary capillary wedge pressure.
   b. Trendelenburg position or application of **pneumatic antishock garment** (unless contraindicated).
   c. If hypotension persists despite fluid challenge, vasopressors may be beneficial:
      (1) Dopamine: Add 200 mg dopamine HCl (Dopastat, Intropin) to a 250 or 500 ml bottle of saline solution or 5% dextrose in water and titrate dose to a rate of 2–50 µg/kg/min, to desired response.
      (2) Norepinephrine bitartrate (Levophed) for dopamine-depleting drugs (antidepressants): Add 4 ml norepinephrine bitartrate solution to 1 L 5% dextrose in saline or water solution and administer IV. Depending on the patient's response to the initial 2–3 ml, adjust rate of flow to 0.5–1.0 ml/min to maintain low normal blood pressure.
      (3) Other pressor agents (e.g., dobutamine) or agents to increase heart rate (atropine, isoproterenol) may also be appropriate in certain situations.
   d. Monitor central venous pressure or pulmonary capillary wedge pressure.
3. Arrhythmias: If treatment is indicated, antiarrhythmic therapy should be specific to the arrhythmia. Some poisonings may not respond to standard ACLS protocols for arrhythmias (see Cardiac Arrest, above).

BIBLIOGRAPHY

Olson KR, Pentel PR, Kelley MT: Physical assessment and differential diagnosis of the poisoned patient. *Med Toxicol* 1987; 2:52–81.
Standards and guidelines for cardiopulmonary resuscitation and emergency cardiac care: American Heart Association. *JAMA* 1986; 255:2841–3044.

11

Necessary Supplies, Equipment, and Drugs

Douglas J. Floccare, M.D.

I. Necessary disposable supplies:
   A. Activated charcoal
   B. Central venous line kit and manometer
   C. Endotracheal tubes
   D. Intravenous equipment
   E. Irrigation fluids
   F. Lubricant jelly
   G. Orogastric lavage tubes
   H. Oropharyngeal airways
   I. Oxygen masks/cannulas
   J. Plastic funnel
   K. Suction catheters (rigid and soft)
   L. Syringes (10 and 60 ml)
   M. Syrup of ipecac
   N. Urethral catheters
II. Necessary equipment:
   A. Ambu-bag
   B. Blankets
   C. Cardiac monitor and defibrillator
   D. Cutdown tray
   E. Cricothyroidotomy tray
   F. Decontamination facilities
   G. Electronic thermometer with rectal probe (range 20–45 C)

    H. Eyelid retractors
    I. Irrigation tray
    J. Mechanical ventilator
    K. Oxygen equipment
    L. Slit lamp
    M. Suction equipment
    N. Warming/cooling blanket unit
III. Drug stocklist for treatment of poisoning

Drug	Use
Activated charcoal	General adsorbent
Aminophylline	Propranolol
Ammonium chloride	Urine acidification
Amyl nitrite	Cyanide
Antivenin (snake, scorpion, black widow spider)	Per regional need
Ascorbic acid	Urine acidification
Atropine	Organophosphates, physostigmine
Botulism antitoxin	Botulism
Bretylium	ACLS*
Calcium chloride	Calcium channel blockers; ethylene glycol, oxalates
Calcium gluconate	Black widow spider bite; fluoride, hydrofluoric acid burns
Dantrolene	Hyperthermia
Deferoxamine	Iron
Dextrose 50% solution	Hypoglycemia
Diazepam	Anticonvulsant
Dimercaprol (BAL)	Arsenic, mercury, gold, lead
Diphenhydramine	Dystonic and allergic reactions
Dopamine	ACLS
Edrophonium	Anticholinergics
Epinephrine	Anaphylaxis, ACLS
Ethanol 10%	Methanol, ethylene glycol
Folinic acid	Methanol
Furosemide	Diuresis
Glucagon	Propranolol
Haloperidol	Severe agitation psychosis
Ipecac syrup	Emetic
Isoproterenol	Propranolol
Lidocaine	ACLS
Magnesium citrate	Oral cathartic
Methylene blue 1%	Methemoglobinemia
N-acetylcysteine (Mucomyst)	Acetaminophen
Naloxone (Narcan)	Narcotics
Nitroprusside	Hypertension
Norepinephrine	ACLS
Penicillamine	Copper, lead, mercury, arsenic

(Continued.)

Drug	Use
Phenobarbital	Anticonvulsant
Phenytoin	Antiarrhythmic, anticonvulsant
Physostigmine	Anticholinergics
Potassium chloride	Hypokalemia
Pralidoxime	Organophosphates
Protamine sulfate	Heparin
Pyridoxine	Ethylene glycol, isoniazid, mushrooms
Sodium bicarbonate	Acidosis, iron, tricyclic antidepressants
Sodium nitrite	Cyanide
Sodium thiosulfate	Cyanide
Starch	Iodine
Thiamine	Malnutrition
Vitamin K_1	Dicumarol, warfarin

*Advanced Cardiac Life Support.

12

Prevention of Absorption

John M. Wogan, M.D.

I. External decontamination:
   A. Skin:
      1. Remove corrosive substances (acids and alkalis) by copious flushing with water. Because insecticides (e.g., organophosphates, carbamates) are absorbed transdermally, skin should be flushed and clothing, including footwear, destroyed.
      2. See Chapter 29, General Protocol for Dermatologic Poisoning.
   B. Eyes:
      1. Begin removal of foreign material from eyes, especially acids or alkalis, immediately after exposure, preferably in the field, with copious amounts (4–6 L) of saline solution or water. Verify neutrality with pH test strip 20 minutes after irrigation. Examine for retained foreign body, corneal abrasion, or globe perforation (especially with propellant injuries, e.g., Mace).
      2. See Chapter 28, Ocular Toxicity.
II. Internal decontamination:
   A. Dilution:
      1. Indications:
         a. Caustic ingestion (acid or alkali).
      2. Contraindications:
         a. Neutralization of ingested acid or alkali by dilution with alkaline or acidic diluent, respectively, could be harmful, causing an exothermic reaction.

3. No value:
   a. Not accepted therapy in ingestions other than caustics. Theoretically could enhance absorption of many drugs.
4. Precautions:
   a. Should not be administered via gastric tube in caustic ingestions.
5. Dosage:
   a. No generally accepted dosage. Too much diluent might provoke emesis and reexposure of the esophagus and oropharynx to caustic; 200 to 300 ml water or milk (demulcent) is a reasonable dose in adults.
6. Efficacy:
   a. Not clearly demonstrated in clinically relevant study.
B. Emesis:
   1. Syrup of ipecac:
      a. Action:
         (1) Gastric irritant (peripheral).
         (2) Stimulates medullary chemoreceptors.
      b. Indications:
         (1) Awake patient with minimal to moderately severe ingestion.
         (2) Awake patient with toxic hydrocarbon ingestion (e.g., halogenated hydrocarbons, aromatic hydrocarbons, hydrocarbons with pesticides or nitrobenzene).
         (3) Emesis of hydrocarbons, which are highly volatile but otherwise nontoxic, is controversial (see below).
      c. Contraindications:
         (1) Alkali or acid.
         (2) Altered level of consciousness.
         (3) Depressed gag reflex or inability to protect airway.
         (4) Seizures; any ingestion with seizure potential; patient with underlying seizure potential.
         (5) Infant <6 months of age.
         (6) Hemorrhagic diathesis.
         (7) Hematemesis.
         (8) Drug ingestions that may lead to rapid change in patient's condition or level of consciousness (e.g., tricyclic antidepressants, β-blockers, propoxyphene, isoniazid, strychnine, camphor, chloroquine, phencyclidine).
      d. No value:
         (1) Usually not helpful in ethanol intoxication (see Chapter 52) and certain hydrocarbon ingestions (see Chapter 104).
      e. Precautions:
         (1) Avoid in any patient who is drowsy.
         (2) Avoid in any poisoning where decreased level of consciousness may occur rapidly (e.g., tricyclic antidepressants).
         (3) If emesis does not occur, the stomach must be evacuated by another means. Ipecac may be cardiotoxic (see below).
         (4) If substance has antiemetic properties, ipecac may not be successful (e.g., prochlorperazine).

(5) Only water should be given with ipecac.

(6) Do not confuse syrup of ipecac with the toxic fluid extract of ipecac.

f. Dosage:

(1) Syrup of ipecac, orally with water:

>12 yr   30 ml

1–12 yr   15 ml

6 mo–1 yr   10 ml (2–4 oz)

<6 mo   Not indicated

If vomiting not induced, repeat dose in 15–30 min.

g. Kinetics:

(1) Onset 15–30 minutes in 95% of patients.

(2) Duration: approximately 2 hours.

h. Efficacy:

(1) In simulated overdoses, ipecac-induced emesis has repeatedly been shown to reduce drug absorption. However, the clinical relevance of these simulated overdoses has been questioned (see Controversies, below).

i. Other considerations:

(1) Ability of emesis to prevent absorption decreases markedly within 1–2 hours of poison ingestion.

(2) However, this should not prevent its use since:

a Some drugs form gastric concretions:

i Salicylates.

ii Meprobamate.

iii Barbiturates.

iv Glutethimide.

b Some drugs delay gastric emptying:

i Tricyclic antidepressants.

ii Narcotics.

iii Salicylates.

iv Conditions producing adynamic ileus.

j. Controversies:

(1) Several authors have recently questioned the use of ipecac as first-line therapy in the emergency department treatment of drug overdoses since:

a Ipecac is not immediately effective.

b Its effects may persist for 2 hours or longer, thereby delaying administration of activated charcoal.

c Its efficacy is probably substantially reduced within several hours of a poison ingestion.

Although ipecac-induced emesis may be controversial, some form of gastric emptying prior to charcoal administration is currently accepted standard of care.

(2) The efficacy of the two methods of gastric emptying (emesis and lavage) have been compared in several studies (Tenenbein, 1987c; Kulig, 1985; Boxer, 1969), but to date neither has been consistently shown to be superior to the other.

    (3) In cases of isolated acetaminophen overdose the use of ipecac may delay administration of effective antidotal therapy (oral *N*-acetyl-cysteine). If there is any doubt as to combination ingestion, current practice is to administer ipecac.

    (4) Use with hydrocarbons is highly controversial (see Chapter 104).

  k. Complications:

    (1) Ipecac-induced emesis is safe therapy with an extremely low incidence of adverse reactions.

    (2) Complications are usually related to injudicious administration.

    (3) No evidence exists that therapeutic doses will lead to cardiac or neurotoxicity.

    (4) Chronic ipecac use (several ounces per day for weeks or months) may produce severe myopathies.

    (5) Drowsiness and diarrhea are the most common side effects.

2. Apomorphine

  a. Indications:

    (1) In the past apomorphine has been indicated as a general emetic. Currently it is rarely, if ever, indicated.

  b. Contraindications:

    (1) Same as for ipecac (see above).

    (2) Especially with any drug ingestion that depresses mental function or respiratory drive.

    (3) Some authors consider apomorphine contraindicated altogether.

  c. Precautions:

    (1) Apomorphine could potentially exacerbate effects of drugs that depress mental function or respiratory drive.

  d. Dosage:

    (1) 70–100 μg/kg SC/IM.

    (2) 10 μg/kg IV.

    (3) See Other considerations, below.

  e. Kinetics:

    (1) Onset within 5 minutes.

    (2) Duration of action 20–30 minutes.

  f. Efficacy:

    (1) Although apomorphine effectively induces vomiting, no controlled trials demonstrate clinically relevant effects in reversing or decreasing drug toxicity.

  g. Other considerations:

    (1) Apomorphine is formulated at the time of use and is therefore inconvenient and time consuming.

    (2) May cause protracted vomiting.

    (3) Because of inconvenience and protracted vomiting and because apomorphine can depress mental functioning and respiratory drive, ipecac has supplanted apomorphine as the emetic of choice.

    (4) Respiratory depression related to apomorphine may be only partially reversed by naloxone.

    h. Complications:
      (1) Respiratory depression.
      (2) Central nervous system depression clouds patient assessment.
      (3) Prolonged vomiting.

C. Gastric lavage:
   1. Indications:
     a. When gastric emptying is indicated but emesis is inappropriate or contraindicated.
     b. Comatose patient or potential to become so within next 30 minutes.
     c. Awake patient in whom delay until emesis may contribute to undue absorption of toxin (i.e., recent ingestion of large quantity of lethal toxin or ingestion of a rapidly absorbed liquid).
     d. Awake patient after ingestion of toxin with serious seizure-causing potential.
   2. Contraindications:
     a. Ingestion of corrosive substance.
     b. Hemorrhagic diathesis.
   3. Precautions:
     a. Do not use standard nasogastric tubes; they are not able to effectively evacuate the stomach due to their small diameter.
   4. Method:
     a. Explain to patient what you will be doing.
     b. Intubate with **cuffed endotracheal** tube if:
      (1) Gag reflex impaired.
      (2) Depressed mental status.
      (3) Seizures or seizure potential.
     c. Pass a large gastric tube (Ewald or Lavaculator) orally (with lubricant):
      (1) Adult: 36–40 F.
      (2) Child: 26–28 F.
     d. Patient in left lateral decubitus position and Trendelenburg position with knees flexed.
     e. Aspirate prior to lavage for toxicologic screening sample and to confirm tube placement.
     f. Lavage with normal saline solution or water in repeated runs of 1.5 ml/kg/run (not to exceed 200 ml/run) until effluent is clear, and then with 1–2 L more.
     g. The patient should be moved gently about during the procedure to enhance removal of the drug(s).
     h. Leave tube in place for instillation of charcoal or neutralizing agent (see p. 41).
   5. Efficacy:
     a. Lavage is roughly as effective as ipecac-induced emesis in removing poison from the stomach (see Controversies, below). Like emesis, lavage is less effective several hours after poison ingestion except with drugs that form gastric concretions or drugs or conditions that decrease or delay gastric emptying.

6. Other considerations:
   a. Can be initiated immediately.
   b. Takes only 15–20 minutes to complete.
   c. Facilitates expeditious administration of charcoal.
   d. If emesis is contraindicated and large nasogastric or orogastric tube cannot be passed, intubate stomach with standard nasogastric tube to allow placement of charcoal.
7. Controversies:
   a. Some studies indicate gastric lavage may be more effective than emesis.
8. Complications:
   a. Esophageal rupture.
   b. Perforation of pharynx.
   c. Perforation of esophagus.
   d. Nasopharyngeal trauma.
   e. Pneumothorax.
   f. Empyema secondary to aspiration of activated charcoal.
   g. Tracheal intubation.
D. Adsorption: Activated charcoal:
   1. Action:
      a. Finely divided black powder, prepared by pyrolysis of carbonaceous material, results in small particles of charcoal with an extensive internal network of pores that absorb substances (brands include Acta-Char, Actidose-Aqua, Insta-Char, Liqui-Char).
      b. Recently a new form of charcoal, superactivated charcoal (Super-Char, previously known as PX-21) has become available, with a surface area of 2,500–3,500 sq m/gm. It can adsorb two to three times the amount of drug or poison as can standard charcoal.
      c. May enhance elimination of drugs by capture during enterohepatic circulation.
   2. Indications:
      a. Use after gastric emptying procedures.
      b. Use after failed gastric emptying procedures.
      c. For many substances with enterohepatic circulation administer every 2–4 hours (gastric dialysis). Especially useful for theophylline, phenobarbital.
   3. Precautions:
      a. The longer the delay between ingestion of poison and administration of activated charcoal the less effective it will be. May want to give charcoal immediately after ipecac. Recent work indicates it may not render conventional doses of syrup of ipecac ineffective, as previously thought.
      b. Use of agents such as ice cream and syrup to improve palatability of activated charcoal may compromise its adsorptive capacity.
   4. Contraindications
      a. Caustic acids and alkalis. Ineffective and may obscure injured areas, making endoscopy difficult or impossible.

5. Ineffective against:
    a. Elemental metals (e.g., iron, lithium).
    b. Some pesticides (malathion, DDT).
    c. Strong acids and alkalis.
    d. Cyanide.
    e. Ethanol and methanol.
    f. Electrolytes.
6. Precautions:
    a. Airway management.
7. Dosage:
    a. Dose of activated charcoal should be roughly 10 times the weight of the ingested drug. Reasonable initial dosages are:
        (1) Child: 15–30 gm.
        (2) Adult: 30–100 gm.
    b. Dose of charcoal should be followed by a cathartic to speed elimination of charcoal-toxin complex. Typical cathartic dosages:
        (1) Sorbitol: 50 ml 70% solution.
        (2) Magnesium sulfate: Adult, 30 gm; child, 250 mg/kg.
8. Administration:
    a. Slurry of charcoal and cathartic (see below) is administered orally or via gastric tube immediately after lavage.
    b. If administered after ipecac, may need to wait until vomiting has subsided.
    c. May need to give multiple doses over hours to days, up to every 4 hours in certain ingestions.
9. Efficacy:
    a. Activated charcoal adsorbs most drugs, thereby decreasing their absorption. It is at least as effective and possibly more effective than gastric emptying in decreasing drug absorption.
    b. Multiple-dose activated charcoal: Repeated administration over hours to days of activated charcoal–cathartic slurry enhances elimination kinetics of several drugs. Proposed mechanisms for this effect (gastrointestinal dialysis) include:
        (1) "Dialysis" of already absorbed drug from the blood across the gastrointestinal surface back into the intestinal lumen, where it is adsorbed to charcoal.
        (2) Adsorption and trapping of drugs during the enteral phase of enterohepatic circulation.
        (3) Drugs with elimination kinetics improved by multiple doses of activated charcoal includes:

Phenobarbital	Salicylic acid
Theophylline	Nadolol
Digoxin	Dapsone
Nortriptyline	Carbamazepine
Meprobamate	Phenylbutazone
Amitriptyline	Chlordecone
Methotrexate	Benzodiazepines
Salicylates	Phenytoin

(4) Whether multiple doses of activated charcoal are clinically relevant in drug overdoses with these drugs is not entirely clear. Like hemodialysis, it is likely that multiple doses of activated charcoal will be most useful against drugs with low plasma protein binding, low volume of distribution, and low lipophilicity and are adsorbed well on activated charcoal.

10. Other considerations:
    a. Recently superactivated charcoal formulations have been released (e.g., Super-Char) that have two to three times the adsorptive capacity of conventional activated charcoal preparations.
    b. Persistent vomiting caused by ipecac or other drugs may be controlled by antiemetics or by H_2-receptor antagonists such as ranitidine (Zantac).
    c. In patients intolerant of charcoal because of persistent vomiting, continuous slow nasogastric administration rather than bolus therapy can be tried.
    d. Sorbitol is the cathartic of choice with charcoal administration because:
       (1) Sorbitol carries charcoal (and therefore ingested poisons) through the gut much more rapidly than other cathartics:
           a Activated charcoal plus cathartic transit time:

No cathartic	23.5 hr.
Magnesium sulfate	9.3 hr.
Magnesium citrate	4.2 hr.
Sorbitol	0.9 hr.

       (2) Sweet, palatable taste.
       (3) No reduction in charcoal efficacy.
       (4) Long shelf-life.
    e. In some poisonings a neutralizing agent instead of activated charcoal is indicated:
       (1) **Mercury:** Lavage with sodium formaldehyde sulfoxylate (20 gm ampule). Reported to effectively neutralize mercuric chloride and other mercury salts to the less soluble metallic mercury.
       (2) **Iron:** Lavage with sodium bicarbonate solution, which converts ferrous ion to poorly absorbed ferrous carbonate; 200 to 300 ml of the bicarbonate solution should be left in the stomach after lavage.
       (3) **Iodine:** Lavage with starch solution until gastric aspirate is no longer blue. Solution is prepared by mixing 75 gm starch in 1 L water.
       (4) **Strychnine, nicotine, quinine, physostigmine:** Lavage with 1:10,000 potassium permanganate solution (100 mg tablet dissolved in 1 L water).
11. Controversies:
    a. Whether activated charcoal alone should replace gastric emptying plus activated charcoal is controversial; current standard of care includes both therapies.

      b. Some studies indicate that mixture of activated charcoal and *N*-acetyl-cysteine does not significantly reduce serum *N*-acetyl-cysteine levels. (See Chapter 77.)

      c. Concurrent administration of charcoal and syrup of ipecac has been proposed as the ideal combination because toxins are rapidly adsorbed and eliminated before significant absorption occurs (Freedman, 1987). This would eliminate the long delay of approximately 2 hours that often occurs between their administration. Larger studies need to be conducted to confirm the utility of this treatment method.

  12. Complications:

      a. Charcoal impaction in patients with atonic bowel.

E. Cathartics:

  1. Indications:

      a. After gastric emptying procedures.

      b. Primary application is in the elimination of activated charcoal–toxin complex from GI tract.

      c. Prevention of constipation.

  2. Action:

      a. Catharsis is produced by osmotic retention of fluid in the GI tract. Increased intraluminal bulk of fluid activates GI motility, which leads to propulsion of GI contents.

  3. Contraindications:

      a. Severe diarrhea.

      b. Trauma to abdomen.

      c. Intestinal obstruction.

      d. Relative contraindication: adynamic ileus.

      e. Specific cathartic contraindications:

        (1) Renal failure: magnesium sulfate.

        (2) Congestive heart failure: sodium sulfate.

        (3) Ethylene glycol ingestion: Phospho-Soda.

        (4) Laxatives and nonionic cathartics other than sorbitol.

        (5) Oil cathartics.

  4. Precautions:

      a. **WARNING:** Cathartic should be used only when needed. Sorbitol may produce catharsis for 8–12 hours.

      b. Therefore, if charcoal is being administered at 6-hour intervals, a cathartic may be necessary only with alternative or every third dose of activated charcoal.

      c. Cathartics are not innocuous and should be used judiciously in all patients, especially elderly and pediatric patients, and those receiving multiple-dose charcoal therapy.

  5. Dosage:

      a. Adult:

        (1) Sorbitol: 50 ml 70% solution.

        (2) Magnesium citrate: 4 ml/kg to 300 ml/dose.

        (3) Magnesium sulfate: 30 gm.

        (4) Sodium sulfate: 30 gm.

        (5) Phospho-Soda: 30 ml (diluted 1:4).

    b. Child:

        (1) Sorbitol: Use very judiciously.

        (2) Magnesium citrate: 4 ml/kg.

        (3) Magnesium sulfate: 250 mg/kg body weight.

        (4) Sodium sulfate: 250 mg/kg body weight.

        (5) Phospho-Soda: Contraindicated.

6. Efficacy:

    a. Sorbitol is most rapidly acting cathartic, producing results in less than 1 hour; magnesium sulfate, 9 hours; magnesium citrate, 4 hours.

    b. Qualitatively, sorbitol produces the most voluminous and longest acting catharsis. This suggests that it may be the best cathartic to eliminate activated charcoal and adsorbed toxin (Krenzelok 1985).

7. Other considerations:

    a. Laxatives and nonionic cathartics, with the exception of sorbitol, are often ineffective because they may be adsorbed by activated charcoal.

    b. Oil cathartics are contraindicated because they may be aspirated or may actually increase absorption of hydrocarbons.

8. Complications:

    a. Fluid and electrolyte imbalance resulting from overaggressive use, especially with sorbitol (Krenzelok 1985).

F. Whole-bowel irrigation:

  1. Indications:

    a. Not first-line treatment for overdose.

    b. May be useful in clearing GI tract of iron, delayed-release formulations not adsorbed by activated charcoal, or very delayed onset of treatment when drug may already be in intestine.

  2. Action:

    a. Physical passage of whole or dissolved pills by complete irrigation of bowel.

  3. Contraindications:

    a. Bowel perforation or obstruction.

    b. Ileus.

    c. GI hemorrhage.

  4. Method:

    a. Similar to routine preparative procedure for colonoscopy.

    b. Administer polyethylene glycol lavage solution either orally or via nasogastric tube.

    c. Procedure takes 3–5 hours.

  5. Dosage:

    a. Adult: Infusion rate 2 L/hr.

    b. Child: Infusion rate 0.5 L/hr.

  6. Efficacy:

    a. Ampicillin absorption decreased 67% after whole-bowel irrigation (Tenenbein, 1987b).

    b. Whole-bowel irrigation was used in six patients, aged 2–19 years, who had ingested on average 84 mg/kg elemental iron. In all six, peak serum-iron levels were lower than expected—in negligible toxicity range (Tenenbein, 1987a).

BIBLIOGRAPHY

Amitai Y, Yeung AC, Moye J, et al: Repetitive oral AC and control of emesis in severe theophylline toxicity. *Ann Intern Med* 1986; 105:386–387.

Auerbach PS, Osterloh J, Braun O, et al: Efficacy of gastric emptying: Gastric lavage versus emesis induced with ipecac. *Ann Emerg Med* 1986; 15:692–698.

Baehler RW, Work J, Smith W, et al: Charcoal hemoperfusion in the therapy for methosuximide and phenytoin overdose. *Arch Intern Med* 1980; 140:1466–1468.

Barone JA, Raia JJ, Huang YC: Evaluation of the effects of multiple-dose activated charcoal on the absorption of orally administered salicylate in a simulated toxic ingestion model. *Ann Emerg Med* 1988; 17:34–37.

Boxer L, Anderson FD, Rowoe DS: Comparison of ipepac-induced emesis with gastric lavage in the treatment of acute salicylate ingestion. *J Pediatr* 1969; 74:800.

Chung DC, Murphy JE, Taylor TW: In-vivo comparison of the adsorption capacity of "superactive charcoal" and fructose with activated charcoal and fructose. *J Toxicol Clin Toxicol* 1982; 19:219–224.

Curtis RA, Barone J, Biacona N: Efficacy of ipecac and activated charcoal/cathartic prevention of salicylate absorption in a simulated overdose. *Arch Intern Med* 1984; 144:48–52.

Freedman GE, Pasternak S, Krenzelok EP: A clinical trial using syrup of ipecac and activated charcoal concurrently. *Ann Emerg Med* 1987; 16:164–166.

Krenzelok EP, Keller R, Steward RD: Gastrointestinal transit times of cathartics combined with charcoal. *Ann Emerg Med* 1985; 14:1152–1155.

Krenzelok EP, Heller MB: Effectiveness of commercially available aqueous activated charcoal products. *Ann Emerg Med* 1987; 16:1340–1343.

Kulig K: Interpreting gastric emptying studies. *J Emerg Med* 1984; 1:447–448.

Kulig K, Bar-Or D, Cantrill SV, et al: Management of acutely poisoned patients without gastric emptying. *Ann Emerg Med* 1985; 14:562–567.

Levy G: Gastrointestinal clearance of drugs with activated charcoal. *N Engl J Med* 1982; 307:676–678.

McDougal CB, Maclean MA: Modifications in the technique of gastric lavage. *Ann Emerg Med* 1981; 10:514–517.

Meester WD: Emesis and lavage. *Vet Hum Toxicol* 1980; 8:225–233.

Moldawsky RJ: Myopathy and ipecac abuse in a bulimic patient. *Psychosomatics* 1985; 26:448–449.

Neuvonen PJ: Clinical pharmacokinetics of oral activated charcoal in acute intoxications. *Clin Pharmacokinet* 1982; 7:465–489.

Neuvonen PJ, Vartiainen M, Tokola O: Comparison of activated charcoal and syrup of ipecac in prevention of drug absorption. *Eur J Clin Pharmacol* 1983; 24:557–562.

North DS, Peterson RG, Krenzelok EP: Effect of activated charcoal on acetylcysteine serum levels in human. *Am J Hosp Pharm* 1981; 38:1022–1024.

Ohring BL, Reed MD, Blumer JL: Continuous nasogastric administration of activated charcoal for the treatment of theophylline intoxication. *Pediatr Pharmacol* 1986; 5:241–245.

Park GD, Spector R, Goldberg MJ, et al: Expanded role of charcoal in the poisoned and overdosed patient. *Arch Intern Med* 1986; 146:969–973.

Pond SM: Role of repeated oral doses of activated charcoal in clinical toxicology. *Med Toxicol* 1986; 1:3–11.

Riegel JM, Becker CE: Use of cathartics in toxic ingestions. *Ann Emerg Med* 1981; 10:254–258.

Rumack BJ, et al: Emesis: Safe and effective? *Ann Emerg Med* 1981; 10:551.

Shannon M, Fish SS, Lovejoy FH: Cathartics and laxatives: Do they still have a place in management of the poisoned patient? *Med Toxicol* 1986; 1:247–252.

Stewart JJ: Effects of emetic and cathartic agents on the gastrointestinal tract and the treatment of toxic ingestion. *Clin Toxicol* 1983; 20:199–253.

Tandberg D, Diven BG, McLeod JW: Ipecac-induced emesis versus gastric lavage: A controlled study in normal adults. *Am J Emerg Med* 1986; 4:205–209.

Tenenbein M: Inefficacy of gastric emptying procedures. *J Emerg Med* 1985; 3:133–136.

Tenenbein M: Whole bowel irrigation in iron poisoning. *J Pediatr* 1987a; 111:142–145.

Tenenbein M, Cohen S, Sitar DS: Whole bowel irrigation as a decontamination procedure after acute drug overdose. *Arch Intern Med* 1987b; 147:905.

Tenenbein M, et al: Efficacy of ipecac-induced emesis, orogastric lavage, and activated charcoal for acute drug overdose. *Ann Emerg Med* 1987c: 16:838–841.

Watson WA, Cremer KF, Chapman JA: Gastrointestinal obstruction associated with multiple-dose activated charcoal. *J Emerg Med* 1986; 4:401–407.

13

Enhancement of Elimination

John M. Wogan, M.D.

I. Simple diuresis (without ion-trapping techniques):
  A. Indications:
    1. May be used in mild overdose with lithium and bromide. Probably minimal if any efficacy.
  B. Contraindications:
    1. Any patient with heart or kidney failure or any drug that produces any of the following complications:
      a. Pulmonary edema, cardiogenic or noncardiogenic (e.g., narcotics and tricyclic antidepressants).
      b. Cerebral edema.
      c. Renal failure.
      d. Syndrome of inappropriate secretion of antidiuretic hormone (SIADH).
  C. Ineffective in:
    1. Almost all poisonings.
  D. Precautions:
    1. May precipitate:
      a. Congestive heart failure.
      b. Electrolyte abnormalities.
  E. Dosage/Method:
    1. Administer sufficient fluids and diuretic to maintain urine flow rate of 5 ml/min (300 ml/hr).
  F. Efficacy:
    1. Minimal. Use only in very selected poisonings (see Indications).

G. Controversies:
  1. The clearance of drugs that undergo renal elimination could be substantially augmented by decreasing renal tubular reabsorption. In theory fluid diuresis should decrease a drug's renal tubular concentration, thereby decreasing the osmotic gradient driving tubular reabsorption and promoting drug excretion. In practice this is not the case and simple fluid diuresis is:
     a. At best, probably only marginally effective for a few drugs (e.g., bromine, lithium).
     b. Offers potentially serious complications.
     c. In cases where it may have some effect, alternatives (e.g., hemodialysis) are much more effective in promoting elimination.
H. Complications:
  1. See Precautions.
II. Diuresis with ion-trapping techniques:
  A. Principles:
    1. Only the nonpolar form of a drug undergoes tubular reabsorption; thus increasing the proportion of a drug that is in a polar, ionic form will decrease reabsorption and enhance elimination. For drugs that are weak acids and bases, alkalinization or acidification of the urine will accomplish this goal.
  B. Indications:
    1. Urine alkalinization:
      a. Salicylates.
      b. Barbiturates (phenobarbital, mephobarbital, primidone).
      c. Use of alkalinization has been proposed for other drugs, but these are the only drugs in which it has been demonstrated to be quantitatively significant.
    2. Urine acidification (see Controversies, below).
  C. Ineffective in:
    1. Poisonings other than those above.
  D. Precautions:
    1. See Complications, below.
  E. Dosage/Method:
    1. Urine alkalinization:
      a. Insert a Swan-Ganz catheter if patient at high risk for pulmonary edema (underlying cardiac disease, history of congestive heart failure).
      b. If patient volume depleted, prepare an IV solution composed of 2 ampules sodium bicarbonate in 1 L 5% dextrose in one-half normal saline solution (D5 0.45%, NS + 88 mEq/L) and administer at 2 L/hr for 3 hours.
      c. Once adequate hydration is established, the IV fluids should be changed to D_5W with 1 or 2 ampules (44–88 mEq) sodium bicarbonate/L plus 40 mEq KCl/L at a rate of 2–3 ml/kg/hr, titrating administration to achieve urine pH approximately 7.5.
    2. Urine acidification (See Controversies, below).

F. Efficacy:
   1. Alkalinization of the urine is safe and effective except as noted (see Complications, below).
G. Controversies:
   1. Urine acidification rarely if ever advocated. Has been recommended in the past for: amphetamines, phencyclidine
   2. Acidification of the urine is controversial because amphetamines and phencyclidine can produce rhabdomyolysis, which is more likely to produce nephrotoxicity in the setting of an acid urine.
   3. Recommended dosages to achieve acidification of urine:
      a. Ascorbic acid: Add 4 gm to 1 L normal saline solution and infuse over 1 hour. When urine pH drops to 5.5, furosemide 1 mg/kg is given IV. Alternatively, administer 0.5 to 1.5 gm ascorbic acid IV or PO every 4–6 hours.
      b. Ammonium chloride: 2.75 mEq/kg added to 1 L normal saline solution, administered through a controlled infusion pump. May be repeated every 6 hours as necessary. When urine pH drops below 5.5, administer furosemide, 1 mg/kg, to maintain urine output of 2 ml/kg/hr. Alternatively, administer 1–2 gm IV or by nasogastric tube until urinary pH is less than 5.5.
H. Complications:
   1. Alkalinization:
      a. Fluid overload, especially in presence of congestive heart failure or renal failure.
      b. Hyperosmolar state.
      c. Paradoxical cerebrospinal fluid acidosis.
   2. Acidification (see Controversies, above).
III. Hemodialysis:
   A. Principles:
      1. For hemodialysis to promote clinically relevant drug elimination, characteristics of the target drug should be:
         a. Low molecular weight (less than 500 daltons).
         b. Low plasma protein binding.
         c. Low lipid solubility.
         d. Low volume of distribution.
         e. Readily diffusible across dialysis membrane.
   B. Indications:
      1. Intoxication with:
         Methanol
         Ethylene glycol
         Mushroom (*Amanita phalloides*)
      2. Intoxications with certain drugs that have produced complications (e.g., acid-base disorders, electrolyte abnormalities, hypertension, hypotension, thermoregulatory disorders) that cannot be treated with supportive care:
         Salicylates
         Theophylline
         Lithium

Phenobarbital
Boric acid
3. Intoxications that produce renal failure, whether secondary to direct nephrotoxicity (e.g., ethylene glycol) or secondary to a less direct pathophysiologic mechanism (e.g., acute tubular necrosis following opiate-induced shock).
4. **Heavy metal** poisonings being treated with chelation therapy in which the patient also has renal failure or insufficiency (e.g., iron).
5. See Table 13–1.
C. Contraindications:
 1. See Ineffective in, below.
D. Ineffective in:
 1. **Amphetamines**
 Barbiturates (short acting)
 Benzodiazepines
 Chlordiazepoxide
 Cocaine
 Cyanide
 Digoxin
 Glutethimide
 Hallucinogens
 Iron
 Narcotics
 PCP
 Phenothiazines
 Procainamide
 Quinidine
 Tricyclic antidepressants
 2. The role of hemodialysis is not clear in cases of tricyclic antidepressants, quinine, quinidine, and amphetamines.
E. Efficacy:
 1. Most drug overdoses can be successfully treated with techniques described above and with good supportive care (see Chapters 8, 9, 10, and 12). Hemodialysis is neither uniformly necessary nor routinely useful.
F. Controversies:
 1. There is some controversy as to the indications for dialysis for ethchlorvynol, chloral hydrate.
G. Complications:
 1. Infection, venous thrombosis, hypotension, air embolus, hemorrhage.
IV. Hemoperfusion:
 A. Indications:
 1. Like hemodialysis, hemoperfusion (pumping blood directly through a charcoal or resin adsorbent) is rarely required for management of drug intoxication.
 2. Potentially superior to hemodialysis because drug clearance is less limited by molecular weight, water solubility, or plasma protein binding.

TABLE 13–1.

Choice of Hemodialysis or Hemoperfusion for Certain Drugs

Hemodialysis	Hemoperfusion
Lithium	Lipid-soluble drugs
Bromide	Barbiturates
Ethanol	Nonbarbiturate hypnotics, sedatives,
Methanol	tranquilizers
Ethylene glycol	? Antidepressants
Salicylates	? Digitalis glycosides
	Theophylline
	Phenytoin

From Haddad LM, Winchester JF: *Clinical Management of Poisoning and Drug Overdose.* Philadelphia: WB Saunders Co, 1983, p 166. Used with permission.

3. Hemoperfusion has been successfully used in intoxications with **phenobarbital, theophylline, phenytoin,** and **ethchlorvynol.**
4. See Table 13–1 for a more complete listing.
   B. No value:
   1. Drugs other than those mentioned in Table 13–1.
   C. Efficacy:
   1. Hemoperfusion is limited by the affinity of a drug for the adsorbent and by adverse reactions (see Complications).
   D. Complications:
   1. Thrombocytopenia, bleeding, hypotension, infection, hypoglycemia, hypocalcemia, and infection.
V. Peritoneal dialysis:
   A. Considerations:
   1. Has been used to enhance clearance of many of the same drugs that can be much more effectively removed with hemodialysis or hemoperfusion.
VI. Other methods to enhance removal of toxins from the body:
   A. Exchange transfusion.
   B. Immunopharmacology (e.g., Fab fragments for digitalis toxicity).
   C. Gastric suctioning.
   D. Intestinal lavage.
   E. Oral adsorbents (charcoal, clays, cholestyramine).
   F. Plasmapheresis.
   G. Lymphatic drainage.
   H. Pulmonary lavage.
   I. Cerebrospinal fluid drainage and replacement.

BIBLIOGRAPHY

Rollins DE, Brizgys M: Immunological approach to poisoning. *Ann Emerg Med* 1986; 15:1046–1051.

14

Medications Useful in Poisonings

Douglas J. Floccare, M.D.

I. Antidotes (see Table 14–1).
II. Contraindicated and ineffective agents:
  A. Analeptics:
      Amphetamine
      Caffeine
      Bemegride
      Picrotoxin
    1. These drugs act directly on the central nervous system to stimulate respiration. However, analeptics may also cause generalized seizure activity and therefore may result in significant harm to patients with diminished airway reflexes.
  B. "Universal antidote": charcoal, magnesium oxide, tannic acid.
    1. The so-called universal antidote is burnt toast, tea, and milk when made at home. The rationale is that the charcoal provides adsorption and the magnesium oxide and milk provide neutralization of acidic and alkaline poisons, respectively. However, the universal antidote is less effective at detoxification than is charcoal alone and the tannic acid component is potentially toxic. Use of this combination is not recommended.
  C. Apomorphine:
    1. Apomorphine is an emetic agent that is not effective orally but acts within 3–5 min when given parenterally, via stimulation of the chemoreceptor trigger zone of the area postrema in the medulla. However, it is also a respiratory depressant and adds to the effect of any CNS depressant the patient may have already taken. Inasmuch as the exact na-

TABLE 14–1.

Poisonings for Which Antidotes are Available

Poison	Antidote	Dosage
Acetaminophen	N-acetyl-cysteine	140 mg/kg PO load, then 70 mg/kg q4h × 17 doses
Atropine, anticholinergics	Physostigmine	Adult: 1–2 mg IV slowly (1 mg/min). Child: 0.5 mg IV (0.5 mg over 1 min).
Carbon monoxide	Oxygen	100% Face mask; consider hyperbaric oxygen
Cholinergic agents	Atropine	Adult: 2 mg IV Child: 0.05 mg/kg IV (minimum, 0.1 mg). Repeat until secretions dry.
Clonidine	Naloxone	2 mg (0.01 mg/kg)
Cyanide	Amyl nitrite	Crushed pearl inhaled by patient 30 sec of each min until sodium nitrite administration
	Sodium nitrite	Adult: 300 mg IV (10 ml 3% solution) Child: 10 mg/kg
	Sodium thiosulfate	Adult: 12.5 gm IV (50 ml 25% solution) Child: Dose based on serum hemoglobin levels (see Chapter 101)
Ethylene glycol	Ethyl alcohol	7.5–10 ml/kg 10% ethanol IV over 30 min with maintenance drip 0.8–1.4 ml/kg/hr (see Chapter 53)
Fluoride	Calcium gluconate	(See Chapter 110, Halogens)
Heavy metals	BAL Disodium edetate Penicillamine	(See Chapter 109, Heavy Metals)
Hydrofluoric acid	Calcium gluconate	(See Chapter 110, Halogens)
Iron	Deferoxamine	10–15 mg/kg/hr
Isoniazid	Pyridoxine	2–5 gm IV slowly
Methanol	Ethyl alcohol	Same as ethylene glycol
Narcotics	Naloxone	2 mg IV*
Nitrites	Methylene blue	1–2 ml/kg 1% solution
Organophosphates	Atropine	Adult: 2 mg IV Child: 0.05 mg/kg IV
	Pralidoxime	Adult: 1 gm IV over 2 min Children: 25–50 mg/kg
Phenothiazines	Diphenhydramine	1–2 mg/kg (50 mg max) IV over 2 min

(Continued.)

TABLE 14–1 (cont.).

Poison	Antidote	Dosage
Propranolol	Glucagon	50–150 μg/kg IV bolus, then 1–5 mg/hr IV drip
Tricyclic antidepressants	Sodium bicarbonate	1–3 mEq/kg

*Propoxyphene, pentazocine, and methadone may require 10 mg or more.

ture of an ingestion is rarely known at the time of initial treatment, it is unlikely that apomorphine would be indicated with any clinical frequency (see Chapter 12).

III. Other therapeutic medications and indications:
   A. Ammonium chloride: Acidification of urine. Poisoning from phencyclidine, amphetamines, strychnine. (Controversial: see Chapter 13, p. 50.)
   B. Calcium chloride: Fluorides, ethylene glycol, calcium channel blockers.
   C. Diazepam (Valium): Seizures, severe agitation, stimulants.
   D. Folate: Methyl alcohol.
   E. Haloperidol, droperidol: Severe psychosis, agitation.
   F. Phenytoin: Seizures, dysrhythmia.
   G. Protamine sulfate: Heparin.
   H. Pyridoxine HCl: Ethylene glycol, isoniazid, monomethylhydrazine (MMH), MMH-containing mushrooms.
   I. Starch: Iodine.
   J. Thiamine HCl: Thiamine deficiency, ethylene glycol.
   K. Vitamin K (Aquamephyton): Oral anticoagulants (e.g., Coumadin).

BIBLIOGRAPHY

Daly JS, Cooney DO: Interference by tannic acid with the effectiveness of activated charcoal in "universal antidote." *Clin Toxicol* 1978; 12:515.

Goodman AG, Gilman LS, Gilman A: *The Pharmacological Basis of Therapeutics.* New York, Macmillan, 1980, p 1609.

Picchioni AL, Chin L, Verhulst HL, et al: Activated charcoal vs. "universal antidote" as an antidote for poisons. *Toxicol Appl Pharmacol* 1966; 8:447.

15

Appropriate Use of the Toxicology Laboratory

Harlan A. Stueven, M.D., F.A.C.E.P.

David Roberts, M.D., F.A.C.E.P., A.B.M.T.

I. Introduction:
   A. "Toxicological screens" often are too late or detect drugs whose presence does not impact on management.
   B. Quantitative tests are available for only 5%–10% of drugs that can be detected.
   C. Yet, selected overdoses should be screened for, and common laboratory tests might help in management or following the course of the poisoning.
   D. As a general rule, to be useful the screen should be reported in 2–4 hours.
   E. Emergency drug screening should be performed only when the results are expected to influence the acute management of the overdose.
II. Minimum recommended laboratory workup for unknown or multiple drug poisoning:
   A. Electrolytes:
      1. Increased **anion gap-type metabolic acidosis** suggests:
         a. **Carbon monoxide** (lactate).
         b. **Cyanide** (lactate).
         c. **Ethylene glycol.**
         d. **Iron** (lactate).
         e. **Isoniazid** (lactate).
         f. **Methanol.**
         g. **Paraldehyde.**
         h. **Salicylates.**
         i. **Toluene.**

j. Any overdose causing profound hypotension and poor tissue perfusion (lactic acidosis).

k. Consider diabetic ketoacidosis and renal failure as part of differential.

2. Nonincreased anion gap-type metabolic acidosis suggests:

a. **Carbonic anhydrase inhibitors** (e.g., acetazolamide).

b. **Toluene** (glue sniffing).

3. Hyperkalemia. Consider:

a. **Digoxin.**

b. **Beta-blockers.**

c. **Succinylcholine.**

d. Any drug that causes renal failure (see Chapter 44, p. 199) or hemolysis (see Chapter 48, p. 230).

4. Hypokalemia. Consider:

a. **Theophylline.**

b. **Diuretics.**

c. **Metaproterenol.**

d. **Toluene.**

e. **Terbutaline.**

f. **Sympathomimetics.**

5. Hyperglycemia. Consider:

a. **Iron.**

b. **Sympathomimetics.**

c. **Salicylates.**

d. **Vacor.**

6. Hypoglycemia. Consider:

a. **Alcohol.**

b. **Beta-blockers.**

c. **Insulin.**

d. **Oral hypoglycemics.**

e. **Salicylates.**

B. Urinalysis:

1. Calcium oxalate crystals suggest **ethylene glycol.**

2. Various urine colors may suggest a variety of specific substances (see Chapter 48, p. 230 for listing).

3. Protein (see Chapter 48).

4. Cells (see Chapter 48).

C. ECG rhythm strip (see Chapter 48).

D. **Acetaminophen** levels: Consider obtaining because of wide availability, lack of correlation between history and substance ingested.

E. **Ethanol** level: Commonly found associated with overdoses.

F. Osmolality: Osmolar gap suggests:

1. **Alcohols.**

2. **Acetone.**

3. **Mannitol.**

4. **Sorbitol.**

G. Arterial blood gas: As indicated to assess acid/base status and respiratory function.

1. Note effect of patient temperature for interpretation. (See Table 15–1).

TABLE 15–1.

Temperature Correction for Arterial Blood
Gas Values*

Body Temperature		Correction Factors†		
°F	°C	Pco₂	Po₂	pH
98.6	37.0	1.00	1.00	0.00
95.0	35.0	0.92	0.89	+0.03
90.0	32.2	0.82	0.76	+0.07
88.0	31.1	0.78	0.72	+0.09
86.0	30.0	0.74	0.67	+0.10
84.0	28.9	0.71	0.63	+0.12
82.0	27.8	0.68	0.59	+0.14
80.0	26.7	0.64	0.56	+0.15
78.0	25.6	0.61	0.52	+0.17
76.0	24.4	0.59	0.49	+0.18
74.0	23.3	0.56	0.46	+0.20
72.0	22.2	0.53	0.43	+0.22

*Adapted from Wears RL: Blood gases in hypother-
mia (letter to the editor) *J Am Coll Emerg Physicians* 1979; 8:247. Adapted from data in Bradley
AF, Stupfel M, Severinghaus JW: Effect of temperature on Pco_2 and Po_2 of blood in vitro. *J Appl
Physiol* 1956; 9:201–204.
†Pco_2 decreases 2.4% per °F fall in temperature.
Po_2 decreases 3.3% per °F fall in temperature. pH
increases .006 units per °F fall in temperature.

III. Spot tests available in emergency department for specific poisonings:
  A. **Iron:**
    1. Deferoxamine test: Add deferoxamine to gastric aspirate; red color suggests presence of iron.
  B. **Salicylate:**
    1. Ferric chloride test: Add several drops 10% or 20% ferric chloride to boiled urine.
      a. Purple color suggests presence of **acetylsalicylic acid, acetoacetic acid,** or **phenylpyruvic acid.**
      b. This is only a qualitative test and all positive results must be confirmed with a serum salicylate test. False positive results may occur, but false negative results are rare.
    2. Phenistix: Dip into serum or urine.
      a. Brown color suggests either **salicylates** or **phenothiazines** are present in urine or serum, as opposed to the typical gray-green to blue for phenylketonuria (PKU).
      b. Adding 1 drop of 20N H_2SO_4 to the strip bleaches out the color in the case of **phenothiazines,** but not **salicylates.**
      c. The color change with Phenistix is often difficult to interpret and therefore should only be used when the ferric chloride test is not available.

C. **Carbon monoxide:**
1. Add 2 drops blood to 15 ml water, add 5 drops 25% NaOH; yellow color suggests carboxyhemoglobin >20%.

D. **Methemoglobinemia:**
1. Chocolate-colored blood.
2. Addition of 1 crystal potassium cyanide to 1:1,000 dilution of patient's blood results in color change to pink if methemoglobinemia present.

E. **Cyanide:**
1. Add few crystals of ferrous sulfate to 5 ml gastric aspirate, followed by 5 drops 20% NaOH; boil, then cool; add 8–10 drops 10% HCl.
2. Greenish color suggests **cyanide** or **salicylates.**

F. **Phenothiazines:**
1. Ferric chloride test (see above).

IV. Common toxicology laboratory techniques:

A. Amounts of fluid needed for toxicology screen:
1. Whole blood: 5–10 ml.
2. Serum: 5–10 ml.
3. Urine: 50 ml.
   a. NOTE: Urine is generally more useful for screen than blood or serum: more and varied substances detected in urine.
4. Gastric contents: 25–50 ml.

B. Information required by toxicology laboratory:
1. Agents suspected and probable dose.
2. Probable time of ingestion and time of sampling.
3. Patient's level of consciousness, acid-base status, and clinical condition.
4. Any pills or other evidence found on or near patient.

C. Qualitative tests:
1. No correlation between detection and intensity of drug effect.
2. Used for support or confirmation of suspected overdose.
3. Useful in patients with confusing clinical picture, atypical signs and symptoms, and little or no history.

D. Quantitative tests:
1. Measures levels.
2. Useful only if clinical correlation with drug level exists or if quantification directly relates to treatment or disposition. Examples include ethanol, methanol, acetaminophen, salicylates, iron, theophylline, lithium, ethylene glycol, phenobarbital, phenytoin, carboxyhemoglobin, methemoglobin, heavy metals, digoxin.
   a. Toxic levels may imply:
      (1) Severe toxicity.
      (2) Habituation (e.g., alcohol, sedative-hypnotics).
      (3) Addiction (e.g., narcotics).
   b. Less than toxic levels may imply:
      (1) Mild toxicity.
      (2) Incomplete absorption.
      (3) Drug withdrawal (imminent).
      (4) Drug interaction (e.g., disulfiram displacing phenytoin binding resulting in clinical phenytoin toxicity with therapeutic phenytoin levels).

(5) Poisoning does not explain clinical findings.
3. Delays in gastric emptying (e.g., opiates, anticholinergics, salicylates, long-acting theophylline preparations) may alter "peak" concentrations. Should obtain follow-up samples about 2 hours after collecting initial specimen.
4. Indications for repeat quantitative testing:
   a. Assess effectiveness of therapy (e.g., N-acetyl-cysteine in acetaminophen poisoning).
   b. Determine drug half-life (e.g., drugs that form concretions such as meprobamate, glutethimide, salicylates).
E. Types of tests:
   1. Enzyme multiple immunoassay technique (EMIT): rapid, quantitative and qualitative, widely available. Examples of substances identified by EMIT include barbiturates, benzoyl ecgonine (cocaine metabolite), benzodiazepines, opiates, PCP, propoxyphene, methaqualone.
   2. Radioimmunoassay (RIA): slow, quantitative and qualitative. Based on antibody/drug reaction and resultant precipitate analyzed by gamma counter.
   3. Thin-layer chromatography (TLC): slow, qualitative only. Solvent is placed on plate, separation occurs because of migration of substances.
   4. Gas liquid chromatography (GLC): best for quantification. Specimen is vaporized and carried by inert gas in a column.
F. Types of toxicologic screens:
   1. Complete toxicology screen: both blood and urine.
      a. Blood analyzed by GLC for volatiles (see below), then saved for confirmation or quantification of substances found in urine.
      b. Urine is screened using TLC and other methods (e.g., colorimetry).
   2. GLC blood volatiles screen for:
      a. **Alcohols.**
      b. **Acetone, acetaldehyde.**
   3. Urine screen:
      a. TLC and other qualitative techniques (see above).
      b. Taking a sample before drug metabolism occurs may provide erroneous result.
      c. Patients in shock may have renal hypoperfusion and decreased renal drug clearance.
   4. Gastric screen (same as urine).
V. Poisoning for which quantitative serum levels can be obtained:
   A. **Acetaminophen** at 4 hours after ingestion. Greater than 150 μg/ml is potentially hepatotoxic and suggests a need for *N*-acetyl-cysteine (see acetaminophen nomogram, Chapter 77).
   B. **Carboxyhemoglobin.** Levels greater than 25% suggest need for hyperbaric therapy. NOTE: Symptoms and signs do not necessarily correlate with levels. Decisions should be based on clinical picture if levels are lower. With knowledge of half-life, calculate level back to time of exposure. (See Chapter 100.)

    C. **Digoxin** at 2–4 hours after ingestion. Greater than 10 ng/ml suggests need for antibody therapy (Digibind).

    D. **Ethanol.** Coma with levels less than 200 mg/dl suggests another cause.

    E. **Ethylene glycol.** Levels greater than 25–50 mg/dl require hemodialysis.

    F. **Iron** and **iron binding capacity** 3–5 hours after ingestion. If iron levels exceed iron binding capacity, deferoxamine should be considered.

    G. **Lithium.** Levels greater than 4.0 mEq/L suggest need for hemodialysis.

    H. **Methanol.** Levels greater than 25–50 mg/dl require hemodialysis.

    I. **Methemoglobin** may be caused by a variety of chemicals. Levels guide use of methylene blue (see Chapter 102).

    J. **Phenobarbital.** Levels correlate with clinical picture.

    K. **Phenytoin.** Levels greater than 30 µg/ml can cause CNS symptoms. Levels can be used as guide to admission. Note long half-life.

    L. **Salicylate** at 6 hours after ingestion. Levels greater than 50 mg/ml suggest toxicity.

    M. **Theophylline.** Levels greater than 20 µg/ml are toxic; greater than 50 µg/ml are associated with increasing risk for seizures and arrhythmias. Hemoperfusion may be indicated.

VI. Poisonings to be considered for qualitative screening in sedated, lethargic, or comatose patient:

    A. **Amphetamines.**

    B. **Carbon monoxide.**

    C. **Cocaine.**

    D. **Ethanol.**

    E. **Ethylene glycol** often requires immediate dialysis. **Do not wait for screen to confirm.**

    F. **Heavy metals.**

    G. **Lithium.**

    H. **Methanol** often requires immediate dialysis. **Do not wait for screen to confirm.**

    I. **Opioids.**

    J. **Phencyclidine.**

    K. **Phenothiazines.**

    L. **Phenytoin.**

    M. **Sedative hypnotics:**
        1. Barbiturates.
        2. Benzodiazepines.
        3. Chloral hydrate, glutethimide, methaqualone, ethchlorvynol, meprobamate.

    N. **Tricyclic antidepressants.**

VII. Poisonings to be considered for qualitative screening in stimulated, agitated, or "toxic" patient

    A. **Amphetamines.**

    B. **Cocaine and derivatives.**

    C. **Heavy metals.**

    D. **Methylxanthines** (theophylline and caffeine).

    E. **Phencyclidine.**

    F. **Tricyclic antidepressants.**

BIBLIOGRAPHY

Bailey DN: The role of the laboratory in treatment of the poisoned patient: Laboratory perspective. *J Anal Toxicol* 1983; 7:136.

Bryson PD: *Comprehensive Review in Toxicology.* Rockville, Md, Aspen Systems Corp, 1986.

Epstein FB, Hassan M: Therapeutic drug levels and toxicology screens. *Emerg Med Clin North Am* 1986; 4:367–376.

Flomenbaum N, Goldfrank L: *Diagnostic Testing in the Emergency Department.* Rockville, Md., Aspen Systems Corp, 1984.

Goldfrank LR, et al: *Goldfrank's Toxicologic Emergencies.* New York, Appleton-Century-Crofts, 1986.

Hepler BR, Sutheimer CA, Sunshine I: The role of the toxicology laboratory in emergency medicine. *J Toxicol Clin Toxicol* 1982; 19:353.

Ingelfinger JA, Isakson G, Shine D, et al: Reliability of the toxic screen in drug overdose. *Clin Pharmacol Ther* 1981; 29:570–575.

Kaye F: Bedside toxicology. *Pediatr Clin North Am* 1970; 17:522.

Kellerman AL, Fihn SD, LoGerfo JP, et al: Impact of drug screening in suspected overdose. *Ann Emerg Med* 1987; 16:1206–1216.

Krenzelok EP, Guharoy SL, Johnson DR: Toxicology screening in the emergency department: Ethanol, barbiturates, and salicylates. *Am J Emerg Med* 1984; 2(4):331–332.

Kulig K: Utilization of emergency toxicology screens (editorial). *Am J Emerg Med* 1985; 6:573–574.

Lundberg GD: Operations management in emergency toxicology. *J Anal Toxicol* 1982; 7:152.

McCarron MM: The use of toxicology tests in emergency room diagnosis. *J Anal Toxicol* 1983; 7:131.

McCarron MM: The role of the laboratory in treatment of the poisoned patient: A clinical perspective. *J Anal Toxicol* 1983; 7:154.

Medical toxicology: *Emerg Med Clin North Am* 1984; 2:1.

Poisonings and overdose: *Top Emerg Med* 1979; 1:3.

Sandhu RS, Thind IS: Evaluation of hospital and commercial toxic screens. *J Med Soc NJ* 1983; 80:833.

Stewart MJ: Drug analyses in poisoned patients. The need to be specific. *Ann Clin Biochem* 1982; 19:254–257.

Stewart DC: The use of the clinical laboratory in the diagnosis and treatment of substance abuse. *Pediatr Ann* 1982; 11:669–682.

Sullivan JB, Fisher JG: Proper use of the toxicology laboratory. *Emerg Med Rep* 1984; 5:125–132.

Taylor FL, Cohan SL, White JD: Comprehensive toxicology screening in the emergency department. An aid to clinical diagnosis. *Am J Emerg Med* 1985; 3:504–511.

Teitelbaum DT, Morgan J, Gray G: Nonconcordance between clinical impression and laboratory findings in clinical toxicology. *Clin Toxicol* 1977; 10:417–422.

Walsh MJ: Reliability of drug testing. *JAMA* 1987; 258:2587–2588.

Weisman R, Howland MA: The toxicology laboratory. *Top Emerg Med* 1983; 5:9.

16

Staff Precautions in Toxicologic Emergencies

James L. Baker, M.D., F.A.C.E.P.

I. Introduction. Invasive procedures usually need to be urgently performed during the management and resuscitation of patients who have a serious poisoning or toxic exposure. Also, the intravenous drug abuser is at particular risk for harboring both hepatitis B and human immunodeficiency virus (HIV; acquired immune deficiency syndrome [AIDS] virus). Precautions to reduce the possibility of nosocomial transmission of these and other infectious diseases should be routinely undertaken.

For description of staff precautions to be taken in caring for patients contaminated with hazardous materials see Chapter 111.

II. Risk to health care workers:
   A. Current literature indicates a very low likelihood of transmission of HIV infection to health care workers via occupational exposure. However, there have been several cases of documented and suspected nosocomial transmission:
      1. By needle stick injury (both deep and superficial).
      2. By repeated ungloved contact with blood, secretions, or excretions from infected patients.
      3. By nonparenteral single exposures to infectious blood (that may have involved minor open wounds, such as chapped hands, or mucus membranes, such as a splash in the mouth).
      These events, although rare, provide evidence that occupational exposure can result in acquisition of the virus during the provision of health care.
   B. For emergency care personnel who care for many high-risk patients, such as intravenous drug abusers, and who frequently must perform invasive procedures on actively bleeding or combative patients, this **risk cannot be ignored.**

C. Evidence indicates that traditional risk factors for HIV cannot be used to selectively use infectious disease precautions. Many if not most patients who are infected with HIV will have no readily identifiable characteristics on presentation or during the course of management.

D. After needle stick injury from a hepatitis carrier, the risk of a health care provider acquiring the infection has been shown to be 6% to 30%.

    1. Emergency personnel have been identified as being at significantly greater risk for acquiring hepatitis B infection in the workplace than persons in other medical specialties.

III. Recommended infection control precautions:

    The Centers for Disease Control (CDC) has developed guidelines for the prevention of transmission of infectious disease, clearly intended to be utilized when there is exposure to blood or other bodily fluids, **whether or not suspicion of HIV infection exists.** Updates are issued by the CDC.

A. Sharp items:

    1. Disposable syringes and needles, scalpel blades, and other sharp items should be placed in puncture-resistant containers located as close as practical to the area in which they were used.

    2. To prevent needle stick injuries, needles should not be recapped, purposefully bent, broken, removed from disposable syringes, or otherwise manipulated by hand.

    3. The health care worker should be aware that the intravenous drug abuser may have on his or her person needles that may have been contaminated not only by the patient but by others; utmost care should be exercised when reaching into pockets or in handling clothing.

B. During the rapid resuscitation of critically ill patients, the often crowded bedside provides the possibility for potential needle stick injuries to occur from one health care provider accidentally injuring another; this has resulted in documented cases of acquisition of HIV infection.

C. When the possibility of exposure to blood or other body fluids exists, the following routinely recommended precautions should be followed:

    1. Gloves:

        a. Use when handling any body fluids.

        b. Use with mucous membrane contact.

    2. Gown:

        a. Use in all resuscitations.

        b. Use in all invasive procedures.

        c. Use with potentially aerosolized material.

        d. Use in pelvic examinations.

    3. Mask:

        a. Use in all resuscitations.

        b. Use in all invasive procedures.

        c. Use with potentially aerosolized material.

    4. Eye covering:

        a. Use in all resuscitations.

        b. Use in all invasive procedures.

        c. Use with potentially aerosolized material.

D. Hands should be washed thoroughly and immediately if they accidentally become contaminated with blood.

E. To minimize the need for emergency mouth-to-mouth resuscitation, mouth pieces, resuscitation bags, or other ventilation devices should be strategically located and immediately available for use.

F. No health care provider who has exudative lesions or weeping dermatitis should perform or assist in invasive procedures or other direct patient care activities or handle equipment used in patient care. (An incident occurred in 1986 in which a nurse acquired HIV infection through contact of infective blood and her chapped hands.)

IV. Suggested protocol after possible exposure:

A. Possible HIV exposure:

General procedures to be followed if a significant exposure (such as a needle stick injury) occurs have been outlined by the CDC, specifically addressing HIV.

1. After parenteral (needle stick or cut) or mucus membrane (splash to the eye or mouth) exposure to blood or other bodily fluids, the source patient should be assessed clinically and epidemiologically to determine the likelihood of HIV infection.

2. If the assessment suggests that infection may exist, the patient should be informed of the incident and requested to consent to serologic testing for evidence of HIV infection.

a. If the patient declines testing or tests positive the health care provider should be evaluated clinically and serologically for evidence of HIV infection as soon as possible after the exposure and, if seronegative, retested after 6 weeks and periodically thereafter (e.g., 3, 6, 12 months after exposure) to determine if transmission has occurred. Most infected persons are expected to seroconvert in the first 6–12 weeks.

b. During this follow-up period exposed health care workers should receive counseling about the risk of infection and follow U.S. Public Health Service recommendations for preventing transmission of AIDS.

c. If the source patient is seronegative and has no other evidence of HIV infection, no further follow-up is necessary.

d. If the source patient cannot be identified, decisions regarding appropriate follow-up should be individualized based on the type of exposure and the likelihood that the source patient was infected.

B. Possible hepatitis B exposure:

1. Policies regarding possible exposure to hepatitis B are generally defined by individual institutions.

2. The availability to most health care personnel of an effective vaccine against hepatitis B should help to minimize occupational risk. We recommend that all emergency personnel be vaccinated against hepatitis B.

3. If a significant exposure occurs (such as is described above), the source patient should be tested for the presence of hepatitis B surface antigen and the exposed person should be tested for hepatitis B surface antibody.

a. If the source patient is negative for antigen or if the exposed person is positive for the antibody, no further action is indicated.

b. If the source patient is antigen positive and the exposed person is

antibody negative, the exposed person should receive hepatitis B immune globulin (0.06 ml/kg) as soon as possible after the incident,
with subsequent follow-up at 30 days for a repeat dose. Specific policies of follow-up in these instances should be referred to the hospital infection control personnel.
C. Possible hazardous chemical exposure:
    See Chapter 111 on hazardous chemicals in industry and the environ-
ment.

BIBLIOGRAPHY

Baker JL, Kelen GD, Sivertson KT, et al: Unsuspected human immunodeficiency virus in critically ill emergency patients. *JAMA* 1987; 257:2609–2611.

Centers for Disease Control: Update: Human immunodeficiency virus infections in health
care workers exposed to blood of infected patients. *MMWR* 1987; 36:285–289.

Centers for Disease Control: Recommendations for preventing transmission of infection
with human T-lymphotropic virus type III/lymphadenopathy-associated virus during invasive procedures. *MMWR* 1986; 35:221–223.

Centers for Disease Control: Update: Evaluation of human T-lymphotropic virus type III/
lymphadenopathy-associated virus infection in health-care personnel—United States.
MMWR 1985; 34:575–578.

Gerberding JL, University of California, San Francisco, Task Force on AIDS: Recommended
infection-control policies for patients with human immunodeficiency virus infection. *N
Engl J Med* 1986; 315:1562–1564.

Grady JF, Lee VA, Prince AM, et al: Hepatitis B immune globulin for accidental exposures
among medical personnel: Final report of a multicenter controlled trial. *J Infect Dis* 1978;
138:625–638.

Kelen GD, Fritz S, Qaguish B, et al: Unrecognized human immunodeficiency virus (HIV) in
emergency department patients. *N Engl J Med* 1988; 318:1645–1650.

Seeff LB, Wright EC, Zimmerman HJ, et al: Type B hepatitis after needlestick exposure: Prevention with hepatitis B immune globulin. *Ann Intern Med* 1978; 88:285–293.

17

Disposition Considerations for Pediatric Patients

M. Douglas Baker, M.D.

NOTE: **Child abuse or neglect should be considered in all pediatric poisonings.**

I. Introduction. The bulk of this book deals with specific guidelines for the diagnosis and management of individual toxins. In general these guidelines apply to both the adult and pediatric patient. The purpose of this brief discussion is not to reiterate individual management plans but to review the more universal principles of disposition planning for pediatric patients.

II. General considerations:
   A. Medical considerations (see specific chapters) must be met prior to release from the medical center.
   B. The majority of children who ingest toxins will require close adult supervision following discharge. It is the physician's obligation to ensure that such conditions will be met before releasing the patient from care. Adequacy of the home environment and of parental observation must be assessed before discharging the patient from the emergency department.
   C. If the physician feels unqualified or insecure in making this judgment, help should be obtained from the pediatric social worker.
   D. Regardless of diagnosis related groups (DRGs) or the decisions rendered by hospital review boards, any child who is unable to be discharged to a stable and *safe* home environment (either his own or foster placement) should be hospitalized.

E. All pediatric patients should be assessed for suicide risk. It is preferable that pediatric patients at risk for suicide be evaluated by a specialist in child psychiatry. No child should be discharged from the medical center if suicide risk is ongoing.

F. Discharge from the hospital also implies prior arrangement of adequate follow-up care. The responsible adult accompanying the child must have a clear understanding of the physician's recommendations for ongoing care. These should be in writing.

G. Discharge instructions should include the availability of repeat assessment in the event of a sudden worsening of the child's condition.

H. As always, documentation of the physician's assessment and treatment plans, including discharge instructions and follow-up plans, should be thorough and clearly written.
   1. Follow-up may involve psychiatric evaluation or social work assessment.
   2. Some ingestions in the pediatric age group will require outpatient follow-up the next day, for example, kerosene ingestion in a patient with normal chest x-ray film and no respiratory distress.

I. Although not common, the possibility of child abuse or neglect must be considered in the differential diagnosis (see Chapter 31).
   1. The "poison repeater," a child who has had multiple ingestions, may be an attention-getter, may be defiant, or may not have sufficient supervision. Enlist the aid of a social worker.

J. Poison prevention and home "poison proofing" should be discussed before discharge and is usually warmly received. Parents are usually attentive and appreciative.

BIBLIOGRAPHY

Guzzardi LJ: Role of the emergency physician in the treatment of the poisoned patient. *Emerg Med Clin North Am* 2:3–13.

18

Disposition Considerations for Adult Patients

Keith T. Sivertson, M.D., F.A.C.E.P.

NOTE: **All patients must be assessed for suicide risk before discharge.**

I. Introduction. The decision to discharge the poisoned adult from the hospital or emergency department must address two broad concepts: Is the health of the patient in any further jeopardy? Is anyone else potentially endangered by discharge of the patient?

II. General considerations:

In determining the suitability of the patient for discharge the physician must consider:

  A. The patient's medical condition:

    1. Normal vital signs (e.g., sinus tachycardia should prompt search for hypovolemia, infection, persistence of toxin effect such as amphetamines).

    2. Ability of patient to tolerate oral intake.

  B. The properties of the toxin involved:

    1. Some toxins (e.g., acetaminophen) may have minimal effects initially and devastating consequences at greater than 24 hours.

    2. Certain toxins (e.g., tricyclic antidepressants, carbon monoxide) may have effects not clearly correlated with serum levels.

    3. If the toxin is unknown, observation should be extended and hospitalization may be necessary.

  C. The course of the patient's physical and emotional condition:

    1. Danger to others must be considered.

    2. Danger to self (suicide potential) must be considered.

3. Is the patient still sufficiently impaired as to represent a danger if he or she should attempt to drive or operate equipment?

4. Is this poisoning representative of habits that may endanger co-workers, friends, or family?

D. The probability of reexposure to the toxin:

1. Is this exposure a harbinger of dangerous working conditions? Are toxins being transmitted to the home and family members?

2. Is this exposure indicative of living conditions in a particular environment and therefore suggest hazardous conditions for others in that environment (e.g., public housing, nursing home, apartment complex)?

E. Follow-up:

1. Consider telephone follow-up, home visit by visiting nurse or physician, or return visit.

2. Further contact may be needed between employer, social service workers, occupational health officials, patient's personal physician, and treating physician.

F. Discharge instructions:

1. Written discharge instructions, telephone number for the patient to call if questions arise later.

G. Responsible adult to accompany the patient if indicated. A stable home environment must exist to allow for close observation of the patient's physical and mental status.

H. Transfer of patients (see Chapter 19).

III. General considerations for hospitalization:

A. In-hospital observation of the patient with overdose may be necessary for several reasons:

1. Unconsciousness at any time during drug overdose except in a few specific situations (e.g., iv heroin overdose). Hospitalization should continue for 24 hours after the patient becomes asymptomatic.

2. Hypotension at any time.

3. Potential for respiratory compromise.

4. Underlying disease or injury complicating toxic exposure.

5. Persistent, altered mental status despite appropriate treatment.

6. Poisoning with an unknown toxin.

7. Suicide risk.

8. Drugs with unusual action.

a. Latent phase toxicity:

(1) Drugs such as **iron, acetaminophen, carbon tetrachloride,** or **mercury** have a *latent phase* in which the patient appears to recover from the initial insult, only to decompensate 48–72 hours after ingestion.

b. Delayed toxicity:

(1) Some drugs are associated with *delayed effects:*

a **Acetaminophen** (hepatic necrosis).

b ***Amanita*** mushroom (hepatic necrosis).

c **Mercury** (hemorrhagic colitis).

d **Methanol** (blindness).

        e **Carbon tetrachloride** (hepatic or renal failure).

        f **Paraquat** (pulmonary fibrosis).

        g **PCP** (hypertension).

        h **Thallium** (neurotoxin).

    (2) *Remote effect:* For example, **Tricyclic antidepressant** overdose has been reported to cause fatal arrhythmia several days after ingestion.

  c. Prolonged toxicity: The victim of **methadone HCl** (Dolophine) or **oral hypoglycemic** agent overdose must be admitted for at least 24 hours because of continuous or prolonged effect.

  9. Persistent vomiting or diarrhea.

  10. Inability to observe appropriately or for sufficient time in emergency department.

  11. Social problems that make follow-up unlikely.

  12. Serious withdrawal symptoms imminent.

  13. Cannot be considered for discharge (see Discharge considerations, below).

IV. Consideration for admission to intensive care unit:

  A. Current literature supports the hypothesis that the clinical course of patients with drug overdose can be accurately predicted during the first several hours of observation. At least one retrospective set of clinical criteria, readily available in the emergency department, has been suggested to identify high risk outcomes that necessitate ICU admission:

    1. Arterial carbon dioxide pressure $\geq$ 45 mm.

    2. Seizures.

    3. Unresponsiveness to verbal stimuli or a deeper level of obtundation.

    4. Cardiac dysrhythmia (except asymptomatic sinus tachycardia or sinus bradycardia):

      1. Second- or third-degree atrioventricular block.

      2. QRS $\geq$ 0.12 sec.

    5. Systolic blood pressure <80 mm Hg (Brett AS, et al: *Arch Intern Med* 1987; 146:133–137).

  B. Because these criteria have not been prospectively evaluated, it is probably best at this time to consider in addition the following general criteria for intensive care admission:

    1. The need for respiratory or cardiovascular support or the presence of severe complications (e.g., inadequate airway or potential need for intubation, cardiac arrhythmias).

    2. Unstable vital signs (e.g., persistent hypotension).

    3. Declining level of consciousness or mental status (e.g., coma).

V. Discharge considerations:

  A. Each toxin has specific considerations. Generally patients should be asymptomatic at time of discharge, and without clinical findings.

  B. Clear sensorium.

  C. Drug counseling or education offered.

  D. Appropriate follow-up arranged.

  E. Patient understands discharge instructions.

F. Patient has appropriate disposition environment, including appropriate supervision if applicable.
G. Suicide and psychiatric status have been appropriately evaluated.

BIBLIOGRAPHY

Brett AS, Rothschild N, Gray R, et al: Predicting the clinical course in intentional drug overdose. Implications for use of the ICU. *Arch Intern Med* 1987; 147:133–137.

Guzzardi LJ: Role of the emergency physician in the treatment of the poisoned patient. *Emerg Med Clin North Am* 1984; 2:3–13.

Tintinalli JE, Rothstein RJ, Krome RL: *Emergency Medicine: A comprehensive study guide.* New York, McGraw-Hill Book Co, 1985.

19

Interhospital Transfer of Poisoned or Intoxicated Patients

Dan K. Morhaim, M.D., F.A.C.E.P.

I. Precautions in the interhospital transfer of poisoned patients:
   A. Patients at risk for suicidal, homicidal, or other unexpected behavior.
   B. Patients at risk for unexpected or violent behavior related to ingestion of hallucinogens, phencyclidine, etc.
   C. Patients with narcotic overdoses may require repeated naloxone boluses or continuous naloxone infusion.
   D. Care must be taken to ensure that patients with overdoses are not transferred to a psychiatric facility before they are medically stable.
II. Transfer responsibilities and arrangements: The vast majority of poisoned patients will be able to receive satisfactory care in the local hospital. However, some will require facilities and personnel beyond those locally available (e.g., hemodialysis, charcoal hemoperfusion, hyperbaric oxygen). It is essential for the local physician to recognize this group of patients early and to arrange for their transfer to an institution where optimum care can be provided.
   A. Referring physician: The responsibility for the initiation of patient transfer rests on the local physician or, in the rural setting where no physician is immediately available, on the emergency department nurse. There should be direct contact by the referring physician to the receiving physician to ensure that space and personnel are available for care of the patient.
   B. Receiving physician:
      1. The specifics of patient transfer normally rest with the receiving physician, who must establish what care should be initiated prior to the patient transfer, how that transfer is to be established, and what data should accompany the patient.

73

2. One of the advantages of an established transfer arrangement is that it allows for feedback to the local hospital and physician and suggestions for improving future patient care.
3. It should be remembered that the patient transported to another facility is usually critically ill. Too often this critically ill patient is transported in a substandard vehicle and cared for by personnel not trained to deal with severely ill patients.

III. Protocols for patient transfer:
A. The referring physician should talk to the physician accepting the patient at the receiving hospital. This should not be left to the nurse or emergency department administrator to arrange.
B. Arrangements and details of the transfer, including mode of transportation, are the responsibility of the physician at the receiving hospital. Where local ambulances are to be used for transporting the patient to the receiving facility, approval of the equipment and personnel involved in the transfer should be obtained by the local physician from the receiving physician. It is very important that the referring physician become personally involved with the details of such transfer to ensure optimum care of the patient during transit.
C. Proper equipment (e.g., infusion pumps, suction, 100% oxygen) and trained personnel must be present to handle the problems specific to toxicologic emergencies, whether the transfer is by ground or air.
D. Verbal and written instructions are given to the personnel transporting the patient by the referring physician.
E. Information regarding the patient's condition and needs during transfer must be given to the personnel responsible for transporting the patient and should include:
1. Airway maintenance.
2. Fluid volume.
3. Special procedures or medications (e.g., naloxone) that may be necessary.
F. A written record of the nature of the toxic exposure, treatment rendered at the local hospital, complications, and status at time of transfer is essential, and **must** accompany the patient.
G. Prior to transfer:
1. If possible, obtain written permission from the patient or family for transfer to another institution.
2. Resuscitate and stabilize the patient **before transport.** Determine with the receiving physician what interventions are appropriate and that the patient's condition is favorable for transport.
H. Management during transport:
1. Continue support of respiratory and circulatory systems.
2. Monitor vital signs.
3. Use appropriate medications as ordered by the physician or as provided by written protocol (e.g., naloxone, 50% dextrose solution, ethanol infusion).
4. Maintain communication with the receiving physician or institution during transfer.
5. Maintain accurate records during transfer.

BIBLIOGRAPHY

American College of Emergency Physicians: Guidelines for transfer of patients. *Ann Emerg Med* 1985; 14:1221–1222.

Committee on Trauma, American College of Surgeons: Stabilization and Transfer, in *Advanced Trauma Life Support Course Manual.* Chicago, American College of Surgeons, 1985.

Reed WG, Cawley KA, Anderson RJ: The effect of a public hospital's transfer policy on patient care. *N Engl J Med* 1986; 315:1428–1432.

Relman AS: Texas eliminates dumping: A start toward equity in hospital care. *N Engl J Med* 1986; 314:578–579.

Schiff RL, Ansell DA, Schlosser JE, et al: Transfers to a public hospital: A prospective study of 467 patients. *N Engl J Med* 1986; 314:552–557.

Transfers to a public hospital (letters). *N Engl J Med* 315, 1421–1422.

20

Medical-Legal Issues in Toxicology

Jordan M. Laub, M.D.

Bruce Moskow, M.D., J.D., F.A.C.E.P.

I. False imprisonment:
   A. Defined as the total restraint of a person against that person's will and not conforming with specific societal exceptions.
   B. Potential area of liability for the physician dealing with poisoned patients perceived as having psychiatric, sensory, or chemical impairment. The specific exceptions are in the main defined in each state's mental health code. An example of such an exception is self-defense in the case of violent patients.

II. Implied consent:
   A. Consent is implied from the circumstances and is not actually expressed. In other words, the actions of the patient are deemed sufficient to imply to a reasonable person that the patient has consented to treatment. An example would be lifesaving treatment for an unconscious or mentally incompetent patient. Courts have held that implied consent exists in such situations because it is believed that the patient, if mentally competent, would have given his consent to treatment necessary to save his life.
   B. Consent from the next-of-kin should be obtained if possible. If emergency conditions require immediate treatment, proceed with treatment while simultaneously attempting to contact the patient's nearest relative.

III. Informed consent:
   A. Informed consent requires that the patient be competent to consent to and understand all the risks and benefits inherent in a procedure and the consequence of alternative methods of treatment or of no treatment.
   B. Patients should be informed of the risks and benefits before being asked for consent to procedures such as intravenous pyelogram, suturing, hemodialysis or peritoneal dialysis, hemoperfusion, or any surgical procedure.

C. Failure to obtain proper and informed consent exposes the physician to a charge of technical battery, and the physician may be responsible for all resulting damages if a patient is injured as a result of treatment (and the patient claims he or she would not have consented knowing the risks).

D. Treatment should not be withheld for lack of consent in situations that may cause serious impairment of health, such as in true life-threatening emergencies (see Implied Consent).

IV. Refusal of treatment:

A. Competent patient:

1. A mentally competent adult patient cannot be forced to receive treatment, even in a life-threatening emergency, except by order of a court.

2. Whenever the emergency department staff has questions relating to consent regarding a life-and-death or serious harm situation, the hospital administration should be involved as soon as possible to pursue every available legal avenue.

3. To minimize potential legal reprisal against the hospital and staff, most patients who refuse medically indicated treatment are asked to sign a form stating that they have been informed of their condition and the need for its treatment and that they are refusing treatment or leaving the hospital against medical advice. They must therefore assume any liability that results. The competent, conscious adult thus "signs out" and is allowed to leave the hospital. The physician, however, should not depend solely on an AMA form for protection against subsequent litigation. **The episode should be fully documented in the chart.** This note should include at least the following:

   a. The life- or limb-threatening illness.

   b. The mental competence of the patient as documented by normal vital signs and mental status examination.

   c. That the patient has been advised to return immediately to the hospital should he or she have a change of mind.

B. Incompetent patient:

1. The physician may proceed with treatment against the patient's will (e.g., patient in imminent danger of death or serious impairment if not treated) if the patient can be declared incompetent.

2. Determination of clinical competence is a clinical not a legal decision. Competence to refuse treatment must be assessed in the light of vital signs, mental status (both acute and chronic), age, toxins, and intoxicants. Clinically incompetent patients include those who are intoxicated, victims of head trauma, in shock, or psychotic.

3. If the patient is deemed mentally incompetent and is thus unable to refuse treatment the following actions should be undertaken:

   a. Notify the appropriate hospital administrator and the hospital attorney.

   b. Seek consent from a family member.

   c. Contact the appropriate court or judicial authority responsible for civil commitment. A probate court hearing must be held within 24 hours (this may vary from state to state).

   d. Treatment of overdose and poisoning almost always must be instituted prior to a formal court hearing. The fact that the patient's condition poses an immediate risk of significant morbidity or mortality if treatment is not instituted before a formal court hearing can be arranged should be documented.

V. Blood alcohol test request and police:
  A. On occasion police may request the staff to draw blood specimens for legal blood alcohol analysis. Both state and Supreme Court rulings suggest that this is proper police practice and admissible as court evidence; however, the issue of potential civil liability for the person who takes the blood sample from an unwilling patient remains unsettled in these cases in some states.
  B. An emergency physician, nurse, or technician can be liable for assault and battery for touching a patient without the patient's consent. Therefore written consent must be obtained prior to complying with the police request unless state (or provincial) law is clear. Only a court order can force an individual to do something against his or her will.
  C. Some states provide the physician with immunity from civil liability for blood alcohol tests requested in writing by an appropriate law enforcement official. The motorist's arrest warrant, however, does not constitute such a legal document. In other states, such as New York, immunity will protect the physician only when the motorist willingly agrees to the test. Many states now allow the forced drawing of blood for alcohol level determination from the alleged defendant in a negligent homicide or potential negligent homicide case when drunk driving is the cause. The emergency department staff should be familiar with local laws.
  D. If a blood specimen is to be drawn in such patients the following procedure should be followed:
    1. The patient's consent for blood alcohol testing should be obtained, as well as his or her permission for notifying the authorities of the results of the test. Proper documentation may be provided by having the patient sign a Blood Alcohol Specimen Collection Consent Form.
    2. The patient's skin should be prepared with non-alcohol-containing substances, and the blood should be injected into clearly identified test tubes.
    3. Specimens should be properly labeled and recorded on hospital forms and appropriately witnessed.
    4. The specimen should be handed directly to the appropriate law enforcement official or examining pathologist. A receipt should be obtained from the receiving party.
    5. If no receiving party is available, the specimens should be placed in a locked receptacle and handed over at a subsequent date to prevent a break in the chain of evidence. Preserving the chain of evidence is extremely important if the case goes to trial. If the chain is not preserved the defense will invariably allege that someone tampered with the specimens.
  E. There would seem to be no ethical or medical consideration that requires or forbids a physician to draw blood as legal evidence at the potential defendant's request. On the other hand, there should be no hesitation in determining blood alcohol level if medically indicted.

VI. Drug specimen collection:
   A. Police may physically remove pieces of evidence from the emergency department (e.g., bullets, bags of heroin, weapons, clothing).
   B. Should police confiscate illegal drugs in the emergency department, this should be clearly documented.
   C. Staff should cooperate as much as possible with the authorities, short of infringing on the patient's legal rights. In fact, the staff may be accused of obstructing justice by actively resisting or not cooperating with a police investigation of suspected concealed drugs by an emergency patient.
   D. On the other hand, legal precedent precludes "search of intolerable intensity and scope" even if a legal warrant is obtained. For example, forced gastric emptying to obtain drug-filled balloons constitutes excessive force. On the other hand, collection of the same balloons in passed fecal material does not violate the patient's rights because no excessive force or violent bodily intrusion was used.
VII. Telephone medical advice:
   A. Emergency personnel can be held liable for information, both diagnostic and therapeutic, given over the telephone. This has resulted in lawsuits for negligence.
   B. A patient can also suffer a charge of abandonment over the phone. Abandonment is defined as the premature termination of a patient-physician relationship without the patient's consent and without giving the patient sufficient opportunity to secure the services of another competent physician.
   C. Emergency department personnel should never engage in telephone diagnosis or treatment of poisonings or overdoses if subsequent follow-up is not possible. Such follow-up may consist of a return call or home visit. If either is not possible, the patient should be instructed to seek direct medical attention at the most convenient health care facility.
VIII. Reportable events:
   A. Many states require the reporting of child abuse, persons who are dead on arrival at the hospital, drug addiction, impaired drivers, or drivers who have epilepsy. Violation of reporting laws may result in misdemeanor charges.
      1. Child abuse:
         a. A poisoned child may be the victim of child abuse (see Chapter 31).
         b. All states have statutes or regulations providing for some degree of child abuse reporting. Some of these reporting laws are permissive and allow the physician to use discretion in deciding whether to report; others are mandatory and require reporting under penalty of fine or imprisonment or both.
         c. Some states provide immunity from civil or criminal liability for those who report suspected battered children. The approved reporting party varies among states, but the trend is toward broadened reporting requirements authorizing **any person** who reasonably suspects an abused child to report that suspicion.
         d. Individual state statutes should be read, and the emergency department should have written policy.

2. Dead on arrival:
   a. Almost all states require that a person who arrives in the emergency department dead on arrival (DOA) be reported to the coroner or medical examiner for possible investigation of foul play and to determine the need for postmortem examination.
   b. The physician's professional responsibility in the case of DOA is to pronounce the patient dead. The health care provider may be held liable if a decision not to initiate cardiopulmonary resuscitation (CPR) is arbitrarily made. Since there is presently no reliable means of defining "brain death" during resuscitation, the decision to discontinue resuscitative efforts should be based on "cardiovascular unresponsiveness." When Advanced Cardiac Life Support (ACLS) techniques "have been properly applied, and the cardiovascular system fails to respond, the cardiovascular systems can be said to be unresponsive to standard resuscitative therapy. . . . At this point, the issue of brain viability becomes . . . an academic concern." The absence of pupillary response to light, a single "flat" EEG, and "boxcars" in the fundi are all unreliable as indicators of brain death.
   c. Conditions simulating death:
      (1) **Hypothermia:** Depressed metabolic state in the patient with hypothermia may be mistaken for death.
      (2) Drug overdoses that may be mistaken for DOA in the emergency department include:
      Ethanol
      Opioids
      Phenothiazines
      Butyrophenones
      General anesthetics
      Carbon monoxide
      Tricyclic antidepressants
      Cyanide
      Sedative-hypnotics (e.g., chloral hydrate, barbiturates)
IX. Violent patients:
   A. If a patient threatens hospital staff or others, threatens to destroy property in the emergency department, or actually destroys property or assaults someone, sufficient reason exists to physically restrain or detain that patient for medical evaluation or criminal prosecution.
   B. In many states, the physician who suspects that a patient is mentally deranged and is dangerous to self or others may commit the person to an appropriate mental facility. However, there are occasions when persons who are obviously psychotic must be released. It is best to be familiar with local laws if potential for commiting patients to a hospital exists. Also it is generally wise to consult family members and to ask for their opinions about causes and possible treatments and to keep the family informed.
   C. If a patient assaults you or others and is not mentally or medically ill (including drug intoxication), you may call local law enforcement agents and press criminal charges. If possible, attempt to have family members

assume care for such patients if they are being discharged from the emergency department.

D. See Chapter 27 for treatment of the violent or agitated patient.

BIBLIOGRAPHY

Boisaubin EV, Dresser R: Informed consent in emergency care: Illusion and reform. *Ann Emerg Med* 1987; 16:62–67.

Borak J, Veilluex S: Informed consent in emergency settings. *Ann Emerg Med* 1984(Part I); 13:731–735.

Curran WJ: Breaking off the physician-patient relationship: Another legal hazard. *N Engl J Med* 1982; 307:1058–1060.

Declaration of brain death (Questions and Answers) *JAMA* 1986; 255:3302.

George JE: *Law and Emergency Care.* St Louis, CV Mosby Co, 1980.

Lebegue B, Clark LD: Incompetence to refuse treatment: A necessary condition for civil commitment. *Am J Psychiatry* 1981; 13:1075.

McIntyre KM: Medicolegal aspects of cardiopulmonary resuscitation and emergency cardiac care, in *Textbook of ACLS,* American Heart Association, Chicago, 1983.

Mancini MR, Gale AT: *Emergency Care and the Law.* Rockville, Md, Aspen Systems Corp, 1981.

Purdie FRJ, Honigman B, Rosen P, et al: Prudent handling of patients signing out against medical advice. *ER Rep* 1982; 3:73.

Roth LH: A commitment law for patients, doctors and lawyers. *Am J Psychiatry* 1979; 136:1121.

Rund DA: Emergency management of the difficult patient. *EMS* 1984; 13:17–22.

Schroeder O Jr: Toxicology and law, in Wecht CH (editor): *Legal Medicine—1980.* Philadelphia, WB Saunders Co, 1980.

Steinbrook R, Lo B: Decision making for incompetent patients by designated proxy: California's new law. *N Engl J Med* 1984; 310:1598–1602.

PART THREE

Specific Approaches
in the Poisoned Patient

21

General Approach to Coma

Louis J. Ling, M.D., F.A.C.E.P.

NOTE: **All patients with altered mental status have concomitant *trauma* or *underlying illness* until proved otherwise.**

I. Primary survey:
   A. Follow APTLS (see Chapter 8).
      1. Particular attention should be paid to:
         a. Airway.
         b. Breathing (ventilation and supplemental oxygen).
         c. Circulation (vital signs).
II. Initial therapy (resuscitation):
   A. IV medications:
      1. 50 ml $D_{50}W$ (2 ml/kg $D_{25}W$ in infants).
      2. 2–10 mg naloxone (0.01 mg/kg in infants).
      3. 100 mg thiamine (adults).
   B. Decontamination:
      1. Perform gastric lavage and administer activated charcoal if indicated. (Protect airway during procedure; intubation may be indicated.)
      2. Skin decontamination if indicated.
III. Secondary survey (general examination to search for other causes of coma):
   A. Structural:
      1. Head trauma (with intracranial hemorrhage):
         a. Ecchymosis, abrasions, palpable fracture, unilateral dilated pupil, hemotympanum, CSF rhinorrhea or otorrhea, focal neurological findings.

    2. Subarachnoid hemorrhage:
        a. Stiff neck; note breathing pattern (Kussmaul suggestive of metabolic cause, Cheyne-Stokes suggestive of increased intracranial pressure).
B. Nonstructural:
    1. Infection:
        a. Meningitis (fever, stiff neck).
        b. Encephalitis.
        c. Reye's syndrome (hepatic failure).
        d. Sepsis: tachycardia, hypotension.
    2. Hyper/hypothermia.
    3. Hypertensive encephalopathy:
        a. Hypertension, may have fundoscopic findings (hemorrhages, exudates, decreased or absent venous pulsations, papilledema), hyperreflexia, hematuria.
    4. Hypoxia.
    5. Metabolic encephalopathies:
        a. Diabetic, hepatic, uremic, hyper/hypocalcemia, hyper/hyponatremia.
        b. Hypothyroid (look for thyroid surgery neck scar).
    6. Seizures:
        a. Status epilepticus (from any of the above causes).
        b. Postictal phase: increasing level of consciousness; can be prolonged.
    7. Shock.
    8. Toxins that cause coma*:

Antihistamines	Diquat	Nitrogen dioxide
Antipsychotics	Disulfiram	Opiates
Atropine/hyoscine-	Ethanol	Organophosphates
containing plants	Ethylene glycol	Nonsteroidal anti-
Barbiturates	Hydrogen sulfide	inflammatory
Benzodiazepines	Hypoglycemia	drugs (NSAIDs)
Bromide	Hypnotic agents	Phencyclidine
Carbon monoxide	Isopropanol	Salicylates
Clonidine	Lithium	Tetrahydralazine
Cyanide	Methanol	Triazolam

IV. Neurological examination:
A. Important aspects:
    1. Pupils, fundoscopic examination.
    2. Motor response to pain (appropriate, decorticate, decerebrate, flaccid).
    3. Caloric testing (or testing for "doll's eyes" if cervical spine injury has been ruled out).
    4. Level of consciousness (see Glasgow Coma Scale, p. 168).
B. The neurological examination may be of value in differentiating structural, toxic/metabolic, or functional causes of coma.
    1. Structural (including cerebral edema):
        a. Cushing's response (hypertension with bradycardia).
        b. Focal examination.

*Data from Olson KR, Pentel PR, Kelley MT: *Med Toxicol* 1987; 2:61.

    c. Funduscopic: papilledema (may be delayed up to 24 hours).
    d. Caloric testing: absent reflex.
  2. Nonstructural (without cerebral edema):
    a. Toxic/metabolic:
      (1) Symmetric pupils.
      (2) Funduscopic: venous pulsations present.
      (3) Symmetric motor response.
      (4) Caloric testing: intact reflex.
      (5) Dissociation of clinical findings: normal pupillary response and hypoventilation *or* flaccid motor response *or* absent caloric response.
    b. Functional:
      (1) Symmetric pupils.
      (2) Positive corneal reflex.
      (3) Calorics testing: nystagmus, inconsistent or nonanatomic motor response, active resistance and tensing of muscles.
      (4) Dropping arm avoids face and head.
V. Laboratory tests·
  A. Blood work:
    1. Complete blood count (with spun hematocrit), glucose (with initial dextrose stick estimate), electrolytes, calcium, glucose, osmolality, ketones.
    2. Arterial blood gases, carboxyhemoglobin.
    3. Consider liver function tests, serum ammonia.
  B. Urinalysis.
  C. Toxicology screen (serum, urine, gastric contents).
  D. X-ray studies:
    1. Cervical spine if trauma cannot be excluded.
    2. Head CT:
      a. If any suspicion of structural cause.
      b. Decreasing level of consciousness.
      c. Consider in all patients with Glasgow Coma Score <12.
    3. Chest x-ray (if aspiration suspected or respiratory compromise part of clinical presentation).
VI. Treatment (toxic cause established):
  A. See specific chapters if toxin known.
  B. In most cases of drug- or toxin-induced coma treatment is supportive while the toxin is metabolized or eliminated (see Chapters 12 and 13 for discussion of methods to minimize toxic effects).
VII. Disposition:
  A. See Chapters 17 and 18.
  B. In general, all patients with prolonged coma should be admitted. All patients with history of trauma or those in whom trauma cannot be ruled out should be admitted even if full sensorium is regained.
  C. Most patients with loss of consciousness at any time related to poisoning should be admitted except in a few specific situations (e.g., IV heroin overdose).
  D. Patients who can be considered for discharge from the emergency depart-

ment include stable patients whose comatose state has been completely reversed in the emergency department and who meet the following conditions:

1. Structural cause ruled out.
2. Metabolic causes with serious consequences ruled out (see above).
3. Normal neurologic findings over several hours of observation.
4. If toxic cause, no risk of delayed or prolonged effects.
5. Stable discharge environment exists to allow for close observation of the patient's physical and mental status by reliable observers.

BIBLIOGRAPHY

Approach to the unconscious patient. A clinical regimen for diagnosis and management, in Plum F, Posner JB: *The Diagnosis of Stupor and Coma,* ed 3. Philadelphia, FA Davis, 1980, pp 345–362.

Hahn AL: Stupor and coma: A clinical approach. *Geriatrics* 1983; 38:65.

Sabin T: Coma and the acute confusional state in the emergency room. *Med Clin North Am* 1981; 65:15.

Sullivan JB: Drugs and toxins presenting as neurological disorders, in Earnest M (editor): *Neurologic Emergencies.* New York, Churchill Livingston, 1983, pp 259–273.

22

General Approach to Seizures

Louis J. Ling, M.D., F.A.C.E.P.

NOTE: **Do not assume seizures are solely related to ingestions. Toxic ingestions may lower the seizure threshold in underlying conditions and trauma.**

I. Toxins that can cause seizures*:

Amphetamines
Aminophylline
Anticholinergics
Beta blockers
Boric acid
Camphor
Carbamazepine
Carbon monoxide
Chlorinated hydrocarbons
Cholinergic agents (nicotine, organophosphates)
Cicutoxin in water hemlock
Citrate
Cocaine
Cyanide
Dilantin (high levels)
DET insect repellant
Ethylene glycol
Fluoride
Heavy metals
Isoniazid
Lidocaine
Lithium
Nonsteroidal anti-inflammatory drugs (NSAIDs)
Phencyclidine
Phenol
Phenothiazines
Phenylpropanolamine
Phenytoin
Propoxyphene
Salicylates
Strychnine
Theophylline
Tricyclic antidepressants

*Data from Olson KR, Pentel PR, Kelley MT: *Med Toxicol* 1987; 2:63.

II. Nontoxic causes of seizures:
   A. Discontinuation of anticonvulsant medication.
   B. Metabolic derangements:
      1. Hypoxia
      2. Hypo/hypernatremia
      3. Hypomagnesemia
      4. Hypo/hyperosmolarity
      5. Hypo/hyperglycemia
      6. Hypo/hypercalcemia
   C. Alcohol or sedative withdrawal.
   D. Structural abnormalities:
      1. Cerebrovascular accident
      2. Intracerebral bleed related to trauma
      3. Posttrauma foci
      4. Tumor
      5. Degenerative disorders
   E. Infection or inflammation.
   F. Uremia.
   G. Congenital or perinatal disorders.
III. Treatment:
   A. Follow APTLS (see Chapter 8).
      1. Adequate airway.
      2. Cervical spine immobilization until trauma ruled out.
      3. Establish IV followed by administration of D_{50}, thiamine, naloxone.
      4. In the nontraumatized patient, position on side to avoid aspiration.
      5. Monitor for hyperthermia and rhabdomyolysis.
      6. Initial laboratory tests should include electrolytes, calcium, magnesium, glucose, toxicology screening, anticonvulsant levels if the patient has a history of seizures.
   B. Treatment of status epilepticus:
      1. Diazepam (Valium):
         a. Adult: 5–10 mg IV over 2–3 min. May be repeated q10–15 min.
         b. Children: 0.1–0.4 mg/kg IV over 2–3 min q10–15 min. Children without IV access can be given diazepam 0.5 mg/kg rectally with a plastic syringe and catheter.
         c. Maximum dose: Adult, 30 mg; child, 10 mg.
      2. Lorazepam (Ativan):
         a. Adult: 2–3 mg IV over 2–3 min. May be repeated.
         b. Child: 0.05 mg/kg.
      3. Phenytoin (Dilantin):
         a. Loading dose 15–18 mg/kg IV at a rate not to exceed 25–50 mg/min with cardiac monitoring.
         b. In children, loading dose per kilogram is similar, but infusion rate should not exceed 0.5–1.5 mg/kg/min.
      4. Phenobarbital:
         a. Loading dose 10–15 mg/kg IV at a rate of 25 mg/min.
         b. An additional 5 mg/kg may be given in 30–45 min if seizures are not controlled.

5. For seizures refractory to these measures, consider:
   a. Pancuronium 0.1 mg/kg IV.
   b. Halothane general anesthesia.
   NOTE: Pancuronium and general anesthesia stop motor activity and thus prevent resultant metabolic disturbances but should be accompanied with continuous EEG monitoring to determine continued presence of brain seizure activity.

IV. Disposition:
   A. Admission considerations (see also Chapters 17 and 18):
      1. New-onset seizures (toxin related or otherwise).
      2. Status epilepticus.
      3. Focal seizures.
      4. Focal neurological findings.
      5. Evidence of head trauma.
      6. Persistent altered mental status or decreasing level of consciousness.
   B. Discharge considerations (see also Chapters 17 and 18):
      1. Seizure unchanged from previously described seizures in a patient with known seizures.
      2. Seizure definitely not toxin induced or related.
      3. Identification and correction of precipitating factors (e.g., alcohol withdrawal, nontherapeutic anticonvulsant serum levels).
      4. Neurologic findings remain unchanged over several hours of observation.
      5. No evidence of head trauma.
      6. Counseling and appropriate follow-up have been arranged.

BIBLIOGRAPHY

Carducci B, Hedges JR, Beal JC, et al: Emergency phenytoin loading by constant intravenous infusion. *Ann Emerg Med* 1984; 13:1027–1031.

Delgado-Escueta AV, Wasterlain C, Treiman DM, et al: Current concepts in neurology: Management of status epilepticus. *N Engl J Med* 1982; 306:1337–1340.

Earnest MP, Marx JA, Drury LR: Complications of intravenous phenytoin for acute treatment of seizures. *JAMA* 1983; 249:762–765.

Eisner RF, Turnbull TL, Howes DS, et al: Efficacy of a "standard" seizure workup in the emergency department. *Ann Emerg Med* 1986; 15:33–38.

Leppik IE, Derivan AT, Homan RW, et al: Double-blind study of lorazepam and diazepam in status epilepticus. *JAMA* 1983; 249:1452–1454.

Olson KR, Pentel PR, Kelley MT: Physical assessment and differential diagnosis in the poisoned patient. *Med Toxicol* 1987; 2:63.

Sullivan JB: Drugs and toxins presenting as neurological disorders, in Earnest M (ed): *Neurologic Emergencies.* New York, Churchill Livingston, 1983, pp 259–273.

Walker JE, Homan RW, Vasko MR, et al: Lorazepam in status epilepticus. *Ann Neurol* 1979; 6:207–213.

23

General Approach to Syncope

Richard A. Christoph, M.D., F.A.C.E.P.

I. Cause:
   A. Syncope can be caused by a wide spectrum of disorders, both cardiovascular and noncardiovascular:
      1. Cardiovascular:
         a. Ventricular tachycardia
         b. Sick sinus syndrome
         c. Bradycardia
         d. Supraventricular tachycardia
         e. Complete heart block
         f. Mobitz II atrioventricular block
         g. Pacemaker malfunction
         h. Carotid sinus syncope
         i. Aortic stenosis
         j. Myocardial infarction
         k. Dissecting aortic aneurysm
         l. Pulmonary thromboembolism
         m. Pulmonary hypertension
      2. Noncardiovascular:
         a. Vasodepressor syncope
         b. Situational syncope
         c. Drug-induced syncope
         d. Orthostatic hypotension
         e. Transient ischemic attacks

   f. Subclavian steal syncope
   g. Seizure disorder
   h. Conversion reaction
   i. Metabolic:
      (1) Hypoglycemia
      (2) Hypomagnesemia
      (3) Hypocalcemia
      (4) Hypokalemia
   B. It is important to differentiate cardiac from other causes of syncope because, according to recent prospective studies, patients in this group appear to be at greater risk for mortality or major morbidity within 1 year of emergency department evaluation. Identifying those patients with syncope of cardiac origin can be difficult.
      1. Factors suggesting cardiac cause:
         a. Age greater than 55 years.
         b. Male.
         c. History of chronic heart failure
         d. History of ventricular arrhythmia.
         e. Atrial fibrillation.
         f. Left ventricular hypertrophy.
         g. History of a *short* (less than 10 seconds) warning period prior to syncope: weakness, sweating, nausea, dizziness or lightheadedness, epigastric discomfort, blurring or fading of vision, tinnitus, generalized numbness, pallor, shortness of breath, sighing, aura, palpitations.
II. Evaluation and treatment:
   A. Primary survey and resuscitation:
      1. Follow APTLS (see Chapter 8):
         a. Airway: Stabilize and protect, intubate if indicated (see Chapter 9). Cervical spine immobilization required if trauma has not been ruled out.
         b. Breathing: Assess, provide oxygen, ventilate if necessary.
         c. Circulation: Cardiac monitor, IV access, and stabilize vital signs.
         d. **Glucose, thiamine, naloxone** in all patients with altered mental status.
   B. Secondary survey:
      1. History (important aspects):
         a. Incontinence, tongue biting, postictal state *may suggest* a **seizure,** but incontinence and brief generalized tonic-clonic activity lasting less than 5–10 seconds can occur with simple vasodepressor (vasovagal) syncope or faint.
         b. Palpitations, chest pain, and history of a very short (less than 10 seconds) warning period suggest a **cardiac** cause. A familial history of syncope may suggest one of the familial Q-T prolongation syndromes. A specific history of known cardiac or arteriosclerotic disease should be checked.
         c. **Drug** History: **diuretics, beta blockers, vasodilators** such as prazosin or nitrates, **phenothiazines,** several **antihypertensives, hypoglycemics,** and ʟ-**dopa** may indicate a pharmacologic basis.

    d. Events associated with situational or **vasodepressor** syncope should be screened: postural changes, cough, micturition, trauma, pain, fear, defecation, hyperventilation.

    e. Factors suggesting intravascular **volume depletion** include poor oral intake, polyuria, diarrhea, or occult GI blood loss.

    f. History of **diabetes** or hypoglycemia.

2. Physical examination:

    a. Vital signs, including postural (orthostatic) pulse and blood pressure measurements.

    b. Head and neck:

        (1) Look for evidence of trauma.

        (2) Fundoscopic examination should assist in evaluation of arterio-sclerotic cardiovascular disease and *may* be helpful in evaluating increased intracranial pressure.

        (3) Subclavian or carotid bruit associated with reduced ipsilateral brachial blood pressure may suggest subclavian steal syndrome.

        (4) Examine tongue for bite marks associated with seizure activity.

    c. Cardiac:

        (1) Check for evidence of aortic stenosis, idiopathic hypertrophic subaortic stenosis (IHSS), click-murmur syndrome of mitral valve prolapse, etc.

    d. Abdomen:

        (1) Examine for abdominal aneurysm, ascites.

        (2) Guaiac test of stool for occult blood.

    e. Neurologic (see Chapter 21, p. 86).

3. Laboratory adjuncts:

    a. Hematocrit (volume).

    b. Blood glucose determination (hypoglycemia).

    c. Serum electrolytes:

        (1) Na: diuretic, renal failure, volume.

        (2) K^+: diuretic, arrhythmias, renal failure.

        (3) Decreased HCO_3^-: evidence of recent (within hour) seizure. If persistent, search for other causes, particularly poisoning (see Chapter 48, p. 221).

    d. Serum creatinine and blood urea nitrogen.

    e. ECG (arrhythmia, ischemia).

    f. Toxicology screen.

C. Definitive care:

1. See APTLS, Chapter 8.

2. In most cases drug- or toxin-induced syncope is caused by a physiologic effect of drug. Definitive care is aimed at correcting or blocking this effect. Ultimate management depends on drug neutralization or elimination (see Chapters 12 and 13).

III. Disposition:

A. Admission considerations:

1. Syncope of cardiac origin.

2. Syncope of cardiac origin cannot be ruled out.

3. Syncope secondary to serious underlying condition (e.g., pulmonary em-

bolism, dissecting aortic aneurysm, hypovolemia, drug reactions, peripheral neuropathy).
4. Orthostatic syncope that persists despite adequate fluid replacement.
5. Specific poisonings or toxic exposures (follow Admission Considerations in specific chapter).
6. Physiologic impairment that cannot be corrected and maintained by emergency department therapy.
7. Significant suicide risk.

BIBLIOGRAPHY

Caird FI, Andrews GR, Kennedy RD: Effect of posture on blood pressure in the elderly. *Br Heart J* 1973; 35:527–530.

Day SC, Cook EF, et al: Evaluation and outcome of emergency room patients with transient loss of consciousness. *Am J Med* 1982; 73:15–23.

Eagle KA, Black HR, Cook EF, et al: Evaluation of prognostic classifications for patients with syncope. *Am J Med* 1985; 79:455–460.

Kapoor WN, Karpf M, et al: A prospective evaluation and follow up of patients with syncope. *N Engl J Med* 1983; 309:197–204.

Linzer M, Osborn IIH, et al: Syncope: How to evaluate, when to admit. *Hosp Physician* 1983; 8–33.

Martin GJ, Adams SL, et al: Prospective evaluation of syncope. *Ann Emerg Med* 1984; 13:499–504.

Thames MD, Alpert JS, Dalen JE: Syncope in patients with pulmonary embolism. *JAMA* 1977; 238:2509–2511.

24

Anaphylaxis

Richard A. Christoph, M.D., F.A.C.E.P.

I. Definitions:
  A. Anaphylactic reaction: Described initially by Portier and Richet in 1902; an immune mechanism of the "immediate hypersensitivity" (type 1) type, produced by IgE-mediated release of a pharmacologically active substance.
  B. Anaphylactoid reaction: Clinical syndrome indistinguishable from anaphylaxis but caused by biologic reactions not mediated by IgE.

II. Cause:
  A. Agents causing anaphylaxis and anaphylactoid reactions:
    1. Drugs:
      a. Antibiotics (penicillin* and analogues).
      b. Analgesics (aspirin* and other nonsteroidal anti-inflammatory drugs).
      c. Hormones (insulin, ACTH).
    2. Diagnostic agents:
      a. Iodinated contrast media.*
      b. Sulfobromophthalein.
      c. Biological agents.
      d. Equine antitoxins.*
      e. Egg embryo–grown vaccines.
    3. Local anesthetics:
      a. Procaine.
      b. Lidocaine.
    4. Stinging insects:
      a. Hymenoptera (bee, wasp, yellow jacket, hornet*; fire ant).
    5. Allergic extracts:
      a. Skin testing or desensitization.

*Common cause.

6. Foods:
   a. Eggs.
   b. Milk.
   c. Nuts.
   d. Seafood.
III. Clinical presentation:
   A. Cardiovascular:
      1. Profound hypotension, orthostatic dizziness, altered level of consciousness.
      2. Vasodilation at the capillary and postcapillary venule, resulting in decreased intravascular volume from colloid shifts into interstitial space and resulting in increased capacitance of vascular compartment.
      3. ECG changes:
         a. Nonspecific S-T segment changes.
         b. T-wave changes.
         c. Ventricular fibrillation.
         d. A-V dissociation or asystole may occur.
   B. Respiratory:
      1. Cough, wheeze, tachypnea.
      2. Nasal stuffiness or itching.
      3. Dyspnea, laryngeal stridor from angioneurotic edema; cyanosis or pharyngeal, epiglottic, or glottic edema may occur.
   C. Skin:
      1. Itching, warmth, minor or deep cutaneous swelling, itching of eyes.
      2. Urticaria.
IV. Treatment:
   A. Initial therapy:
      1. Follow APTLS (see Chapter 8).
      2. Discontinue suspected allergen.
   B. Airway maintenance:
      1. Jaw thrust or sniffing position.
      2. Oxygen (100%).
      3. If no improvement consider:
         a. Epinephrine (1:10,000) 0.01 mg/kg (0.1 ml/kg) to a maximum dose of 1.0 mg; route of administration may be IV, IM, or via endotracheal tube.
         b. Epinephrine (1:1,000) 0.01 mg/kg or 0.01 ml/kg to a maximum dose of 1.0 mg; most pediatricians advise a maximum dose of 0.3–0.5 mg in children. May be given SC if no other route is available.
      4. Active airway management:
         a. Indications (also see Chapter 9):
            (1) Patient apneic.
            (2) Head and neck maneuvers fail to open airway because of profound laryngeal edema.
            (3) Hypoxemia resistant to 100% oxygen.
            (4) Bronchospasm or pulmonary edema prohibits adequate air exchange using bag-mask techniques.

b. Techniques:
   (1) Endotracheal intubation.
   (2) Cricothyroidotomy.
C. Breathing:
   1. Assist ventilation if necessary.
   2. Positive end-expiratory pressure if necessary.
D. Cardiovascular:
   1. Check pulse; administer cardiopulmonary resuscitation if necessary.
   2. Epinephrine (1:10,000) 0.01 mg/kg IV or (1:1,000) 0.01 ml/kg SC or IM; repeat every 10–15 min as needed.
   3. Two large bore IVs: normal saline or Ringer's lactate solution wide open. Infuse at least 1–2 L rapidly, more if necessary.
   4. ECG monitor.
   5. Consider pneumatic antishock garment if hypotension persists.
E. Secondary treatment:
   1. Antihistamines:
      a. More effective prophylactically than as a treatment once mediators of anaphylaxis are released. Both H_1 and H_2 receptors must be blocked.
      b. Diphenhydramine 1 mg/kg IV or IM (H_1 blockade).
      c. Cimetidine 4 mg/kg IV (H_2 blockade).
   2. Aminophylline:
      a. May prove useful if bronchospasm persists.
      b. Aminophylline "loading": 5–7 mg/kg over 20–30 min.
      c. Aminophylline maintenance: continuous drip at 0.5–1.0 mg/kg/hr.
   3. Beta adrenergic agents for persistent bronchospasm:
      a. Isoetharine (Bronkosol): 0.5 ml 1% isoetharine diluted with normal saline solution or diluent to 3.0 ml and administered by nebulized inhalation treatment or low-pressure intermittent positive-pressure breathing (IPPB) over 15–20 min.
      b. Metaproterenol (Alupent): 0.3 ml 5% metaproterenol diluted with normal saline solution or diluent to 3.0 ml and administered by nebulized inhalation treatment or low-pressure IPPB over 15–20 min.
   4. Catecholamines:
      a. For persistent hypotension, possibly accompanied by continued bronchospasm.
      b. Epinephrine (1:10,000) 0.1 ml/kg IV every 10–15 min.
      c. Dopamine 2–50 µg/kg/min.
      d. Norepinephrine titrated from 0.1 µg/kg/min to maintain systolic blood pressure 80–100 mm Hg.
   5. Corticosteroids:
      a. Hydrocortisone 0.5–1.0 gm IV
      b. Methylprednisolone 10–35 mg IV
V. Disposition:
   A. Observe in emergency department for no more than 4 hours. If even mild symptoms persist, admit.
   B. Admit to suitable hospital unit if cardiovascular or pulmonary factors require IV bronchodilators or vasopressors beyond the initial treatment phase.

C. If reaction is milder, consider discharge from emergency department if patient becomes asymptomatic within 4 hours. Observe for another 2–4 hours after symptoms abate prior to discharge.
D. If patient is to be discharged home after observation period, consider:
1. Diphenhydramine 25 mg PO every 6 hours for 2–3 days.
2. Prednisone 40–60 mg PO each morning for 5 days. (For a short course of therapy, tapered withdrawal is not necessary.)
3. Patient education regarding anaphylaxis prevention, especially if event was caused by Hymenoptera sting (Epi-Kit, Anakit).
4. Referral to allergist.

BIBLIOGRAPHY

Barach EM, Nowak RM, Lee TG, et al: Epinephrine for treatment of anaphylactic shock. *JAMA* 1984; 251:2118.

Boxer M, Greenberger PA, Patterson R: Clinical summary and course of idiopathic anaphylaxis in 73 patients. *Arch Intern Med* 147:269–272.

Claman HN: The biology of the immune response. *JAMA* 1987; 258:2834–2840.

Fath JJ, Cerra FB: The therapy of anaphylactic shock. *Drug Intell Clin Pharm* 1984; 18:14.

Levy JH, Roizen MF, Morris JM: Anaphylactic and anaphylactoid reactions: A review. *Spine* 1986; 11:282–291.

Matthews KP: Mediators of anaphylaxis, anaphylactoid reactions, and rhinitis. *Am J Rhinol* 1987; 1:17–26.

Sheffer AL: Anaphylaxis. *J Allergy Clin Immunol* 1986; 75:227–233.

Valentine MD, Lichtenstein LM: Anaphylaxis and stinging insect hypersensitivity. *JAMA* 1987; 258:2881–2885.

25

General Approach to the Intoxicated or Alcoholic Patient

Christopher T. Morrow, M.D., F.A.C.E.P

NOTE: Like anyone else, alcoholics and intoxicated patients can be seriously ill from other causes. Their complaints should be taken seriously.

NOTE: Anyone with altered mental status has a serious underlying condition until proved otherwise.

NOTE: There is no such thing as signing out "against medical advice" (AMA) for a patient with altered mental status.

NOTE: Alcoholism is one of the few chronic diseases whose progression can be arrested or reversed.

I. Introduction. Dealing with intoxicated or alcoholic patients is a daily challenge in acute care medicine. Between 15%–50% of emergency department and office visits relate directly or indirectly to alcohol abuse. Careful evaluation and treatment of these individuals are essential.
   A. Definitions:
      1. Alcoholism: physiologic or psychosocial impairment of well-being related to ethanol consumption (B, C, D, or E below).
      2. Tolerance: decreasing tissue effect of a "given dose" of ethanol over time (i.e., greater "dose" required to produce the desired effect). Tolerance involves increased metabolism, decreased tissue sensitivity, and

behavioral adaptation; however, it does not imply reduced susceptibility to the toxic effects.

3. Physiologic dependence: precipitation of withdrawal signs or symptoms on reduction of ethanol intake.
4. Psychosocial maladaptation: Problems with personal care, family structure, or job or legal difficulties or development of psychiatric disease related to ethanol consumption.
5. Physical illness or injury: includes sleep disorders, minor trauma, GI irritation, nutritional disorders. Coincidence of intoxication should alert the physician to the probability of ethanol abuse.

II. Clinical presentation:
   A. Alcoholic or intoxicated patients frequently come to the emergency department with:
      1. Minor trauma (including fractures and burns).
      2. GI complaints (vomiting, abdominal pain, bleeding).
      3. Vague physical or psychiatric complaints.
      4. Seizures.
      5. Hypertension.
      6. Social upheaval or violence.
      7. Motor vehicle accidents.
      8. Pneumonia.
      9. Volume depletion (with or without alcoholic ketoacidosis).
      10. Altered mental status.
   B. Some may also **ask for help** with their drinking problem.

III. Evaluation and treatment of intoxicated patient:
   A. Primary survey:
      1. Follow APTLS (see Chapter 8).
      2. Particular attention to:
         a. Adequate airway; avoid aspiration.
         b. Cervical spine precautions until trauma ruled out.
         c. Circulation (volume status).
         d. Level of consciousness.
   B. Initial treatment (if appropriate):
      1. Start IV with 5% dextrose in normal saline solution (D_5NSS): many intoxicated patients have intravascular volume depletion and are prone to hypoglycemia related to poor liver reserve of glycogen. D_5NSS is also the fluid of choice for alcoholic ketoacidosis (AKA).
      2. Glucose: all patients with altered mental status should be given 50 ml 50% dextrose solution.
      3. Naloxone will transiently arouse some ethanol intoxicated patients, but this response is not reliable. It is still indicated, however, for any patient with altered mental status.
      4. Most alcoholics have total body magnesium depletion (with or without hypomagnesemia). Give magnesium sulfate 1–2 gm diluted in IV fluid or given IM; may be repeated every 4 hours. NOTE: **Contraindications** to IV bolus dosing are hypotension, renal insufficiency, severe hypokalemia.
      5. Thiamine 100 mg IV, IM, or PO and multivitamins.

6. Gastric emptying: emesis or lavage, and charcoal are indicated if it is suspected that the patient has also used other drugs (charcoal does not effectively bind ethanol alone).
C. Secondary survey:
   1. Complete history:
      a. Deal with the chief complaint first! Do not modify a standard work-up just because "the patient is drunk." Many physicians subconsciously (or consciously) punish intoxicated patients by making them wait or anger them by ignoring the chief complaint and thus losing any possible rapport.
      b. Consider alternate etiologic explanations for the patient's condition and plan evaluation in consideration of them. Other major considerations:
         (1) Other toxins (e.g., methanol, ethylene glycol).
         (2) Trauma.
         (3) Hypoglycemia.
         (4) Hypoxia.
         (5) Sepsis, hyperthermia.
         (6) Postictal state.
         (7) Also see Chapter 26.
   2. Complete physical examination:
      a. Vital signs: May have tachycardia, hypotension, fever, hypothermia (only rectal temperature is reliable).
      b. Neurologic examination:
         (1) Careful examination of mental status:
            a Apply Glasgow Coma Scale if level of functioning is significantly altered (p. 168).
            b Assess current level of function:
               i. Can the patient walk unassisted safely?
               ii. Can the patient speak clearly?
               iii. Can the patient think clearly?
            c Cranial nerve examination (II–VII is a basic screen).
            d Motor (grip strength, pronator drift, gait).
            e Reflexes (symmetry or lack thereof).
      c. Head and neck:
         (1) Evidence of trauma: hemotympanum, CSF rhinorrhea or otorrhea, ecchymoses, lacerations, raccoon eyes, battle sign, palpable skull or facial fractures.
         (2) Breath odor.
         (3) Abdominal examination:
            a Tenderness, bruises, bowel sounds.
            b Occult blood in stools.
   3. Laboratory tests:
      a. Serum ethanol levels:
         (1) Also called blood alcohol concentration (BAC). Usually expressed as milligrams or grams per deciliter (0.1 gm/dl = 100 mg/dl, which is the legal limit in most states). NOTE: milligram

percent is not equivalent to milligrams per deciliter because ethanol weighs less than water (specific gravity, .79).

(2) High individual variation of intoxicated behavior at given ethanol level, dependent on tolerance and other factors; thus levels may be misleading.

(3) Caution must be exercised in ordering blood ethanol levels for "medical reasons." Unless the patient has specifically consented to the test or unless sufficient medical justification is written in the medical record, subsequent reading of the medical record by law enforcement officials or employers might place both the physician and patient in significant legal jeopardy.

(4) Ethanol concentrations should decrease between 10–20 mg/dl per hour (up to 50 mg/dl in tolerant individuals).

  b. Other diagnostic adjuncts:

(1) Arterial blood gases (consider for assessment of metabolic acidosis or ventilatory failure).

(2) Blood glucose.

(3) Electrolytes (detection of anion and osmolal gap).

(4) BUN and creatinine (assess renal function. May be important in ethylene glycol poisoning or if patient is receiving magnesium therapy).

(5) Blood or urine ketone tests.

(6) Calcium, phosphorus, magnesium, if indicated.

(7) Toxicology screen if diagnosis at all in doubt.

(8) Osmolality (only of value to prove that alcohol was taken. In some hospitals this can be obtained faster than an ethanol level).

(9) Urinalysis (Check for crystals if ethylene glycol intoxication suspected).

(10) ECG (intoxication or withdrawal may precipitate a supraventricular tachycardia).

IV. Special considerations in intoxicated patient:

  A. Observe the patient for as long as necessary to ensure recovery from intoxication. Admit if emergency department observation is not feasible.

  B. Use passive restraint liberally by recruiting family members, friends, nursing personnel, counselors, social workers to aid in the observation/recovery period. Do not allow intoxicated patients to dictate own care.

  C. Use active restraint if necessary: large security guards at doorways; soft two- or four-point restraints with the patient in the *prone* position (to prevent aspiration) if all else fails. Avoid sedation of any intoxicated patient. (See chapter 27 for discussion regarding appropriate restraints.)

  D. Documentation of why patient was restrained or detained is essential and should provide protection for the physician.

  E. Intoxicated patients may refuse procedures (e.g., laceration repair). These refusals can be honored temporarily if the patient's health is not jeopardized. The doctrine of "implied consent," however, applies to those critical procedures that are necessary to save life or limb. For minor procedures, the patient should be kept for observation and the patient's cooperation sought later when he or she is mentating more clearly.

V. Disposition (also see Chapter 26):
  A. Admission considerations (also see Chapters 17 and 18):
    1. Complicating illness or injury, especially one which will worsen with continued drinking (e.g., alcoholic hepatitis).
    2. Patients manifesting signs and symptoms of major withdrawal (hallucinations, agitation, tachycardia, fever, confusion) need admission.
    3. Seizures:
       a. First-time seizures.
       b. Status epilepticus.
       c. Focal seizures.
    4. Patients with acute pancreatitis should be admitted for parenteral hydration.
    5. Inability to observe patient sufficiently.
    6. Abnormal psychiatric state.
    7. Inability to establish diagnosis as simply alcohol intoxication.
  B. Discharge considerations:
    1. General discharge considerations have been met (Chapter 18).
    2. Significant illness or injury has been definitively ruled out.
    3. The patient is fully functional (can walk, talk, and think independently).
    4. Suicide potential and psychiatric state has been appropriately evaluated.
    5. A plan for follow-up care is formulated that the patient understands.
    6. The patient has sober escort.
    7. Patient has appropriate disposition environment. **Do not send patients out into the cold.**
    8. Patients with mild alcohol withdrawal should be treated and observed in the emergency department for 4–6 hours before discharged to outpatient treatment.
    9. Patients with mild exacerbations of chronic pancreatitis may be discharged if:
       a. They can tolerate oral intake.
       b. Pain has subsided.
       c. Close follow-up can be arranged.
    10. Patients with mild withdrawal and one or two isolated seizures (with history of previous withdrawal seizures) do not necessarily require admission. These patients should be observed for a reasonable period (6 hours). If seizure free after 6 hours and all other considerations met, patient may be discharged.
    11. Extended liability means the physician may be held liable for subsequent injuries or death in an intoxicated patient who has been allowed to leave or sign out against medical advice (AMA). For this reason intoxicated patients should be kept for observation until discharge criteria are met. **There is no such thing as "signing out AMA" for a patient with altered mental status.** Family members **cannot** sign a patient out AMA unless legal guardian status can be established.

C. Follow-up care for alcoholic patient:
  1. Counseling, Alcoholics Anonymous, and outpatient detoxification should be offered to all ethanol abusers.
  2. Alcoholic patients who undergo outpatient treatment need close supervision; a follow-up appointment within 24–48 hours should be considered.
  3. These patients also need arrangements for regular medical care and for definitive care of the disease of *alcoholism.*

BIBLIOGRAPHY

Becker CE: The alcoholic patient as a toxic emergency. *Emerg Med Clin North Am* 1984; 2:47–61.
Tabakoff B, Cornell N, Hoffman PL: Alcohol tolerance. *Ann Emerg Med* 1986; 15:1005–1012.

26

Head Injury vs. Intoxication

Christopher T. Morrow, M.D., F.A.C.E.P.

NOTE: **No patient is "just drunk" except in retrospect.**

NOTE: **Altered mental status should not be explained on the basis of blood alcohol concentration (BAC) until trauma and other underlying causes have been confidently ruled out.**

I. Introduction:
   A. Acute head injury and acute alcohol intoxication are frequently encountered emergency department presentations, accounting for 10% and 25% of emergency visits, respectively.
   B. Head injury in the intoxicated patient is not well addressed in the toxicology literature.
   C. The diagnosis of significant brain injury is often delayed or missed completely in intoxicated patients, resulting in increased morbidity and mortality.
   D. Studies show ethanol intoxication plays a role in 40% to 60% of motor vehicle accident (MVA) fatalities and in 35% to 65% of admitted trauma patients, 58% of concussions, 30% neurosurgery admissions, 75% of severe motorcycle accidents. Home accidents, assault, drownings, suicide, and pedestrian trauma victims all demonstrate a high incidence of premorbid drinking.
   E. Both alcohol intoxication and head injury can lead to altered level of consciousness. This level should be measured by the Glasgow Coma Scale (GCS; Chapter 37, p. 168) at initial examination. The initial GCS score is well correlated with outcome for all types of head injury. The GCS can also be used to follow changes in mental status.

II. Subdural hematoma (SDH):
   A. Present in 3% of trauma admissions and 11% of patients in coma.
   B. Carries worst prognosis of all blunt head injuries, accounting for about 20,000 deaths per year in the United States.
   C. Alcoholics are at high risk for acute SDH related to frequent trauma, cortical atrophy, coagulopathy, and cranial osteoporosis. Fifty percent of patients with SDH have been drinking alcohol.
   D. Rapid diagnosis and surgical intervention can markedly improve the percentage of patients with good functional outcome from 10% to 60%, if evacuation of hematoma occurs within 4 hours.
   E. Signs and symptoms:
      1. Usually follows a significant blow to the head; however, in chronic alcoholics or in those with clotting disorders, subdural hematomas have been reported following minor trauma or no history of trauma at all.
      2. Skull fracture accompanying SDH is not a typical finding.
      3. Altered mental status develops either immediately or after an intervening "lucid" interval.
      4. Although a GCS score less than 13 is common, it is not unusual to have an initial score of 13–15.
      5. Classic findings of anisocoria and hemiparesis are not reliably present. In fact, both signs together are seen in fewer than 50% of patients with SDH.
         a. Anisocoria alone is seen in only 58% of patients with SDH. In only 78% of patients is anisocoria the classic ipsilateral finding.
         b. Hemiparesis alone occurs in only 34% of patients with SDH. Only 60% of patients with hemiparesis have this as the classic contralateral finding.
      6. In 50% of patients with SDH alcohol intoxication confuses the initial evaluation. In 22% SDH is not diagnosed before death, principally because of diagnostic confusion secondary to alcohol. A larger percentage have a delayed diagnosis, affecting outcome.
III. Differentiating between intoxication and CNS injury (Table 26–1):
   A. No currently accepted criteria exist for differentiating the similar clinical presentation of alcohol intoxication and CNS injury.
   B. Initial GCS 9–12: risk of SDH 35%.
   C. Initial GCS 13–15: low risk for SDH.
   D. Value of blood alcohol concentration (BAC):
      1. Several authors feel that serum ethanol level may correlate with GCS levels. Our extensive experience is that levels **are not** reliably correlated with neurologic function. This is probably related to wide variation in individual tolerance. Awaiting a blood alcohol level in the face of a potentially lethal CNS injury is not justified. Coma should not be assumed to be related to a high blood alcohol level until trauma and other underlying causes have been confidently ruled out. When initial GCS score is below 13 SDH must be actively ruled out, along with other significant brain injury, regardless of breath odor, blood alcohol level or other findings of intoxication.
      2. Zero blood alcohol level is valuable information.

TABLE 26–1.

Brain Injury vs. Alcohol Intoxication

Clinical Findings	Significant Brain Injury	Significant Alcohol Intoxication/Overdose
Alcohol by-products on breath	Occasionally	Yes
Conjunctival injection	Occasionally	Often
Slurred speech	Occasionally	Often
Altered mental status:		
Initial GCS 3–8	Some*	Some
Initial GCS 9–12	Many†	Many
Initial GCS 13–15	Few	Many
Anisocoria	58% of SDH‡	15% incidence§
Nystagmus	Unusual	Variable‖
Motor asymmetry	Less than 50%	Rare
Posturing	Sometimes	Sometimes
Respiratory drive insufficiency	Common	Common

*Associated with 50% mortality.
†Associated with 20% mortality.
‡"Classic" finding of ipsilateral anisocoria seen in only 78% of patients with anisocoria.
§Incidence in normal population.
‖Unreliable physical findings.

E. Skull films are not a reliable means of differentiation. Only 45% of SDH are associated with skull fractures. Therefore normal skull films are not reassuring. Skull films are not diagnostic of brain injury and may waste valuable time; thus it is probably better to obtain a head CT scan as soon as possible if significant brain injury is suspected.

F. CT scan will detect acute subdural, epidural, and intracerebral bleeding in 95% of cases. Therefore a normal head CT provides good evidence against brain injury in patients with nonfocal neurologic signs and symptoms. NOTE: **Underlying nontraumatic conditions must still be ruled out.**

G. Definitive treatment in any patient with rapidly deteriorating neurologic status should not be delayed for diagnostic studies. It is imperative that early neurosurgical evaluation be obtained.

H. Suspect significant brain injury in any patient who does not improve over time or deteriorates neurologically, even though the initial head CT was normal. (Occasionally the CT is obtained too early.) The cause in such cases is usually diffuse brain injury or secondary cerebral edema. Such patients require aggressive supportive care and follow-up head CT scans.

IV. Management:

  A. Primary survey: Follow APTLS (see Chapter 8).

    1. Attention to:

      a. Airway management.

      b. Disability.

B. Resuscitation:
1. Oxygen, ECG monitor: supplemental oxygen therapy is instituted in all patients with altered mental status.
2. IV: intravenous access should be established in all intoxicated patients whenever other causes (including head injury) have not been ruled out. Draw blood (see Useful laboratory tests, below).
3. Administer **glucose** (all patients with altered mental status should be given 50 ml 50% dextrose solution).
4. Administer **naloxone** (2 mg); will transiently arouse some ethanol intoxicated patients, but this response is not reliable.
5. Most alcoholics have total body **magnesium** depletion (with or without hypomagnesemia). Give magnesium sulfate 1–2 gm diluted in IV fluid, or IM; may be repeated every 4 hours. NOTE: **Contraindications** to magnesium sulfate are hypotension, renal insufficiency, severe hypo kalemia. **Do not give as IV bolus.**
6. Add **thiamine** and multivitamins to IV.
7. If head injury established during primary survey or strongly suspected:
   a. Intubate and hyperventilate (goal is Pco_2 25–30 mm Hg).
   b. Consider dexamethasone, phenytoin, furosemide, or mannitol if patient has focal neurologic findings or severely depressed level of consciousness (e.g., GCS 3–8).
   c. Urgent neurosurgical consultation and intervention is indicated, particularly if patient has focal neurologic findings or severely depressed level of consciousness.
C. Secondary survey:
1. See Chapter 8.
2. Attention to:
   a. Evidence of trauma about head and neck (e.g., battle sign, raccoon sign, hemotympanum, CSF leak, laceration, depressions on skull).
   b. Detailed and **repeated** neurologic evaluation.
3. Useful laboratory tests:
   a. Blood tests:
      (1) Arterial blood gas (assess ventilation, acidosis).
      (2) Blood glucose (altered mental status).
      (3) Electrolytes (detection of increased anion gap).
      (4) BUN and creatinine.
      (5) Serum/urine ketone tests (diabetes, alcoholic ketoacidosis).
      (6) Calcium, phosphorus, magnesium (seizures, altered mental status).
      (7) Baseline blood alcohol level.
      (8) Osmolality (only of value to prove that alcohol was taken. In some hospitals this can be obtained faster than an ethanol level). Can be predictive of level (see Chapter 48, p. 224).
   b. Head CT: Obtain with clinical findings and **if any doubt** regarding head injury,
D. Definitive care:
1. Continuous reevaluation: a constant process of reevaluation of the head-injured, intoxicated patient should be performed so that clinical deterioration is not overlooked.

2. Close observation with **frequent abbreviated neurologic examinations:**
   a. Particularly mental status examination and evidence of focal findings.
   b. May need as often as every 15–20 min, particularly during initial stages of observation.
   c. Never less frequent than hourly even during later stages of observation.
3. If sedation is required, neurological consultation or CT scan is indicated.
4. No head-injured, intoxicated patient should be unattended until sensorium clear (GCS 15), patient can walk and talk appropriately, and potential head injury has been evaluated and treated.
5. Passive restraint, using family or friends or even active physical restraint, may be required on occasion and is preferable to allowing an intoxicated and potentially brain-injured patient to leave (see Chapter 27, pp. 112–113 for restraining techniques).

V. Disposition:
   A. Admission considerations:
      1. See general admission considerations (Chapter 18).
      2. Any evidence of brain injury by physical examination (e.g., focal neurologic findings, seizures, penetrating head trauma) or diagnostic tests (e.g., head CT).
      3. Complications related to alcohol alone (including alcoholic hepatitis, pancreatitis, withdrawal, aspiration, multiple seizures).
      4. Persistent depressed level of consciousness or altered mental status.
      5. Inability to establish diagnosis as simply alcohol intoxication (i.e., failure to rule out serious head injury).
      6. Inability to observe patient sufficiently.
      7. Inability to find appropriate disposition environment.
      8. Suicide risk.
   B. Observation period:
      1. Difficult to make recommendations because of variable individual metabolism of ethanol, role of underlying diseases.
      2. Expected metabolism of ethanol results in an hourly decrease in blood alcohol level of 10–20 mg/dl/hr.
      3. Discharge should not be based on blood alcohol level but on the patient's clinical condition.
      4. At minimum, all intoxicated persons with evidence of head trauma (by history or examination) should be observed for several hours in the emergency department. Depressed sensorium is expected to slowly improve each hour.
      5. Observation implies ability to perform repeated neurologic tests. In some cases this means as often as every 20 minutes.
   C. Discharge considerations:
      1. See general disposition considerations (Chapters 17 and 18) and disposition of the intoxicated patient, Chapter 25).
      2. Trauma has been ruled out.
      3. Associated conditions related to alcohol have been evaluated and appropriately managed.

4. Patient is alert with clear sensorium (GCS score 15), can walk with steady gait, tolerate oral fluids, has normal vital signs.
5. Patient has been observed sufficiently (see above).
6. Counseling has been offered.
7. Patient understands instructions.
8. Patient has appropriate disposition environment.

NOTE: **Patients with altered mental status cannot sign out against medical advice (AMA).**

NOTE: **The patient's family or friends cannot sign an AMA form on behalf of the patient unless they are the patient's legal guardians.**

D. Follow-up care for the alcoholic:
1. Counseling, Alcoholics Anonymous, and outpatient detoxification should be offered to all abusers.
2. Alcoholic patients who undergo outpatient treatment need close supervision; a follow-up appointment within 24–48 hours should be considered.
3. These patients also need arrangements for regular medical care and for definitive care of the disease of **alcoholism.**

BIBLIOGRAPHY

Fisher RP, Carlson J, Perry JP: Postconcussive hospital observation of alert patients in a primary trauma center. *J Trauma* 1981; 81:920–924.

Jagger J, Fife D, Vernberg K, et al: Effect of alcohol intoxication on the diagnosis and apparent severity of brain injury. *Neurosurgery* 1984; 15:303.

Lowenfels AB, Miller TT: Alcohol and trauma. *Ann Emerg Med* 1984; 13:1056.

Mendelow AD, Teasdale G, Jennett P, et al: Risks of intracranial hematoma in head injured adults. *Br Med J* 1983; 287:1173.

Rimel RW, Giordani B, Barth JT, et al: Moderate head injury: Completing the clinical spectrum of brain trauma. *Neurosurgery* 1982; 11:244.

Roberts JR: Pathophysiology, diagnosis and treatment of head trauma. *Topics Emerg Med* 1979, p 41.

Seelig JM, et al: Traumatic acute subdural hematoma. *N Engl J Med* 1981; 304:1511.

27

Violent or Agitated Patient

Louis J. Ling, M.D., F.A.C.E.P.

I. Cause:
   A. Intoxication with the following drugs can present as violent behavior:
      1. Amphetamines
      2. Anticholinergics
      3. Cocaine
      4. Ethanol
      5. Hallucinogens
      6. Marijuana
      7. Phencyclidine
      8. Phenylpropanolamine
      9. Any toxin resulting in hypoxia
      10. Any toxin resulting in hypoglycemia
   B. Beware of underlying organic disorders because confusion and violence may be manifestations of hypoxia, hypoglycemia, encephalitis, and temporal lobe seizures.
II. Treatment:
   A. Follow APTLS as soon as possible (see Chapter 8).
   B. Call for additional assistance to stand by. Adequate personnel from police or security officers should be present before the patient is approached.
   C. Talk-down approach:
      1. Do not approach within striking distance.
      2. Stay between patient and door.
      3. Avoid sudden, rapid movement or loud sounds.
   D. Physical restraints if necessary:
      1. Indications:
         a. Dangerous, uncontrolled behavior.
         b. Uncooperative with necessary evaluation.
         c. Uncooperative with necessary treatment.

2. Method:
   a. Should be done quickly with all limbs restrained simultaneously.
   b. Two-point alternating restraints if necessary, or four-point restraints, ideally applied by security personnel to prevent physicians from playing an adversary role against the patient.
   c. Patient should be restrained in the prone position, and can be lavaged in this position.
   d. Monitor restrained patient to prevent self-injury or vascular impairment of restrained limbs.
   e. Once restrained, patients should not be released until evaluation and treatment are well under way with demonstrated cooperation.
   f. Watch for rhabdomyolysis (elevated CPK, heme-positive urine).
   g. Undetected injury possible with PCP.
E. Chemical restraints if necessary:
   1. Indications:
      a. Physical restraints inadequate.
   2. Useful medications:
      a. Haloperidol 5–10 mg IM or IV; may repeat every 30 minutes as necessary to achieve control of extremely violent patient.
         (1) Alternatively, may use droperidol (Inapsine).
      b. Diazepam: 10 mg IV; may repeat if necessary until patient is calm.
         (1) IM benzodiazepines are unpredictably absorbed.
      c. Precautions/limitations:
         (1) Constant monitoring of patient after chemical restraint is essential, with attention to decreasing level of consciousness and respiratory failure from drugs or toxins.
F. Patients who are violent usually become calm after a short period of restraint and are more cooperative for examination; others become more cooperative as the drug intoxication subsides.
III. Special considerations:
A. There may be a psychiatric disorder concomitant with a drug intoxication, such as mania or schizophrenia, that may predispose to violence.
B. Condition may not be toxin related; consider other diagnoses during evaluation.
IV. Disposition:
A. Admission considerations (also see Chapter 18):
   1. Patient potentially dangerous to self or others.
   2. Patient requests hospitalization because he or she is afraid of losing control of impulses.
B. Discharge considerations (also see Chapter 18):
   1. Discharge should only be allowed after psychiatric evaluation.

BIBLIOGRAPHY

Conn LM, Lion JR: Pharmacologic approaches to violence. *Psychiatr Clin North Am* 1984; 7:879.

Dickens BM: Legal issues in medical management of violent and threatening patients. *Can J Psychiatry* 1986; 31:772.

Dubin WR: Evaluating and managing the violent patient. *Ann Emerg Med* 1981; 10:481–484.

Jacobs D: Evaluation and management of violent patients in emergency settings. *Psychiatr Clin North Am* 1983; 6:259–260.

Lakovics M: Evaluation of the emergency patient: Suicide, violence and panic, in Oken D, Lakovics M (eds). *A Clinical Manual of Psychiatry.* New York, Elsevier, 1982.

Lehman LS, Padilla M, Clark S, et al: Training personnel in the prevention and management of violent behavior. *Hosp Commun Psychiatry* 1983; 34:40.

Lion JR, Boch-y-Rita G, Ervin FR: Violent patients in the emergency room. *Am J Psychiatry* 1969; 125:1706.

Monahan J: Clinical prediction of violent behavior. *Psychiatr Ann* 1982; 5:509–513.

Perry S: Effective management of the violent patient. *ER Rep* 1983; 4:31–36.

Phillips MA, Nasr SJ: Seclusion and restraint and prediction of violence. *Am J Psychiatry* 1983; 140:229.

Rada R: The violent patient: Rapid assessment and management. *Psychosomatics* 1981; 22:101.

Salzman C, Green AI, Rodriguez-Villa F, et al: Benzodiazepines combined with neuroleptics for management of severe disruptive behavior. *Psychosomatics* 1986; 27:suppl 17.

Tupin JP: The violent patient: A strategy for management and diagnosis. *Hosp Commun Psychiatry* 1983; 34:37.

Weissberg MP: Safe strategies for recognizing and managing violent patients. *Emerg Med Rep* 1987; 8:169–176.

28

Ocular Toxicity

Keith T. Sivertson, M.D., F.A.C.E.P.

NOTE: **Patients with ocular exposure also have other injuries until proved otherwise.**

I. Introduction: When considering agents toxic to the eye several factors must be considered, including route of exposure, structures of the eye likely to be injured, and the temporal nature of the toxic effects.
II. Route of exposure:
   A. Splash contamination:
      1. Most frequent form of toxic exposure to eye.
      2. Lid, lashes, conjunctiva, and cornea are most likely to be exposed.
   B. Vapor contact:
      1. Less frequent than splash contamination.
      2. Most often affects the conjunctiva and cornea.
      3. Toxic effects may be immediate, delayed, or both. It may be difficult to relate symptoms to a vapor exposure with delayed effects unless a meticulous history is taken.
   C. Particulate matter:
      1. May be embedded.
      2. May have mechanical effect (e.g., corneal abrasion) as well as toxic effects.
      3. Most often affects the conjunctiva and cornea.
   D. Systemic exposure:
      1. Many ingestants have ocular effects (see Chapter 40).
      2. For certain toxins, ocular effects may be the primary symptom complex.

III. Temporal nature of toxic effects:
   A. Immediate effects:
   1. Caustics (e.g., acids and alkalis), solvents, and surfactants require the most rapid therapeutic response.
   2. Alkali (e.g., sodium hydroxide, concentrated ammonia) and strong acids (e.g., hydrochloric, hydrosulfuric acids) are believed to cause saponification of corneal epithelial lipids, resulting in rapid and deep penetration.
   3. Weak acids (e.g., acetic acid) denature corneal protein and thus their penetration appears to be somewhat self-limited.
   4. Solvents (e.g., alcohols, ketones, and chlorinated hydrocarbons) and surfactants (e.g., detergents) may also have severe immediate effects.
   B. Delayed effects:
   1. Ultraviolet light typically causes corneal injury hours after exposure. Patients typically have bilateral tearing and foreign body ("sandlike") sensation in eyes.
   2. Certain amines (e.g., ethylenediamine, diisopropylamine) that occur in vapor form can cause corneal epithelial swelling hours after exposure, resulting in painless blurred vision and halos that resolve spontaneously.
   3. Other agents occurring as gases, vapors, or dust (e.g., ethylene glycol, osmic acid, hypochlorite-ammonia mixtures) may cause corneal epithelial cell death hours after exposure, resulting in painful tearing, halos, and blepharospasm similar to ultraviolet keratitis.
   4. Chronic industrial exposure in the manufacture of aniline and hydroquinone is reported to cause corneal discoloration, scarring, and distortion years after exposure.
IV. Treatment:
   A. Treatment of immediate effects:
   1. All exposures:
      a. Irrigation with water or saline solution is critical and **should be started by the patient, bystanders, or paramedics at the site of contamination** and continued during transport and in the emergency department. Time of irrigation is the critical component, not the volume of solution (as long as the irrigant fills the eye continuously). Suggested irrigation times: solvents, 30 minutes; alkalis, 1–2 hours continuously.
      b. Irrigation should flow from the nasal side of the eye toward the temporal side to decrease contamination of the other eye.
      c. Application of topical **ophthalmic anesthetic** such as 0.5% tetracaine may be necessary to relieve blepharospasm and lid retractors may be necessary to adequately irrigate under the lid.
      d. Disposable contact lens specially designed for eye irrigation is available.
      e. **Cycloplegic/mydriatics** such as atropine or homatropine and topical antibiotics should be instituted in collaboration with the physician who will provide follow-up care for the patient.
      f. Once under the care of an ophthalmologist, other techniques may be

required to maximize reepithelialization, minimize chances of symblephara formation, and maximize residual visual acuity.

2. Alkali:
   a. Irrigation with normal saline solution should continue for 1–2 hours after exposure until the pH of tears in the conjunctival sac has stabilized at <8. The pH of tears is normally slightly acidic. The pH of sterile normal saline solution is 5–6. Equilibration must be allowed before determination of pH with litmus paper to avoid artificially low pH determinations.
   b. **Anterior chamber paracentesis** has shown some promise in rapidly lowering the pH of the anterior chamber after alkali contamination and may be considered by physicians familiar with the technique.

3. Surfactants and solvents:
   a. Length of time for irrigation of the conjunctiva and cornea by irrigation are less clear (20–30 min), but erring on the side of excess irrigation appears prudent (up to 1–1.5 hr).

4. Particulate matter:
   a. May be removed with a 25-gauge needle on a tuberculin syringe or by using a special spud.
   b. Removal of particles containing calcium hydroxide (e.g., lime, mortar, plaster) from the cornea or conjuctiva may be facilitated by the use of 0.05 mol/L EDTA on cotton swabs (Grant, 1985).
   c. Other particles imbedded in the conjunctiva may require the use of toothless forceps for removal.

B. After immediate treatment:
   After thorough decontamination of the eye, minimum examination should include:
   1. Visual acuity testing.
   2. Careful inspection with hand lamp or, if available, a slit lamp to confirm that all particulate matter has been removed.
   3. Funduscopic examination and tonometry are important in establishing a baseline for comparison with follow-up examinations.

V. Disposition:
   Necessity for admission should be determined in consultation with the opthalmologist who will provide subsequent care.
   A. Admission considerations:
      1. Visual acuity loss, especially bilateral.
      2. Preexisting ophthalmologic or medical conditions (e.g., glaucoma, diabetes mellitus, cataracts).
      3. Previous eye surgery (e.g., corneal transplantation, lens implantation).
      4. Toxicity of the presumed toxin and the likelihood of reexposure.
      5. Patient's social situation, particularly ability for self-care.
   B. Observation in emergency department:
      1. Repeat pH testing 1 hour after irrigation may be useful in the patient with alkali exposure to confirm that the pH of the conjunctival sac is not rising.

2. If decontamination is deemed complete and the patient does not require admission, discharge is appropriate after the following discharge criteria have been satisfied.

C. Discharge considerations:

1. Toxin is known and the effects have been terminated by treatment in the emergency department.
2. Reexposure has been determined to be unlikely.
3. Ophthalmologic consultation (by telephone or in person) has been obtained if necessary and careful written instructions concerning follow-up care (e.g., appointment with ophthalmologist) have been given to the patient.

BIBLIOGRAPHY

Grant WM: *Toxicology of the Eye.* Springfield, Ill, Charles C Thomas, 1985.

Saari KM, Leinonen J, Aine E: Management of chemical eye injuries with prolonged irrigation. *Acta Ophthalmol [Suppl] (Copenh)* 1984; 161:52–59.

29

General Protocol for Dermatologic Poisoning

Richard A. Christoph, M.D., F.A.C.E.P.

NOTE: **In victims of unknown poisoning, consider the possibility of transdermal entry. Personnel should take appropriate precautions to prevent dermal exposure to themselves when handling clothes and materials from a patient with possibility of transdermal exposure.**

I. Introduction:
   A. Absorption through the skin of toxins, organic chemicals, and industrial compounds is generally the rule rather than the exception.
   B. Among those agents for which transdermal absorption causing systemic toxicity is possible, the most notable would include:
      Organophosphate insecticides
      Organochlorines
      Nitrates
      Industrial aromatic hydrocarbons
   C. Of special note is the speed with which **organophosphate insecticides** can pass through intact skin to cause systemic toxicity. This can and does occur without causing any specific skin sensation of burning or itching.
II. Treatment:
   A. Follow APTLS (see Chapter 8).
   B. Rapid removal of all clothes is critical.
   C. Wash skin *thoroughly* with warm soapy water. It may be worthwhile to use an industrial shower (as is used for corrosive exposure) to thoroughly rinse entire body. *Be generous* with irrigation volume and velocity!

    D. A rare exception to immediate decontamination with water would be exposure to agents that react violently with water (e.g., the chemical may ignite, explode, or produce toxic fumes with water), such as chlorosulfonic acid, titanium tetrachloride, or calcium oxide. Another consideration would be agents insoluble in water such as phosphorus.

    E. Do not replace clothing or footwear until they also have been adequately decontaminated.

    F. For treatment of specific dermatologic exposures see the following:
       1. Acids and alkalis: Chapter 73.
       2. Hydrofluoric acid: Chapters 73 and 110.
       3. Formaldehyde: Chapter 74.
       4. Phenols: Chapter 75.
       5. Nitrates: Chapter 102.
       6. Sulfides/sulfites: Chapter 103.
       7. Hydrocarbons: Chapter 104.
       8. Organophosphates: Chapter 106.
       9. Industrial chemicals: Chapter 111.

III. Disposition:
    A. Admission considerations:
       1. Dermatologic exposure resulting in systemic manifestations.
       2. Full-thickness chemical burns covering more than 2% body surface area.
       3. Partial-thickness burn exceeding 10% body surface area.
       4. Serious burns of the face, hands, or feet.
       5. Burns of the perianal or genital areas.
       6. Burns that cross flexion creases.
       7. Severe pain.
       8. Suicide risk.
    B. Consultation criteria:
       1. Dermatology consultation may be required.
       2. Severe burns may require referral to a burn unit or plastic surgeon.
       3. Skin toxicity or burns associated with trauma may require general surgical consultation.
    C. Discharge criteria:
       1. Follow recommendations for specific poisonings.
       2. In general, patients should be considered for discharge from the emergency department only if they show no systemic toxicity from the toxic skin exposure after several hours of observation and treatment.
    D. Patient transfer:
       1. Some types of burn injuries should be considered for referral to a burn unit or burn center:
          a. Burns that involve more than 25% body surface area (20% in children younger than 10 years of age and adults over 40 years).
          b. Full-thickness or third-degree burns involving more than 10% of the total body surface.
          c. Partial-thickness or second-degree burns exceeding 20% of the body surface.
          d. All burns involving the face, eyes, ears, hands, feet, or perineum.
          e. Burns associated with significant trauma.

    f. Inhalation injury.

    g. Lesser burns in patients with preexistent disease.

2. Care must be taken to ensure that patients with severe burns are not transferred to a burn center before they are medically stable. All questions regarding treatment prior to transfer and care during transportation en route to the receiving hospital should be discussed by the referring physician at the first hospital and the accepting burn unit physician (see Chapter 19).

BIBLIOGRAPHY

Committee on Trauma, American College of Surgeons, in *Advanced Trauma Life Support Instructor Manual.* 1985, pp 283–291.

Edlich RF, Haynes BW, Allen MS, et al: Emergency department treatment, triage and transfer protocols for the burn patient. *JACEP* 1978; 7:152–158.

Jelenko C: Chemicals that "burn." *J Trauma* 1974; 14:65–72.

Rodcheaver GT, Hiebert JM, Edlich RF: Initial treatment of chemical skin and eye burns. *Compr Ther* 1982; 8:37–43.

Skiendzielewski JJ: Cement burns. *Ann Emerg Med* 9:316–318.

30

General Approach to the Pregnant Patient

Christopher T. Morrow, M.D., F.A.C.E.P.

I. Introduction:
   A. The safety of most drugs during pregnancy is poorly defined (Table 30–1). All drugs should be avoided unless the benefits to maternal health are carefully considered in light of any risks. Therapy for chronic disease (seizures, heart disease, asthma) may require medications with some risk to the fetus.
   B. Acute illness and injury represents a great threat to the fetus. Hypoxia, hypoperfusion, and hypoglycemia are major pathophysiologic threats to the fetus and the mother. Therefore **treat the pregnant woman as aggressively as any other patient.**
   C. Depression and adjustment disorders can be precipitated by the stresses of pregnancy. It is a time of **high risk for suicide attempt.**
   D. The period of greatest vulnerability and teratogenicity is thought to be up to 10 weeks' gestation. Therefore contraindications to medications are strongest during the early weeks (see Table 30–1).
   E. **Quinine** and **pennyroyal oil** are street remedies for inducing abortion.
II. Management of poisoning in the pregnant patient:
   A. General considerations:
      1. In general, a successful outcome for both mother and baby is most dependent on optimum management of the mother.
      2. One should be especially careful not to withhold proven effective treatment for a (potentially) serious overdose based on theoretical concerns regarding the fetus.
      3. There is little data on the use of antidotes in pregnancy. In general, antidotes should not be used if indications for their use are equivocal,

TABLE 30–1.

Drug Use During Pregnancy

Drug	Fetal Risk	Therapeutic Use Contraindicated	Comments
Antidotes			
Ipecac	±		
Charcoal	±		
N-acetyl cysteine	±		
Atropine	±		
Deferoxamine	+ +		Skeletal abnormalities
Penicillamine	+ + +		
Naloxone	±		
Physostigmine	+		
Disulfiram		x	Multiple congenital malformations
Drugs of Abuse			
Caffeine	+ to + +		Birth defects in rats; with moderate ingestion low risk in humans
Nicotine	+ + to + + +		Low birth weight, placental abnormality
Ethanol	+ + to + + +		Fetal alcohol syndrome
Heroin	+ + +		Acquired immune deficiency syndrome (AIDS), hepatitis, withdrawal, low birth weight
Methadone	±		
Marijuana	+ to + +		
Amphetamines	+ + +	x	Cardiac abnormalities, microcephaly, dysmorphia
Cocaine	+ +	x	
Antibiotics			
Pencillins	±		
Cephalosporins	±		
Sulfa	+	x	Contraindicated near term (kernicterus)
Trimethoprim (TMP)– sulfamethoxazole		x	Folate inhibitor (TMP)
Tetracycline		x	Bone and teeth deformities, maternal hepatotoxicity
Erythromycin	±	x	Estolate form contraindicated
Chloramphenicol	+ to + +		Rare "gray baby" syndrome
Aminoglycosides	+ to + +		Dose-dependent ototoxicity
Metronidazole	+ +		Teratogenic in animals
Nitrofurantoin	+ + +		
Clotrimazole	±		
Spectinomycin	+		
Acyclovir	±		
Isoniazid	±		

(Continued.)

TABLE 30–1 (cont.).

Drug	Fetal Risk	Therapeutic Use Contraindicated	Comments
Vaccines			
Live		x	Rubella, measles, mumps, oral polio, smallpox
Other	±		Tetanus, rabies, hepatitis B, gammaglobulin
Analgesics			
Acetylsalicylic acid	+ to + +	x	Coagulation effects; adverse effects on labor, contraindicated near term
Acetaminophen	±		
Codeine	+		
Meperidine	+		Respiratory depression at delivery
Ibuprofen	+	x	Contraindicated near term
Morphine	+		
Nitrous oxide	*		Chronic exposure contraindicated
GI medications			
Antacids	±		
Bicarbonate		x	pH imbalance in fetus
Bendectine		x	Probably safe but now off market
Methobenzamide (Tigan)	±		
Prochlorperazine (Compazine)	+ to + +		
Sulcrafate	±		
Cimetidine	+		
Hormones			
Estrogens		x	
Birth control pills		x	
Thyroid replacement	±		
Propylthiouracil	+ + +		
Sedative/psychiatric			
Barbiturates	±		
Benzodiazepines	+ + +		Fourfold increase in congenital malformations, neonatal withdrawal
Chloral hydrate	±		
Haloperidol	+		
Lithium	+ + +		Ebstein's cardiac anomaly
Tricyclic antidepressants	+ +		Limb abnormalities reported
Doxepin	±		
Anti-asthma			
Epinephrine	+ +		
Terbutaline	+		Delay of labor

(Continued.)

TABLE 30–1 (cont.).

Metaproterenol	+		As inhaler
Theophylline	+		Theophylline toxicity can manifest in neonate
Steroids	+		Aerosol preferred
Anti-seizure			
Phenytoin	+ +		Fetal hydantoin syndrome; should take supplemental folate
Phenobarbital	+ +		Developmental abnormalities reported in animals only
Valproic Acid	+ + +		Spina Bifida
Trimethadione		x	
Carbamazepine	+		May be safest single agent
Cardiovascular			
Beta blockers	+ to + +		Preferably use low doses only; high doses may lead to hypoglycemia, growth retardation
Thiazide diuretics	+ to +	x	Fetal electrolyte disorders
Furosemide	+		
Digitalis	+		
Methyldopa	±		
Hydralazine	±		
Reserpine		x	
Lidocaine	±		
Nifedipine	±		
Verapamil			
Other			
Coumadin		x	
Heparin	±		
Insulin	±		
Oral hypoglycemic agents		x	
Antihistamines	+ to + +	x	Brompheniramine contraindicated
Diphenhydramine	+		
Phenylephrine	+		
Pseudoephedrine	+ +		

Fetal Risk: ± Probably safe, + Low risk, + + Moderate risk, + + + High risk.

but they should not be withheld if they would be likely to make a difference in the woman's health and survival.

4. Early notification of the obstetrician and close cooperation between the primary clinician and the obstetrician are essential for the best results.

B. Physiologic changes that may affect management or disposition (Table 30-2):

1. During pregnancy the circulatory system supports an expanded blood volume and cardiac output that may mask significant blood loss. The volume increases as much as 35%, allowing blood loss of more than

TABLE 30–2.

Pregnancy Alterations of Baseline Laboratory Values

Study	Pregnancy Effect	Comments
Glucose	Increase	May become gestational diabetic
Total CO_2	Decrease	From relative hyperventilation
Lipids	Increase	
Ketonuria	Increase	Lower threshold for spilling ketones with starvation
Hematocrit	Decrease	Relatively greater increase in serum, despite increased erythrocyte production
White blood cell count	Increase	Usually 9,000–13,000 range; marked increase during labor
Erythrocyte sedimentation rate	Increase	
Fibrinogen	Increase	
Prothrombin time	Decrease	
Partial thromboplastin time	Decrease	
Blood urea nitrogen	Decrease	Increase glomerular filtration
Creatinine	Decrease	Increase glomerular filtration
Alkaline phosphatase	Increase	May be twice normal
Bilirubin	Increase	May increase in third trimester
Total protein	Decrease	May alter calcium and magnesium measurements
Albumin	Decrease	3.0 is mean
Albumin/globulin ratio	Decrease	Globulins increase slightly
Thyroxine	Increase	
Thyroid stimulation hormone	Increase	
Triiodothyronine Uptake	Decrease	

30% before vital signs falter. Therefore signs of hypoperfusion and hypotension will manifest later than they would in the nonpregnant patient, at which point uterine blood flow might already be compromised. The physician must therefore be that much more **aggressive in treating hypotension.**

2. Blood pressure is usually low during pregnancy, averaging 110/70 mm Hg, but a systolic pressure of 80 mm Hg or less should be considered potentially abnormal.

3. Because plasma volume usually rises more than red blood cell volume, there is a normal decrease in hematocrit. The value of a specific hematocrit is not as important as evidence of a recent decrease. Regarding other hematologic changes, there is a normal increase in white blood count (normal full-term value is 10,500/μl).

    4. Patients beyond 30 weeks' gestation should be treated in a **left oblique or left lateral decubitus position** to maximize uterine blood flow. The left lateral decubitus position will prevent impaired systemic venous return and is compatible with gastric lavage.

    5. Gastric emptying may be prolonged. Reflux is more common.

    6. Liver function may be altered (e.g., increased alkaline phosphatase).

    7. Tidal volume is increased at the expense of both inspiratory and expiratory reserve, and respiratory rate (and hence minute ventilation) is also increased to 18–20 per minute. The net effect is lower P_{CO_2} and a rise in pH (respiratory alkalosis). Therefore appropriate adjustment should be made when interpreting arterial blood gas values.

C. Treatment of the poisoned pregnant patient:

    1. Follow APTLS (see Chapter 8).

    2. Particular attention to correction of:

        a. Hypoxia.

        b. Hypotension and evidence of hypoperfusion (see above).

        c. Hypoglycemia.

    3. Fetal monitoring: Should be considered for patients beyond 23–24 weeks' gestation.

    4. Early consultation with obstetrician.

    5. Careful assessment of depression and **suicide potential.**

III. Special considerations:

A. Opioids:

    1. If the woman is an opioid addict, naloxone may precipitate acute withdrawal, one component of which may be uterine cramps, and possible induction of labor.

    2. Use naloxone sparingly, in small doses (e.g., 0.2–0.4 mg IV or less), just enough for reversal but not enough to precipitate acute withdrawal.

    3. See Chapter 67.

B. Carbon monoxide:

    1. Particularly threatening to fetal survival. The normal P_{O_2} of blood supplying the fetus is about 15–20 mm Hg. Oxygen delivery to fetal tissues is optimized by the presence of fetal hemoglobin, which shifts the oxyhemoglobin dissociation curve to the left, but CO further shifts the curve to the left, potentially compromising an already tenuous balance.

    2. Many authorities recommend aggressive use of **hyperbaric oxygen** in pregnancy, **regardless of the carboxyhemoglobin level.**

    3. See Chapter 100.

BIBLIOGRAPHY

Berkowitz RL, Coustan DR, Michizuki TK (eds): *Handbook for Prescribing Medications During Pregnancy.* Boston, Little, Brown & Co, 1981.

Briggs GG, Freeman RK, Yaffe SJ: *Drugs in Pregnancy and Lactation,* ed 2, 1986.

Lewis BV: Drug therapy in pregnancy. *Practitioner* 1978; 221:566–873.

Safety of antimicrobial drugs in pregnancy. *Med Lett Drugs Ther* 1987; 29:61–64.

Whipkey RR, Paris PM, Stewart RD: Drug use in pregnancy. *Ann Emerg Med* 1984; 13:346–354.

31

Risk Factors for Child Abuse and Neglect

Patricia D. Fosarelli, M.D.

NOTE: **Abuse can be psychological as well as physical; overdosing on a drug might be the only way a child can obtain help to extricate himself from a destructive situation.**

I. Introduction. Whenever a pediatric patient presents with an ingestion or overdose, the possibility of child abuse or neglect must be considered. Poisonings caused by direct parental action (abuse) **are not common** and reflect a psychotic or criminal parent. Poisonings caused by parental inaction or lack of concern (neglect) are much more common.

II. General considerations:
- A. Older infants and toddlers explore their environments by climbing and placing objects in their mouths.
  1. When a parent leaves medications or harmful household products in easy reach of a child a harmful ingestion is likely.
  2. When medications or household products are in a cupboard or drawer to which the child has easy access a harmful ingestion may occur.
  3. When medications or household products are stored in food containers a harmful ingestion is likely.

  All of these scenarios reflect parental lack of understanding of normal child behaviors and ignorance about common household safety practices.
- B. Ingestion in an older child or adolescent should raise the possibility of an intentional overdose (suicide gesture or attempt).
  1. The precipitating episode might seem trivial (e.g., child swallows pills because parent won't let him go to the movies), but the attempt is real and may reflect intrafamilial conflict.

2. In general, happy children and adolescents from supportive families do not resolve conflicts by overdosing (no matter how harmless the ingested substance). Thus the attempt should be taken seriously; a psychiatric consult is indicated.
3. Older children and adolescents, especially boys, may ingest a substance on a dare or to prove that they are not "chicken."

III. Children at high risk for abuse or neglect:
  A. Infant incapable of independent locomotion presenting with overdose.
  B. Young child with:
     1. Unknown ingestion.
     2. Significant time lapse between ingestion and presentation.
     3. Evidence of neglect (dirty, unkempt).
     4. Evidence of abuse (bruises, burns, lacerations, bite marks, belt marks, fractures).
     5. Disinterested parent.
     6. Hostile or inebriated parent.
     7. Parent who "blames" ingestion on child or sibling.
     8. Parent who is abused, depressed, overwhelmed, or has psychiatric disorder.
     9. Evidence of poor parent-child bonding (e.g., child would rather be held by examiner than by parent).
     10. Evidence of poor self-esteem (e.g., eyes downcast, crying).
     11. Evidence of malnutrition.
     12. Past history of burns, fractures, significant lacerations, head trauma, other poorly explained injuries.
     13. Past history of protective services referral or a past history of abuse or neglect.
     14. No regular physician.
     15. Delinquent immunizations.
     16. Family lacking adequate social supports.
  C. Older children or adolescents with:
     1. Unknown ingestion.
     2. Significant time lapse between ingestion and presentation.
     3. Evidence of abuse or neglect (as described above).
     4. Parent who acts inappropriately for the situation.
     5. Poor parental-child relationship (e.g., arguing, yelling, hitting).
     6. Evidence of poor self-esteem (child may be withdrawn or frankly belligerent).
     7. Significant past history of injuries, hospitalizations (especially psychiatric), and trouble with the law.
     8. Past history of protective services referral or past history of abuse or neglect.
     9. Scholastic difficulties.
     10. No trusted adult contact.
     11. No regular physician.
     12. Parent who is depressed, abused, overwhelmed, or has a psychiatric problem.
     13. Story that doesn't match the patient's condition.

IV. Consultation considerations:
   A. Social worker consultation is necessary for **all** pediatric ingestion victims and their parents.
   B. Psychiatric consultation is mandatory for children with suicide gestures or attempts.
 V. Admission considerations:
   A. See Chapter 17.

32

Street-Drug Abuser

Richard Cantor, M.D.

I. Introduction. The "street drug" abuser poses a special problem for emergency department personnel in that a myriad of easily obtainable illicit drugs are available. Most physicians are not well trained in the area of drug abuse. The street vocabulary (Table 32–1) is unfamiliar and many physicians may not recognize the drug abuser.

II. Recognition of drug abuse:
   A. Behavioral signs:
      1. Chronic lying about whereabouts.
      2. Sudden disappearance of money or valuables from home.
      3. Marked dysphoric mood changes that occur without good reason.
      4. Abusive behavior toward self or others.
      5. Frequent outbursts of poorly controlled hostility with lack of insight or remorse for this behavior.
   B. Social signs:
      1. Driving while impaired, auto accidents.
      2. Frequent truancy.
      3. Definite deterioration of academic performance over past 6–12 months.
   C. Circumstantial evidence:
      1. Drugs or drug paraphernalia in room, clothes, or automobile.
      2. Drug terminology in school notebooks or in school yearbook.
      3. Definitive change in peer group preference to those who lack purpose, are unmotivated, and may be known to use illicit drugs.
   D. Physical symptoms:
      1. Chronic fatigue.
      2. Chronic dry irritating cough, chronic sore throat.
      3. Chronic conjunctivitis (red eyes) otherwise unexplained.

III. Complications of street-drug abuse (Table 32–2).

TABLE 32–1.

Language of Street Drugs

Street Name	Definition
Acapulco gold	Mexican marijuana (extremely potent)
Acid	Lysergic acid diethylamide (LSD) or other hallucinogens
Alley juice	Methyl alcohol
Amidone	Methadone
Angel dust	Phencyclidine hydrochloride, sprinkled on parsley or marijuana
Barbs	Barbiturates
Beans	Amphetamine
Benn	Amphetamine sulfate
Bennies	Benzedrine (amphetamine sulfate)
Bernies flake	Cocaine
Bitter	Paregoric
Black beauties	Amphetamines
Black hash	Hashish containing opium
Black Russian	Hashish (potent, dark)
Black stuff	Opium, prepared for smoking
Blackjack	Paregoric that has been prepared for injection
Blotter acid	LSD on paper
Blue birds	Amobarbital capsules
Blue devils	Amobarbital capsules
Blue heaven	Amobarbital capsules
Bombido	Injectable amphetamine
Bombita	Methamphetamine
Boy	Heroin
Brick	Marijuana compressed, usually for purposes of transport
Brody	A fit of spasm staged by an addict to elicit sympathy
Browns	Amphetamine tablets
Bull jive	Marijuana heavily cut with tea, catnip, or other impurities
Bush	Marijuana
Button	Peyote button; top of marijuana plant flower
C	Cocaine
Caballo	Heroin
Cactus	Peyote
Cadet	New addict
California sunshine	LSD (hallucinogen)
Canary	Pentobarbital
Cartwheels	Amphetamine tablets
CD	Glutethimide tablet
Cecil	Cocaine
Charlie	Cocaine

(Continued.)

TABLE 32–1 (cont.).

Chief	Mescaline
Cohobe	DMT in powdered seeds (hallucinogen)
Coke	Cocaine
Cokomo (Kokomo)	Cocaine
Copilots	Amphetamines
Courage pills	Barbiturates
Crack	Extremely concentrated cocaine, smoked or injected
Cracks	Methamphetamine
Crystal	Methamphetamine
Cube (The)	LSD
D (Big)	LSD
DET	Diethyltryptamine (hallucinogen)
Dexies	Dextroamphetamine sulfate (Dexedrine)
Diane	Meperidine hydrochloride
DMT	Dimethyltryptamine (Businessman's special; hallucinogen)
DMZ	Baenactyzine (hallucinogen)
Doe	Methamphetamine
Dolls, dollies	Methadone
DOM	4-Methyl-2,5-dimethoxyamphetamine (STP; stimulant)
DooJee	Heroin
Double trouble	Amobarbital sodium plus secobarbital sodium
Downers	Sedatives, usually barbiturates
Dust	Heroin; cocaine
Dust of angels	Phencyclidine base (hallucinogen)
Emma (Miss)	Morphine
Emsel	Morphine
Eye openers	Amphetamines
F-40s	Secobarbital
Fag	Tobacco
Fizzies	Methadone tablets
Flake	Cocaine
Flower	Marijuana
Flying saucers	PCP (hallucinogen)
Footballs	Amphetamine tablets
Ganja	Jamaican marijuana
Gift of the Sun God	Cocaine
Glad rag	Cloth or handkerchief saturated with a material to be inhaled (e.g., for use in glue sniffing)
Gold dust	Cocaine
Goofballs	Amphetamine
Griffo	Marijuana

(Continued.)

TABLE 32–1 (cont.).

Street Name	Definition
H	Heroin
Hacus	Morphine
Happy trails	Cocaine
Hard stuff	Morphine
Harry, Big Harry, Hairy	Heroin
Hash	Hashish (THC), resin from top of *Cannabis sativa*
Hash oil	Concentrated extract of hashish
Hearts	Amphetamine
Heavenly blue	LSD (hallucinogen)
Hemp	Marijuana *(Cannabis sativa* or *C. indica)*
Hog	PCP mixed with vegetable material; veterinary tranquilizer
Horror drug	Belladonna preparations
Horse	Heroin
Huatari	Peyote
Idiot pills	Barbiturates
In-betweens	Barbiturates in combination with amphetamines
Indian hay	Marijuana
J	Marijuana cigarette
Jelly babies	Amphetamine
Joy juice	Chloral hydrate
Joy powder	Heroin
Jugs	Injectable amphetamines
Juice	Alcohol
Junkie	Heroin abuser
Kif	Marijuana
Kikuli, Kilorik	Peyote
Leaf (The)	Cocaine
Licorice	Paregoric
Lid pollers	Amphetamines
Lords	Hydromorphone hydrochloride
Love drug	MDA (methylenedioxyamphetamine)
LSD	Lysergic acid diethylamide (hallucinogen)
M	Morphine
Mary Jane	Marijuana
MDA	3,4-Methylenedioxyamphetamine (hallucinogen)
Mesc	Mescaline (hallucinogen)
Mescal button, mescal beans	Peyote; mescaline
Meth, Methedrine	Methamphetamine
Mickey Finn	Choral hydrate and alcohol

(Continued.)

TABLE 32–1 (cont.).

Mohasky	Marijuana
Monkey, Morf, Morpho	Morphine
Moonshine	Ethyl alcohol
Mooters	Marijuana
Mu	Marijuana
Mud	Stramonium preparation mixed with carbonated beverage
Mushrooms, sacred mushrooms, magic mushrooms	Psilocybin (hallucinogen)
Mutah	Marijuana
Nemmies	Yellow capsules of pentobarbital
Nimbie, Nimbles	Barbiturates
Nose	Cocaine
Panama red	Hachish; marijuana
PCP, peace pill	Phencyclidine (hallucinogen)
Peace	STP
Peaches	Amphetamine tablets
Peanuts	Barbiturates
Pearly gates	Morning glory seeds
Pep pills	Amphetamines
Pethidine	Meperidine hydrochloride
PG, PO	Paregoric
Phennies	Barbiturates
Pimp's drug	Cocaine
Poppy	Flowering plant from which opium is derived
Rainbow	Amobarbital and secobarbital capsule (red and blue)
Reds, red devils, red birds (capsules)	Barbiturates, secobarbital
Roses	Amphetamine tablets
Royal blue	LSD
Scag, Scat, Smack, Stuff	Heroin
Schoolboy	Codeine
Seggy, Seccy	Barbiturates
Seni	Peyote
Serenity	STP
Sleepers	Barbiturates
Snappers	Amyl nitrate ampules
Snow	Cocaine
Sopors	Methaqualone
Speed	Methamphetamine usually, but may be any stimulant
Speedball	Heroin and cocaine mixture; also percodan and methedrine
Splash	Methamphetamine
Star spangled powder	Cocaine
Stardust	Heroin with cocaine

(Continued.)

TABLE 32–1   (cont.).

Street Name	Definition
Stick	Marijuana cigarette
STP	Dimethoxymethylamphetamine (DOM; hallucinogen)
Straw, Smoke, Splim	Marijuana
Sugar	LSD; heroin
Syndicate acid	STP (hallucinogen)
Synthetic marijuana	PCP (hallucinogen)
Sweeties	Phenmetrazine hydrochloride (stimulant)
T & B's (blues)	Pentazocine (Talwin) and tripelennamine
Tab	General term to describe drug of solid dosage
Texas tea	Marijuana
THC	Tetrahydrocannabinol (hallucinogen in marijuana and hashish)
Tops	Peyote
Track drivers	Amphetamines
Tranquility	STP (hallucinogen)
Travel agent	LSD seller
Trips, Trippin'	High mediated by LSD
Wedding bells	LSD
Weed	Marijuana
White lady	Heroin
White lightning	Ethyl alcohol; also name for a specific speed drug (or amphetamine)
White stuff	Morphine; heroin
Whites	Amphetamine tablets
Windowpane	LSD
Wokouri	Peyote
Yellows, yellow jackets	Pentobarbital capsules

TABLE 32–2.

Complications of Street Drug Abuse

Organ System	Clinical Problem
Skin	Hypertrophic lesions
	Nonpitting edema
Infections	Skin abscess, cellulitis, thrombophlebitis
	Endocarditis
	Osteomyelitis
	Septic arthritis
	Marlaria
	Tetanus
	AIDS
Pulmonary	Pneumonia
	Pulmonary edema
	Pulmonary hypertension
Hepatic	Chronic hepatitis (A and B)
	Alcoholic hepatitis
Gastrointestinal	Pseudo-obstruction (ileus)
	Hemorrhoids
	Fecal impaction
Central nervous system	Seizures
	Subarachnoid hemorrhage
	Traumatic mononeuritis
	Nontraumatic mononeuropathy
	Transverse myelitis
Muscular	Compartment syndromes
	Necrotizing fasciitis
	Rhabdomyolysis syndrome
Gynecologic	Amenorrhea
	Concomitant pregnancy
Cardiovascular	Hypertensive crisis
	Acute myocardial infarction
	Arrhythmias
	Sudden death

BIBLIOGRAPHY

Cherubin CE: The medical sequelae of narcotic addiction. *Ann Intern Med* 1967; 67:23–33.
Evens RP, Clementi W: Compendium of drug abuse jargon. *J Fam Pract* 1977; 4:67.
Litt IF, Schonberg SK: Medical complications of drug abuse in adolescents. *Med Clin North Am* 1975; 59:1445–1452.

33

Withdrawal States

Christopher T. Morrow, M.D., F.A.C.E.P.

NOTE: **Several medical conditions may have signs and symptoms similar to those of withdrawal states. Careful evaluation is imperative.**

I. Introduction:
   A. Abuse of **opiates, ethanol, and sedative/hypnotic drugs** accounts for the vast majority of toxicologic illnesses. These abuses also carry the dangerous backlash of withdrawal syndromes.
   B. Withdrawal implies physiologic dependence, which in turn implies abuse or therapeutic dependence. Tolerance for higher than usual drug doses almost always accompanies withdrawal; not all tolerant individuals necessarily manifest withdrawal.
   C. Conditions that may mimic signs and symptoms of drug withdrawal syndromes include:
      1. Hypoglycemia.
      2. Thyrotoxicosis.
      3. Drug toxicity: **theophylline, aspirin** (early), and **sympathomimetics** (cocaine and amphetamine).
      4. Psychiatric conditions such as **mania.**
II. Opiate withdrawal:
   A. Pathophysiology:
      All narcotics produce both physical and psychological dependence. Physical dependence refers to an alteration of normal functions of the body, necessitating the continued presence of narcotics to prevent withdrawal or abstinence syndrome. In other words, body tissues have adapted to require a drug's continued presence to maintain normal physiologic

functioning. Abrupt discontinuance or lowering of narcotic levels precipitates withdrawal symptoms.

B. Clinical Features (Table 33–1):
C. Symptoms:
1. Frequent symptoms: agitation, anxiety, piloerection, tachycardia, hypertension, mydriasis
2. Occasional symptoms: yawning, lacrimation, rhinorrhea, vomiting, diarrhea, cramps.
3. Atypical symptoms: fever, hallucinations, delirium, seizures, hyperreflexia.
4. May be precipitated by naloxone (Narcan).
D. Laboratory tests:
1. Immediate Dextrostix (glucose reagent stick) test.
2. Infection workup: Complete blood cell count with differential, urinalysis, chest x-ray, blood cultures (implies admission has been decided).
3. For excessive sympathetic effects see Chapter 68 for guidelines as to laboratory tests.
4. Toxicology screen if cause of symptoms not clear (look for stimulants, sympathomimetics, theophylline, salicylates).
E. Management:
1. Mild withdrawal: reassurance, counseling.
    NOTE: **Do not confuse mild withdrawal with early withdrawal (symptoms of early withdrawal may also be mild).**
2. Significant withdrawal:
    a. Methadone:
        (1) **Methadone should never be given to addicts in the emergency department for any reason except acute withdrawal and then the initial dose should be 10 mg.**
        (2) For those in treatment programs, a daily dose of 40 mg methadone will prevent withdrawal in a chronic addict; 80 mg will prevent heroin-induced euphoria.
        (3) Methadone should be given in divided doses, using no more than 40 mg daily in these patients (e.g., 10 mg PO three to four times a day during the first 24 hours, followed by lower doses). In any case, heroin addicts should never be given more than 20 mg methadone at one time.

TABLE 33–1.

Withdrawal Syndrome

	Onset After Last Dose	Peak Symptoms	Duration
Morphine, heroin	8–14 hr	48–72 hr	7–10 day
Methadone	24–48 hr	3 day–3 wk	3–7 wk
Meperidine	3 hr	8–12 hr	4–5 days
Opiate antagonist induced	Immediate	30 min	90–150 min

(4) If a patient comes to the emergency department requesting methadone, the following should be done before giving methadone to the patient:

    a Confirm the patient's participation in a methadone treatment program.

    b Attempt to verify the patient's maintenance dose by contacting his or her drug counselor.

    c As stated above, methadone should never be given to addicts in the emergency department for any reason except acute withdrawal.

  b. Clonidine: Dose: 6 μg/kg PO, then 10–17 μg/kg/day PO for 10 days.

3. Outpatient detoxification: Goal is to eliminate need for self-injection and criminal acquisition of drug money:

  a. Clonidine for short-term detoxification.

  b. Methadone maintenance: federally controlled programs (see above).

  c. Naltrexone (Trexan), an opioid antagonist, is a nonaddicting, long-acting adjunctive medication for the treatment of patients recently detoxified from methadone programs. By blocking the usual euphoric effect of opioids and preventing the redevelopment of opioid dependence, proper use of naltrexone in a treatment program may help to prevent readdiction in the postaddiction period.

4. Counseling programs.

F. Prognosis:

1. Expected response to treatment:

  a. Prognosis for medical recovery from opioid withdrawal is excellent.

  b. Prognosis for long-term abstinence depends on patient's commitment to a life-style free of opioid abuse, whether he or she is employed, married, or in a stable relationship.

2. Expected complications and long-term effects:

  a. For a list of complications of parenteral drug abuse see Chapter 32.

  b. Untreated withdrawal is generally nonfatal; however, rarely it may result in complications related to excessive sympathetic stimulation, adrenergic drive, volume depletion (secondary to vomiting), and even death. These complications are rare, and opioid withdrawal is one of the least life threatening of the withdrawal states.

G. Disposition:

1. Admission considerations:

  a. See general admissions considerations (Chapters 17 and 18).

  b. Significant intravenous drug abuse complications (e.g., endocarditis, pulmonary edema, abscesses of skin or organ, AIDS, thrombosis).

  c. Multiple-drug withdrawal states.

  d. Significant withdrawal symptoms or complications.

  e. Poorly motivated individuals or poor response to outpatient detoxification.

  f. Inability to arrange appropriate outpatient detoxification in a highly motivated person.

  g. Intensive care admission considerations:

    (1) Major symptoms, complications, or unstable vital signs (see Complications, above).

2. Consultation considerations:
   a. Drug counselor.
3. Observation period:
   a. Guidelines for the admission of suspected opioid withdrawal are not clear. If the patient is stable in the emergency department after a period of observation of 6–8 hours and can receive reliable observation at home, and if there are no psychiatric contraindications, the patient can be discharged with appropriate follow-up.
4. Discharge considerations:
   a. General discharge considerations have been met (see Chapters 17 and 18).
   b. Medical conditions with similar symptoms have been ruled out.
   c. Complications from drug abuse have been ruled out (see Chapter 32).
   d. Counseling and follow-up have been offered and arranged.

III. Acute ethanol withdrawal:
   A. Pathophysiology:
      1. Reduction of intake unmasks compensatory chronic CNS hyperactivity and increased circulating catecholamines.
      2. Total body magnesium depletion, a concomitant of chronic ethanol consumption, with or without hypomagnesemia, can exacerbate seizures and tremor. Delirium tremens pathophysiology poorly understood; does not seem to be magnesium related.
      3. Nutritional factors, fluctuations in acid-base balance, and possibly other circulating factors also play a role.
   B. Clinical features:
      1. Stage I (acute withdrawal state: minor syndrome):
         a. Onset 6–24 hours after reduction of intake in physiologically dependent drinkers.
         b. Symptoms: agitation, startle reaction, anxiety, tachycardia, tachypnea, hypertension, diaphoresis, tremor, hyperreflexia, insomnia, nausea, vomiting.
         c. May not correlate with low blood alcohol levels; dependent on degree of tolerance.
         d. May present subclinically after resumption of drinking.
         e. Will abate without treatment or complications in most patients in 3–5 days.
         f. Approximately 25% progress to stage II, 10% to stage III.
      2. Stage II (withdrawal hallucinosis: minor syndrome):
         a. Stage I symptoms with the addition of hallucinosis.
         b. Hallucinations are usually visual (animals, bugs) or auditory (accusatory voices) and are sensed as threatening.
         c. Illusions may precede hallucinations.
         d. Underlying sensorium is clear.
         e. Presence of stage II is not a negative prognostic indicator.
      3. Stage III (withdrawal seizures: minor syndrome):
         a. Usually coincident or closely followed by stage I symptoms.
         b. Seizures are grand mal, brief, tonic-clonic or tonic events. Focal seizures or status epilepticus are not typical.

    c. Most patients will have only one or two seizures, each lasting less than a few minutes. Almost all will have fewer than six such short seizures within 6 hours.

    d. Postictal phase is short (usually less than 15 min) followed by a return to the agitated, tremulous, alert, stage I phase. A postictal phase lasting beyond an hour should not be ascribed to withdrawal until other important causes of altered mental status have been ruled out (see Chapter 21, 22, and 34).

4. Stage IV (delirium tremens: major syndrome):

    a. Relatively uncommon finding in alcohol withdrawal related to development of effective treatment methods; however, may still occur in 5% to 10% of untreated alcoholics in withdrawal.

    b. Onset usually 3–7 days after ethanol reduction.

    c. Virtually always following some degree of stage I (±stage II or III) withdrawal.

    d. Symptoms:

        (1) Adrenergic overdrive: tachycardia, elevated blood pressure, increased minute ventilation and temperature.

        (2) Global disorientation and delirium.

        (3) Psychomotor agitation.

        (4) Diaphoresis and tremor may be extreme.

C. Diagnostic tests:

1. Dextrostix (glucose reagent stick) test.

2. ECG if signs and symptoms of major syndrome present.

3. Seizures:

    a. See Chapter 22.

    b. Have high index of suspicion for other causes of seizures (e.g., trauma, infection).

    c. Consider checking serum **magnesium** concentration.

4. With significant symptoms consider infection workup (see above under Diagnostic tests for narcotic withdrawal).

D. Management:

1. Search for medical conditions that may mimic withdrawal.

2. Check for serious medical conditions associated with alcohol intake (e.g., pancreatitis, alcoholic hepatitis, coagulopathy, myocardiopathy, pneumonia, Wernicke-Korsakoff's syndrome, trauma, cardiac arrhythmia).

3. Stages I and II:

    a. Administer:

        (1) Thiamine 100 mg (PO or IM): ensure glucose supply (PO or IV).

        (2) Multivitamins (PO or IV).

        (3) Folate 1–5 mg (PO, IM, or IV).

        (4) Magnesium sulfate (up to 1 gm/hr IV or up to 4 gm IM). In patients with significant magnesium depletion it may take up to 20 gm magnesium to replete body stores (about 10 gm of which are wasted in the urine).

        (5) Correct electrolyte abnormalities as indicated. NOTE: Metabolic acidosis following seizures should self-correct within 1 hour. Beyond that time frame, another cause must be searched for.

b. Place patient in quiet lighted area. (Darkness potentiates illusions and visual hallucinations)
c. Mild withdrawal signs and symptoms:
   (1) **Chlordiazepoxide** (Librium) 200–400 mg PO in four divided doses on first day (some patients require as much as 1,600 mg). Should then be rapidly tapered over 4 days to minimize risk of cumulative sedation and dependency.
   (2) Agents such as **clorazepate** and **oxazepam** are gaining in popularity because their shorter half-life reduces potential for dependency and cumulative sedation:
      a **Oxazepam** (Serax) 15–30 mg PO every hour, titrating to relief of symptoms.
      b **Clorazepate** is a good choice because it has a high margin of safety, does not cause euphoria, and is reported to be nonaddictive. Dose: 15 mg PO four times on day 1, three times on day 2, twice on day 3, and at bedtime on day 4. On day 5 dosage is reduced to 7.5 mg at bedtime. If patient shows symptoms of withdrawal on this schedule, can give 15 mg supplements every 4–6 hours during first 3 days.
d. Moderate or severe withdrawal signs and symptoms:
   (1) **Diazepam** (Valium) 2–5 mg/min IV initially, titrating upward to desired sedative response. Generally 10 mg or less is adequate; however, up to 20 mg may be given. Pulse, blood pressure, and respirations should be closely monitored.
   (2) Avoid giving benzodiazepines intramuscularly because of irratic absorption and sterile abscess formation.
e. Other therapeutic considerations:
   (1) Beta blockers (propranolol or atenolol):
      a May be used as adjuncts to the benzodiazepines to reduce tachycardia, tremor, and diaphoresis.
      b Should not be used alone, and must be carefully titrated for effect.
      c **Propranolol** 0.1–0.5 mg IV initially, followed by 40 mg/day PO.
      d **Atenolol** 50–100 mg/day PO in divided doses.
   (2) **Clonidine:**
      a May be effective in managing the physical and psychological effects of withdrawal; however, questions remain about its ability to prevent withdrawal seizures.
      b Dose: 6 μg/kg PO followed by 10–17 μg/kg/day.
f. Contraindicated or dangerous therapy:
   (1) **Phenothiazines, butyrophenones, antihistamines:** Altered temperature regulation and lowered seizure threshold.
   (2) **Paraldehyde:** Difficult titration; problems with all delivery routes.
   (3) **Barbiturates:** Although intravenous phenobarbital for alcohol withdrawal and convulsions has been suggested by some, barbiturate therapy carries significant withdrawal risk.

(4) Intramuscular injection: Erratic absorption and difficult to titrate. Furthermore, many alcoholic patients have impaired clotting abilities.

4. Stage III: Seizures:
   a. See Chapter 22.
   b. Protect patient from harm from subsequent seizures (e.g., aspiration, falling off stretcher).
   c. Consider more serious causes for seizures: meningitis, hypoxia, hypoglycemia, electrolyte imbalance, CNS mass lesion or bleeding.
   d. Aggressively treat Stage I/II effects.
   e. Most alcohol withdrawal seizures do not require pharmacologic intervention.
   f. If seizure prophylaxis is indicated, may administer phenytoin (loading dose 15–18 mg/kg IV at maximum rate of 50 mg/min with careful monitoring). Oral phenytoin is less reliably absorbed. Although oral loading is widely practiced, risk of aspiration with subsequent seizure may be a complication.

5. Stage IV (delirium tremens):
   a. Recognize the gravity of the diagnosis.
   b. Arrange for intensive care.
   c. Support vital signs and volume status.
   d. Aggressively treat as for Stages, I, II, and III.
   e. Restrain patient carefully, preferably in prone position (see Chapter 27 for suggestions on restraining techniques).

E. Prognosis:
   1. Expected response to treatment:
      a. Excellent with appropriate treatment.
      b. Seventy-five percent to 88% of patients with diagnosis of alcohol withdrawal have mild symptoms only.
      c. Five percent to 6% progress to delirium tremens, which has mortality of 5% to 10%.
      d. Aggressive management of Stages I and II has been reported to prevent progression to delirium tremens.
   2. Expected complications and long-term effects:
      a. Significant morbidity and mortality may arise from the complications of poorly controlled excessive sympathetic stimulation.
      b. Aspiration secondary to seizures.

F. Special considerations:
   1. **Alcoholism may be the most "curable" chronic disease. It is worth the health care provider's time to offer counseling to these patients.**

G. Disposition:
   1. Admission considerations:
      a. See general admission considerations (Chapters 17 and 18).
      b. Alcohol-dependent patients with seizures:
         (1) Patients with first-time seizures should be admitted for thorough workup.
         (2) Status epilepticus.
         (3) Focal seizures.

        (4) More than six short seizures.

        (5) Occurrence of seizures after 6 hours of observation.

        (6) Confusion, stupor, or coma.

        (7) Focal neurologic deficits.

        (8) Evidence of significant head trauma.

    c. Atypical presentation or unclear diagnosis.

    d. Stage IV: Imminent or present evidence of delirium tremens.

    e. Stages I to III with the following symptoms that are unresponsive to initial sedation and fluid resuscitation:

        (1) Tachycardia >100/min.

        (2) Fever >38.5° C.

        (3) Severe tremor or extreme agitation.

        (4) Confusion or delirium.

    f. Inability to observe progress of withdrawal in emergency department for whatever reason (e.g., lack of sufficient staff to closely monitor patient).

    g. Poor social supports:

        (1) Inability of patient to care for self at home.

        (2) Admit homeless persons during the winter if disposition to sheltered environment cannot be found. Many such patients freeze to death each winter.

  2. Consultation considerations:

    a. Intensive care unit for patients with signs and symptoms of major syndrome (delirium tremens).

  3. Observation period:

    a. Withdrawal seizures: If patient with history of alcohol-related seizures is seizure free for at least 6 hours from last convulsion, he or she may be discharged.

    b. Patients in Stage I should respond to treatment within 2–4 hours.

  4. Discharge considerations:

    a. All general discharge considerations have been met (see Chapter 18).

    b. Associated medical or surgical illnesses have been ruled out.

    c. Assure that patient or family understands gravity of diagnosis of alcohol dependence.

    d. Arrangements for follow-up medical care have been made.

    e. Adequate supply (5–7 days) of short-acting benzodiazepines to counter mild withdrawal as outpatient, if indicated.

    f. Counseling or referral to detoxification center has been offered.

    g. Discharge patient only if appropriate environment and care assured (e.g., homeless patient in winter cannot simply be returned to the street; ensure a sheltered location.

IV. Other withdrawal syndromes:

  A. **Amphetamine** withdrawal: Characterized by drowsiness, lethargy, hunger, tremor, chills; potential for long-term depression and suicide.

  B. **Cocaine** withdrawal: Characterized by irritability, paranoid ideation, delayed depression. Generally milder than amphetamine withdrawal.

  C. **Tricyclic antidepressant** withdrawal: Characterized by nausea, cramps, diarrhea, chills, insomnia, anxiety, and rarely mania. Usually seen 4–7 days after abupt cessation from high doses.

D. **Benzodiazepine** withdrawal: Characterized by findings similar to ethanol withdrawal but with onset 3–14 days after cessation. The shorter acting benzodiazepines have more severe and earlier presentations. Tapering benzodiazepines is always recommended.

E. **Barbiturate** withdrawal:
1. Characterized by protracted withdrawal state with similarities to ethanol and benzodiazepine withdrawal.
2. Auditory hallucinations and status epilepticus are common and a source of serious mortality.
3. Treatment is indicated with pentobarbital 100–200 mg or phenobarbital 30–60 mg every 6 hours to achieve mild sedation.
4. Admission is indicated.
5. Other drugs with similar withdrawal presentation: **ethchlorvynol** (Placidyl), **glutethemide** (Doriden), **meprobamate** (Equanil, Miltown), **methaqualone** (Quaalude), **methyprylon** (Noludar).

BIBLIOGRAPHY

Abraham E, Shoemaker WC, McCartney SF: Cardiorespiratory patterns in severe delirium tremens. *Arch Intern Med* 1985; 145:1057–1059.

Ashton H: Benzodiazepine withdrawal: An unfinished story. *Br Med J* 1984; 288:1135–1140.

Baumgartner GR, Rowen RC: Clonidine vs. chlordiazepoxide in the management of acute alcohol withdrawal syndrome. *Arch Intern Med* 1987; 147:1223–1226.

Brown CG: The alcohol withdrawal syndrome. *Ann Emerg Med* 1982; 11:276–280.

Busto U, Sellers EM, Naranjo CA, et al: Withdrawal reaction after long-term therapeutic use of benzodiazepines. *N Engl J Med* 1986; 315:854–859.

Callahan EJ, Rawson RA, McCleave B, et al: The treatment of heroin addiction: Naltrexone alone with behavior therapy. *Am J Drug Alcohol Abuse* 1980; 7:795–807.

Gold MS, Pottash AC, Sweeney Dr: Opiate withdrawal using clonidine. *JAMA* 1980; 243:343–346.

Hillbom ME, Hjelm-Jager M: Should alcohol withdrawal seizures be treated with anti-epileptic drugs? *Acta Neurol Scand* 1984; 69:39–42.

Jasinski DR, Johnson RE, Kocher TR: Clonidine in morphine withdrawal. *Arch Gen Psychiatry* 1985; 42:1063–1066.

Kleber HD, Riordan CE, Rounsaville B, et al: Clonidine in outpatient detoxification from methadone maintenance. *Arch Gen Psychiatry* 1985; 42:391–394.

Kraus ML, Gottlieb LD, Horwitz RI, et al: Randomized clinical trial of atenolol in patients with alcohol withdrawal. *N Engl J Med* 1985; 313:905–909.

Lerner WD, Fallon HJ: The alcohol withdrawal syndrome. *N Engl J Med* 1985; 313:951–952.

Robinson GM, Sellers EM, Janacek E: Barbiturate and hypnosedative withdrawal by a multiple oral phenobarbital loading dose technique. *Clin Pharmacol Ther* 1981; 30:71–76.

Sellers EM, Naranjo CA, Harrison M, et al: Diazepam loading: Simplifed treatment of alcohol withdrawal. *Clin Pharmacol Ther* 1983; 34:822–826.

Tabakoff B, Cornell N, Hoffman PL: Alcohol tolerance. *Ann Emerg Med* 1986; 15:1005–1012.

Winokur A, Rickels K, Greenblatt DJ, et al: Withdrawal reaction from long-term, low-dosage administration of diazepam. *Arch Gen Psychiatry* 1980; 37:101–105.

Young GP, Rores C, Murphy C, et al: Intravenous phenobarbital for alcohol withdrawal and convulsions. *Ann Emerg Med* 1987; 16:847–850.

34

Psychiatric Considerations in Poisonings and Overdoses

Mary L. Dunne, M.D.

NOTE: **Many successful suicides are failed parasuicides.**

I. Introduction. The following is considered to be the minimum psychological/ psychosocial evaluation that should be performed in all poisoned and over-dosed patients. It is assumed that advanced poisoning treatment and life sup-port (APTLS) principles have been followed in the medical evaluation and treatment of the patient. It is best to initially focus on the medical manage-ment, keeping in mind only basic psychologic considerations such as protect-ing the patient and others from harm and dealing with the patient with sym-pathy and understanding. Later a more detailed psychological assessment can be done. Particular attention must be placed on disposition decisions.

II. Primary psychological patient evaluation and treatment:
   A. APTLS (see Chapter 8).
   B. History:
      1. Consider all sources of history (see the 10 Ps, Chapter 8).
      2. Cause of harmful exposure:
         a. Accident or error in judgment.
         b. Compromised judgment (confusion, youth, retardation): consider acute organic cause (e.g., hypoglycemia), adequacy of home environ-ment and supervision, possibility of abuse or neglect.
         c. Suicidal intent.

C. Continued monitoring:
  1. Written orders should specify appropriate behavioral monitoring.
  2. Continuous supervision:
     a. To prevent patient from harming self or others.
     b. To prevent patient from leaving emergency department prior to discharge by physician.
  3. Physical restraint:
     a. Degree and type of restraint (e.g., Posey, leather) must be individualized.
     b. Consider medical condition (risk of deterioration, aspiration).
     c. See Chapter 27.
  4. Frequent vital signs.
D. Repeat medical examinations: Even though psychologic assessment is in progress, the patient's medical condition and potentially changing status should be kept in mind.
III. Patient interview:
A. General considerations:
  1. Patient's condition:
     a. Prolonged interview must be deferred until medically stable.
     b. Drugs or alcohol may influence cooperation and validity of information.
     c. Always reinterview patient after effects of intoxications have abated.
  2. Interview is facilitated by:
     a. Nonjudgmental demeanor, helpful attitude.
     b. Maximizing patient comfort and dignity.
     c. Limiting extraneous distractions.
  3. If interviewer is considered at risk of violence, stay between patient and open door. Restrain appropriately (see above). See Chapter 27.
B. History:
  1. Important information to elicit and document:
     a. Intent to harm self or others.
     b. Precipitating events.
     c. Patient's perception of problem.
     d. Hallucinations:
        (1) Specific nature.
        (2) Any commands.
     e. Depression:
        (1) Perceived cause.
        (2) Duration.
        (3) Vegetative function: sleep pattern, appetite, libido.
     f. Drug or alcohol use (including over-the-counter drugs and home remedies).
     g. Social factors:
        (1) Living situation.
        (2) Interactions with family, friends.
        (3) Work status.
     h. Previous psychiatric illness.
     i. Past medical history.

C. Mental status examination:
1. In the context of toxicologic emergencies the mental status examination is directed toward:
   a. Assessing suicide risk.
   b. Establishing level of competence.
   c. Differentiating organic conditions (especially acute toxicity) from functional psychiatric illness (Table 34–1).
2. Much information may be gained by attentive observation alone; a directed interview will complete the mental status examination.
3. Elements of mental status examination:
   a. Appearance (appropriateness).
   b. Orientation.
   c. Attention and cooperation.
   d. Affect (e.g., flat, depressed, spontaneous, agitated).
   e. Speech.
   f. Thought.
      (1) Content:
         a Suicidal ideation.
         b Harm to others.
         c Lack of control or telegraphic control.
         d Ideas of reference.
         e Hallucinations.
         f Delusions.
         g Obsessions.
      (2) Process:
         a Pressure of speech.
         b Tangential.

TABLE 34–1.

Differentiation of Functional (Psychiatric) and Organic (Toxicologic, Metabolic, Neurologic) Causes in Confused or Delirious Patients

	Functional	Organic
Level of consciousness	Stable	Fluctuating
Attention	Variable	Inattentive
Orientation	Present × 3	Disoriented
Memory	Intact	Deficient
Thought	Delusions, if present, often bizarre and complex	Delusions, if present, not as bizarre
Perception	Hallucinations, if present, auditory	Hallucinations, if present, visual or tactile
Motor	Usually normal except for mild catecholamine tremor	Focal findings, asterixis, tremor, myoclonus

        c Flight of ideas.

        d Perseveration.

    f. Memory (consistency with expected abilities).

    g. Judgment (consistency with expected abilities).

    h. Intelligence (consistency with expected abilities).

    i. Insight (consistency with expected abilities).

4. Method of administering mental status examination:

    a. A brief formal screening examination may help identify those patients who require further evaluation of organic pathology.

    b. Cognitive Capacity Screening Examination (e.g., Table 34–2), takes about 5 minutes to administer. Some patients will be unwilling or unable to cooperate and a qualitative description of their level of cooperation and ability must suffice.

TABLE 34–2.

Cognitive Capacity Screening Examination*

Examiner_____ Date_____

Instructions: Check items answered correctly. Write incorrect or unusual answers in space provided. If necessary, urge patient once to complete task.

Introduction to patient: "I would like to ask you a few questions. Some you will find very easy, and others may be very hard. Just do your best."

1. What day of the week is this? _____
2. What month? _____
3. What day of the month? _____
4. What year? _____
5. What place is this? _____
6. Repeat the numbers 8 7 2. _____
7. Say them backward. _____
8. Repeat the numbers 6 3 7 1. _____
9. Listen to these numbers: 6 9 4. Count 1 through 10 out loud, _____
    then repeat 6 9 4. (Help if needed. Then use numbers 5 7 3.)
10. Listen to these numbers: 8 1 4 3. Count 1 through 10 out _____
    loud, then repeat 8 1 4 3.
11. Beginning with Sunday, say the days of the week backward. _____
12. 9 + 3 is: _____
13. Add 6 (to the previous answer or 12). _____
14. Take away 5 (from 18). _____
    Repeat these words after me and remember them; I will ask
    for them later: hat, car, tree, 26.
15. The opposite of fast is slow. The opposite of up is: _____
16. The opposite of large is: _____
17. The opposite of hard is: _____
18. An orange and a banana are both fruits. Red and blue are _____
    both:
19. A penny and a dime are both: _____
20. What were those words I asked you to remember? (Hat). _____
21. (car). _____

22. (tree).   ———————
23. (26).   ———————
24. Take away 7 from 100; then take away 7 from what is left,   ———————
    and keep going: 100 − 7 is:
25. Minus 7:   ———————
26. Minus 7 (write down answers; check correct subtraction of 7):   ———————
27. Minus 7:   ———————
28. Minus 7:   ———————
29. Minus 7:   ———————
30. Minus 7:   ———————
Total correct (maximum score = 30)
Patient's occupation (previous, if not employed)——————————————————————
Education————————————————————————— Age——————————
Estimated intelligence (based on education, occupation, and history, not on test score):
Below average, average, above average—————————————————————————
Patient was: Cooperative———————   Uncooperative———————   Depressed———————
              Lethargic———————   Other———————
Emergency department chief complaint:———————————————————————————

If patient's score is less than 20, the existence of diminished cognitive capacity is
present. Therefore, an organic mental syndrome should be suspected and the following
information obtained or considered:

CBC———————   LFTs———————
Electrolytes———————   ABG———————
Glucose———————   EKG———————
Calcium———————   CXR———————
Creatinine/BUN———————   CT brain———————
Urinalysis———————
Medication use:————————————————————————————————————
    (Especially steroids, digitalis, antihypertensives, antimicrobials, anticonvulsives,
    anticholinergics, antihistamines, L-dopa, aminophylline, disulfiram, indomethacin,
    salicylates, sedative-hypnotics, psychiatric and abused drugs)
Possible endocrine dysfunction: ————————————————————————————
                        (T_3, T_4, Ca, P, etc.)
Neurologic consultation————————————————————————————————
Psychiatric consultation————————————————————————————————

*Modified from Jacobs JW, Bernhard M, Delgado A, et al: Screening for organic mental syndromes in
the medically ill. *Ann Intern Med* 1977; 86:40–46.

IV. Recognition of suicide risk
    A. Epidemiology:
        1. Social demographics:
            a. Age:
                (1) Adolescents are at high risk.
                (2) Adults: older at higher risk (especially white Protestant males
                    over 40 years).

      b. Sex:
          (1) Men more often commit suicide.
          (2) Women more often attempt suicide.
      c. Formerly married.
      d. Living alone.
      e. Foreigner.
  2. Past history:
      a. Previous suicide attempt.
      b. Recent medical care, surgery.
      c. Alcoholism or drug addiction.
      d. Family history of suicide.
      e. Psychiatric history (particularly schizophrenia).
  3. Life stress:
      a. Recent loss of job, loved one.
      b. Disturbed interpersonal relationships.
      c. Physical illness.
      d. Financial difficulties.
  4. Symptoms:
      a. Definite death intention.
      b. Suicide plan.
      c. Pessimism, hopelessness, depression.
B. Adult risk associations:
  1. Affirmation of suicidal intent:
      a. Wish to die.
      b. Detailed plan and preparation.
      c. Lethal method.
      d. Suicide note.
      e. Giving away property.
  2. History:
      a. Impairment:
          (1) Alcohol or drug (ab)use or dependence.
          (2) Poor employment or school history.
      b. Psychiatric:
          (1) Psychosis (especially schizophrenia).
          (2) Major depression.
          (3) Previous suicide attempt.
      c. Medical:
          (1) Chronic disease (especially, painful or incurable).
          (2) Recent surgery or childbirth.
          (3) Hypochondriasis.
  3. Life circumstances:
      a. Advancing age.
      b. Homosexuality.
      c. Social isolation.
      d. Bankrupt resources.
      e. Recent serious loss.
  4. Family history:
      a. Suicide.
      b. Affective disorder.

      5. Foreigners.
- C. Adolescent risk association:
  1. More common in late than early adolescence. Although more females attempt suicide, more males actually die. Suicide rate among adolescents older than 15 years approximately 12 per 100,000; however, incidence of suicide attempts may be 5 to 15 times higher. Second leading cause of death among 15- to 19-year-olds.
  2. Depression, loss of self-esteem.
  3. Impulsive, often don't have plans.
  4. Previous acting out behavior:
     a. Sexually precocious.
     b. Drug abuse.
     c. Delinquent or criminal behavior.
  5. May have talked about suicide but was not taken seriously.
  6. Dare.
  7. Recent media attention to suicide with occurrence of "epidemics."
  8. Family disruption, recent loss of friend, feeling (often false) of being unwanted, exposure to repeated violence within household.
  9. Frequent method of suicide attempt is taking parent's medication.
- D. Children:
  1. Suicide rare (0.4 per 100,000) among prepubertal children and teenagers younger than 15 years.
  2. Unlike adolescents, more male than female children attempt suicide, and more also die of suicide.
  3. Childhood suicide victims frequently come from disturbed families where marital discord and abuse are common.
- V. "Parasuicide" (suicide gesture):
  1. Definition: action intended to achieve secondary gain rather than actual self-destruction.
  2. Differentiation may not be clear-cut. Remember, **suicide "gestures" can kill.**
  3. Criteria to help differentiate gesture from suicide attempt:
     a. No or few risk factors for suicide (see above).
     b. Action is a response to a readily defined interpersonal crisis.
     c. Action is of low intended lethality undertaken to provoke an anticipated (or fantasized) outcome.
     d. Patient engineers own discovery and rescue.
  4. Emergency department intervention:
     a. Medical evaluation as for any overdose or toxic exposure.
     b. Psychiatric evaluation and crisis intervention:
        (1) Facilitate understanding of incident for those involved.
        (2) Develop alternative, direct, constructive modes of communication.
        (3) Develop plan that includes protection for patient and initiates ongoing therapy.
- VI. Disposition:
  - A. Implications of "medical clearance"
    NOTE: **The term has no uniformly accepted definition or set of applied criteria.**

1. Specific implications of medical clearance in the emergency department:
   a. The patient's medical status has been assessed with regard to both specific presentation and general health.
   b. The patient requires no further acute evaluation or treatment and no test results pertinent to emergency treatment are outstanding.
   c. An acute organic cause for any psychiatric symptoms has been reasonably excluded. (Beware the patient without previous psychiatric history).
   d. There is no medical problem that prevents or compromises psychiatric evaluation.
B. Psychiatric consultation considerations:
   1. Optimal resource use:
      a. Emergency department policy and procedure manual should delineate available resources and their appropriate use.
      b. Clear communication is essential:
         (1) Concise case summary provided to consultant.
         (2) Goal of consultation request defined.
         (3) After consultation is completed, consultant and emergency department physician must confer to plan appropriate disposition.
   2. Indications for psychiatric consultation in the emergency department:
      a. If the treating physician cannot make appropriate assessment for any reason.
      b. Patient has (or possibly has) serious underlying psychiological problems.
      c. Patient's suicidal or homicidal risk is established or unclear.
      d. Poor family dynamics or home environment may contribute to continued risk.
      e. Patient request.
      f. All adolescents and children.
   3. Precautions:
      a. It is inappropriate to send or transfer such patients to a referral or tertiary care center before medical stability has been assured.
      b. All questions regarding treatment prior to transfer, and care during transportation to the receiving hospital should be discussed between the patient's physician at the first hospital and the accepting physician at the receiving hospital.
      c. Primary responsibility rests with ED staff until consultant or admitting physician has clearly indicated acceptance of responsibility for care of patient.
      d. Do not transfer patient to other facility for psychiatric treatment without appropriate medical escort. Patient's family and friends are not appropriate guardians in this case (See Chapter 19 Interhospital Transfer of Poisoned or Overdosed Patients).
C. Commitability:
   1. Although each jurisdiction may have different statutes, it is generally not enough to be "mentally ill" (psychotic or delusional) to be committed (see Chapter 20).

    2. The following generalities are usually held:
        a. Underlying medical illness as an explanation for behavior has been ruled out.
        b. The patient has been clinically diagnosed as having a debilitating mental illness (e.g., inadequate reality testing, delusional).
        c. The patient is a danger to self or others.
        d. The patient refuses voluntary admission for assessment.

D. Psychiatric admission considerations:
    1. The patient's acute medical evaluation and treatment is completed, with an organic etiology of the patient's behavior ruled out.
    2. Admission for purely psychiatric reasons should be decided in conjunction with a specialty consultation, if possible.
    3. Indications for psychiatric hospitalization after suicide attempt:
        a. Continued suicide risk is established or unclear.
        b. Patient is elderly, debilitated, or has chronic medical condition that may compromise self-care or psychological stability.
        c. Major depression.
        d. Psychosis.
        e. No social support.
        f. Repeat suicide attempt.
        g. Physician uncertain.
    4. Patient meets criteria for involuntary commission (absolute criteria for admission).
    5. Poor family environment or home dynamics that may contribute to continued risk.
    6. Consider strongly for all adolescents and children.
    7. Treating physician cannot make clear assessment; consultation unavailable (absolute criteria for admission).

E. Discharge considerations:
    1. Appropriate psychological evaluation has taken place, including consultation if indicated:
        a. No significant potential for self-harm.
        b. Low suicide potential.
        c. Adequate home environment and supervision.
    2. Medical evaluation and treatment completed.
    3. Admission considerations not met (see above).
    4. Appropriate medical, psychological, or social follow-up has been arranged:
        a. Patient or responsible adult given written instructions.
        b. Patient or responsible adult understands instructions.
        c. As part of follow-up, patient or responsible adult knows what to do (including where to seek help) if situation (medical or psychological) should deteriorate:
            (1) Transportation available (phone number of ambulance or 911).
            (2) Phone number of crisis line.
    5. Psychological considerations, including suicide and homicide risk, are clearly documented, as well as follow-up arrangements.

BIBLIOGRAPHY

Beck AT, Beck R, Kovacs M: Classification of suicidal behaviors. I. Quantifying intent and medical lethality. *Am J Psychiatry* 1975; 132:285.

Dubin WR, Weiss KJ, Zeccardi JA: Organic brain syndrome: The psychiatric imposter. *JAMA* 1983; 249:60–62.

Fauman MA, Fauman BJ: The differential diagnosis of organic-based psychiatric disturbance in the emergency department. *JACEP* 1977; 6:315–323.

Hodgman CH: Recent findings in adolescent depression and suicide: A review article. *Dev Behav Pediatr* 1985; 6:162–170.

Jacobs JW, Bernhard M, Delgado A, et al: Screening for organic mental syndromes in the medically ill. *Ann Intern Med* 1977; 86:40–46.

Litt IF, Cuskey WR, Rudd S: Emergency room evaluation of the adolescent who attempts suicide: Compliance with follow-up. *J Adolesc Health Care* 1983; 4(2):106–108.

Pfeffer C: Self-destructive behavior in children and adolescents. *Psychiatr Clin North Am* 1985; 8:215–226.

Pfeffer C: Elements of treatment for suicidal pre-adolescents. *Am J Psychother* 1987; 41:172–184.

Pfeffer C: Clinical aspects of childhood suicidal behavior. *Ped XX Annals* 1984; 13:56–61.

Rosenberg M, Smith J, Davidson L, et al: The emergence of youth suicide: An epidemiologic analysis and public health perspective. *Ann Rev Pub Health* 1987; 8:417–440.

Rosenthal P, Rosenthal S: Suicidal behavior by preschool children. *Am J Psychiatry* 1984; 141:520–525.

Roth LH: A commitment law for patients, doctors and lawyers. *Am J Psychiatry* 1979; 136:1121.

Rund DA: Emergency management of the difficult patient. *EMS* 1984; 13:17–22.

Solomon P, Patch VD (eds): *Handbook of Psychiatry,* ed 3. Los Altos, Lange Publications, 1974.

Weissberg MP: Emergency room medical clearance: An educational problem. *Am J Psychiatry* 1979; 136:787–790.

Williams PW: New developments in the civil commitment of the mentally ill. *JAMA* 1979; 242:2307.

Zun L, Gold I: A survey of the form of the mental status examination administered by emergency physicians. *Ann Emerg Med* 1986; 15:916–922.

PART FOUR

Diagnostic Evaluation of the Poisoned Patient

35

Introduction

Stuart R. Fritz, M.D.

NOTE: **Poisoning should not be considered simply as an isolated event separate from other disease process or injury.**

When confronted with a severely poisoned or overdosed patient, "classic" Oslerian diagnostic methods may prove inefficient and perhaps even dangerous. Emergency physicians managing life-threatening illness or injury must often initiate therapeutic intervention based on scant history and a brief physical examination well before arriving at a definitive diagnosis. It does not benefit the patient (or the physician) to have correctly diagnosed the cause of illness after the fact if the patient has otherwise reversible morbidity or mortality.

The physician treating a potentially poisoned patient must quickly synthesize a differential diagnosis that includes the possibility of trauma or medical illness masking, mimicking, or exacerbating poisoning. A striking example of this is found in data reported by the National Safety Council, which estimates that in 1986 alcohol was a major contributing factor in 21,000 fatal motor vehicle accidents.

Even in instances where a poisoning can be diagnosed with relative certainty, the severity or extent of the toxic exposure often cannot be immediately determined. Studies evaluating the clinician's ability to immediately predict agents involved in poisoning range from 25% to 60% compared with later laboratory analysis (i.e., complete toxicology screen). If a toxic substance is not suspected or if the severity of a poisoning is underestimated, serious and potentially life-threatening delayed sequelae may result.

Because toxic ingestion may be difficult to diagnose with certainty, it is essential that each potentially poisoned patient be managed in a consistent, systematic fashion. Management must always begin with resuscitation and stabilization of vital signs (see APTLS, Chapter 8), followed by identification of the toxin (if possible) and determination of severity of poisoning. The physician must then determine the type of supportive care necessary, indications for specific therapy, and whether active elimination of the toxin is appropriate. Finally, the physician must determine the proper disposition of the patient regarding admission, need for intensive care, appropriate consultation, transfer to another facility, or discharge (see Chapter 17 and 18).

During patient assessment "universal precautions" should be taken by **all** of the health care providers, as well as precautions against hazardous materials and safety from potential violence (see Chapter 16).

BIBLIOGRAPHY

Accident Facts. Chicago, National Safety Council, 1987, p. 52.

Hepler BR, Sutheimer CA, Sunshine I: The role of the toxicology laboratory in emergency medicine. II. Study of an integrated approach. *Clin Toxicol* 1984–85; 22:503–528.

36

Obtaining the History

Stuart R. Fritz, M.D.

I. Introduction. When managing a critically ill patient the initial history of necessity should be brief and directed toward gathering information that may assist in resuscitation (See APTLS, Chapter 8). Detailed histories are never part of primary surveys. Consider alternative sources of information (see below) if the patient is disoriented, obtunded, or unable to speak.

NOTE: **Obtaining the history should never take precedence over the primary survey and resuscitation.**

Once the patient is stabilized and the secondary assessment is progressing, the treating physician can obtain a detailed history. The history is aimed at not only identification of the poison but toward identifying all concomitant or complicating underlying medical *and* psychological conditions. Other useful information includes age and weight of the patient (particularly in the pediatric age group), time since ingestion or exposure, amount ingested, history of trauma, and known medicines and allergies.

If the patient is alert and cooperative, he or she can usually supply the necessary information. Unfortunately, the patient is often comatose, stuporous, or an infant. Other factors that may influence the amount of information available from the patient include level of education, intelligence, or cooperation (e.g., the patient who is still actively suicidal may resist the physician's help or purposefully give a deceptive history).

NOTE: **Always be suspicious of inaccurate history from patients claiming to have taken only a few pills.**

II. Alternate sources of information ("Ten Ps"):

When a satisfactory history cannot be obtained from the patient (for reasons mentioned above), one of the following sources can often supply vital

161

information. Even when information can be obtained from the patient, confirmation from these sources is useful.

A. **Patient:**
   1. Look for medical alert bracelet.
   2. Identify evidence of illicit drug use such as a coke spoon or other drug paraphernalia worn as jewelry, track marks on the skin, or ice in the groin or axilla (home remedy for opioid overdose).
B. **Pockets** (shoes, billfold, purse):
   1. Look for **pill** containers.
   2. Look for job identification (hazardous chemical exposure).
   3. Look for **phone numbers** that can be used to contact friends, family, or the patient's private physician.
   4. Read all recent sales receipts, looking for the name of any pharmacy, medication, or purchase of hazardous materials.
   5. When searching a patient's belongings be careful to avoid accidental injury from needles and other sharp objects (see Chapter 16).
C. **Prehospital** personnel, **Police, Paramedics:**
   1. These personnel often have access to the scene of the poisoning and, if radio contact has been established, may still be at that location.
   2. Police can be sent to the scene to retrieve information or question witnesses and neighbors.
D. **Parents, Partner, Pals:**
   1. These persons can be sent to the scene to identify and return with pill bottles or other information.
   2. Always have parents, spouses, or friends phone the emergency department with information from the scene or send them back to retrieve this information. Instruct them to bring pill bottles or other suspect containers to the emergency department to confirm their verbal report (assuming there is no danger in doing so).
E. **Pedestrians** and bystanders.
F. **Personal Physician, Psychiatrist:**
   1. If known, call **at any hour.**
G. **Pharmacist, Poisindex, Physician's** Desk Reference:
   1. Pill bottles have pharmacy identification numbers.
   2. Unidentified pills can sometimes be analyzed by hospital pharmacies, Poisindex, or identified by size, color, and shape.
4. **Poison** information center:
   1. See Chapter 4.
I. **Past** medical records (**Previous** hospitalizations):
   1. Always obtain the hospital medical records. Surprising information can often be found even when it seems everything is already known.
   2. Call medical records department of other facilities that have treated the patient in the past.
J. **Pill** bottles:
   1. Routinely listed data include the name and address of the person for whom the prescription was written; the prescribing physician; the type, strength, and **number of pills originally in the bottle;** and the date of distribution. The name of the pharmacy filling the prescription and a

prescription number (usually located in the upper left) are required by law.

NOTE: **Never assume that the label on the container describes the pills that were stored in the bottle.**

III. Organization of the history:

As the secondary survey progresses, an expedient but thorough history should be obtained regarding every poisoned or overdosed patient.

A. History of present illness:
  1. Personal data:
     a. Names, address, phone number.
     b. Age, sex, weight.
  2. Method of arrival:
     a. Type of transportation to the emergency department.
     b. Where the patient was brought from and with whom.
  3. Patient symptoms:
     a. Chief complaint.
     b. Other ongoing symptoms. Be especially alert for symptom complexes (toxindromes) suggestive of a specific poisoning (see Chapter 47).
  4. Type of poisoning:
     a. Identify the poison or toxic exposure.
     b. Quantify the amount or estimate maximal exposure.
     c. Method of exposure (e.g., inhalation, ingestion, injection, transdermal, ocular).
     d. Time since exposure.
  5. Circumstances of poisoning:
     a. Accidental.
     b. Possible assault or attempted homicide.
     c. Child abuse or neglect.
     d. Self-inflicted, suicide attempt.
  6. Verify suspicion of attempted suicide:
     a. Intentional drug ingestion is the most frequent method used to attempt suicide (O'Brien JP, 1977).
     b. Expect multiple-drug overdoses in instances of acute self-poisoning. Fifty-nine percent of cases involving self-poisoning involved two or more drugs in a series of 265 patients studied (Rygnestad T, 1984).
  7. History of pre-hospital interventions:
     a. Antidotes used. Results of administration.
     b. Decontamination procedures (induced or spontaneous emesis, ocular or cutaneous irrigation).
  8. Associated conditions:
     a. Associated trauma.
     b. Actively suicidal patient.
     c. Underlying medical or psychiatric illness.
  9. Current medications, including over-the-counter (OTC) preparations.

B. Past medical history:
  1. Known allergies, history of anaphylaxis.
  2. Previous significant medical disease, especially liver or kidney disease.
  3. Surgical history (including tetanus immunization status).

C. Psychiatric history:
   1. See Chapter 34 for detailed psychiatric evaluation.
   2. Underlying psychiatric illness, especially depression, schizophrenia, mania.
   3. Previous psychiatric hospitalizations.
   4. History of prior suicide attempts:
      a. Intentional drug ingestion is the most frequent method used to attempt suicide.
      b. In one series of 255 patients requiring admission to the intensive care unit for treatment of drug overdose (Stern TA, 1984):
         (1) Seventy-five percent had received prior psychiatric treatment.
         (2) Seventy percent used alcohol regularly.
         (3) Fifty-four percent had been seen by a physician shortly before the overdose.
         (4) Twenty-six percent had a history of substance abuse.
         (5) Fifty-seven percent had made a prior suicide attempt.
D. Social history (if indicated)
   1. Occupational hazards.
   2. Possible exposure from exotic hobbies or travel.
   3. Alcohol and illicit drug use habits.

BIBLIOGRAPHY

O'Brien JP: Increase in suicide attempts by drug ingestion: The Boston experience, 1964–74. *Arch Gen Psychiatry* 1977; 34:1165–1169.

Rygnestad T, Berg KJ: Evaluation of benefits of drug analysis in the routine clinical management of self-poisoning. *Clin Toxicol* 1984; 22:51–61.

Stern TA, Mulley AG, Thibault GE: Life-threatening drug overdose: Precipitants and prognosis. *JAMA* 1984; 251:1983–1985.

37

Physical Examination

Stuart R. Fritz, M.D.

I. Introduction. In this chapter the basic physical examination required to evaluate the poisoned patient and to aid in the identification of the toxic substance
is outlined. An attempt has been made to prioritize the examination such that
life-threatening problems are discovered and corrected early in the assessment.
In subsequent chapters the diagnostic value of specific findings is discussed.

II. General principles:
   A. Always start with a primary survey assessment (see APTLS, Chapter 8) si-
   multaneous with resuscitation.
   B. Once the patient's condition has been stabilized, a more thorough secondary survey may begin (see Minimal complete examination, below).
   C. Because so many toxic substances affect the cardiovascular and autonomic
   nervous systems, continuous monitoring of respiration, pulse, blood pressure, and temperature is required until the patient is proved to be at no
   further risk.
   D. The presence of an intoxicating agent does not necessarily account for
   abnormal vital signs; always consider concomitant medical illness or
   trauma.

III. Minimal complete examination: (interpretation of findings related to specific
poisonings are discussed later in this chapter).
   A. Vital signs:
      1. Pulse:
         a. Quality.
         b. Rate.
         c. Regularity.
         d. Peripheral pulses present and equal bilaterally.

2. Blood pressure.
3. Respiratory rate.
4. Body temperature:
   a. Oral routinely.
   b. Rectal:
      (1) If hyperthermia is suspected (use rectal thermometer with low scale capacity).
      (2) In unconscious patients.
      (3) In hyperventilating or tachypneic patients (artificially lowered oral temperature reading).
      (4) In pediatric patients.
B. Head and Neck:
   1. Evidence of trauma:
      a. Lacerations, contusions, hematomas.
      b. Basilar skull fracture:
         (1) Hemotympanum.
         (2) Battle's sign (ecchymosis behind ear).
         (3) CSF rhinorrhea or otorrhea.
         (4) Periorbital ecchymoses.
   2. Eyes:
      a. Neurologic examination as outlined below.
      b. Visual acuity.
      c. Funduscopic examination.
   3. Mouth and throat:
      a. Breath odor.
      b. Mucosal discoloration.
      c. Caustic ulceration.
      d. Pharyngeal edema.
      e. Status of gag reflex (stabilize neck before checking if evidence of head or neck trauma and have suction available).
   4. Neck:
      a. Suppleness, presence of nuchal rigidity.
      b. Lymphadenopathy?
C. Pulmonary:
   1. Confirm adequate air exchange:
      a. Equal thoracic excursion.
      b. Equal bilateral breath sounds.
      c. Quality of respirations: record hypoventilation, hyperventilation, or irregular breathing patterns.
   2. Lung function:
      a. Work of breathing (e.g., intercostal retractions or accessory muscle use).
      b. Quality of breath sounds (e.g., wheezing, rhonchi, rales).
D. Cardiovascular:
   1. Pulse and blood pressure (see Vital signs, above).
   2. Volume status:
      a. Suspected hypovolemia:
         (1) Blood pressure (hypotension).

(2) Orthostatic changes.

(3) Pulse (tachycardia).

   b. Suspected venous congestion:

     (1) Jugular venous distention.

3. Cyanosis:

   a. Central.

   b. Peripheral.

4. Auscultation of heart:

   a. Murmurs.

   b. Gallops and rubs.

   c. Ectopy.

E. Abdomen:

1. Pain or tenderness on palpation.

2. Guarding.

3. Peritoneal signs.

4. Stomach, intestinal, or bladder distension.

5. Bowel sounds: hypoactive, hyperactive, silent.

6. Rectal examination: melena, bright red blood.

7. Stool: occult blood (guaiac examination).

F. Skin:

1. Color and evidence of flushing.

2. Moisture: dry or diaphoretic.

3. Temperature.

4. Piloerection.

5. Urticaria or target lesions.

6. Bullae or exfoliative dermatitis.

7. Needle tracks.

8. Trauma (including penetrating wounds).

G. Neurologic:

1. Level of consciousness: requires constant monitoring.

   a. Initial assessment:

     (1) Alert, follows verbal commands.

     (2) Responds to noise.

     (3) Responds to painful stimuli only.

     (4) Unconscious, unresponsive.

   b. Repeat assessment:

     (1) Glasgow Coma Scale (Table 37–1) is the most sensitive, easily used tool to identify changing level of consciousness.

2. Cranial nerves:

   a. Conscious patient:

     (1) Pupils: size, symmetry, reaction to light.

     (2) Extraocular motions; record diplopia, ophthalmoplegia, nystagmus.

     (3) Hearing: equal auditory acuity, presence of tinnitus.

     (4) Facial symmetry, strength, sensation.

     (5) Tongue midline, status of gag reflex.

   b. Unconscious patient:

     (1) Pupils: size, symmetry, reaction to light.

TABLE 37–1.

Glasgow Coma Scale

Activity	Score
Best eye-opening response	
Spontaneous	4
In response to voice command	3
In response to pain	2
Does not occur	1
Best motor response	
Follows commands	6
Removes noxious stimulus	5
Withdraws from noxious stimulus	4
Has decorticate posturing	3
Has decerebrate posturing	2
Has no motor response	1
Best verbal response	
Coherent, oriented conversation	5
Confused, disoriented conversation	4
Understandable but nonsensical speech	3
Unintelligible sounds	2
No speech	1

(2) Corneal reflexes.
(3) Oculocephalic reflex (doll's eyes maneuver) or cold caloric stimulation.
(4) Facial symmetry.
(5) Intact gag reflex.
3. Upper and lower sensory motor neuron integration and function:
   a. Conscious patient:
      (1) Strength and tone as tested by hand grip and flexion/extension of the lower extremities.
      (2) Intact sensation to light touch.
      (3) Coordination: speech, gait, finger-to-nose test.
      (4) Proprioception; test for pronator drift.
   b. Unconscious patient:
      (1) Muscle tone and activity: tremor, rigidity, myoclonus.
      (2) Deep tendon reflex response.
      (3) Response to plantar stimulation.
      (4) Response to deep pain:
          a Equal movement or flaccidity in all extremities.
          b Posturing or purposeful movement.
          c See Glasgow Coma Scale (Table 37–1).
H. Mental status examination:
   1. See Chapter 34.

BIBLIOGRAPHY

Accident Facts. Chicago, National Safety Council, 1987, p 52.

Hepler BR, Sutheimer CA, Sunshine I: The role of the toxicology laboratory in emergency medicine. II. Study of an integrated approach. *Clin Toxicol* 1984–85; 22:503–528.

O'Brien JP: Increase in suicide attempts by drug ingestion: The Boston experience 1964–74. *Arch Gen Psychiatry* 1977; 34:1165–1169.

Rygnestad T, Berg KJ: Evaluation of benefits of drug analysis in the routine clinical management of self-poisoning. *Clin Toxicol* 1984; 22:51–61.

Stern TA, Mulley AG, Thibault GE: Life-threatening drug overdose: Precipitants and prognosis. *JAMA* 1984; 251:1983–1985.

General Signs and Symptoms, and Vital Signs

Donald R. Chabot, M.D.

I. General signs and symptoms:
  A. Weight loss: Any chronic poisoning, but especially:

Arsenic	Lead
Chlorinated	Mercury
hydrocarbons	Thyroid
Dinitrophenol	

  B. Lethargy, weakness:

Arsenic	Thiazide diuretics	Nicotine
Botulism	Fluorides	Nitrites
Chlorinated	Lead	Organophosphates
compounds	Mercury	Thallium

  C. Loss of appetite:
    Trinitrotoluene

  D. Alcohol intolerance:

Carbamate	Fungicides	Herbicides
insecticides	Furazolidone	Metronidazole
Disulfiram		

  E. Chills:

Copper fumes	Metal oxides (several)	Vacor
	Spectinomycin	Zinc

II. Vital signs:
  A. Respiration:
    1. Bradypnea/hypoventilation:

Anesthetics	Carbon monoxide	Clonidine
Barbiturates (late)	(late)	Cyanide (late)

Ethanol   Insecticides   Sedative-hypnotics
Fluorides   Opioids   Snake venom (late)

2. Tachypnea/hyperpnea/hyperventilation:

Amphetamines   Clonidine   Methanol
Atropine   CNS stimulants   Salicylates
Barbiturates (early) Cocaine   Snake venom (early)
Camphor   Cyanide (early)   Strychnine
Carbon dioxide   Ethanol   Theophylline
Carbon monoxide   Ethylene glycol   Withdrawal states
   (early)   Hydrocarbons

B. Pulse:

1. Bradycardia:

Aconitine   Ethyl gasoline   Nicotine
Anticholinesterases   Guanethidine   Nitrite
Barium   Haloperidol   Oleander
Beta blockers   Hydrogen sulfide   Opioids
Calcium channel   Isopropanol   Parasympathomi-
   blockers   Lead   metics
Carbon monoxide   Local anesthetics   Pilocarpine
Chloroquine   Minor/major   Quinacrine
Cholinergics   tranquilizers   Quinidine
Cimetidine   Mistletoe   Quinine
Clonidine   Morphine   Reserpine
Cyanide   Mushrooms   Rhododendron
Digitalis   (cholinergics)   Sedatives/hypnotics
Ethchlorvynol   Nasal decongestants   Squill

2. Tachycardia:

Anticholinergics   Dinitrophenol   Phenol
Alcohols   Doxepin   Phenothiazines
Amanita   Ethanol   Potassium bromate
   mushrooms   Glutethimide   Primidone
Amphetamines   Hydrogen sulfide   Procainamide
Antihistamines   Hypoglycemics   Salicylates
Arsenicals   Iron salts   Sympathomimetics
Atropine   Lithium   Theophylline
Caffeine   Loxapine   Thyroid supplements
Carbon monoxide   *Muscaria* mushrooms   Tricyclic
Cimetidine   Nicotine   antidepressants
Cocaine   Phencyclidine   Withdrawal states
Cyanide (early)

3. Irregular pulse:

Digitalis   Nitrite   Veratrum
Mushrooms   Oleander   Zygadenus

C. Blood pressure:

1. Hypertension:

Amphetamines   Carbon monoxide   Cocaine
Anticholinergics   Cadmium   Corticosteroids
Barium   Clonidine   Ephedrine

Ergot
Fenfluramine
Lead
Lobeline
Loxapine
Mercury

Monoamine oxidase
  inhibitors
Nicotine
Phencyclidine
Phenmetrazine
Pseudoephedrine
Sympathomimetics

Thallium
Thyroid supplements
Tricyclic
  antidepressants
Xanthines
Withdrawal states

2. Hypotension:

Amanita
  phalloides
  mushrooms
Antihypertensives
Antipsychotics
Arsenicals
Barbiturates
Beta blockers
Boric acid
Bromides.
Calcium channel
  blockers
Carbon
  tetrachloride
Carbon monoxide
Cholinergics
Cicutoxin
Clonidine
Cobalt
Copper
Cyanide
Disulfiram
  (Antabuse)
Diuretics
Ethanol
Ethchlorvynol
Fluorides
Glutethimide

Herbicides
Hexachlorophene
Hydrogen sulfide
Insecticides
Iodine
Iron salts (second-
  degree
  hemorrhage)
Isoniazid
Isopropanol
Local anesthetics
LSD
Magnesium
Meprobamate
Mercury
Methaqualone
Methyl bromide
Minor/major
  tranquilizers
Mistletoe
Monkshood
Monoamine oxidase
  inhibitors (late)
Nalidixic acid
Narcotics
Nicotine
Nitrates
Nitrites

Nitroglycerin
Oleander
Oxalate
Paraldehyde
Phenols
Phenothiazines
Phosphine
Phosphorus
Procainamide
Procaine
Propoxyphene
Pufferfish
Quinidine
Quinine
Reserpine
Sedatives/hypnotics
Selenium
Silver nitrate
Theophylline
Thioxanthines
Tolbutamide
Tricyclic
  antidepressants
Vacor
Vancomycin
Verapamil

D. Temperature:
  1. Hyperthermia, fever:

Amphetamines
Anticholinergics
Antihistamines
Arsenicals
Benzodiazepines
Boric acid
Camphor
Cimetidine
Cocaine

Cogentin
Copper fumes
Cotton dust
Dinitrocresol
Dinitrophenol
Ethanol
Fenfluramine
Fluoroacetate
Glutethimide

Herbicides
Hexachlorobenzene
Iron
Laxative abuse in
  elderly
LSD
Metal fumes
Methaqualone
Methyl chloride

Methyl bromide	Phenothiazines	Theophyllines
Methyprylon	Polymer fumes	Thyroid supplements
Monoamine oxidase	Propranolol	Tricyclic
inhibitors	Salicylates	antidepressants
Nalidixic acid	Snake venom	Withdrawal states
Pentachlorophenol	Spectinomycin	Xanthines
Petroleum distillates	Sympathomimetics	Zinc fumes
Phencyclidine		

2. Hypothermia:

Alcohol	Ethanol	Opioids
Barbiturates	Ethchlorvynol	Phenols
Benzodiazepines	General anesthetics	Phenothiazines
Butyrophenones	Glutethimide	Pine oil
Carbon monoxide	Haloperidol	Sedatives/hypnotics
Chloral hydrate	Hydrogen sulfide	Tetracyclines
Clonidine	Hypoglycemics	Vacor
CNS depressants	Minor/major	
Cyanide	tranquilizers	

BIBLIOGRAPHY

Goldfrank LR, Kulberg AG: Vital signs and toxic syndromes, in Goldfrank LR (ed): *Goldfrank's Toxicologic Emergencies.* Norwalk, Conn, Appleton-Century-Crofts, 1986, pp 58–68.

Johns Hopkins Hospital: *The Harriet Lane Manual* (Rowe PC, ed). Chicago, Year Book Medical Publishers, 1987.

Done A: Signs, symptoms and sources. *Emerg Med* January 15, 1982, pp 42–77.

39

Skin

Thomas P. Gross, M.D.

I. Skin findings:
 A. Hot, dry:
 Anticholinergics
 Botulinus toxin
 B. Gray:
 Lead
 Phenacetin
 C. Jaundice:
 1. From liver injury:

Acetominophen	Chromates	Nitric acid
Aniline	Diuretics	Phenothiazines
Carbon	Heavy metals (e.g.,	Phosphorus
tetrachloride	arsenic, iron)	Sulfonamides
Chlorinated	Isoniazid	Thiazides
compounds	Mushrooms	Trinitrotoluene
Chlorpromazine	Naphthalene	

 2. From hemolysis:

Aniline	Castor beans	Pamaquine
Arsine	Fava beans	Pentaquine
Benzene	Nickel	Phosphine
Nickel	Nitrobenzene	Primaquine
carbonyl		

 D. Cyanosis (O_2 resistant):

Benzocaine	Nitrates	Phenacetin
Methemoglobin	Nitrites	Sulfhemoglobin

 E. Diaphoresis:

Amphetamines	Anticholinesterases	Arsenic

Bismuth
Cholinergic agents
Ciguatera
Cimetidine
Cocaine
Dinitrophenols
Fluorides
Hexachlorobenzene

Hydrogen sulfide
Hypoglycemics
LSD
Mercurials
Mushrooms
 (muscarinic)
Naphthalene
Nicotine

Pentachlorophenol
Phencyclidine
Pokeweed
Quinine
Salicylates
Snake bite
Sympathomimetics

F. Flushing:

Acetaldehyde
 (Asians/American
 Indians)
Amphetamines
Anticholinergics
Antihistamines
Beryllium
Boric acid
Carbamazepine
Carbon monoxide
Chloral hydrate
Cobalt
Cocaine

Cyanide
Dinitrophenol
Disulfiram
Ethanol (intoxication,
 withdrawal)
Iodide
LSD
Metaldehyde (face)
Monosodium
 glutamate
Mushrooms
Niacin
Nicotinamide

Nitrites
Phenothiazines
Reserpine
Saccharin
Scromboid fish
Poisoning
Snake bite
Sympathomimetic
 agents
Tyramine reaction
 (associated with
 monoamine oxidase
 inhibitors

G. Sclerosed veins:
   Amphetamines
   Cocaine
   Opioids, Phencyclidine
H. Purpura:
   Quinine
   Salicylates
   Snake bite
   Spider bite
   Warfarin
I. Discoloration:
   1. Yellow:
      Carotenoids
      Epoxy resins
      Quinacrine
      Rifampin
      Vitamin A
   2. Bronze:
      Arsine
   3. Red:

Anticholinergics
Antihistamines
Boric acid ("boiled
 lobster"
 appearance)

Belladonna
Carbon monoxide
Cyanide

Mercury
Rifampin

4. Orange:
   Nitric acid
   Tetrylchlorine
5. Green:
   Copper salts
6. Blue:
   Oxalic acid
7. Brown:

Bromides	Local anesthetics	Nitrates/nitrites
Iodine	Mushrooms	(methemoglobinemia)
		Phenytoin

8. Gray-black:
   Chloramphenicol
   Osmium trioxide
   Silver (chronic)

J. Pallor:

Benzene	Fava beans	Naphthalene
Chlorates	Fluorides	Phenols
Clonidine	Lead	Solanine plant poisons
Ergot	Methysergide	

K. Pruritus

Belladonnas	Gold salts	Rifampin
Boric acid	Jimson weed	Scombroid
Ciguatera	Narcotics	Thiocyanates
Cobalt	Phenytoin	

L. Piloerection:
   Withdrawal states
M. Fingernail lines:
   Arsenic
   Thallium
N. Keratinization:
   Arsenic
   Thallium
O. Characteristic skin odors:
   See Chapter 40
P. Chloracne: Chlorinated aromatic compounds and contaminants in their manufacture, such as PCB, PBB, TCDDioxin, 245-T (Agent Orange).
Q. Erythema multiforme:

Anticonvulsants	Hydralazine
Arsenic	Mercurials
Barbiturates	Penicillins
Cimetidine	Phenolphthalein
Dapsone	Phenylbutazone
Gold salts	Salicylates
Halogenated steroids	Sulfanilamides

R. Burns:

Acids	Alkali

Carbamate (strong)
Carbon disulfide
Detergents (some)
Dieffenbachia plants
Dimethyl sulfate
Fluorides
Formaldehyde
Herbicides (strong)
Hydrogen sulfide
Hypochlorite
Iodine
Iron
Mercury

Nicotine
Oxalate
Permanganate
Peroxides
Persulfate
Phenols
Phosphorus
Pine oil
Selenium
Silver nitrate
Sodium bisulfate
Thioglycolate
Toluene

S. Photosensitizers:

Anthracene
Asphalt
Benoxaprofen
Coal tar
Fluorescein
Nalidixic acid

Perfumes derived from citrus
Phenothiazines
Porphyrins
Sulfanilamides
Tetracyclines

T. Bullae/vesicles:

Alkyl mercurials
Barbiturates
Carbon monoxide
Caustic agents
Diphenoxylate
Insect bites
Dimethyl sulfate
Ethylene oxide
Hexachlorobenzene

Scombroid
Snake bite
Sulfonamides
Tetracyclines
Ethchlovynol
Glutethimide
Meprobamate
Methaqualone

U. Toxic epidermal necrolysis:

AlkaSeltzer
Allopurinol
Anti-tuberculosis drugs
Barbiturates
Phenytoin

Penicillin
Pentazocine
Sulfa drugs
Tetracycline

V. Pressure sores:

Barbiturates
Carbon monoxide

W. Generalized skin edema:

Anabolic agents
Androgens
Antifertility agents
Estrogens

Glucocorticoids
Indomethacin
Methaqualone

X. Dryness:

Alcohols
Anticholinergics

Boric acid
Ephedrine

Glutethimide
Mushrooms
Nutmeg

Sympathomimetics
Thallium
Thiocyanates

Y. Rash:

Antibiotics
Atropine
Beryllium
Boric acid
Bromide (chronic)
Bromides
Carbamates
Chlorinated compounds
Chromium
Dinitrophenols
Glutethimide
Gold Salts

Hair preparations
Herbicides
Indomethacin
Iodine
Nalidixic acid
Phenothiazines
Photo developers
Poison ivy/oak
Polymyxins
Salicylates
Sulfonamides

Z. Hair loss:

Arsenic
Boric acid
Chemotherapy agents
Chloral hydrate
Chloroquine
Gold salts
Hexachlorobenzene

Lead
Mercury
Radioelements
Selenium
Thallium
Thiocyanates

AA. Desquamation:

Arsenic
Boric acid

40

Head and Neck

Edward S. Wang, M.D.

I. Hair:
   A. Alopecia:
      1. See Chapter 39, p. 178).
II. Eyes:
   A. Pupillary dilation:

Alkaloids
Aminophylline
Anticholinergics
Antihistamines
Atropine
Barbiturates (coma)
Belladonna alkaloids
Benzene
Botulinus toxin
Camphor
Carbamazepine
Carbon monoxide
Cimetidine
Cocaine
Cyanide
Cyclopentolate
Ergot
Ethanol
Ethylene glycol
Fluoride
Fluoroacetate
Glutethimide
Hemlock
Homatropine
Jimsonweed
LSD
Meperidine
Mescaline
Methaqualone
Mushrooms
Nicotine
Nutmeg
Oleander
Parasympatholytics
Phenothiazines
Phenylephrine
Phenytoin
Quinine
Reserpine
Substance withdrawal

Sympathomimetics

Thallium

Toluene

Tricyclic antidepressants

Tropicamide

Withdrawal states

Yew

B. Pupillary constriction:

Acetone

Barbiturates

Benzodiazepines

Caffeine

Chloral hydrate

Cholinergics

Cholinesterase inhibitors

Clonidine

Codeine

Ethanol

Hexachlorophene

Meprobamate

Nicotine

Opiates (except meperidine)

Organophosphates

Parasympathomimetics

Phencyclidine

Pentazocine

Phenothiazines

Propoxyphene

Sympatholytics

C. Nystagmus:

Arsenic

Barbiturates

Benzodiazepines

Carbamazepine

Carbon monoxide

Cocaine

Cyanides

Carbon disulfide

Ethanol (acute)

Ethylene glycol (chronic)

Fenfluramine

Fluoroacetate

Glutethimide

Methaqualone

Mcthyl halides

Nitrofurans

Phencyclidine

Phenytoin

Primidone

Tricyclic antidepressants

Propoxyphene

D. Ptosis:

Botulinus toxin

Phenytoin

Propoxyphene

Thallium

E. Cataracts:

Busulfan

Chloroquinones

Chlorpromazine

Dinitrocresol

Dinitrophenol

Naphthalene

Steroids

Thallium

F. Extraocular palsy:

Botulinus toxin

Ethanol

Lead

Thallium

G. Open-angle glaucoma:

Corticosteroids

H. Conjunctivitis:

Marijuana

I. Blurred vision:

Atropine

Botulinus toxin

Cocaine

Digitalis

Dinitrophenol

Emboli (IV drug abuse)

Indomethacin

Insecticides

Methanol
Nicotine
Organophosphates

Physostigmine
Quinidine
Solvents
Vitamin A

J. Papilledema:
Lead
Vitamin A toxicity
K. Strabismus:
Botulinus toxin
Thallium
L. Hyperemic retina:
Methanol
M. Distorted color vision:
Barbiturates
Bromides
Carbon monoxide
Digitalis
Ethambutol (loss of green)
Ethanol
Hydrogen sulfide
Isoniazid

Lead
LSD
Marijuana
Mercury
Methanol
Organic solvents
Quinine

N. Optic disk pallor:
Carbon disulfide
Nicotine
Quinine
O. Pigmented sclera:
Carotene
Rifampin
Vitamin A
P. Lacrimation:
Anticholinesterases
Arsenic
Cholinergics
Irritant gases
Insecticides

Mushrooms
Nicotine
Organophosphates
Thallium
Withdrawal states

Q. Peripheral field constriction:
Carbon dioxide
Carbon monoxide
Methanol

Methyl mercury
Naphthalene

R. Choked optic disks, optic neuritis:
Arsenic
Carbon disulfide
Carbon tetrachloride
Chloramphenicol
Dinitrobenzene
Dinitrotoluene
Ethambutol
Ethanol

Ethylene glycol
Glutethimide
Isoniazid
Lead (chronic)
Mercury (chronic)
Methanol
Methylacetate
Morphine

Nalidixic acid
Naphthalene
Nicotine
Phosphorus
S. Retinal hemorrhages:
  Benzene
  Carbon monoxide
  Lead
T. Retinal edema:
  Cyanide
  Methanol
U. Photophobia:
  Anything causing mydriasis
  Ciguatera
  Mercury
V. Acute myopia:
  Diuretics
  Phenothiazines

III. Ears:
A. Tinnitus:
  Aminoglycosides
  Caffeine
  Camphor
  Ethacrynic acid
  Furosemide
  Heavy metals
B. Deafness:
  Aminoglycosides
  Arsenic
  Atropine
  Benzene
  Carbon monoxide
  Cobalt
  Cocaine
C. Disturbances of equilibrium:
  Quinine
D. Hyperacusis:
  Chlorinated hydrocarbons
  Phencyclidine

IV. Nose:
A. Smell:
  1. Dysosmia,* cacosmia,† parosmia‡:
    Allopurinol
    Antihistamines

Quinine
Tetracyclines
Thallium
Theophyllines

Methaqualone
Methyl bromide
Warfarin (chronic)

Quinine
Trimethadione

Sulfonamides
Tetracyclines

Indomethacin
Methanol
Nicotine
Quinidine
Quinine
Salicylates

Cyanide
Digitalis
Methanol
Quinidine
Quinine
Salicylates
Vancomycin

Streptomycin

Strychnine
Toluene

Antithyroid agents
Captopril

*Distorted perception of smell.
†Foul smell sensation.
‡Sensation of smell without stimulus.

Carbamazepine   Methylthiouracil
Colchicine   Metronidazole
Diazoxide   Nicotine
DMSO (dimethylsulfoxide)   Opioids
Ethacrynic acid   D-Penicillamine
Gold salts   Phenylbutazone
Insecticides   Phenytoin
Levodopa   Propylthiouracil
Lithium   Sympathomimetics
Local anesthetics   Vitamin D
Methimazole

2. Hyposmia, anosmia
  Cadmium   Hydrogen sulfide
  Chromium   Phenol nose drops

B. Nasal septal perforations:
  Cocaine snorting
  Chromium

C. Fetor nasalis:
  Chromium

V. Mouth:

A. Salivation:
  Ammonia   Mercury (chronic)
  Anticholinesterases   Methaqualone
  Arsenic   Muscarinic mushrooms
  Bismuth   Nicotine
  Caustics   Organophosphates
  Cholinergics   Phencyclidine
  Cocaine   Rhododendron
  Copper   Saccharin
  Fluoride   Salicylates
  Heavy metals   Strychnine
  Iodide   Thallium
  Lead
  Local effects of plant or
    chemical irritants

B. Dry mouth:
  Alkaloids   Ephedrine
  Amphetamines   Ergot
  Anticholinergics   Narcotics
  Antihistamines   Phenytoin
  Atropine   Sympathomimetics
  Barium   Thallium
  Botulinus toxin

C. Teeth:

1. Loose:
  Mercury
  Lead
  Phosphorus

    2. Painful:

Bismuth	Mercury
Ciguatera	Phosphorus

D. Gums:
    1. Black line:

Arsenic	Lead
Bismuth	Mercury

    2. Discoloration:

Arsenic	Lead
Bismuth	Mercury
Hypervitaminosis A	

    3. Gray color:

Lead	Phenacetin

E. Burns:
    1. See Chapter 39, p. 176.

F. Stomatitis:
    Chemotherapeutic agents
    Corrosives
    Thallium

G. Gingivitis:

Arsenic	Lead
Bismuth	Mercury
Heavy metals	

H. Numb tongue:
    Pyrethrins
    Shellfish

I. Taste:
    1. Hypogeusia,* ageusia†:

Carbon monoxide	Penicillamine
Cocaine	Smoking
DMSO (dimethylsulfoxide)	Spironolactone
Gasoline	

    2. Cacogeusia‡

Acetaldehyde	Ferrous salts
Arsenicals	Iodine
Cadmium	Lead
Copper	Mercuric chloride
Disulfiram	Metoclopropamide

    3. Dysgeusia§

Captopril	Nicotine
DMSO	Quinine
Griseofulvin	

*Decreased perception of taste.
†Absence of taste.
‡Bad taste.
§Distorted or bad taste.

   J. Dysphagia, dysphonia
       Extrapyramidal syndrome   Effects of plant or chemical
                                               irritant

VI. Breath odor:
   A. Acetone:
      Acetone   Ketoacidosis
      Chloroform   Lacquer
      Ethanol   Phenol
      Isopropyl alcohol   Salicylates
   B. Alcohol congeners:
      Chloral hydrate
      Ethanol
      Isopropanol
      Phenols
   C. Ammoniacal:
      Uremia
   D. Aromatic essential oils:
      Acetone   Paraldehyde
      Alcohols   Phenols
      Ethylene glycol
   E. Automobile exhaust:
      Carbon monoxide (odorless, but associated with exhaust)
   F. Bitter almond:
      Cyanides (See Chapter 101 for list of substances containing cyanide.)
   G. Burned rope:
      Marijuana
   H. Carrots:
      Cicutoxin
   I. Coal gas:
      Carbon monoxide (odorless but associated with coal gas)
   J. Disinfectants:
      Creosote
      Phenol
   K. Eggs (rotten):
      Disulfiram   Mercaptans
      Hydrogen sulfide   Sewer gas
   L. Fish or raw liver (musty):
      Hepatic failure
      Zinc phosphide
   M. Fruity:
      Amyl nitrite
      Ethanol
      Isopropyl alcohol
   N. Garlic:
      Arsine   DMSO
      Arsenic   Organophosphates

      Phosphorus   Tellurium
      Selenium   Thallium
  O. Mothballs
      Camphor
      p-Dichlorobenzene
      Naphthalene
  P. Pear:
      Chloral hydrate
      Paraldehyde
  Q. Peanuts:
      Vacor (RH-787)
  R. Pepper:
      O-chlorobenzylidene
      Malononitrile
  S. Pine:
      Pine oil
  T. Pungent aromatic:
      Ethchlorvynol (Placidyl)
  U. Shoe polish:
      Nitrobenzene
  V. Sweet distillates:
      Acetone   Ether
      Chloroform   Petroleum
  W. Tobacco (stale):
      Nicotine
  X. Wintergreen:
      Methyl salicylates
  Y. Violets:
      Turpentine
VII. Neck
  A. Stiffness:
      Cocaine
      Phenothiazines
      Strychnine

BIBLIOGRAPHY

Arena JM: *Poisoning.* Springfield, Ill, Charles C Thomas, Publisher, 1979, pp 6–9.

Johns Hopkins Hospital, *The Harriet Lane Handbook,* (Cole C, ed). Chicago, Year Book Medical Publishers, 1984, pp 230–233.

Klassen CD, Amdur MO, Doule J: *Casarett and Doule's Toxicology.* New York, Macmillan Publishing Co, 1986, pp 478–518.

Rosen P, et al: *Emergency medicine: Concepts and Clinical Practice.* St Louis, CV Mosby Co, 1983, pp 215–253.

41

Chest/Pulmonary System

Christopher J. Knuth, M.D.

I. Dyspnea:
- Aminophylline
- Anticholinesterases
- Beta blockers
- Carbon monoxide
- Chlorine gas
- Cyanide
- Ethylene glycol
- Guanethidine
- Herbicides
- Hydrogen sulfide
- Mercury vapor
- Metaproterenol
- Methanol
- Methaqualone
- Methyl bromide
- Methyl chloride
- Methylene chloride
- Naphtha
- Nitrites
- Paraldehyde
- Paraquat (late)
- Perchloroethylene
- Physostigmine
- Puffer fish
- Scorpion sting
- Selenium
- Strychnine
- Thiocyanates
- Toluene
- Trichloroethane
- Trichloroethylene
- Turpentine

II. Tachypnea:
- Alcohol
- Amphetamines and other stimulants
- Atropine
- Carbon dioxide
- Carbon monoxide
- Cocaine
- Cyanide
- Dinitrophenol
- Mushrooms
- Salicylates

III. Central respiratory stimulation:

Acetanilid
Amphetamines
Aniline
Atropine
Benzocaine
Boric acid
Botulinus toxin
Caffeine
Calcium cyanamide
Carbon disulfide
Carbon monoxide
Chloral hydrate
Chlorinated hydrocarbons
Cholinergics
Cocaine
Cyanide
Digitalis
Dinitrophenols

Ethanol
Fluoroacetate
Food poisoning
Herbicides
Hexachlorobenzene
Hydrogen sulfide
LSD
Methanol
Methemoglobinemia
Nitrobenzene
Paraldehyde
Pentachlorophenol
Phenacetin
Salicylates
Strychnine
Sympathomimetics
Withdrawal states
Xanthines

IV. Hyperpnea:

Dinitrophenol
Ethylene glycol
Fluoroacetate

Methanol
Paraldehyde
Salicylates

V. Respiratory depression (bradypnea, apnea):

Acetylcholine
Alcohols
Anesthetics
Anticholinesterases
Antihistamines
Aromatic hydrocarbons
Barbiturates
Benzodiazepines
Botulinus toxin
Carbon monoxide
Clonidine
CNS depressants
Colchicine
Cyanide
Fluorides
Food poisoning
Glutethimide

Hypnotics/sedatives
Insulin
Mushroom poisoning
Neuromuscular blockers
Nickel
Nitrofurantoin
Opiates/narcotics
Organophosphates
Phencyclidine
Pilocarpine
Salicylates
Snake venom
Snake bite
Strychnine
Thallium
Thiazides
Tricyclic antidepressants

VI. Bronchospasm:

Anticholinesterases
Beta blockers
Carbamates
Cholinergics
Insecticides
Mushroom poisoning

Neostigmine
Organophosphates
Penicillin
Physostigmine
Salicylates
Sulfites

VII. Laryngospasm or stridor:
    Anaphylaxis
    Caustics
    Irritant gases and smoke
    Obstruction (pill fragment)
    Phenothiazines

VIII. Kussmaul breathing:
    Acetanilid
    Beryllium
    Cyanide
    Hydrocarbons
    Mercury vapor
    Salicylates
    Silica
    Smoke inhalation

IX. Coryza and sneezing:
    Chlorine
    Chromates
    Rhododendron plants
    Riot control agents

X. Pulmonary edema:
    Ammonia
    Amphetamines
    Beta blockers
    Carbon monoxide
    Chlorine gas
    Cocaine
    Colchicine
    Dimethyl sulfate
    Disopyramide
    Halothane
    Hydrocarbons
    Hydrochlorthiazide
    Hydrogen sulfide
    Insulin
    Irritant gases
    IV contrast medium
    Mercury vapor
    Metal fumes
    Methyl halides
    Nitrofurantoin
    Nitrogen oxides
    Opiates/narcotics
      Heroin (IV)
      Methadone (PO)
      Propoxyphene (PO)
    Organophosphates
    Ozone
    Paraldehyde
    Paraquat
    Petroleum distillates
    Salicylates
    Sedatives/hypnotics
      Ethchlorvynol
      Methaqualone
    Smoke inhalation
    Tricyclic antidepressants

XI. Aspiration pneumonia:
    Any drug that causes depressed sensorium (see Chapter 45, p. 204)

XII. Chest pain (noncardiac):
    Carbon disulfide (burned)
    Irritant gases
    Monosodium glutamate (MSG)
    Vacor

BIBLIOGRAPHY

Done A: Signs, symptoms and sources. *Emerg Med* January 15, 1982, pp 42–77.

Goldfrank LR, Kulberg AG: Vital signs and toxic syndromes, in Goldfrank LR (ed): *Goldfrank's Toxicologic Emergencies.* Norwalk, Conn, Appleton-Century-Crofts, 1986, pp 58–68.

Johns Hopkins Hospital: *The Harriet Lane Manual* (Cole C, ed). Chicago, Year Book Medical Publishers, 1984.

42

Cardiovascular System

Carol Jack Scott, M.D.

I. Anginal pain:
   Carbon monoxide
   Emetine
   Guanethidine
   Ipecac
   Methylene chloride
   Nicotine
II. Palpitation:
   Nitrites
   Nitroglycerin
   Organic nitrates
   Potassium bromate
III. Pulse:
   1. See Chapter 37, p. 171.
IV. Arrhythmia:
   A. Bradyarrhythmia:
      Anticholinesterases
      Beta blockers
      Calcium channel blockers
      Cholinergics
      Cyanide
      Digitalis
      Sedatives/hypnotics (e.g.,
         ethchlorvynol, chloral hydrate)
   B. Tachyarrhythmia:
      Anticholinergics (including over-
         the-counter sleep preparations)
      Antihistamines (anticholinergic
         effect)
      Ethanol
      Hallucinogens
        PCP
        TCH
      Methylphenidate (Ritalin)
      Plants (*Amanita muscaria,*
         Amanita pantherina)
      Sedatives/hypnotics
         (Chloral hydrate)
      Stimulants
        Cocaine
        Amphetamines
        Dextroamphetamine
        Methamphetamine
      Sympathomimetics
      Tricyclic antidepressants
      Withdrawal states

C. Nonspecific:
  Cyanide
  Dinitrophenols
  Ethanol
  Hydrocarbons
  Benzene

V. Blood pressure:
  A. Hypertension:
    Caffeine
    Hallucinogens
      LSD
      PCP
    Monoamine oxide inhibitors
      (MAOIs) (early)
    Nicotine
  B. Hypotension:
    Antihypertensive agents
    Antipsychotics
    Beta blockers
    Calcium channel blockers
    Diuretics
    Ethanol
    Iron
    Lead
    MAOI (late)
    Nitrates
    Nitrites
  C. Orthostatic hypotension:
    Antihypertensives
      Alpha blocker
      Alpha methyldopa
      Ganglionic blockers
      Vasodilators
    Antiparkinson drugs
      Bromocriptine
    Antipsychotic drugs

Toluene
Phenols
Phenothiazines
Physostigmine

Sympathomimetics
  Amphetamines
  Cocaine
  Phencyclidine (PCP)
Thyroid supplements
Tricyclic antidepressants

Sedatives/hypnotics
  Barbiturates
  Glutethimide (Doriden)
  Methaqualone
  Quinazolione
  Piperidinediones
  Methyprylon
  Ethchlorvynol (Placidyl)
  Meprobamate
Theophylline
Thiamine depletion

CNS depressants
  Ethanol
  Opioids
  Sedatives/hypnotics
Diuretics
Monoamine oxidase inhibitors
Narcotics
Tricyclic antidepressants

BIBLIOGRAPHY

Benowitz N, et al: Cardiopulmonary castastrophies in drug-overdose patients. Med Clin North Am 1979; 63:267–296.

Goldberg R, et al: Cardiac complications following TCA overdose: Issues for monitoring policy. *JAMA* 1985; 254:1772–1775.

Goldfrank L, et al: *Toxicologic Emergencies,* ed 3. Norwalk, Conn, Appleton-Century-Crofts, 1986.

Haddad L, Winchester J: *Clinical Management of Poisoning and Drug Overdose.* Philadelphia, WB Saunders Co, 1983.

Pentel P, Peterson CD: Asystole complicating physostigmine treatment of TCA overdose. *Ann Emerg Med* 1980; 9:588–590.

Rosen P, et al (eds): *Emergency Medicine: Concepts and Clinical Practice.* St. Louis, CV Mosby Co, 1983.

Schweitzer P, Teichholz LE: Carotid sinus massage: Its diagnostic and therapeutic value in arythmias. Am J Med 1985; 78:645–654.

Tintinalli J, et al (eds): *Emergency Medicine: A Comprehensive Study Guide.* New York, McGraw-Hill Book Co, 1985.

Wellens W, et al: The value of the electrocardiogram in differential diagnosis of tachycardia with widened QRS complex. Am J Med 1978; 64:27–33.

43

Gastrointestinal Tract

Luis F. Eljaik, M.D.

I. Upper esophageal symptoms:
  A. Dysphagia:
   Aldehydes
   Antiseptics
   Camphor
   Corrosives
   Diquat
   Esters
   Ethers (acetaldehyde,
     metaldehyde)
   Food poisoning (botulism)
   Halogenated hydrocarbons
     (tear gas, mace)
   Hydrogen sulfide
   Ketones
   Marine animal bites (jellyfish,
     Portuguese man-of-war)
   Paraquat
   Scorpion sting
   Soaps and detergents (anionic,
     nonionic, cationic)
   Volatile oils
  B. Odynophagia:
   Antiseptics (boric acid and
     derivatives, silver nitrate)
   Bleaches (hypochloric acid)
   Camphor
   Corrosives
   Diquat
   Hydrogen sulfide
   Paraquat
   Scorpion sting
   Soaps and detergents (anionic,
     nonionic, cationic)
   Volatile oils
 II. Nausea:
   Virtually any overdose or toxin
III. Vomiting:
   Virtually any overdose or toxin

IV. Hematemesis:

Aminophylline

Anticoagulants (e.g., Coumadin)

Corrosives

Iron

Fluorides

V. Abdominal pain

Alcohols and glycols

Anticancer agents

Antiseptics

Aspartic acid

Beta blockers

Bleaches

Bromides

Cantharidin (Spanish fly)

Cathartics

Chloral hydrate

Cocaine

Colchicine

Corrosives

Corticosteroids (peptic ulcer disease, perforation)

Diquat

Erythromycin

Food poisoning

Hydrocarbons

Iron

Marine animals (jellyfish, Portuguese man-of-war)

Metallics

Methaqualone

Mushrooms

Organophosphates

Paraquat

Plants (many)

Reptile bites

Rodenticides

Salicylates

Soaps and detergents

Spider bites (brown recluse, black widow)

Tetracycline

Tricyclic antidepressants

Volatile oils

VI. Colic:

Arsenic

Botanical irritant toxins

Caffeine

Colchicine

Food poisoning

Laxatives

Lead

Mushrooms

Organophosphates

Thallium

Withdrawal states

VII. Rigidity:

Marine animals (jellyfish, Portuguese man-of-war)

Metallics (lead)

Spider bites (black widow)

VIII. Abdominal distention:

Corrosives

Anticholinergic syndrome

IX. Diarrhea:

Acrylonitrile

Alcohol and glycols

Aminocaproic acid

Amrinone

Antibiotics

Anticancer agents

Antiseptics

Arsenic

Aspartic acid

Beta blockers

Cantharidin (Spanish fly)

Cathartics

Clofibrate

Colchicine

Cyanide

Digitalis

Diquat

Ergots

Food poisoning
Gold
Hydrocarbons
Iron
Lithium salts
Metallics
Nicotine
Organophosphates
Paraquat

X. Constipation:
Amiloride
Antihistamines
Beta blockers
Cholestyramine
Colestipol
Diltiazem
Lead

XI. Ileus:
Anticholinergics
Antihistamines
Barium sulfate
Botulinus toxin
Cicutoxin
Clonidine
Infantile botulism

XII. Activation of peptic ulcer:
Adrenal corticosteroids
Indomethacin

XIII. Jaundice (hepatocellular, cholestatic):
Alcohols and glycols
Antimicrobials (e.g., sulfonamides,
  penicillin, chloramphenicol,
  erythromycin, isoniazid)
Anticancer agents (e.g.,
  methotrexate, asparagine)
Antiepileptics (e.g., carbamazepine, valproic acid)
Antiseptics (boric acid and
  derivatives, potassium
  permanganate)

XIV. Hepatitis:
A. High likelihood:
Acetaminophen
Alcohol
Carbon tetrachloride
B. Reported in literature:
Aminosalicyclic acid

Parasympathomimetics (involuntary
  defecation)
Plants (castor bean)
Quinidine
Saccharin
Thiazides
Vitamin C (≥ 10 gm)
Vitamin D
Volatile oils

Narcotic opioids
Nifedipine
Phenothiazines
Thallium
Tricyclic antidepressants
Verapamil

Lead
Mushrooms
Narcotics
Phenothiazines
Thallium
Tricyclic antidepressants

Phenylbutazone
Salicylates

Diquat
Gold compounds
Halogenated hydrocarbons
Iron compounds
Nitrogen compounds
Paraquat
Phenothiazines
Thiazide diuretics
Tricyclic antidepressants
Volatile and gaseous anesthetics
  (e.g., halothane, fluoroxene)

Methotrexate
6-Mercaptopurine

Amitriptyline

Aspirin
Chlorambucil
Chloramphenicol
Clindamycin
Phenytoin
Ethionamide
Flurazepam
Gold
Halothane
Imipramine
Indomethacin

Isoniazid
Methyldopa
Nitrofurantoin
Oxacillin
Quinidine
Rifampin
Sulfonamides
Sulfonylureas
Tetracycline
Valproate sodium

XV. Pancreatitis:

Acetaminophen

Methanol

XVI. Melena:

Alcohol and glycols
Anticoagulants (e.g., dicoumarol, heparin, warfarin)
Antiseptics (e.g., potassium permanganate)
Bleaches

Cathartics (e.g., sodium sulfate, aloe, senna, cascara)
Corrosives
Iron compounds
Metallics (e.g., lead)
Nonsteroidal anti-inflammatory drugs

XVII. Hematochezia:

Anticoagulants (rare)
Cathartics (e.g., sodium sulfate, aloe, senna, cascara)
Iron compounds

Nonsteroidal anti-inflammatory agents (rare)
Salicylates

XVIII. Occult blood in stools:

See XVI and XVII above.

XIX. Luminescent vomitus and flatus:

Phosphorus

XX. Involuntary or uncontrolled defecation:

Cholinesterase inhibitors

Cholinergic agents

XXI. Gastroenteritis:

Acetaminophen
Aluminum
Amanita mushrooms
Antihistamines
Benzene
Bromates
Carbamate
Carbamazepine
Carbon monoxide
Carbon tetrachloride
Chlorinated hydrocarbons
Ciguatera
Clonidine
Cobalt
Colchicine

Copper
Dapsone
Death camas plants
Detergents
Dinitrophenols
Diquat
Equinidine
Ergot
Ethambutol
Ethanol
Ethylene glycol
Food poisoning
Guanethidine
Herbicides
Hexachlorophenol

Hyacinth plants
Hypochlorite
Iodine
Iris plants
Isopropanol
Jetberry bush
LSD (vomiting)
Lead (vomiting)
Leander plants
Mescaline
Metaldehyde
Methanol
Methaqualone
Methyprylon
Methysergide
Mushrooms
Nalidixic acid
Naphtha
Naphthalene
Narcissus plants
Nicotine
Nitrites
Paradichlorobenzene
Paraldehyde
Paraquat
Perchloroethylene

Phenolphthalein
Phenols
Phenylbutazone
Pine oil
Pokeweed
Primidone
Reserpine
Rhododendron
Rifampin (hyperemesis)
Salicylates (vomiting)
Sassafras oil (vomiting)
Scromboid
Sedatives, nonbarbiturate
Selenium
Silver nitrate
Theophyllines (vomiting)
Thiazides
Thiocyanates
Tolbutamide
Toluene
Turpentine
Water hemlock
Wisteria
Withdrawal states
Yew
Zinc

XXII. Hemorrhagic gastroenteritis:

Ammonia
Arsenic
Borates
Cadmium
Caustics
Chromates
Cicutoxin (hematemesis)

Fluorides
Formaldehyde
Ipecac
Iron
Mercury
Oxalate
Phosphor
Thallium

XXIII. Hemorrhagic enterocolitis (including pseudomembranous enterocolitis):

Amanita phalloides
Ampicillin
Cephalosporins
Chloramphenicol

Lincosamide
Macrolide antibiotics
Tetracyclines

XXIV. Anorexia:

Acetaminophen
Amphetamines
Bismuth
Cadmium
Carbon monoxide
Cocaine
Digitalis

Ethanol
Fluoride (chronic)
Infantile botulism
Lead
Mercury
Narcotics
Theophyllines

XXV. Thirst:

Antimony	Fluorides
Arsenic	Lead
Atropine	Morphine
Chloral hydrate	Salicylates

BIBLIOGRAPHY

Johns Hopkins Hospital: *The Harriet Lane Manual* (Cole C, ed). Chicago, Year Book Medical Publishers, 1984, pp 230–233.

Matthews SJ, Schneiweiss F, Cersosimo RJ: *A Clinical Manual of Adverse Drug Reactions,* ed 1. East Norwalk, Conn, Appleton-Century-Crofts, 1986.

Done A: Signs, symptoms and sources. *Emerg Med* January 15, 1982, pp. 42–77.

44

Genitourinary System

Jordan M. Laub, M.D.

I. Acute renal failure (anuria, oliguria):
  A. Therapeutic drugs:

Acetaminophen	Deferoxamine
Acyclovir	Demeclocycline
Allopurinol	Dextran 40
Aminocaproic acid	Dicloxacillin
Aminoglycosides	Diltiazem
Amphotericin B	Diphenhydramine
Anything causing hemoglobinuria	Disodium edetate
or myoglobinuria	Disopyramide
Ascorbic acid	Edetic acid
Aspirin	Enalapril
Bacitracin	Enflurane
Barium sulfate	Erythromycin
Boric acid	Fenoprofen
Captopril	Furosemide
Carbamazepine	Gold salts
Cephalosporins	Halothane
Cholera vaccine	Hydralazine
Colchicine	Hydrochlorthiazide
Colistin mesilate	Ibuprofen
Contrast medium	Indomethacin
Clotrimazole	Interleukin-2
Cyclosporin	Iodine

Isoniazid
Mannitol
Mercuric acid
Methaqualone
Methotrexate
Methylphenidate
Metrizimide
Mitomycin
Nifedipine
Nonsteroidal anti-inflammatory
  drugs
Opioids
Paraldehyde
Penicillamine
Penicillins
Pennyroyal
Pentamidine

Phenacetin
Phencyclidine
Phenylbutazone
Polymyxins
Potassium bromide
Retinol (overdose)
Rifampicin
Streptokinase
Sulfamethizole
Sulfonamides
Theophylline (overdose)
Thiazide
Thiopental sodium
Tolmetin
Triamterene
Warfarin
Zomepirac

B. Biologic poisons:
  Mushrooms   Rattlesnake venom
C. Miscellaneous:
  Bismuth   Mercurials
  Bromates   Mercury
  Carbon monoxide   Methanol
  Carbon tetrachloride   Methyl halides
  Chlorates   Naphthalene
  Chlordane   Organic solvents
  Copper   Oxalates
  DDT   Oxalic acid
  Dimethyl sulfate   Paraquat
  Dinitrophenols   Petroleum distillates
  Ethylene glycol   Phosphorus
  Formaldehyde   Thallium
  Heavy metals   Trinitrotoluene
  Inorganic phosphorus   Turpentine
  Iron   Urethane
  Isopropanol
  Lead
II. Hematuria:
  Allopurinol   Indomethacin
  Ascorbic acid   Methanol
  Bacille Calmette-Guérin vaccine Mitomycin
  Busulfan   Naphthalene
  Chlorates   Nitrates
  Corrosives   Penicillamine
  Cyclophosphamide   Phenol
  Doxorubicin   Sulfonamides
  Gold salts   Turpentine
  Heavy metals

III. Hemoglobinuria:
   Drugs causing hemolysis (arsine, cephalosporins, snake venoms, primaquin, copper, nitrites, sulfonamides)
   Heroin

IV. Myoglobinuria:
   Phencyclidine
   Water hemlock

V. Polyuria:

Amphotericin B	Nifedipine
Halothane	Xanthines
Lithium salt	

VI. Urinary retention:

Atropine	Levodopa
Baclofen	Lindane
Disopyramide	Neuroleptics
Guanethidine	Opioids
Intraspinal anesthetics	Silver nitrate
Isoniazid	Tricyclic antidepressants

VII. Dysuria:

Anticholinergics	Arsenic
	Mushrooms

XIII. Sexual dysfunction: Table 44–1.

TABLE 44–1.

Sexual Dysfunction*

Drug	Loss or Deceased Libido	Impotence (Erectile Difficulty)	Ejaculatory Difficulty	Hormonal Alteration
Anticholinergics				
Atropine		+		
Benztropine		+		
Propantheline		+		
Scopolamine		+		
Trihexylphenidyl		+		
Antidepressants				
Amitriptyline	+	+	+	
Doxepin	+		+	
Isocarboxazid		+	+	
Phenelzine		+	+	
Tranylcypromine		+	+	
Antihistamines				
Diphenhydramine	+	+		
Hydroxyzine	+	+		
Antihypertensives				
Clonidine	+	+	+	
Guanethidine	+	+	+	
Hydralazine		?		

(Continued.)

TABLE 44–1 (cont.).

Drug	Loss or Deceased Libido	Impotence (Erectile Difficulty)	Ejaculatory Difficulty	Hormonal Alteration
Methyldopa	+	+	+	
Phenoxybenzamine			+	
Phentolamine			+	
Prazosin			+	
Propranolol	+	+		
Reserpine	+	+	+	
Spironolactone	+	+	+	+
Thiazides	+	+		
Antipsychotics				
Chlorpromazine	+	+		+
Haloperidol		+	+	+
Thioridazine	+	+	+	+
Narcotics				
Methadone	+	+		+
Morphine sulfate	+	+		+
Sedatives/hypnotics				
Barbiturates	±			?
Benzodiazepines	±		?	
Miscellaneous				
Alcohol	±	+		
Aminocaproic acid			+	
Baclofen	+	+		
Cimetidine	+	+		+
Clofibrate	+	+		
Disopyramide		+		
Levodopa			+	
Lithium carbonate		+		
Marijuana	±	+		?
Metoclopramide				+
Oral contraceptives	+			+

*From Aldridge SA: *Clin Pharm* 1982; 1:141–146. Used by permission.

IX. Involuntary/uncontrolled urination:
   Cholinergic syndrome (see Chapter 47, p. 218)
X. Menstrual irregularities:
   Bismuth   Lead
   Estrogens   Mercurials
   Heavy metals

BIBLIOGRAPHY

Aldridge SA: Drug-induced sexual dysfunction. *Clin Pharm* 1982; 1:141–146.
Arena JM, Drew RH: *Poisoning: Toxicology, Symptoms, Treatments.* Springfield, Ill, Charles C Thomas, 1986.

DeGowin EL, DeGowin RL: *Bedside Diagnostic Examination,* ed 4. New York, Macmillan Publishing Co, 1981.

Dukes MNG: *Meyler's Side Effects of Drugs,* ed 10. New York, Elsevier North-Holland, 1984.

Goldfrank LR, et al: *Goldfrank's Toxicologic Emergencies.* East Norwalk, Conn, Appleton-Century-Crofts, 1986.

Rosen P, et al: *Emergency Medicine.* St Louis, CV Mosby Co, 1983.

45

Neurological System

Gerald R. Schwartz, M.D.

I. Altered mental status:
  A. Depressed level of consciousness:

Acetaldehyde
Acetone
Alcohols
Aldehydes
Ammonia
Amphetamines
Aniline dyes
Anticholinergics
Antidepressants
Antihistamines
Aromatic hydrocarbon solvents
    (i.e., toluene, xylene, benzene)
Arsenic
Barbiturates
Benzene
Benzodiazepines
Boric acid
Bromides
Camphor
Carbamazepine
Carbon dioxide
Carbon disulfide

Carbon monoxide
Carbon tetrachloride
Cationic detergents
Chloral hydrate
Chloroquine
Chlorothiazides
Cholinergics
Chromium
Cimetidine
Clonidine
Copper salts
Cyanide
Digitalis
Dimethyl sulfoxide
Ergot
Disopyramide
Ethylene glycol
Ethylene oxide
Glutethimide
Glycols
Hydrocarbons
Hydrogen sulfide

Hypoglycemics
Ibuprofen
Iron
Isoniazid
Kerosene
Lead
Lithium
Meprobamate
Mercury
Methaqualone
Methyl halides
Methylene chloride
Methaprylon
Methysergide
Mushrooms
Narcotics
Nitrites
Organophosphates
Oxalate
Paraldehyde
Pentazocine

Perchloroethylene
Phencyclidine
Phenols
Phenothiazines
Phenylbutazone
Phenytoin
Phosphorus
Pokeweed
Quinine
Reserpine
Salicylates
Sedatives/hypnotics
Silver nitrate
Snake venom
Solvents
Thallium
Theophylline
Thiocyanates
Tricyclic antidepressants
Turpentine

B. Delayed-onset coma:
  Acetaminophen
  Botulinus toxin
  Carbon monoxide
  Glutethimide

  Methanol
  Methsuximide
  Mushrooms

C. Depressed reflexes:
  Antidepressants
  Barbiturates
  Benzodiazepines
  Chloral hydrate
  Clonidine
  Ethanol
  Ethchlorvynol

  Glutethimide
  Meprobamate
  Narcotics
  Phenothiazines
  Tricyclic antidepressants
  Valproic acid

D. Hyperreflexia:
  Amphetamines
  Carbamazepine
  Carbon monoxide
  Cocaine
  Cyanide
  Haloperidol
  Isoniazid
  Methaqualone

  Metoprolol
  Phencyclidine
  Phenothiazines
  Phenytoin
  Propoxyphene
  Propranolol
  Strychnine
  Tricyclic antidepressants

E. Coma with pulmonary edema:
  Ethchlorvynol
  Glutethimide
  Narcotics

  Organophosphates
  Propoxyphene
  Salicylates

F. Coma with cardiac dysrhythmias:

Amphetamines
Arsenic
Caffeine
Carbamazepine
Chloral hydrate
Clonidine
Cocaine
Digoxin

Lead
Lithium
Phencyclidine
Phenothiazines
Propranolol
Theophylline
Tricyclic antidepressants

G. Delirium:

Alcohol
Amphetamines
Aniline derivatives
Anticholinergics
Antihistamines
Arsenic
Barbiturates
Benzene
Camphor
Cocaine
DDT
Digitalis
Fluorides
Hallucinogens

Hydrocarbons
Lead
Marijuana
Mercury
Narcotics
Nerve gases
Phenothiazines
Phenytoin
Salicylates
Sedatives/hypnotics
Sympathomimetics
Thallium
Tricyclic antidepressants

II. Headache:

Acetone
Alcohols
Alpha agonists
Amyl nitrite
Anilines
Anticholinergics
Antimony
Barbiturates
Benzene
Bromide (chronic)
Cadmium
Caffeine
Carbon disulfide
Carbon monoxide
Carbon tetrachloride
Chlorinated hydrocarbons
Cocaine
Copper
Cyanide
Digitalis
Ergotamine
Hydrogen sulfide

Hydralazine
Indomethacin
Lead
Methemoglobinemia
Methyl bromide
Monoamine oxidase inhibitors
Monosodium glutamate
Nalidixic acid
Nicotine
Nitrates/nitrites
Nitrofurans
Organophosphates
Paraldehyde
Quinidine
Selenium
Steroids
Tellurium
Tetracycline
Theophyllines
Trinitrotoluene
Vitamin A
Withdrawal from ergotamine

III. Seizures:

Ammonia
Amphetamines
Antihistamines
Arsenic
Atropine
Barium
Belladonna
Benzodiazepines
Boric acid
Caffeine
Camphor
Carbon disulfide
Carbon monoxide
Carbon tetrachloride
Chlorinated hydrocarbon
Chloroquine
Cicutoxin
Clonidine
Cocaine
Copper salts
Cyanide
Digitalis
Diquat
Ergot
Ethanol
Ethychlorvynol
Fluoride
Glutethimide
Heavy metals
Herbicides
Hydrocarbons
Hypoglycemics
Insecticides
Isoniazid
Lead

Lithium
Local anesthetics
LSD
Manganese
Meperidine
Meprobamate
Mercury
Methotrexate
Methyl chloride
Methylbromide
Methylphenidate
Monomethylhydrazine
Mushrooms
Nickel
Nicotine
Organophosphates
Phencyclidine
Phenmetrazine
Phenol
Phenothiazines
Phenytoin
Pokeweed
Propoxyphene
Rhododendron plants
Salicylates
Scorpion sting
Shellfish
Snake bite
Strychnine
Tetanus toxin
Thallium
Theophylline
Thiocyanates
Tricyclic antidepressants
Withdrawal states

IV. Eye findings: See Chapter 40, p. 179.
V. Neurotoxicologic states:
   A. Ataxia:

Alcohols
Aminoglycoside antibiotics
Antihistamines
Arsenic
Barbiturates
Belladonna alkaloids
Benzene
Benzodiazepines

Bromides
Carbamate herbicides
Carbamazepine
Carbon monoxide
Chlorinated hydrocarbons
Cimetidine
Cocaine
Dextromethorphan

Dinitrobenzene
Ethanol
Glutethimide
Hallucinogens
Hemlock
Hexachlorobenzene
Hypoglycemics
Isoniazid
Lead
Lithium
Manganese
Mercury
Methaqualone
Methyl halides
Methyprylon
Narcotics

Nicotine
Organophosphates
Phenothiazines
Phenylbutazone
Phenytoin
Polymyxin
Primidone
Propoxyphene
Puffer fish
Rhododendron plants
Shellfish
Spectinomycin
Thallium
Tricyclic antidepressants
Trimethadione
Volatile hydrocarbons

B. Choreoathetoid movements with myoclonus:

Amphetamines
Anticholinergics
Cadmium
Carbamazepine
Chlorinated chlorophenoxy
    herbicides
Hydrocarbons
Hypoglycemics

Isoniazid
Levodopa
Lithium
Metaldehyde
Methaqualone
Nicotine
Phencyclidine
Phenytoin
Strychnine

C. Muscle atrophy:

Arsenic
Carbon monoxide
Lead

Manganese
Mercury (chronic)
Tricresyl phosphate

D. Opisthotonos:

Caffeine
Carbamazepine
Carbon monoxide
Cocaine
Codeine
Cyanide (trismus)
Haloperidol
Hypocalcemia (secondary to
    methanol, ethylene glycol,
    mithramycin)
Hypoglycemics
Local anesthetics (newborn)
Manganese
Mercury (chronic)

Metaldehyde
Metoclopramide
Mushrooms
Nicotine
Phencyclidine
Phenol
Phenothiazines
Phenytoin
Scopolamine
Strychnine
Tetanus toxin
Tricyclic antidepressants
Water hemlock

E. Fasciculations:

Amphetamines
Atropine

Barium salts
Black widow spider bite

Camphor
Cholinergics
Cocaine
Ergot
Ethanol
Fluorides
Heavy metals
Herbicides
Hypoglycemics
Lithium
Manganese
Mercury
Methanol

Methaqualone
Mushrooms
Nicotine
Organophosphates
Phencyclidine
Phenol
Scorpion venom
Shellfish poisoning
Strychnine
Thallium
Thiocyanates
Xanthines

VI. Peripheral neuropathy:

Arsenic (chronic)
Benzene
Carbon monoxide
Chloramphenicol
Dinitrophenols
Ethambutol
Ethanol
Gold salts
Herbicides
Hexane

Hydrogen sulfide
Isoniazid
Lead
Mercury
Methanol
Methaqualone
Narcotics
Nicotine
Paralytic shellfish
Thallium

VII. Muscle spasms:

Aconitine
Antidepressants
Atropine
Barium
Cadmium
Camphor
Chromates
Dinitrophenols
Emetine
Ethylene glycol
Fluoride
Herbicides
Hydrogen sulfide

Ipecac
Manganese
Metaldehyde
Monkshood
Phencyclidine
Phenothiazines
Saccharin
Scorpion sting
Spider bite
Strychnine
Tricyclic antidepressants
Withdrawal states

VIII. Muscular weakness or paralysis:

Alcoholism
Aminoglycosides
Arsenic
Barbiturates
Botulism
Bromide
Carbamate herbicides
Carbon disulfide
Carbon dioxide

Carbon monoxide
Chlordane
Chlorinated hydrocarbons
Cholinergics
Ciguatera
Clonidine
Cresyl phosphate
Cyanide
DDT

Emetine
Ethylene glycol
Fluoride
Ipecac
Lead
LSD
Manganese
Mercury
Methanol
Methaqualone
Methyl bromide
Nalidixic acid
Narcotics
Nicotine
Nitrofurantoin
Organic mercurials

Organophosphates
Pine oil
Poison hemlock
Polymyxin
Propranolol
Puffer fish
Quinine
Rhododendron plants
Selenium
Shellfish
Spider bite
Tetracyclines
Thallium
Thiocyanates
Vincristine

IX. Muscle pain, myalgias:

Antimony
Ciguatera
Emetine
Ipecac

Methanol
Monosodium glutamate
Thallium
Thiazides

X. Muscle cramps:

Black widow spider bite

Lead
Thiazide diuretics

XI. Tremors:

Amphetamines
Arsenic
Bromide (chronic)
Caffeine
Carbamazepine
Carbon disulfide
Carbon monoxide
Chlorinated hydrocarbons
Cicutoxin
Ciguatera
Cocaine
DDT
Digitalis
Ephedrine
Ethanol
Fluoride
Glutethimide
Hydrocarbons
Hypoglycemic agents
Lead
Lithium
Local anesthetics

LSD
Manganese
Mercury (chronic)
Methyl bromide
Methylene chloride
Parathion
Phenothiazines
Phenytoin
Phosphorus
Propoxyphene
Puffer fish
Reserpine
Sedatives/hypnotics
Selenium
Sympathomimetics
Thallium
Theophylline
Thiocyanates
Thyroid medication
Tin
Tricyclic antidepressants
Withdrawal states

XII. Deafness: See Chapter 40, p. 182.

XIII. Anesthesia:

Arsenic	Ethanol
Barbiturates	Mercury
Benzene	Methanol
Bromides	Nitrofurantoin
Carbon monoxide	Perchloroethylene
Carbon disulfide	Shellfish
Cocaine	Vincristine

XIV. Paresthesia:

Alcohols	Mercury (alkyl)
Arsenic	Methanol
Barbiturates	Methyl bromide
Benzene	Methyl chloride
Botulinus toxin	Methysergide
Bromides	Monosodium glutamate
Camphor	Nicotine
Carbon monoxide	Organophosphates
Carbon disulfide	Polymyxins
Chlorinated hydrocarbons	Propranolol
Ciguatera	Puffer fish
Cocaine	Quinine
Cresyl phosphate	Scorpion sting
Cyanide	Stringray bites
DDT	Strychnine
Dimercaprol	Thallium
Fluoride	Vancomycin
Lead	Vincristine
Lidocaine	

XV. Reversed temperature sensation:

Ciguatera	Shellfish

XVI. Dysphagia:

Botulinus toxin	Phenols
Caustics	Phenothiazines
Cholinergics	Scromboid
Fluoride	Shellfish
Hemlock	Strychnine
Mercury	Vacor

BIBLIOGRAPHY

Done A: Signs, symptoms and sources. *Emerg Med* January 15, 1982, pp 42–77.

Drugs for epilepsy. *Med Lett Drugs Ther* 1986; 28:91–94.

Fernandez RJ, Samuels MA: Epilepsy, in Samuels MA (ed): *Manual of Neurologic Therapeutics.* Boston, Little, Brown & Co, pp 75–117.

Goldfrank LR, et al: *Goldfrank's Toxicologic Emergencies,* ed 3. Norwalk, Conn, Appleton-Century-Crofts, 1986.

Johns Hopkins Hospital, *The Harriet Lane Handbook* (Cole C, ed). Chicago, Year Book Medical Publishers, 1984, pp 230–233.

46

Behavior

M. Douglas Baker, M.D.
Edward S. Wang, M.D.

I. Aggression/violence:
   Alcohol
   Phencyclidine
II. Agitation:
   Amphetamine
   Methaqualone
   Narcotics
   Phencyclidine
   Petroleum distillates
   Theophylline
III. Anxiety/panic:
   Barbiturates
   Hallucinogens
   Indolealkylamines (e.g., psilocybin)
   Morning glory seeds
   Phenylethylamines (e.g., mescaline)
   Sedatives/hypnotics
   Stimulants
IV. Delirium:
   See Chapter 44, p. 206.
V. Depression/worthlessness:
   Alcohol

Antihypertensives (e.g., reserpine, clonidine, hydralazine, methyldopa, propranolol, timolol)
Anti-inflammatory agents
Benzodiazepines
Cimetidine
Corticosteroids
Disopyramide
Disulfiram
Hallucinogens
Hormones (e.g., estrogen, progesterone)
Indolealkylamines (e.g., psilocybin)
Levodopa
Morning glory seeds
Phenylephrine
Phenylethylamines (e.g., mescaline)

VI. Disorientation:
Alcohol
Anticholinergics
Antihistamines
Belladonna alkaloids
Narcotics
Phenothiazines
Tricyclic antidepressants

VII. Euphoria:
Alcohol
Aromatic hydrocarbon solvents
Narcotics
Petroleum distillates (e.g., kerosene)

VIII. Hallucinations:
Alcohol
Amphetamines
Anticholinergics
Antihistamines
Aromatic hydrocarbon solvents
Belladonna alkaloids
Cocaine
Hashish
Hallucinogens
Indolealkylamines (e.g., psilocybin)
Isoniazid
Marijuana
Mephentermine (Wyamine)
Methamphetamine
Morning glory seeds
Narcotics
Phencyclidine
Phenmetrazine (Preludin)
Phenylethylamines (e.g., mescaline)

Salicylates
Tetrahydrocannabinols
Theophylline
Tricyclic antidepressants
IX. Hallucinations (lilliputian):
Anticholinergics
Antihistamines
Belladonna alkaloids
Cocaine
Tricyclic antidepressants
X. Homicidal/suicidal intent:
Amphetamines
LSD
Mephentermine (Wyamine)
Metamphetamines
Phencyclidine
Phenmetrazine (Preludin)
XI. Hyperalertness/stimulation:
Amphetamines
Hallucinogens
Indolealkylamines (e.g., psilocybin)
Mephentermine (Wyamine)
Metamphetamines
Morning glory seeds
Phenmetrazine (Preludin)
Phenylethylamines (e.g., mescaline)
Sympathomimetics
Theophylline
XII. Hyperexcitability:
Anticholinergics
Antihistamines
Belladonna alkaloids
Organochlorine insecticides
Tricyclic antidepressants
XIII. Insomnia:
Amphetamines
Methamphetamine
Mercury
Theophylline
XIV. Irritability:
Amphetamines
Anticholinergics
Antihistamines
Sympathomimetics
Lead
Mercury
Methamphetamine

Salicylates
Theophylline
Thyroid hormones
Vitamins A, D
XV. Lethargy/sedation:
Alcohol
Barbiturates
Hashish
Iron
Marijuana
Phenothiazines
Salicylates
Sedatives/hypnotics
Tetrahydrocannabinols
Tricyclic antidepressants
Vitamin A
XVI. Mania:
Amphetamines
Anticholinergics
Antihistamines
Belladonna alkaloids
Cocaine
Salicylates
Tricyclic antidepressants
XVII. Omnipotence:
Hallucinogens
Indolealkylamines (e.g., psilocybin)
Morning glory seeds
Phenylethylamines (e.g., mescaline)
XVIII. Paranoia:
Amphetamines
Anticholinergics
Antihistamines
Belladonna alkaloids
Cocaine
Mephentermine (Wyamine)
Methamphetamine
Phenmetrazine (Preludin)
Tricyclic antidepressants
XIX. Psychosis:
Amphetamines
Anticholinergics
Antihistamines
Barbiturates
LSD
Methamphetamine
Phenothiazines

BIBLIOGRAPHY

Goldfrank LR, Kirstein RH: Amphetamines, in Goldfrank LR, Flomenbaum NE, Weissman RS, et al (eds): *Goldfrank's Toxicologic Emergencies.* Norwalk, Conn, Appleton-Century-Crofts, 1986, pp 383–390.

Goldfrank LR, Kulberg AG: Vital signs and toxic syndromes, in Goldfrank LR, Flomenbaum NE, Weissman RS, et al (eds): *Goldfrank's Toxicologic Emergencies,* Norwalk, Conn, Appleton-Century-Crofts, 1986, pp 60–63.

Henretig FM: Poisoning in children, in Hanson W (ed): *Toxic Emergencies.* New York, Churchill Livingstone, 1974, pp 20–21.

Kaplan HI, Sadock BJ: *Comprehensive Textbook of Psychiatry.* Baltimore, Williams & Wilkins Co, pp 1315–1329.

Mofenson HC, Greensher J: The unknown poison. *Pediatrics* 1974; 54:336–342.

47

Toxicologic Syndromes (Toxindromes)

Thomas P. Gross, M.D.

I. Anticholinergic syndrome:
   A. Causes:
   > *Amanita muscaria*
   > Antihistamines
   > Antiparkinson agents
   > Atropine
   > Henbane
   > Jimsonweed
   > Mydriatics (e.g., homatropine, tropicamide)
   > Nightshade
   > Phenothiazines
   > Scopolamine
   > Tricyclic antidepressants

   B. Signs and symptoms:
   1. Mnemonic:
      Mad as a hatter;
      Dry as a bone;
      Hot as a hare;
      Blind as a bat;
      Red as a beet.
   2. Manifestations:
      a. General:
         (1) Dry skin and mucous membranes.
         (2) Hoarseness.
         (3) Thirst.

217

(4) Dysphagia.
(5) Visual blurring.
(6) Fixed dilated pupils.
(7) Hyperthermia.
(8) Flushed skin.
b. Neurologic:
(1) Altered mental status (depressed or excited).
(2) Ataxia, hyperreflexia.
(3) Psychosis (manic or schizophreniform).
(4) Hallucinations (visual lilliputian, tactile).
e. Cardiovascular:
(1) Tachycardia.
(2) Hypertension.
(3) Cardiovascular collapse.
d. Pulmonary:
(1) Respiratory failure.
e. Gastrointestinal:
(1) Abdominal distention.
(2) Decreased bowel sounds.
f. Genitourinary:
(1) Urinary urgency and retention.
3. Laboratory findings:
a. ECG: Supraventricular arrhythmia, QRS and QT prolongation.
II. Cholinergic syndrome:
A. Causes:

Acetylcholine
Anticholinesterases
Amanita mushrooms
Betel nut
Bethanechol

Carbamates
Organophosphates (e.g., parathion, malathion)
Pilocarpine

B. Signs and symptoms:
1. Mnemonic: "sludge":
*S*alivation
*L*acrimation
*U*rination
*D*efecation
*G*astrointestinal symptoms, cramps
*E*mesis
2. Manifestations
a. Muscarinic effects:
(1) General: sweating.
(2) Eye findings: constricted pupils, lacrimination, blurred vision.
(3) Pulmonary: wheezing, rales, bronchorrhea.
(4) Gastrointestinal: excessive salivation, cramps, nausea, vomiting, diarrhea, tenesmus.
(5) Cardiovascular: bradycardia, hypotension.
(6) Genitourinary: urinary incontinence.

    b. Nicotinic effects:
      (1) Muscle: fasciculations, cramps, weakness, twitching, paralysis, respiratory insufficiency or arrest, cyanosis.
      (2) Sympathetic ganglia: tachycardia, hypertension.
      (3) CNS effects: anxiety, restlessness, confusion, ataxia, coma, seizures, insomnia, hyporeflexia, Cheyne-Stokes respirations

III. Extrapyramidal syndrome:
  A. Causes:

Chlorpromazine	Prochlorperazine
Droperidol	Thioridazine
Haloperidol	Thiothixene
Perphenazine	Trifluoperazine

  B. Signs and symptoms:
    1. Extrapyramidal movements (parkinsonism): rigidity, tremors, torticollis, oculogyric crisis, trismus, shrieking, dysphonia, dysphagia, tremor, opisthotonos, laryngospasm.

IV. Metal fume fever·
  A. Causes:
    1. Fumes of oxides from:

Brass	Mercury
Cadmium	Nickel
Copper	Titanium
Iron	Tungsten
Magnesium	Zinc

  B. Signs and symptoms:
    1. Fever, chills, nausea, vomiting, myalgia, headache, fatigue, weakness, dyspnea, leukocytosis.

V. Opiate/narcotic syndrome:
  A. Causes:
    1. All synthetic and natural opiates (see Chapter 67).
  B. Signs and symptoms:
    1. CNS depression, hypoventilation, hypotension, pinpoint pupils (except meperidine, codeine, methadone, pentazocine).
    2. Response to naloxone (may require 10–20 mg for some drugs).
    3. May have needle track marks if intravenous drug abuser.

VI. Sympathomimetic syndrome:
  A. Causes:

Aminophylline	Epinephrine
Amphetamines	Methylphenidate (Ritalin)
Caffeine	Phencyclidine
Cocaine	Phenmetrazine
Dopamine	Phentermine
Ephedrine	

  B. Signs and symptoms:
    1. CNS:
      a. Excitation, seizures, anxiety, hyperactivity, tremors, increased deep tendon reflexes, emotional lability.

　　b. Toxic psychosis:
　　　　(1) Paranoia and delusions with a notable restlessness, hyperactivity, irritability, hostility.
　　　　(2) Visual and auditory hallucinations are frequent and often of a threatening nature.
　　　　(3) NOTE: **Disorientation and clouding of memory are not usual.**
　2. Cardiovascular: hypertension, tachycardia, arrhythmia.
　3. Gastrointestinal: nausea, vomiting, hyperactive bowel sounds, abdominal pain.
　4. General: Sweating, hyperthermia, track marks (clue), dilated pupils (reactive), dry mouth.

VII. Withdrawal syndrome:
　A. Caused by withdrawal from:

Alcohol	Meprobamate
Barbiturates	Methaqualone
Benzodiazepines	Methyprylon
Chloral hydrate	Narcotics
Cocaine	Opioids
Ethchlorvynol	Paraldehyde
Glutethimide	

　B. Signs and symptoms:
　　1. Piloerection (probably most reliable sign).
　　2. Neurologic: mydriasis, insomnia, muscle cramps, hallucinosis, restlessness, yawning.
　　3. Other: diarrhea, lacrimation, fever, hypertension, tachycardia.

VIII. Hemoglobinopathies:
　A. Classification:
　　1. Carboxyhemoglobin (from carbon monoxide).
　　2. Methemoglobin (e.g., from nitrates, nitrites).
　　3. Sulfhemoglobin (e.g., from hydrogen sulfide).
　B. Signs and symptoms:
　　1. Most findings are nonspecific and related to tissue hypoxia.
　　2. CNS: headache, disorientation, coma.
　　3. Cardiovascular: arrhythmias, congestive heart failure, shock, hypotension.
　　4. Respiratory: cyanosis, dyspnea.
　　5. Other: Cutaneous bullae, gastroenteritis, epidemic occurrence.

BIBLIOGRAPHY

Tintinalli JE, Rothstein RJ, Krome RL: *Emergency Medicine: A Comprehensive Study Guide.* New York, McGraw-Hill Book Co, 1985, pp 262–263.

48

Laboratory Findings

J. Ward Donovan, M.D.

I. Blood serum:
  A. Acid-base disturbances:
  To determine type of disturbance and differential diagnosis, measure arterial blood gas levels, serum osmolality, blood urea nitrogen, glucose, electrolytes, and calculate anion gap. Determine acid-base disturbance. For those unfamiliar with basic calculations, the acid-base map (Fig 48-1) may be of value. Plot Pco_2 and H^+ ion concentration. If values fall within one of the labeled confidence bands a pure disturbance exists. If outside the bands a mixed disturbance is present.

  The acid-base map has limited utility in mixed acid-base problems because it will fail to detect important disturbances. This is particularly the case with increased anion gap metabolic acidosis with accompanying metabolic alkalosis (as can easily occur with all of the substances that are known to produce increased anion gap metabolic acidosis). The metabolic alkalosis may cancel the effect of the metabolic acidosis, leaving normal or only slightly altered pH. The only clue that a serious problem exists is from the increased anion gap, which the map does not account for. Further, the map will not distinguish between increased anion gap–type metabolic acidosis and normal anion gap–type (hyperchloremic), metabolic acidosis and is incapable of determining triple acid-base disturbances. Therefore it is best to be familiar with the basic acid-base calculations to determine disturbances rather than to rely on the map.

  1. Metabolic acidosis with increased anion gap:
    a. Definition: accumulation of organic acids and unmeasured anions; calculated as $AG = Na - (Cl + HCO_3)$. Normal: 14 ± 2 mEq/L.

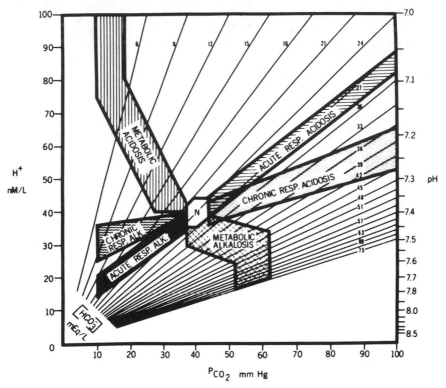

FIG 48–1.
Acid-base map. (From Goldberg M, et al: Computer-based instruction and diagnosis of acid-base disorders. *JAMA* 1973; 223:269–275. Used with permission.)

  b. Pathophysiologic classification:
      (1) Ketoacidosis: diabetic, alcoholic, starvation.
      (2) Lactic acidosis: Tissue hypoxia, shock (insufficient tissue perfusion), liver failure, fasting obese.
          a Drugs: alcohol, isoniazid, phenphormin, cyanide, carbon monoxide, formaldehyde, iron, methemeglobinemia.
      (3) Renal failure: (see Chapter 44, p. 199 for list of poisons).
      (4) Ingestants:
          Salicylates
          Methanol (metabolized to formate)
          Ethylene glycol (metabolized to oxalate)
          Paraldehyde (metabolized to acetate)
          Toluene (mechanism unknown)
  c. Mnemonic: Mud Piles:
      M (methanol)
      U (uremia)
      D (diabetic and alcoholic or starvation ketoacidosis)

P (paraldehyde, phenformin)
I (iron, isoniazid)
L (lactic acidosis; see above)
E (ethylene glycol)
S (salicylates)
d. Increased anion gap without acidosis:
a. Increased anion load:
Carbenicillin some types of hyperalimentation.
2. Normal anion gap metabolic acidosis (hyperchloremic acidosis):
a. Renal tubular acidosis:

Cadmium	Lead
Carbonic anhydrase inhibitors	Lithium
(e.g., acetazolamide)	Mercury
Copper	Tetracycline
	Toluene

b. Gastrointestinal:
Diarrhea (see Chapter 43, p. 194, for list of poisons that cause diarrhea).
Ileus
Pancreatic fistula
Ureterosigmoidostomy
Vomiting
c. Ingestants:
Ammonium chloride
Arginine chloride
Calcium chloride
Hydrogen chloride
Lysine chloride
Magnesium chloride
Some types of hyperalimentation
d. Rapid restoration of extracellular fluid volume contraction.
e. Ketone dump.
3. Classification of narrow anion gap:
a. Increased unmeasured cations:
(1) Calcium, lithium, magnesium, potassium, TRIS buffer.
(2) Increased protein (e.g., multiple myeloma).
b. Decreased unmeasured anions: hypoalbuminemia.
c. Laboratory error: hyponatremia, hyperchloremia.
d. Narrow anion gap disturbances are not in and of themselves related to acidosis.
4. Alcohol and acidosis:
Ethanol is frequently mentioned in texts as a cause of acidosis. In and of itself ethyl alcohol does not cause metabolic acidosis. Alcoholic ketoacidosis occurs in alcoholics usually 24–48 hours after a drinking binge. In the face of impaired liver function ethyl alcohol can lead to acidosis via lactic acidosis. However, **acidosis should never simply be attributed to ethanol intoxication!** An important diagnosis with potentially fatal outcome may be missed.

5. Metabolic alkalosis:
   a. Volume contraction (with chloride depletion).
      (1) Vomiting.
      (2) Diuretics: includes all diuretics except carbonic anhydrase inhibitors. Usually associated with K^+ deficit (except K^+-sparing diuretics).
   b. Adrenal (volume status usually increased):
      (1) Steroid excess.
      (2) Licorice.
   c. Alkali administration:
      (1) HCO_3.
      (2) Milk alkali syndrome.
      (3) Rapid volume administration (dilutes fixed amount of base).
   d. Drugs/toxins:

Carbenicillin	Penicillin
Citrate	Steroids
Excess antacids	

6. Respiratory acidosis:
   a. Cause: Anything that decreases ventilation either directly or by obstruction, aspiration, pulmonary edema, or bronchospasm (see Chapter 41, p. 188, for poisons that cause hypoventilation).
7. Respiratory alkalosis:
   a. Drugs/toxins:

Amphetamines	**Phencyclidine**
Cocaine	**Salicylates**
Marijuana	**Sympathomimetics**

B. Osmolality changes:
   1. Osmolal gap:
      a. Definition: Difference between measured and calculated osmolality. Calculated osmolality is:

$$(2 \text{ Na mEq/L } + \frac{\text{Glucose} > 100}{18} + \frac{\text{BUN (mq/dl)}}{2.8}$$

   b. Pathophysiology: Low molecular weight substances present in high levels in blood.
   c. Normal: <10 mOsm/kg H_2O.
   d. Cause:
      Acetone
      Ethanol
      Ethyl ether
      Ethylene/propylene glycol
      Isopropyl alcohol
      Mannitol
      Methanol
      Sorbitol
      Trichloroethane
      Some salts

C. Electrolyte disorders:
   1. Hyperkalemia:
      a. Drugs/toxins:

Beta blockers	Nonsteroidal anti-inflammatory
Captopril	agents
Digitalis	Penicillin
Fluoride	Potassium supplements
Glycosides	Potassium-sparing diuretics
Heparin	Rhabdomyolysis
Isoniazid	Salt substitutes
Nifedipine	Succinylcholine

      b. Metabolic causes:
         (1) Acidemia.
         (2) Tissue catabolism (surgery, crush injury, rhabdomyolysis, hemolysis).
         (3) Renal failure (see Chapter 44).
         (4) Renal tubular acidosis type IV.
         (5) Adrenal insufficiency.
      c. False positive laboratory results:
         (1) Hemolized sample.
         (2) Thrombocytosis.
         (3) Prolonged tourniquet placement.
   2. Hypokalemia:
      a. Drugs/toxins:

Amphotericin	Lithium
Barium	Polymyxin
Beta adrenergic agents	Potassium salt substitutes
Cadmium	Quinine
Caffeine	Salicylates
Carbenicillin	Steroids
Cesium	Sympathomimetic agents
Chloroquine	Theophylline
Diuretics	Toluene
Laxatives	

      b. Other causes:
         (1) Osmotic diuresis.
         (2) Renal (acute renal failure, renal tubular acidosis, nephrocalcinosis, post-obstruction).
         (3) Endocrine (hyperaldosterone, Cushing's syndrome).
         (4) Gastrointestinal (suction, vomiting, fistula, diarrhea).
         (5) Alkalemia (related to shift of K^+ from extracellular to intracellular space; see above).
         (6) Burns.
   3. Hypernatremia:
      a. Drugs/toxins:
         Excess salt
         Diaphoresis (e.g., salicylates, organophosphates)
         Diarrhea (e.g., organophosphates, antibiotics)

$NaHCO_3$ (excessive administration)
Lithium (measured as Na^+)
Some types of hyperalimentation
Diuretics
Steroids
Osmotic diuresis (e.g., glucose, mannitol, dye)
   b. Other causes:
      a. Nephropathies.
      b. Acute tubular necrosis (diuretic phase).
      c. Post-obstructive uropathy.
      d. Diabetes insipidus (true and nephrogenic).
4. Hyponatremia:
   a. Causes:
      (1) Factitious: hyperlipidemia, hyperproteinemia.
      (2) Osmotic: glucose, mannitol.
   b. Volume depletion present:
      (1) Gastrointestinal:
         a Vomiting, diarrhea (see Chapter 43, p. 194).
      (2) Renal:
         a Acute renal failure (diuretic phase; see Chapter 44, p. 00).
         b Chronic renal failure (salt wasting).
         c Diuretics.
         d Analgesic nephropathy.
         e Obstruction.
      (3) Adrenal insufficiency.
      (4) Skin: burns, cystic fibrosis.
   c. Volume overload present:
      (1) Nephrosis.
      (2) Liver failure.
      (3) Congestive heart failure.
   d. Normal volume status:
      (1) Drugs acting via anti-diuretic hormone (ADH)–related mechanisms:

ADH-receptor stimulus	Cyclophosphamide
(e.g., narcotics, tricyclic	Oxytocin
antidepressants, pain)	Phosphodiesterase inhibitors
Beta receptor stimulus	(e.g., aminophylline)
Chlorpropramide,	Tegretol
Clofibrate	Tolbutamine
	Vincristine

      (2) Syndrome of inappropriate secretion of antidiuretic hormone (SIADH).
      (3) Drugs that cause hyponatremia independent of ADH-related mechanism:
         Cortisol
         Diuretics
         Alcohol

        Nicotine
        Barbiturates
        Salicylates
    (4) Polydipsia (psychogenic).
5. Hypocalcemia:
    a. Drugs/toxins:

Barium	Manganese
Ethylene glycol	Phenytoin (chronic)
Fluoride	Phosphate
Oxalate	Phosphorus
Massive transfusions (citrate toxicity)	

6. Hypercalcemia:
    a. Causes:
        Hypervitaminosis A
        Hypervitaminosis D
        Milk-alkali syndrome
        Diuretic usage (thiazides, chlorthalidone)
        Antacids
        Calcium carbonate
D. Glucose alterations:
  1. Hyperglycemia:
    a. Drugs:

Acetone	Nicotine
Birth control pills	Organophosphates
Caffeine	Phenothiazines
Corticosteroids	Phenytoin
Diazoxide	Salicylates
Dopamine	Sympathomimetics
Epinephrine	Theophylline
Ethacrynic acid	Thiazides
Glucagon	Thyroid replacement
Growth hormone	Vacor
Haloperidol	Verapamil
Isoniazid	

  2. Hypoglycemia:
    a. Drugs:

Acetaminophen	Iron (children)
Acetone	Isoniazid
Amatoxin (*Amanita*) mushrooms	Leucine
Marijuana	Monoamine oxidase inhibitors
Chlorpromazine	Methanol
Clonidine	Methysergide
Ethanol	Oral hypoglycemics
Guanethidine	Phentolamine
Haloperidol	Propranolol
Insulin	Propoxyphene
	Reserpine

        Salicylates   Theophylline
        Tetracyclines   Thioglycolate
                                  Verapamil

    b. Factitious hypoglycemia:
        Acetylsalicylic acid
        Monoamine oxidase inhibitors
        Phenobarbital
        Narcotics
    c. Other (possibly drug related):
        (1) Liver failure (see Chapter 43).
E. Hyperamylasemia:
    Acetaminophen
    Acetophenetidin
    Vacor
F. Hematologic disorders:
    1. Anemia:
        a. Aplastic anemia:
            Allopurinol   Methyldopa
            Ampicillin   NSAIDs
            Arsenicals   Phenytoin
            Benzene   Primidone
            Chloramphenicol   Prochlorperazine
            Chlordane   Quinidine
            DDT   Salicylates
            Ethosuximide   Sulfadiazine
            Gold   Sulfonamides
            Isoniazid   Trimethadione
                                  Trinitrotoluene

        b. Megaloblasic anemia:
            Arsenic   Ethanol
            Barbiturates   Glutethimide
            Benzene   Neomycin
            Colchicine   Oral contraceptives
            Phenytoin   Primidone
        c. Hemolytic anemia:
            Cephalosporins   Methyldopa
            Chlorpromazine   Phenacetin
            Envenomation   Probenecid
            Fava bean   Quinidine
            Lead (chronic)   Quinine
                                  Salicylates
                                  Sulfonamides

    2. Agranulocytosis:
        Benzene   Chlorpromazine
        Carbamazepine   Hydantoins
        Carbamazole   Indomethacin
        Chloramphenicol   Phenylbutazone

Procainamide
Sulfonamide

3. Thrombocytopenia:
    Acetaminophen
    Acetylsalicylic acid
    Chloramphenicol
    Chlorpropamide
    Envenomation

Thioridazine
Tricyclic antidepressants

Furosemide
Gold
Methyldopa
Quinidine
Quinine
Sulfonomides

4. Leukocytosis:
    Any severe poisoning

5. Leukopenia:
    Antimony
    Arsenic
    Benzene
    Cancer chemotherapeutics
    Carbamazepine
    Carbon monoxide
    Chloramphenicol

Hydantoins
Isoniazid
Manganese
Methicillin
Methotrexate
Phenol

6. Polycythemia:
    Cobalt (chronic)

Manganese

G. Methemoglobinemia:
    Acetanilid
    Acetophenetidin
    Amyl nitrite
    Aniline dyes
    Benzocaine
    Bismuth subnitrate
    Bitter almond oil
    Chlorates
    Cobalt preparations
    Crayons, wax (e.g., red or
        orange)
    Dapsone
    Diesel fuel
    Dinitrobenzenes
    Lidocaine
    Menthol

Nitrates
Nitrobenzene
Nitrofurans
Nitroglycerin
Phenacetin
Phenazopyridine
Phenols
Phenytoin
Pyridine
Quinones
Shoe dye or polish
Sodium nitrite
Spinach
Sulfonamides
Sulfones
Toluidine
Trinitrotoluene (TNT)

H. Color of blood:
    1. Bright red: Carbon monoxide, cyanide.
    2. Brown: Methemoglobinemia (see above).

I. Coagulopathy:
    Antibiotics
    Envenomation
    Anticoagulants
    Salicylates

J. Prothrombin decrease (prolonged prothrombin time):
   Anticoagulants
   Salicylates
   Anything causing liver disease
K. Hemolysis:

Arsine	Nalidixic acid
Cephalosporin antibiotics	Naphthalene
Copper	Nitrite
Dimethyl sulfoxide	Nitrofurans
Envenomation	Primaquin
Favism	Sulfonamides

II. Urine findings:
   A. Color changes:
      1. Colorless:
         a. Osmotic diuresis (e.g., diabetes mellitus, diabetes insipidus).
         b. Dilution of urine.
      2. Milky: Chyluria, pyuria.
      3. Intense yellow:

Carrots	Phenacetin
Cascara	Quinacrine
Fluorescein	Riboflavin

      4. Black:

Cresols	Phenacetin
Levodopa	Phenazopyridine
Methocarbamol	Phenol
Naphthalene	Quinine

      5. Blue:

Amitriptyline	Methocarbamol
Anthraquinone	Methylene blue
Boric acid	Tetrahydronaphthalene

      6. Brown:

Benzene	Metronidazole
Carbon tetrachloride	Naphthalene
Chloroquine	Niridazole
Cresols	Nitrofurantoin
Dinitrophenol	Phenacetin
Fava beans	Phenols
Hydroquinone	Phenothiazine
Lead	Phenytoin
Levodopa	Primaquine
Mercury	Quinines
Methemoglobinemia	Sulfonamides
Methocarbamol	

      7. Green:

Amitriptyline	Carbolic acid
Anthraquinone	Creosote
Boric acid	Hydroquinone

Indomethacin
Methocarbamol
8. Orange:
Chlorzoxazone
Dantrolene
Dehydration (concentrated urine)
Fluorescein
9. Red/pink:
Ampicillin
Aniline
Anthocyanin (in beets and blackberries)
Betaine (fresh beets)
Deferoxamine
Hematuria (see p. 200)
Ibuprofen
Lead (chronic)
Lycopene (in tomatoes, watermelon)

Methylene blue
Phenols

Phenazopyridine
Rifampin
Santonin
Sulfaxalazine
Warfarin

Mercury (chronic)
Myoglobinuria (see p. 232)
Naphthalene
Phenacetin
Phenazopyridine
Phenothiazines
Phenytoin
Porphyrins
Quinines
Rifampin

10. Red/purple: Chlorzoxazone.
11. Vin rose: Ferrioxamine.
12. Smoky: Phenols.
B. Protein or cells:
Arsenic
Benzene
Bismuth
Bromates
Carbon tetrachloride
Chlorates
Daphne plants
Dimethyl sulfoxide
Dinitrophenols
Ethylene glycol
Fluoride
Formaldehyde
Hydrogen sulfide
Iodine
Iron
Mercury
Methanol

Methaqualone
Methyl bromide
Methyl chloride
Mushrooms
Naphtha
Naphthalene
Nitrofurans
Nutmeg
Oxalate
Paraldehyde
Phosphorus
Pine oil
Rifampin
Selenium
Thallium
Toluene
Turpentine
Xanthines

C. Crystals:
Antimony
Arsenic
Ethylene glycol

Gold
Oxalate
Sulfonamides

D. Ketones:

Acetone	Paraldehyde
Isopropanol	Salicylates
Methanol	

E. Luminescent: phosphorus.
F. Myoglobinuria:
  1. Causes:
    a. Muscle catabolism:
      (1) Extreme muscle contraction/seizures:

Amphetamines	Nicotine
Benzene	Phencyclidine
Tricyclic antidepressants	Strychnine
Hexachloride	Water hemlock

      (2) Metabolic depression:

Barbiturates	Isopropanol
Carbon monoxide	Opiates
Ethanol	Sedatives/hypnotics

      (3) Malignant hyperthermia:

Succinylcholine	Halothane

      (4) Direct toxic effect on muscles:

Ethanol	Copper sulfate
Opiates	Zinc phosphide
Snake venom	Toluene

G. Albuminuria: Mercury poisoning.
III. Cerebrospinal fluid changes:
  A. Increased protein: Lead, mercury.
  B. Increased pressure:

Bromide	Nalidixic acid
Corticosteroids	Tetracyclines
Hypoxia	Thallium
Lead	Theophylline
Methanol	Toluene
Mushrooms	Vitamin A

IV. Radiologic manifestations:
  A. Radiopaque drugs:
    1. Mnemonic for differential diagnosis of radiopaque ingestants: CHIPES:
      Chloral hydrate, CC14
      Heavy metals (e.g., arsenic, lead, iron)
      Health foods (e.g., vitamins, bone meal)
      Iodides, iron
      Phenothiazines
      Enteric-coated medications (e.g., salicylates, KCl)
      Solvents: CHC13 (e.g., chloroform), CC14 (e.g., carbon tetrachloride)
    2. Other radiopaque drugs/toxins:

Acetazolamide	Busulfan
Barium	Calcium carbonate
Batteries	Cocaine packets
Bismuth	Dimetapp

Drixoral   Sodium chloride
Phosphorus   Thiamine
Potassium chloride

B. Bone metaphyseal densities: **Lead** (child), **vitamin A.**

V. Electrocardiographic abnormalities:

A. Sinus tachycardia:

Amphetamines   Drug-induced hypoxia
Antihistamines   Drug withdrawal
Anticholinergics   Ephedrine
Caffeine   Theophylline
Tricyclic antidepressants   Thyroid preparations
Cocaine

B. Ventricular tachycardia:

Amphetamines   Digitalis glycosides
Caffeine   Fluoride
Chloral hydrate   Phenothiazines
Chlorinated hydrocarbons   Solvents
Cocaine   Theophylline
Tricyclic antidepressants

C. Bradycardia:

Beta blockers   Physostigmine
Calcium channel blockers   Quinidine
Digitalis glycosides   Tricyclic antidepressants
Organophosphate insecticides Narcotics

D. AV block:

Beta blockers   Phenytoin
Calcium channel blockers   Procainamide
Clonidine   Tricyclic antidepressants
Digitalis glycosides

E. Heart block and other conduction disturbances:

Antimony   Nicotine
Barium   Phosphates
Beta blockers   Procainamide
Carbon monoxide   Propranolol
Chloroquine   Quinidine (increased QRS)
Clonidine (AV block)   Quinine
Digitalis   Shellfish
Disopyramide   Tricyclic antidepressants (increased
Emetine   QRS)
Local anesthetics   Verapamil
Methaqualone

F. QRS/QT prolongation:

Amantadine   Procainamide
Tricyclic antidepressants   Quinidine
Disopyramide   Quinine
Fluoride   Thallium
Lithium
Phenothiazines

G. Torsade de pointes:
  1. Antiarrhythmics:
     a. Group 1a: quinidine, procainamide, disopyramide.
     b. Group 1b: lidocaine, mexilitene.
     c. Group 1c: encainide.
     d. Group 2: amiodarone.
     e. Group 3: nifedipine.
  2. Psychotropics: thiorizadine.
  3. Toxins:
     Arsenic
     Organophosphates
     Liquid protein diets
  4. Miscellaneous:
     Atropine
     Chloral hydrate
     Diuretics
     Steroids
H. ST segment depression: **ergots.**
I. Nonspecific ST-T wave changes:
   a. Bites: **scorpions, spiders, hymenoptera.**
   b. Other: **lithium.**
J. Junctional rhythm: **tricyclic antidepressants, digoxin.**
K. Asystole: drugs with **anticholinergic** effects.
L. Frequent premature ventricular contractions:
   a. Sympathomimetic syndrome (see Chapter 47, p. 219).

BIBLIOGRAPHY

Done AK: The toxic emergency: Signs, symptoms and sources. *Emerg Med* 1982; 14:42–77.

Goldberg M, Green SB, Moss ML, et al: Computer-based instruction and diagnosis of acid-base disorders. *JAMA* 1973; 223:269–275.

Olson KR, Pentel PR, Kelley MT: Physical assessment and differential diagnosis of the poisoned patient. *Med Toxicol* 1987; 2:52–81.

Proudfoot AT: *Diagnosis and management of acute poisoning.* Oxford, England, Blackwell, 1982.

Savitt DL, Hawkins HH, Roberts JR: The radiopacity of ingested medications. *Ann Emerg Med* 1987; 16:331–339.

Stratman HG, et al: Torsade de pointes associated with drugs and toxins: Recognition and management. *Am Heart J* 1987; 113:1470–1480.

Thorton JR: Atrial fibrillation in healthy nonalcoholic people after an alcoholic binge. *Lancet* 1984; 2:1013–1014.

PART FIVE

Specific Poisonings and Toxic Exposures

Nontoxic Ingestions

49

Nontoxic Ingestants

Patricia D. Fosarelli, M.D.

I. Nontoxic ingestions:

Abrasives
Adhesives
Antacids
Antibiotics
Baby product cosmetics
Ballpoint pen inks
Bathtub floating toys
Battery (dry cell)
Bath oil (caster oil and perfume)
Bleach (less than 5% sodium hypochlorite)
Body conditioners
Bubble bath soaps/detergents
Calamine lotion (beeswax or paraffin)
Caps (toy pistols)
Chalk (calcium carbonate)
Cigarettes or cigars (nicotine)
Clay (modeling)
Colognes
Contraceptives
Corticosteroids
Cosmetics
Crayons (marked AP, CP)
Dehumidifying packets (silica, charcoal)
Detergents (phosphate, anionic)
Deodorants
Deodorizers (spray and refrigerant)
Elmer's glue
Etch-A-Sketch
Eye makeup
Fabric softeners
Fertilizer (without insecticides, herbicides)
Fish bowl additives
Glues and pastes
Golf ball (core may cause mechanical injury)
Greases
Hair products (dyes, sprays, tonics)
Hand lotions, creams
Hydrogen peroxide (medicinal 3%)
Incense
Indelible markers
Ink (black, blue)
Iodophil disinfectant

Laxatives
Lipstick
Lubricant
Lubricating oils
Lysol disinfectant (**not** toilet bowl cleaner)
Magic markers
Makeup (eye, liquid facial)
Mineral oil
Motor oil
Newspaper
Paint (indoor or latex)
Pencil (lead, graphite, candle coloring)
Perfumes
Petroleum jelly (Vaseline)
Phenolphthalein laxatives (Ex-Lax)
Play-Doh
Polaroid picture coating fluid
Porous-tip ink marking pens
Prussian blue (ferricyanide)
Putty (less than 2 oz)
Rouge

Rubber cement
Sachets (essential oils, powder)
Shampoos
Shaving creams, lotions
Shoe polish (most do not contain aniline dyes)
Silly Putty (99% silicones)
Soap and soap products
Spackles
Suntan preparations
Sweetening agents (saccharin, cyclamate, aspartame)
Teething rings (water sterility?)
Thermometers (mercury)
Thyroid hormone
Toilet water
Tooth paste (with/without fluoride)
Vaseline
Vitamins
Warfarin
Water colors
Zinc oxide
Zirconium oxide

II. Nontoxic house plants*

African Violet *(Saintpaulia ionantha)*
Aluminum plant *(Pilea)*
Aralia False *(Dizygotheca elegantissima)*
Bloodleaf plant (Iresine)
Boston fern *(Nephrolepis exaltata bostoniensis*
Cattail *Typha latifolia*
Christmas cactus *(Zygocactus truncatus)*
Coleus
Corn plant *(Dracaena)*
Creeping Charlie (moneywort, *Lysimachia nummularia* or *Plectranthus australis*)
Crocus *(spring blooming, Crocus* spp)
Dandelion *(Taraxacum officinale)*
Devil's walking stick *(Aralia spinosa)*

Donkey tail *(Sedum morganianum)*
Dracaena spp (corn plant)
Dusty miller (rose campion, *Lychnis coronaria*)
Dwarf cactus *(Epiphyl Hybrid elegantissiumum)*
Gardenia
Geranium *(Pelargonium)*
Grape hyacinth *(Muscari)*
Hawaiian ti *(Cordyline terminalis)*
Hen and chickens *(Escheveria; Sempervivum tectorum)*
Hibiscus
Honeysuckle *(Lonicera)*
Impatiens
Inch plant (spiderwort, *Tradescantia*)
Jade plant *(Crassula)*
Kalanchoe (pregnant plant)
Lady's slipper *(Cypripedium)*

*Modified from Crain EF, Gershel JC (eds): *A Clinical Manual of Emergency Pediatrics.* Norwalk, Conn, Appleton-Century-Crofts, 1986, pp 328–329. Used by permission.

Lilac *(Syringa pedula)*
Lipstick plant *(Aeschynanthus lobbianus)*
Magnolia bush
Monkey plant *(Rulla makoyana)*
Moses-in-a-boat *(Rhoea begonia spathacea)*
Mother-in-law's tongue *(Sansevieria trifascianta)*
Palm
Patient Lucy
Peperomia
Piggyback plant *(Tolmia menziestii)*
Pilea (botanical name)
Pink polka dot plant *(Hypoestes sanquinolenta)*
Plextranthus
Prayer plant *(Maranta leuconeura kerchoveana)*
Primrose *(Primula)*
Rattle snake plant *(Calathea insignis)*

Rose (*Rosa* spp)
Rose begonia *(semperflorens)*
Rose of Sharon (St. John's-wort, *Hypericum calycinum; Hibiscus syriacus)*
Rubber plant *(Ficus elastica)*
Scheffelera *(Brassaia actiniphylla;* Umbrella plant, *Cyperus alternifolius)*
Sensitive plant *(Mimosa pudica)*
Snake plant (sansevieria)
Snapdragon *(Antirrhinum)*
Spider plant *(Anthericum* or *Chlorophytum cosmosum)*
Swedish ivy *(Plextranthus australis)*
Violet *(Viola)*
Wandering Jew *(Zebrina; Tradescantia)*
Wax plant *(Hoya)*
Weeping fig *(Ficus benjamina)*

Alcohols

50

General Introduction to Alcohols

Mark S. Smith, M.D., F.A.C.E.P.

I. General comments:
  A. Alcohols **(ethanol, methanol, isopropanol, and ethylene glycol)** are water-soluble compounds that have substantial target organ toxicity.
  B. Because of their small molecular weight, alcohols can substantially elevate serum osmolality. All four distribute primarily in total body water (volume of distribution 0.6–1.0 L/kg).
  C. Toxicity:
     1. All alcohols produce nonspecific central nervous system and gastrointestinal symptoms.
     2. The metabolic lesion each produces is part of their toxic fingerprint:
        a. Methanol and ethylene glycol produce profound anion gap metabolic acidosis.
        b. Isopropanol produces acetonemia without acidosis.
        c. Ethanol may be associated with ketoacidosis or lactic acidosis.
     3. Onset of effect:
        a. Ethanol and isopropanol: immediately after ingestion.
        b. Methanol and ethylene glycol: may be delayed for up to 48 hours after ingestion. It is the toxic metabolites, not the parent compound, that cause the most damage.
  D. Hemodialysis is the treatment of choice for significant alcohol poisoning.
II. Osmolal gap:
  A. Serum osmolality is a measure of the number of molecules of solute per kilogram solvent.
  B. Normal osmolality is 280–290 mOsm/kg body water.

C. The molecules that contribute most to serum osmolality are sodium, chloride, bicarbonate, glucose, and urea. Serum osmolality may be approximated as: Osm (calculated) = (2 × Na) + BUN/2.8 + (Glucose >100/18) Serum osmolality is measured directly by the method of freezing point depression.

D. Ordinarily the calculated serum osmolality is within 5–10 mOsm of measured osmolality. When measured serum osmolality is more than 10 mOsm/L greater than calculated osmolality, an "osmolal gap" exists.

E. Osmolal gap is the presence of large numbers of other low molecular weight molecules. Exogenous substances that can elevate serum osmolality are methanol, ethanol, isopropanol, and ethylene glycol (Table 50–1), and **mannitol,** and **sorbitol.**

F. High serum lipids may also result in osmolal gap.

III. Administration of ethanol:

A. Rationale: Both methanol and ethylene glycol are metabolized by hepatic alcohol dehydrogenase to substances much more toxic than the parent compound. The treatment strategy is to saturate alcohol dehydrogenase with ethanol, for which the enzyme has a higher affinity, thus blocking conversion of either methanol or ethylene glycol to toxic byproducts and permitting the parent compound to be excreted in an unchanged and relatively nontoxic form.

B. Loading dose:

1. Orally or intravenously.

2. At a serum ethanol level of **100 mg/dl,** alcohol dehydrogenase is completely saturated.

   a. The specific gravity of ethanol is 0.79; thus 1 L 100% ethanol contains 790 gm.

   b. Standard hospital pharmacy stock solution is 95% ethanol (0.75 gm/ml), thus 10% ethanol solution contains 0.079 gm/ml.

   c. The volume of distribution of ethanol is 0.6 L/kg; the theoretical dose of ethanol required to obtain a serum level of 100 mg/dl (1 gm/L) is 0.6 gm ethanol per kilogram body weight.

   d. Oral loading dose: **20%–30% concentration** via nasogastric tube. One ml/kg 95% ethanol can be mixed in twice its volume of orange juice to obtain an approximately 30% solution.

   e. Intravenous loading dose: **Usually 0.7–0.8 gm/kg is required,** that is, **1 ml/kg 95% ethanol** (0.75 gm/ml) or **10 ml/kg 10% ethanol**

TABLE 50–I.

Interpretation of Osmolal Gap
Related to Alcohols

100 mg/dL	Raises osmolal gap
Ethanol	22
Methanol	31
Ethylene glycol	16
Isopropanol	17

(0.75 gm/10 ml). **Must be diluted to 5%–10% concentration for safe IV administration.**
3. Precautions:
  a. IV administration of ethanol poses potential fluid overload in some patients because **no greater than 10% concentration can be safely administered.** A 70 kg patient would require a 700 ml intravenous loading dose.
  b. Greater than 30% concentration for oral administration may lead to gastritis.
C. Maintenance dose:
  1. Maintenance dose depends on the patient's alcohol dehydrogenase activity. Chronic alcoholics need a higher maintenance dose of ethanol to **maintain serum levels 100 mg/dl.**
  2. Average maintenance dose of ethanol is **0.1 gm/kg/hr,** that is, **0.15 ml/kg/hr 95% ethanol** or **1.4 ml/kg/hr 10% ethanol** in D_5W.
  3. Maintenance dosing **must be increased during dialysis** or ethanol must be added to the dialysate at a concentration of 100 mg/dl.
  4. Serum ethanol levels need to be checked after ethanol loading and then three times daily (more frequently in the pediatric patient) and the ethanol dose appropriately adjusted.

BIBLIOGRAPHY

Becker CE: The alcoholic patient as a toxic emergency. *Emerg Med Clin North Am* 1984; 2:47–61.

51

Methanol

Mark S. Smith, M.D., F.A.C.E.P.

I. Composition:
   A. Formula: CH_3OH.
   B. Molecular weight 32.
   C. Appearance: Liquid with unpleasant taste and odor when impure; nearly odorless clear liquid when pure.
II. Route of exposure: Oral, transdermal, inhaled.
III. Generic name: Wood alcohol.
IV. Uses: Found in carburetor fluid, glass cleaner, duplicator fluid, gasohol, gas line antifreeze, model airplane fuel, paint stripper, pipe sweetener, windshield deicer, windshield washing solution.
V. Pharmacokinetics:
   A. Onset: Usual pattern is **delayed toxicity** 12–24 hours after exposure.
   B. Peak: Peak serum level **30–60 minutes** after exposure.
   C. Half-life: 8 hours. With ethanol blocking, 30–35 hours. With hemodialysis, 2.5 hours.
   D. Elimination: Most is metabolized. Kidney (5%–10%), lung (10%–70%).
   E. Active: metabolites: formaldehyde (HCHO), formic acid (HCOOH).
   F. Volume of distribution: 0.6 L/kg (total body water)
VI. Toxic mechanism:
   A. Methanol per se is only mildly toxic.
   B. Active metabolites (formaldehyde and formate) have severe toxicity:
      1. Necrosis of putamen.
      2. Optic nerve demyelination.
VII. Range of toxicity:
   A. Toxic dose: ≥4 ml (100% methanol).
   B. Fatal dose: Varies widely. As little as 6 ml (15 ml 40% methanol) has caused death.

VIII. Clinical features:
  A. Latent period lasting 6–24 hours characterized by mild inebriation.
  B. Eye: Blurry vision, cloudiness, mistiness, snowstorm, decreased acuity, fundoscopic examination may show disc/retina edema and hyperemia.
  C. CNS: Headache, dizziness, weakness, confusion, seizures, coma, nuchal rigidity.
  D. GI: Abdominal pain, nausea, vomiting, pancreatitis.
  E. Metabolic: Profound increased anion gap metabolic acidosis (unmeasured anion is formate).
IX. Laboratory findings and evaluation:
  A. Blood:
     1. Serum levels: 20 mg/dl associated with toxicity; should be obtainable from most clinical laboratories.
     2. Osmolality: Calculate osmolal gap (see Chapter 50, p. 244).
     3. Electrolytes: Calculate anion gap.
     4. Amylase: Pancreatitis.
     5. Arterial blood gas: Profound anion gap metabolic acidosis.
X. General treatment:
  A. Follow APTLS (see Chapter 8).
  B. General management (Table 51–1): see Chapter 12 for details.
XI. Specific treatment:
  A. Administration of ethanol:
     1. Indications:
        a. Methanol level >20 mg/dl.
        b. Presence of methanol toxicity symptoms.
     2. Method (see Chapter 50, p. 244).
  B. Hemodialysis:
     1. Indications:
        a. Methanol >25–50 mg/dl.
        b. Metabolic acidosis.

TABLE 51–1.

General Treatment

Treatment	Indicated	Of No Value	Contraindicated
O_2	±		
IV	+		
ECG monitor	+		
Forced diuresis		×	
Acidification			×
Alkalinization*	+		
Emesis/	+ or		
lavage†	+		
Charcoal		×	
Cathartic	+		
Dialysis	+		

*May be needed to combat acidosis; keep pH >7.25.
†Methanol is liquid and can be lavaged through small-bore nasogastric tube.

      c. CNS, visual, or fundoscopic abnormality.

      d. Consumption of >30 ml methanol.

      e. When in doubt, institute dialysis.

    2. Some authorities suggest that dialysis be started as soon as diagnosis is established, even if patient has no symptoms.

  C. Folate therapy:

    1. Promotes rapid metabolism of formate.

    2. Dose: 1 mg/kg (up to 50 mg) IV every 4 hours for 6 doses.

XII. Prognosis:

  A. Expected response to treatment:

    1. Good if recognized and treated early.

    2. Mortality related to degree of acidosis.

  B. Expected complications:

    1. Visual deficit.

    2. Extrapyramidal symptoms (parkinsonism).

XIII. Disposition:

  A. Admission considerations:

    1. See General Admission Considerations (Chapters 17 and 18).

    2. Symptomatic.

    3. Any ingestion ≥4 ml 100% methanol.

    4. Level ≥10 mg/dl.

    5. Consider admitting anyone with established or suspected diagnosis.

  B. Consultation considerations:

    1. Nephrology consultation if dialysis indicated.

  C. Observation period:

    1. If admission criteria not immediately met; until 3 hour level returns.

  D. Discharge considerations:

    1. General discharge considerations are met (see Chapter 18).

    2. No symptoms after sufficient observation.

    3. Serum level <10 mg/dl 3 hours after ingestion.

    4. Because of risk of delayed toxicity, **decision to discharge must be made with great caution.**

    5. Suicide potential and psychiatric status appropriately evaluated.

BIBLIOGRAPHY

Becker CE: Acute methanol poisoning: "The blind drunk" *West J Med* 1981; 135:122–128.

Gonda A, Gault H, Churchill D, et al: Hemodialysis for methanol intoxication. *Am J Med* 1978; 64:749–758.

Litovitz T: The alcohols: Ethanol, methanol, isopropanol, ethylene glycol. *Pediatr Clin North Am* 1986; 3(2):311–323.

Smith M: Solvent toxicity: Isopropanol, methanol, and ethylene glycol. *Ear Nose Throat J* 1983; 62:126–135.

Swartz RD, Millman RP, Billi JE: Epidemic methanol poisoning: Clinical and biochemical analysis of a recent episode. *Medicine* 1981; 60:373–382.

52

Ethanol

Mark S. Smith, M.D., F.A.C.E.P.

I. Composition:
  A. Formula: CH_3CH_2OH.
  B. Molecular weight: 46.
  C. Appearance: Colorless liquid with characteristic taste and odor augmented by impurities (alcohols and aldehydes).
  D. Specific gravity: 0.79 gm/ml.
II. Route of exposure: Oral.
III. Pharmacokinetics:
  A. Onset: Immediate absorption from stomach (5–10 minutes).
  B. Peak: Peak serum concentration 30–90 minutes after ingestion.
  C. Duration: Metabolized at 150 mg/kg body weight per hour, or decrease in serum ethanol concentration 15–25 mg/dl/hr. Chronic alcoholics without significant liver impairment have enhanced metabolism and decrease serum concentration by 50 mg/dl/hr.
  D. Elimination: Liver (alcohol dehydrogenase).
  E. Volume of distribution: 0.6–0.8 L/kg.
IV. Actions and uses:
  A. Found in alcoholic beverages, medicines, colognes, mouthwash, solvents, aftershave, hair tonics, variety of household products.
V. Toxic mechanism: Direct CNS depressant and toxin.
VI. Range of toxicity:
  A. Toxic dose:
    1. 1 ml/kg 100% ethanol produces a serum level of 100 mg/dl. One ounce of whiskey, one glass of wine, or one bottle of beer raises serum ethanol 25 mg/dl in the average adult.
    2. Serum levels <50 mg/dl rarely associated with toxic effects in adults.

B. Fatal dose:
  1. Varies greatly: adult 5–8 gm/kg; child: 3 gm/kg.
  2. 1 ml 100% ethanol equals 0.79 gm.
  3. Most deaths occur at serum levels >400 mg/dl; 300–400 ml (600–800 ml 100 proof whiskey) if consumed in less than 1 hour.
  4. Potentiation by concomitant ingestion, particularly of drugs with sedative effects.

VII. Clinical features:
  A. Inebriation/intoxication syndrome consisting of slurred speech, muscular incoordination, ataxia; progressing to stupor, coma, and respiratory depression in massive intoxications. Pupils often miotic in ethanol-induced coma.
  B. Syndrome of pathologic intoxication: Combative and destructive behavior, often with propensity to spit.
  C. Metabolic: Hypothermia, hypoglycemia (especially in children). Lactic acidosis secondary to ethanol-induced increase in NADH/NAD ratio.
  D. GI: Nausea, vomiting, abdominal pain secondary to gastritis or pancreatitis.
  E. Respiratory depression:
    1. Respiratory depression from severe intoxication is **usual cause of death.**
    2. Potentiated by other sedative/hypnotics (e.g., benzodiazepines).
  F. Correlation of blood alcohol level with clinical findings (Table 52–1).

TABLE 52–1.

Correlation of Blood Alcohol Level With Clinical Findings in Nontolerant Individuals*

Blood Alcohol Concentration (mg/dl)	Clinical Findings
<50	Limited muscular incoordination
	Driving not seriously impaired
50–100	Driving increasingly dangerous
	Incoordination
	Impaired sensory function
100–150	Mood, personality, and behavioral changes
	Driving is dangerous (legally drunk in most states)
	Marked mental impairment, incoordination, ataxia
150–200	Prolonged reaction time
	Driving is very dangerous (legally drunk in all states)
200–300	Nausea, vomiting, diplopia, marked ataxia
300–400	Hypothermia, dysarthria, amnesia
400–700	Coma, respiratory failure, death

*Most applicable to those without development of tolerance.

VIII. Laboratory findings and evaluation:
   A. Blood:
      1. Blood alcohol concentration: a good approximation to blood ethanol can be obtained by measuring ethanol concentration of expired air using a breathalyzer. Correlates well with clinical findings in nonalcohol-tolerant individuals.
      2. Osmolal gap: 100 mg/dL alcohol raises osmolal gap by 22 (see Chapter 50, p. 244).
      3. Glucose: May cause hypoglycemia (especially in children).
      4. Arterial blood gas: Ethanol intoxication may (rarely) cause increased anion gap–type metabolic acidosis (lactic acidosis).
      5. Electrolytes: Patients with chronic alcoholism may be hypokalemic.
   B. CT head scan: If clinical findings not consistent with serum ethanol level, consider intracerebral hematoma or contusion (see Chapter 26).
IX. General treatment:
   A. Follow APTLS (see Chapter 8).
   B. General management (Table 52–2; see Chapter 12 for details).
   C. Consider in the differential diagnosis:
      1. Severe CNS depression:
         a. Acute methanol, ethylene glycol, or isopropanol intoxication.
         b. Head injury.
      2. Seizures (see Chapter 22).
         a. Subdural or epidural hematoma.
         b. Hepatic encephalopathy.
         c. Sepsis or meningitis.
         d. Hypoglycemia.

TABLE 52–2

General Treatment

Treatment	Indicated	Of No Value	Contraindicated
O$_2$	±		
IV*	+		
ECG monitor	±		
Forced diuresis		×	
Acidification			×
Alkalinization			×
Emesis†/	+ or		
lavage	±		
Charcoal‡		×	
Cathartic		×	
Other: Add thiamine, multivitamins, magnesium to IV			

*Indicated in those with decreased level of consciousness or if diagnosis in doubt.

†Use with precaution only. Potential for altered mental status or multidrug ingestion is great. Gastric emptying generally not recognized as treatment for only ethanol. Because of rapid absorption, effective only if done within 90 minutes of ingestion.

‡Not effective because of need for massive amounts, but may still be helpful, especially if multidrug ingestion suspected.

     3. Hypothermia.
     4. Wernicke's syndrome.
     5. Severe metabolic acidosis (lactic acidosis or ketoacidosis).
     6. Severe delirium tremens.
  X. Specific management (also follow recommendations in Chapter 25):
    A. Supportive, with attention to:
     1. Prevention of aspiration.
     2. Observe; declining serum ethanol level should correspond to improvement in sensorium.
    B. Many patients are volume depleted. Assess and replete with D_5N/S.
    C. There are no accepted enhancements to more rapid metabolism of ethanol; patients "sleep it off." Naloxone has unproved benefit in reversing acute ethanol intoxication in some.
    D. If appropriate, treatment of problem of chronic alcoholism must be considered once acute intoxication is managed (see Chapter 25).
    E. Assess all patients for suicide risk.
  XI. Prognosis:
    A. Expected response to treatment:
     1. Uncomplicated; survival for 24 hours is ordinarily followed by recovery.
     2. In alcoholic psychosis, survival is likely but complete recovery is rare. In the presence of mental deterioration, complete withdrawal from ethanol may be followed by minimal improvement.
    B. Expected complications and long-term effects:
     1. None from a single overdose: Short-term effect is "hangover."
     2. Alcohol withdrawal symptoms (see Chapter 33).
     3. Chronic ethanol abuse has numerous target organs of toxicity, including liver (cirrhosis, acute hepatitis), CNS (Wernicke-Korsakoff syndrome, peripheral neuropathy, alcoholic myopathy), bone marrow depression, nutritional deficiencies, heart (cardiomyopathy).
     4. Pulmonary complications: Aspiration pneumonia, pneumonia, pulmonary edema, septic pulmonary emboli, coma-respiratory depression, lung abscess, atelectasis, pneumomediastinum/pneumothorax, pulmonary fibrosis/pulmonary vascular granulomatosis.
     5. Tetanus-induced respiratory muscle dysfunction.
  XII. Special considerations:
    A. Drugs with disulfiram-like reactions (see Chapter 95).
    B. Potential concomitant head injury (see Chapter 26).
    C. Consider possibility of multidrug ingestion.
  XIII. Disposition considerations:
    A. Admission considerations:
     1. See General Admission Considerations (Chapters 17 and 18).
     2. Inability to observe.
     3. Severe overdose (takes too long to observe appropriately in emergency department).
     4. Complications (e.g., hypoglycemia, seizures, hypothermia).
     5. All pediatric and preadolescent patients.
     6. Adolescent with unstable home environment.
     7. Suicide risk.

B. Consultation considerations:
  1. Psychiatry: Suicidal risk, repeated self-destructive behavior.
  2. Neurosurgery: Significant head injury established or cannot be ruled out.
  3. Alcohol counselor or social worker when sober.
  4. Other consultants, depending on complications.
C. Observation period:
  1. Based on expected metabolism of substance and concomitant improvement in medical status.
  2. Based on ability to observe in emergency department. If cannot observe for sufficient time, must admit.
D. Discharge considerations:
  1. General discharge considerations have been met (see Chapter 18).
  2. NOTE: **Patients with altered mental status cannot sign out against medical advice.**
  3. NOTE: **Patient's family or friends cannot sign "against medical advice" form for patient unless patient's legal guardian.**
  4. Patient can walk with steady gait without assistance and talk coherently.
  5. No evidence of withdrawal.
  6. Alcohol counseling has been offered.
  7. A stable disposition environment must exist. **Do not send patient out in the cold without a destination arranged.**

BIBLIOGRAPHY

Sellers, Kallant: Alcohol intoxication and withdrawal. *N Engl J Med* 1976; 294:757–767.
Thorn GW, Adams RA, Braunwald E, et al: *Harrison's Principles of Internal Medicine,* ed 8. New York, McGraw-Hill Book Co, 1977.

53

Ethylene Glycol

Mark S. Smith, M.D., F.A.C.E.P.

I. Properties:
   A. Chemical formula: CH_2OHCH_2OH.
   B. Molecular weight: 62.
   C. Appearance: Colorless and almost odorless liquid that is warm and sweet to taste (opalescent blue color of automobile antifreeze is added to identify the liquid as nonpotable).
II. Route of exposure: Oral.
III. Common name: Antifreeze.
IV. Pharmacokinetics:
   A. Onset:
      1. Inebriation after 30–60 minutes.
      2. Serious toxicity can be delayed up to 12 hours.
   B. Half-life:
      1. 3–8 hours.
      2. 17 hours with ethanol blocking.
      3. 2.5 hours with hemodialysis.
   C. Elimination: Kidneys.
   D. Active metabolites:
      1. Metabolites are responsible for toxicity and may have half-lives up to 12 hours.
      2. Hepatic metabolism produces glycolaldehyde, glycolic acid, glyoxylic acid, glycine, oxalic acid.
   E. Volume of distribution: 0.6–0.8 L/kg.

V. Action: See Toxic mechanism.

VI. Uses: Found in automobile antifreeze, coolant, paint solvent, hydraulic brake fluid, inks.

VII. Toxic mechanism:

    A. Ethylene glycol has inebriation toxicity equivalent to that of ethanol; no other action.

    B. Aldehydes: Direct CNS toxins.

    C. Glycolates and oxalates cause renal and CNS toxicity and cause metabolic acidosis. Widespread petechial hemorrhages occur.

VIII. Range of toxicity:

    A. Toxic dose:

        1. Serum levels >50 mg/dl indicate substantial toxicity.

        2. A 3 ml swallow of 100% ethylene glycol in 10 kg child can produce a serum level of 50 mg/dl.

    B. Fatal dose:

        1. One-fourth ml/kg of 95% ethylene glycol, although survival has occurred with much higher doses.

        2. 2 ml/kg, or about 100 ml.

IX. Clinical features:

    A. Three clinical stages:

        1. Initial toxicity: prodrome of CNS inebriation with the smell of alcohol that results from the ethylene glycol.

        2. First-stage delayed toxicity (30 minutes–12 hours):

            a. CNS: confusion, ataxia, stupor, seizures, coma, myoclonus, nystagmus.

            b. GI: nausea and vomiting.

            c. Metabolic: severe anion gap metabolic acidosis.

            d. Cardiovascular: congestive heart failure (usually occurs later than other symptoms, 12–24 hours after ingestion).

        3. Second-stage delayed toxicity (36–72 hours):

            a. Renal: flank pain, hematuria, pyuria, crystalluria, albuminuria, renal insufficiency, renal failure.

X. Laboratory findings and evaluation:

    A. Blood:

        1. Serum levels: 50 mg/dl prognostic of serious toxicity (serum levels often unobtainable by clinical laboratory and are not included in routine alcohol screens).

        2. Osmolality: Osmolal gap (see Chapter 50, p. 244).

        3. White blood cell count: Often substantial leukocytosis.

        4. Calcium: Hypocalcemia from chelation with oxalate.

        5. Arterial blood gas: profound anion gap metabolic acidosis; unmeasured anion is glycolate.

    B. Urinanalysis: pyuria; hematuria; albuminuria; calcium oxalate; crystalluria, either envelope shaped dihydrate crystals or needle-shaped monohydrate crystals.

    C. Cerebrospinal fluid: Increased pressure, increased protein, few polymorphonuclear cells.

XI. General treatment:
A. Follow APTLS (see Chapter 8).
B. General management (Table 53–1; see Chapter 12 for details).
XII. Specific management:
A. Ethanol administration:
1. Indications:
a. Serum ethylene glycol >20 mg/dl.
b. Presence of metabolic acidosis.
c. Presence of symptoms.
d. Concomitant ingestion of ethanol, which masks symptoms.
2. Method (see Chapter 50, p. 244).
B. Sodium bicarbonate for metabolic acidosis (keep pH >7.25).
C. Thiamine 100 mg to stimulate conversion of glyoxalate to nontoxic metabolite.
D. Pyridoxine 100 mg to help convert glyoxalate to nontoxic glycine.
E. May need to administer calcium if patient hypocalcemic, magnesium if hypomagnesemic.
F. Hemodialysis:
1. Indications:
a. Ethylene glycol >50 mg/dl.
b. 2 ml/kg ingested.
c. Severe acid-base abnormalities.
d. CNS toxicity.
e. Renal failure.
2. Some authorities suggest that dialysis be started as soon as diagnosis is established, even if patient has no symptoms.
G. Forced diuresis: Saline, mannitol, or furosemide diuresis to maintain brisk urine flow and prevent crystal precipitation (must be tempered by concerns of pulmonary edema).

TABLE 53–1.

General Treatment

Treatment	Indicated	Of No Value	Contraindicated
O_2	±		
IV	+		
ECG monitor	+		
Forced diuresis*	+		
Acidification			X
Alkalinization		X	
Emesis/lavage	+/+		
Charcoal†	+		
Dialysis	Effective‡		

*See Specific management.
†Unproved benefit but recommended.
‡See indications below.

XIII. Prognosis:
    A. Expected response to treatment: Good.
        1. Complete recovery of renal function may follow 2 weeks of complete anuria.
    B. Expected complications and long-term effects:
        1. Seizures.
        2. Cerebral damage may be permanent.
        3. Calcium oxaluria may lead to renal insufficiency, cyanosis, pulmonary edema.
XIV. Disposition:
    A. Admission considerations:
        1. See General Admission Considerations (Chapter 18).
        2. Any suspected ingestion.
        3. Symptoms.
        4. Serum levels >20 mg/dl.
    B. Consultation considerations:
        1. Nephrology consultation if dialysis indicated.
    C. Observation period:
        1. If admission criteria not met, 6 hours. See Discharge considerations.
    D. Discharge considerations:
        1. General discharge considerations are met (see Chapter 18).
        2. Asymptomatic after 6 hours and blood level <10 mg/dl 2 hours after ingestion. **Be wary of discharging patient.** See Admission considerations.

BIBLIOGRAPHY

Bryson PD: *Comprehensive Review in Toxicology.* Rockville, Md, Aspen Systems Corp, 1986.

Freed CR, Bobbit WH, Williams RM, et al: Ethanol for ethylene glycol poisoning. *N Engl J Med* 1981; 304:977.

Parry MF, Wallach R: Ethylene glycol poisoning. *Am J Med* 1974; 57:143–150.

Peterson CD, Collis AJ, Himes JM, et al: Ethylene glycol poisoning. *N Engl J Med* 1981; 304:21–23.

54

Isopropyl Alcohol

Mark S. Smith, M.D., F.A.C.E.P.

I. Route of exposure: Oral, inhalation.
II. Generic name: Rubbing alcohol.
III. Pharmacokinetics:
   A. Onset of action: 15–30 minutes after ingestion.
   B. Peak effect: One hour after ingestion.
   C. Plasma half-life: 2.5 to 3 hours.
   D. Duration of action: At same serum level, symptoms of isopropanol last two to four times as long as ethanol.
   E. Elimination: Mostly via kidney; some via lung.
   F. Rate of metabolism: Zero order kinetics at a rate one half that of ethanol.
   G. Active metabolites: Acetone (80% of isopropanol is converted to acetone by hepatic alcohol dehydrogenase).
IV. Action: See Toxic mechanism.
V. Uses:
   A. Found in rubbing alcohol (mostly 70% isopropanol), alcohol sponges, windshield deicer, glass cleaner, aftershave lotion.
VI. Toxic mechanism:
   A. Both isopropanol and acetone are CNS depressants.
   B. General rule of two: At same serum level, isopropanol has twice the CNS toxicity as ethanol and is metabolized half as fast.
VII. Range of toxicity:
   A. Toxic dose:
      1. Approximately twice as toxic as ethanol, with doses as low as 20 ml producing intoxication.
      2. 90 ml of 70% isopropanol can produce levels of 100 mg/dl in 70 kg adult.

B. Fatal dose:
    1. No substantial data available.
    2. Reported lethal dose is 3 ml/kg. Deaths have been reported after ingestions of 250 ml.
    3. Death may occur with serum levels >250 mg/dl.

VIII. Clinical features:
    A. CNS: CNS depression, confusion, ataxia, coma.
    B. GI: Vomiting, abdominal pain, melena, hematemesis secondary to gastritis (more than ethanol).
    C. Cardiovascular: Hypotension.
    D. lmonary: Pneumonia, pulmonary edema.
    E. Metabolic: Ketosis and acetonemia without acidemia. Hypothermia in serious overdose.

IX. Laboratory findings and evaluation:
    A. Blood:
        1. Serum levels: Symptoms occur at 50 mg/dl, with coma noted at levels >150 mg/dl.
        2. Serum osmolality: Increase in osmolality times 6 equals serum isopropanol level (see Table 50–1).
        3. Positive serum and urine acetone.
        4. Arterial blood gas:
            a. Presence of metabolic acidosis variable.
            b. Acute respiratory acidosis in severe ingestion.
    B. Other laboratory tests:
        1. Complete blood cell count. Decrease in hematocrit related to hemolysis.
        2. Blood sugar. Rule out hyperglycemia in presence of ketosis. May see hypoglycemia.
        3. Electrolytes, particularly if vomiting is severe.
        4. Liver function studies. Transaminase levels may be elevated.

X. General treatment:
    A. Follow APTLS (see Chapter 8).
    B. General management (Table 54–1; see Chapter 12 for details).

TABLE 54–1.

General Treatment

Treatment	Indicated	Of No Value	Contraindicated
O$_2$	±		
IV	+		
ECG monitor	±		
Forced diuresis	−		
Acidification			X
Alkalinization	−		
Emesis*/lavage*	+/+		
Charcoal	+		
*Most effective if done early.			

XI. Specific management:
  A. Symptomatic unless hypotension.
  B. Hypotension:
    1. See Chapter 10.
    2. If hypotension persistent, consider hemodialysis.
XII. Prognosis:
  A. Expected response to treatment:
    1. At same serum level, symptoms of isopropanol last two to four times as long as those of ethanol.
    2. Even in serious ingestions, survival for 48–72 hours after ingestion is associated with good prognosis, provided good supportive care is given.
    3. Persistent hypotension indicative of poor prognosis.
  B. Expected complications and long-term effects:
    1. Aspiration.
XIII. Special considerations:
  A. Isopropanol frequently ingested along with other toxic substances such as camphor, methyl salicylate, and methanol.
XIV. Disposition considerations:
  A. Admission considerations:
    1. See General Admission Considerations (Chapter 18).
    2. Symptomatic after appropriate treatment.
    3. Serum isopropanol level >100 mg/dl.
    4. ICU: Persistent hypotension.
  B. Consultation considerations:
    1. Consultation with dialysis service if patient is hypotensive.
  C. Observation period:
    1. Observe for at least 3 hours in the emergency department.
  D. Discharge considerations:
    1. General discharge considerations are met (Chapter 18).
    2. Asymptomatic after 3 hours of observation.
    3. Stable disposition environment exists.
    4. Alcohol counseling has been offered.

BIBLIOGRAPHY

Lacouture PG, Wason S, Abrams A, et al: Acute isopropyl alcohol intoxication: Diagnosis and management. *Am J Med* 1983; 75:680–686.
Rosansky SJ: Isopropyl alcohol poisoning treated with hemodialysis. Kinetics of isopropyl alcohol and acetone removal. *J Toxicol Clin Toxicol* 1982; 19:265–271.

Sedatives/Hypnotics

55

Barbiturates

V. Gail Ray, M.D., F.A.C.E.P.

I. Route of exposure: Oral, intravenous.
II. Common names: See Table 55–1.
III. Pharmacokinetics:
    A. Onset of action:
        1. Long-acting barbiturates: 1 hour (approximate).
        2. Short-acting barbiturates: 3–30 minutes
    B. Duration of action: Clinical effects generally last 6–8 hours.
    C. Half-life: See Table 55–2.
    D. Elimination:
        1. Long-acting barbiturates:
            a. In general, long-acting barbiturates have a low pKa (more acidic), lower degree of protein binding, low lipid solubility, low percentage metabolized, and appreciable amounts (20%) are excreted unchanged in the urine.
            b. Slowly metabolized by the liver, but because of low protein binding, more easily filtered and eliminated by the kidney than are short-acting drugs.
        2. Short-acting barbiturates:
            a. Being highly lipid soluble and protein bound, they are not easily filtered by the kidney and must be almost totally degraded by the liver.
IV. Uses:
    A. History:
        1. Sedative/hypnotic (sleeping pill).
        2. Most frequently used drug in suicide by drug ingestion.

TABLE 55–1.

Barbiturates

Action	Generic Name	Trade Name
Long acting	Phenobarbital	Barbital, Luminal
	Barbital	
	Primidone	Mysoline
Intermediate acting	Amobarbital	Tuinal, Amytal
	Butabarbital	Butisol Sodium
	Butalbital	Fiorinal, Esgic
Short acting	Hexobarbital	
	Pentobarbital	Nembutal
	Secobarbital	Seconal

B. Therapeutic:
   1. Still being used in combination drugs for sedative effect in agents for analgesia, functional gastrointestinal disorders, urethral inflammation, hypertension, asthma, and coronary artery disease.
   2. Specialized uses still include ultrashort-acting barbiturates for anesthesia induction, intermediate-acting (amobarbital) for narcoanalysis and narcotherapy, and long-acting as anticonvulsant.
   3. Phenobarbital also has efficacy in induction of hepatic and microsomal enzyme activity in treatment of kernicterus and hyperbilirubinemia.
   4. Newest use of phenobarbital has been to reduce cerebral blood flow

TABLE 55–2.

Half-Life and Metabolites of Barbiturates

Barbiturates			
Generic Name	Trade Name	Half-Life* (hr)	Metabolites
Amobarbital	Amytal	8–42	Inactive
Aprobarbital	Alurate	14–34	Inactive
Butabarbital	Butisol	34–42	Inactive
Butalbital	Fiorinal, Esgic	29–43	Inactive
Mephobarbital	Mebaral	11–67	Phenobarbital
Pentobarbital	Nembutal	15–48	Inactive
Phenobarbital†	Luminal	80–120	Inactive
Secobarbital	Seconal	15–40	Inactive

*Elimination half-time is increased in hepatic and renal disorders, pregnancy, elderly, and infants.
†Half-life of phenobarbital in children is 50% that in adults.

and oxygen consumption in the presence of cerebral edema (e.g., severe head trauma, conditions with increased intracranial pressure).

5. Barbiturate coma has been used in treatment of Reye's syndrome.
6. No longer recommended as sedative/hypnotic because benzodiazepines have been found to be more specific, with less toxicity, less potential for abuse, and fewer drug interactions.

V. Toxic mechanism:
   A. General depression of all excitable tissues, muscle, and especially CNS.
      1. Produces mild sedation to general anesthesia.
      2. Therapeutic doses have little effect on skeletal, cardiac, or smooth muscle.
      3. Anticonvulsant activity.
      4. Respiratory stimulating mechanisms are depressed with progressively higher doses.
   B. Major site of action appears to be at synaptic junctions. Mechanism of action at these junctions is not fully appreciated. Barbiturates depress excitatory postsynaptic potentials.
   C. Action of barbiturates on the reticular activating system is responsible for their sedative/hyponotic properties.
      1. Because of molecular changes necessary to lower lipid solubility, long-acting barbiturates will have less hypnotic and more anticonvulsant effect.
      2. The opposite characteristics are true for the short-acting barbiturates, which have a potent hypnotic effect.
   D. Poor antianxiolytic. No analgesic effect; may even potentiate pain perception.
   E. Vasodilation of peripheral capacitance vessels, negative inotropic effect on the myocardium, depression of medullary vasomotor centers.
   F. Effects potentiated by alcohol, hepatic disease, hypoalbuminemia, old age.

VI. Range of toxicity:
   A. Fatal dose: Drug ingestions of 6–10 gm long-acting and 2–3 gm short-acting barbiturates are potentially fatal.

VII. Clinical features:
   A. Signs and symptoms:
      1. CNS:
         a. Impairment of consciousness.
         b. Loss of motor reflex activity.
         c. Loss of thermoregulatory control: **Hypothermia.**
         d. Absent oculocephalic reflexes or forced downward ocular deviation.
         e. Pupillary findings normal.
         f. Flexor and extensor posturing may rarely be present.
         g. Euphoric effect.
         h. With severe coma and EEG findings, patient may actually appear brain dead; therefore cannot be declared so unless drug free for 24 hours. Improvement in EEG before clinical improvement.
         i. Respiratory depression to apnea. Apnea may be caused by administration of oxygen.

2. Cardiac:
   a. **Shock:** Hypotension related to increased venous capacity.
   b. Direct depression of myocardial contractility.
   c. Arrhythmias rare and probably secondary to other effects.
3. GI:
   a. Decreased gastrointestinal tone and motility.
   b. Cyclical reabsorption of drug.
4. Dermatologic:
   a. "Barbiturate burns" of bullous skin lesions occur over pressure points and over areas of increased skin tension such as wrists, knees, ankles.

B. Level of toxicity graded using Reed's classification of coma:
   1. Grade I:
      a. Responds to painful stimuli.
      b. Deep tendon reflexes present.
      c. Gag reflex present.
      d. Blood pressure normal and stable.
      e. Respirations of adequate rate and depth.
   2. Grade II:
      a. No response to painful stimuli.
      b. Deep tendon reflexes present.
      c. Gag reflex present.
      d. Blood pressure normal and stable.
      e. Respirations of adequate depth but may be slow.
   3. Grade III:
      a. No response to painful stimuli.
      b. Deep tendon and gag reflexes absent.
      c. Blood pressure stable but may be low.
      d. Respirations adequate but decreased.
   4. Grade IV:
      a. No response to painful stimuli.
      b. Deep tendon and gag reflexes absent.
      c. Blood pressure unstable and requires support.
      d. Respirations unstable and require support.

VIII. Laboratory findings and evaluation:
   A. Blood:
      1. Serum barbiturate levels:
         a. May be misleading because levels of intoxication and rate of elimination vary enormously from person to person, depending on prior drug use and patient's physical state.
         b. Delayed serum drug levels help to establish the individual's metabolic half-life of the drug and may identify further absorption from concretions.
         c. In general, serum level 30 µg/ml short-acting barbiturates or 80 µg/ml long-acting barbiturates indicates severe toxicity in the non-habituated patient.
      2. Arterial blood gas: Respiratory acidosis.
      3. Toxicology screen: Include ethanol.

    4. Blood glucose or Dextrostix: Altered mental status.

    5. CPK: Myoglobinuria.

    6. SGOT if indicated.

  B. Urinalysis.

IX. General treatment:

  A. Follow APTLS (see Chapter 8).

  B. General treatment: Table 55–3 (see Chapter 12 for details).

X. Specific management:

  A. Primarily supportive:

    1. Airway protection and ventilation (see Chapter 9).

    2. Hypotension: Fluids to support circulation related to vasodilation (see Chapter 10).

    3. Beginning in the emergency department, care should be taken to avoid skin and muscle necrosis by frequent turning of patient and padding of pressure points.

  B. Shock (see Chapter 10):

    1. Digoxin may be required to help support circulation in severe cases.

    2. Correct hypothermia.

  C. Treat barbiturate blisters as burns.

  D. Alkaline diuresis enhancement of elimination:

    1. Only effective for long-acting barbiturates.

    2. Detoxification increased by 30% to 180%.

    3. Must establish adequate hydration and renal function before initiation.

    4. Achieve diuresis of 3–6 ml/kg/hr.

    5. Give initial bolus of sodium bicarbonate (see Chapter 13).

    6. Give furosemide 0.5–2.0 mg/kg IV to maintain urine output.

    7. Add 2 ampules sodium bicarbonate to 1 L of D_5W, IV.

TABLE 55–3.

General Treatment

Treatment	Indicated	Of No Value	Contraindicated
O_2	+		
IV	+		
Forced diuresis*	±		
Acidification			X
Alkalinization*	+		
Emesis†	Caution		
Lavage†	+		
Charcoal	Repeated doses		
Cathartic†	+		
Dialysis	±		

*See specific management below.

†Because of potential delayed gastric motility, gastric emptying and catharsis are recommended regardless of time of ingestion. Concretions may have formed and endoscopic gastric lavage may be indicated.

8. Add additional sodium bicarbonate to IV as needed to achieve urinary pH 7.50–8.0.
9. Beware of cardiac and pulmonary overload even in young.
10. Use of forced alkaline diuresis may be controversial, but most authorities agree it is effective. However, it should be reserved for severely poisoned patients because of risks associated.

E. Dialysis:
1. Charcoal hemoperfusion:
   a. Most effective means of drug detoxification.
   b. Generally necessary if drug level >50 µg/ml short-acting barbiturates in nonhabituated patient and grade IV coma present with other complicating factors.
2. Hemodialysis:
   a. Useful for long-acting barbiturates, much less so for short-acting.
   b. Indications:
      (1) Generally necessary for drug level >100 µg/ml long-acting barbiturates in nonhabituated patient with grade IV coma.
      (2) Elderly.
      (3) Decreased renal, hepatic, or cardiovascular function.
      (4) No response to conventional therapy.
      (5) Deterioration of clinical condition.
3. Peritoneal dialysis:
   a. Not effective, especially for short-acting barbiturates.

XI. Prognosis:
A. Expected response to treatment:
1. Mortality ranges from 1% to 10% with higher rates associated with short-acting barbiturates.
2. Determine prognosis by severity of the clinical findings:
   a. Mild: Patient recovers without treatment.
   b. Moderate: Patient cannot be roused; respiration full and regular; no cyanosis or pulmonary edema present; blood pressure normal. Recovery in 24–48 hours with good nursing care and adequate fluid balance.
   c. Severe: Coma with shallow, irregular respiration; cyanosis; absence of all reflexes; low blood pressure; hypothermia of 0.5°–2° C; dilated pupils; absence of response to painful stimuli. Mortality should be less than 5%. Recovery of consciousness may require 3–5 days.
3. Prognosis on basis of serum levels alone is not possible. Serum levels of 30 µg/ml for short-acting barbiturates or 80 µg/ml for long-acting barbiturates indicate severe toxicity in the nonhabituated patient.
4. Prognosis with appropriate treatment is excellent if complications can be avoided:

B. Expected complications and long-term effects:
1. Morbidity and mortality directly increased by complicating factors:
   a. Pulmonary:
      (1) Infection: Pneumonia or pneumonitis (commonly related to *Staphylococcus* or gram-negative organisms), aspiration pneumonia, lung abscess.

(2) Atelectasis.
(3) Pulmonary edema.
(4) Septic pulmonary emboli.
(5) Pneumomediastinum, pneumothorax.
(6) Pulmonary fibrosis, pulmonary vascular granulomatosis
   b. Concurrent illness:
(1) Acute renal failure.
(2) Pulmonary edema.
(3) Deep venous thrombosis or pulmonary embolism.
(4) Withdrawal seizures in habituated patient.
(5) Pyrexia in convalescence.
   c. Aggressive forced diuresis when renal injury has occurred.
2. Long-term complications:
   a. Physiologic and psychologic dependence occur when the drugs are used in excess of sedative dose over 1–2 months.
   b. Abrupt discontinuance will precipitate withdrawal; hyperexcitable state, seizures, psychosis, and hyperpyrexia are possible.
   c. Hepatic enzyme induction with long-term use will enhance metabolism of other drugs (e.g., phenytoin, coumadin, tricyclic antidepressants). These drugs may become toxic on discontinuance of nonbenzodiazepine sedatives.
3. Withdrawl symptoms and pyrexia may occur during recovery from acute overdose by nonhabitual user.
XII. Special considerations:
   A. Drug interactions:
1. Increased CNS depression with ethanol, antihistamines, isoniazid, methylphenidate, and monoamine oxidase inhibitors.
2. Induction of hepatic microsomal enzymes accelerates metabolism of corticosteroids, oral anticoagulants, digitoxin, β-adrenergic antagonists, doxycycline, oral contraceptives, griseofulvin, quinidine, phenytoin, sulfa drugs, testosterone, tricyclic antidepressants, zoxazolamine, and vitamins D and K.
3. Hepatic enzyme metabolism may also induce toxic metabolite formation of acetaminophen, carbon tetrachloride, and hydrocarbon anesthetics.
4. Decreases absorption of dicoumerol and griseofulvin.
5. Protein binding competitively displaces thyroxine.
6. Untoward effects occur when other enzyme systems are induced, such as δ-amino levulinic acid synthetase, which exacerbates pain in porphyria.
   B. Drug abuse:
1. Abuse potential is great because of the euphoric effect but not as great as with other sedative/hypnotics such as methaqualone.
2. Tolerance:
   a. Develops quickly to sedative/hypnotic effects, thus requiring increasing doses continually to acquire the level of effect.
   b. Tolerance by the body's enzyme activation system peaks in a few days. Thus the therapeutic index decreases, as well as the margin

of safety, because the amount of drug required may be six times greater than the initial theapeutic dose.

3. Habituation is both physical and psychological and occurs as early as within 1 month.
4. Withdrawal:
   a. Sudden withdrawal in habitual users may precipitate hyperactivity manifested by tremor, anorexia, insomnia, abnormal sleep patterns, delirium, hyperpyrexia, and progressive seizures. Autonomic symptoms are also characteristic. Severe withdrawal may be life threatening.
   b. Seizures:
      1. Diazepam should be used in acute withdrawal to treat seizures, but benzodiazepines will not prevent this activity.
      2. The barbiturate must be reinstituted and then slowly withdrawn.

XIII. Controversies: Use of forced alkaline diuresis may be controversial, but most authorities agree it is effective. Its use, however, should be reserved for severely poisoned patients because of associated risks.

XIV. Disposition considerations:
   A. Admission considerations:
      1. See General Admission Considerations (Chapter 18).
      2. Depression of vital reflexes.
      3. Underlying illness potentiating drug effect.
      4. Complications.
      5. Grade II–IV coma 1 hour after ingestion.
      6. Symptoms persist after emergency department treatment.
   B. Consultation considerations:
      1. ICU admission with immediate (20–30 minutes) consultation by an internist is indicated in any patient with persistent altered level of consciousness or complications.
      2. Consider psychiatric consultation for all patients because use for suicide may be frequent.
   C. Observation period:
      1. Difficult to make recommendations because of great variety of barbiturate preparations with different half-lives, variable individual metabolism, and unpredictable response to treatment.
   D. Discharge considerations:
      1. General discharge considerations are met (see Chapter 18).
      2. No symptoms remain after observation period.
      3. Suicide potential and psychiatric status have been appropriately evaluated.
   E. Transfer considerations:
      1. Recommendations for barbiturate detoxification should be made, and if necessary patients should be transported by trained paramedical personnel to an appropriate detoxification facility.

XV. Similar acting drugs:
   A. Primidone (Mysoline):
      1. Primary anticonvulsant with active metabolites phenobarbital and phenylethylmalonamide.

2. Peak level 3 hours. Plasma half-life 8 hours.
3. Treatment as for long-acting barbiturates.
4. Crystalluria.

BIBLIOGRAPHY

Barbiturates: Short-acting. Barbiturates: Long-acting. *Poisindex,* vol 47. Micromedex, Inc, 1987.

Berg MJ, et al: Acceleration of the body clearance of phenobarbital by oral activated charcoal. *N Engl J Med* 1982; 307:642–644.

Byatt C, Volans G: Sedative and hypnotic drugs. *Br Med J* 1984; 289:1214–1217.

Gary N, Tresznewsky O: Barbiturates and a potpourri of other sedatives, hypnotics, and tranquilizers. *Heart Lung* 1983; 12:122–127.

Gilman AG, Goodman LS, Rall TW, et al: *The Pharmacological Basis of Therapeutics,* ed 7. New York, Macmillan Publishing Co, 1985.

Goldberg MJ, Berlinger WG: Treatment of phenobarbital overdose with activated charcoal. *JAMA* 1982; 247:2400–2401.

Goldfrank LR, Flomenbaum NE, Lewin NA, et al: *Toxicologic Emergencies,* ed 3. Norwalk, Conn, Appleton-Century-Crofts, 1986.

Greenberg D, Simon R: Flexor and extensor postures in sedative drug–induced coma. *Neurology* 1982; 32:448–451.

Haddad LM, Winchester JF: *Clinical Management of Poisoning and Drug Overdose.* Philadelphia, WB Saunders Co, 1983.

Hadden J, Johnson K, Smith S, et al: Acute barbiturate intoxication. *JAMA* 1969; 209:893–900.

McCarron M, Schulze B, Walberg C, et al: Short-acting barbiturate overdosage. Correlation of intoxication score with serum barbiturate concentration. *JAMA* 1982; 248:55–61.

56

Benzodiazepines

V. Gail Ray, M.D., F.A.C.E.P.

I. Route of exposure: Oral, intravenous, intramuscular.
II. Common generic and trade names: See Table 56–1.
III. Pharmacokinetics:
   A. Absorption: All formulations are virtually 100% absorbed from gut.
   B. Onset of action: Onset within seconds when given IV; see Table 56–2.
   C. Plasma half-life: See Table 56–2.
   D. Peak effect: Peak plasma concentration (correlates with peak effect) varies from 0.5–8 hours; see Table 56–2.
   E. Duration of action:
      1. Short acting: e.g., triazolam, midazolam, brotizolam.
      2. Intermediate acting: e.g., oxazepam, lorazepam.
      3. Long acting: e.g., chlordiazepoxide, diazepam, flurazepam, clonazepam, clorazepate.
   F. Elimination: All parent compounds and active metabolites metabolized in the liver by either desmethylation or conjugation with glucuronide, then excreted by kidney. Renal elimination of free parent and active metabolites negligible. Enterohepatic circulation resecretes drug into gut.
   G. Metabolites: See Table 56–2.
IV. Actions and uses:
   A. Widely prescribed sedative/hypnotic, anxiolytic, muscle relaxant, amnestic, anticonvulsant.
   B. Some abuse potential but low in relation to other sedative/hypnotics.
V. Toxic mechanism:
   A. Actual drug effect determined by active metabolites and their half-lives.
   B. Mechanism of action proposed to be potentiation of neural inhibition by GABA in the CNS. GABA inhibition of neurons in the spinal cord is prob-

TABLE 56–1.

Benzodiazepines

Generic Name	Trade Name	Oral Dosage (mg)
Alprazolam	Xanax	0.25, 0.5, 1
Chlordiazepoxide	Librium	5, 10, 25
Clonazepam	Clonopin	0.5, 1,0, 2
Clorazepate dipotassium	Tranxene	3.75, 7.5, 15
Clorazepate monopotassium	Azene	3.25, 6.5, 13
Diazepam	Valium	2, 5, 10, 15
	Valrelease	
Flurazepam	Dalmane	15, 30
Halazepam	Paxipam	20, 40
Lorazepam	Ativan	0.5, 1, 2
Oxazepam	Serax	10, 15, 30
Prazepam	Centrax	5, 10
	Verstran	
Temazepam	Restoril	15, 30
Triazolam	Halcion	0.125, 0.25, 0.5

ably the mechanism of muscle relaxation. Suppresses spread of seizure activity.
- C. Has a specific CNS site of action with good therapeutic (sedative) effect but minimal generalized CNS depression or toxicity.
- D. Anticholinergic effects.
- E. Most toxicity results when used in combination with other CNS depressants.
- F. Rapid IV administration may produce coronary vasodilation, neuromuscular blockade, and respiratory arrest (particularly in infants).
- VI. Range of toxicity:
  - A. Toxic dose: Least toxic of all sedative/hypnotics; no established toxic dose.
  - B. Fatal dose:
    1. Used alone, even high oral doses not fatal. No well-substantiated fatalities reported from single drug oral ingestions.
    2. Combination of benzodiazepine and ethanol can be fatal.
    3. IV administration has been associated with life-threatening conditions, including hypotension and cardiopulmonary arrest.
- VII. Clinical features:
  - A. Progressive CNS depression including sedation, hypnosis, stupor, and delirium.
  - B. Side effects include weakness, headache, ataxia, dizziness, impaired motor function, confusion.
  - C. Major symptoms rarely include seizure, hyperthermia, psychosis, hypotension, and respiratory depression.
  - D. Anticholinergic effects include dry mouth, dilated pupils, and tachycardia.

TABLE 56–2.
Pharmacodynamics of Benzodiazepines

	Absorption (following ingestion)	Peak Effect (hr)	Half-Life (hr)	Elimination	Metabolites
Diazepam	Rapid	1–2	24	2–3 hr (rapid phase) 2–3 days (slow phase) Renal 70%	Oxazepam (active)
Chlordiazepoxide	Slow	2–4	24–48*	Renal	Two active
Oxazepam	Rapid	4	3–21†	Renal	Inactive
Chlorazepate	Rapid	0.5–3+	48–96	Renal	Active
Flurazepam	Rapid	1–4+	50–100†	Renal	Glucuronide conjugate
Lorazepam	Rapid	2	12		

*Slower in elderly and patients with hepatic disease.
†Biotransformation.

    E. Presence of other CNS depressants is usually responsible for coma, respiratory depression, hypothermia, and hypotension.

    F. Withdrawal symptoms are infrequent, usually manifesting as increased anxiety, insomnia, and anorexia approximately 5 days after last benzodiazepine intake. At times withdrawal reactions can be severe (see Special considerations below).

VIII. Laboratory findings and evaluation:

    A. Serum levels: Not helpful because of numerous active metabolites with varying half-lives and individual rates of elimination.

    B. Toxicology screen. NOTE: **May fail to diagnose ingestions of alprazolam, clonazepam, temazepam, and triazolam.**

    C. Routine laboratory tests not helpful in making specific diagnoses.

IX. General treatment:

    A. Follow APTLS (see Chapter 8).

    B. General Management: See Table 56–3 (see Chapter 12 for details).

    C. Ventilatory support may be necessary to avoid atelectasis.

X. Specific treatment:

    A. Hypotension: Should respond to volume expansion alone.

    B. Forced diuresis and hemodialysis are ineffective because of high degree of protein binding.

    C. Physostigmine will reverse CNS depression but should not be used because risks far outweigh toxicity of benzodiazepines (see Chapter 91).

    D. A specific antagonist, RO15-1788 (not currently approved in the United States) has been reported to result in immediate reversal of CNS depression when administered intravenously.

    E. Contraindicated therapy: Stimulants.

XI. Prognosis:

    A. Expected response to treatment: Most patients do well with only careful observation.

    B. Expected complications and long-term effects: No significant long-term medical complications if good supportive care provided (e.g., prevention of aspiration in patients with temporarily depressed level of consciousness).

TABLE 56–3.

General Treatment

Treatment	Indicated	Of No Value	Contraindicated
O_2	±		
IV	±		
ECG monitor	±		
Forced diuresis		X	
Acidification		X	
Alkalinization		X	
Emesis/lavage	+/+		
Charcoal	Repeated doses		
Cathartic	+		
Dialysis		X	

XII. Special considerations:
   A. Crossover occurs in placenta and breast milk. Possibility of increased risk for malformations when benzodiazepines used in first trimester.
   B. Severe withdrawal reactions can be seen after prolonged or excessive use of benzodiazepines. Signs and symptoms include psychosis and seizures. With long-acting benzodiazepines, such as diazepam, withdrawal symptoms may be delayed for days to weeks.
   C. A new potent intravenously administered benzodiazepine, midazolam HCl (Versed) has been used for sedation. Midazolam is three to four times as potent as diazepam. Reported adverse reactions include respiratory depression, apnea, and cardiac arrest.
XIII. Disposition considerations:
   A. Admission considerations:
      1. See General Admission Considerations (Chapter 18).
      2. Patients with depression of vital reflexes (e.g., respiration, gag reflex).
      3. Altered sensorium, especially with intermediate- and long-acting preparations or when multiple drugs are involved.
      4. Suicide risk.
   B. Consultation considerations: Consider psychiatric consultation for any patient who attempted suicide.
   C. Observation period. Difficult to make recommendations because of great variety of benzodiazepine preparations with different half-lives, active metabolites also with different half-lives, and variable individual metabolism.
   D. Discharge considerations:
      1. General discharge considerations have been met (see Chapter 18).
      2. Asymptomatic with normal examination and mental status.
      3. Suicide potential and psychiatric status have been appropriately evaluated.
      4. Stable discharge environment exists, to allow for close observation of the patient's mental status and level of consciousness.

BIBLIOGRAPHY

Benzodiazepines. *Poisindex,* vol 47. Micromedex, Inc, 1987.

Divoll M, Greenblatt D, Lacasse Y, et al: Benzodiazepine overdose: Plasma concentration and clinical outcome. *Psychopharmacology* 1981; 73:381–383.

Gilman AG, Goodman LS, Rall RW, et al: *The Pharmacological Basis of Therapeutics,* ed 7. New York, Macmillan Publishing Co, 1985, pp 339–351.

Haddad LM, Winchester JF: *Clinical Management of Poisoning and Drug Overdose.* Philadelphia, WB Saunders Co, 1983, pp 475–482.

Havasi G, Gintautas J, et al: Reversibility of diazepam overdose by physostigmine. *Proc West Pharmacol Soc* 1981; 24:109–112.

Hofer P, Scollo-Lavizzari G: Benzodiazepine antagonist Ro 15-1788 in self poisoning. *Arch Intern Med* 1985; 145:663–667.

Scollo-Lavizzari G: First clinical investigation of the benzodiazepine antagonist Ro 15-1788 in comatose patients. *Eur Neurol* 1983; 22:7–11.

57

Paraldehyde

V. Gail Ray, M.D., F.A.C.E.P.

I. Route of exposure: Oral, rectal, intravenous, intramuscular.
II. Common names: Paraldehyde.
III. Pharmacokinetics:
    A. Absorption: Rapid absorption from gut.
    B. Onset of action: Rapidly acting in 10–15 minutes.
    C. Half-life:
        1. 7 hours for parent compound.
        2. 30 hours or more in presence of liver disease.
    D. Peak concentration: 30 minutes.
    E. Duration of action: Hypnotic effect may last 8–12 hours but is greatly dependent on amount taken and patient's tolerance.
    F. Elimination: 70% to 80% metabolized in liver, remainder exhaled by lung; negligible excretion by kidney.
    G. Active metabolites: Metabolized to acetaldehyde, then oxidizes to acetic acid, which converts to carbon dioxide and water.
IV. Actions:
    A. Global depression of CNS function.
    B. No analgesic properties; may even increase pain perception.
    C. Addiction similar to alcohol addiction may occur with chronic use, and withdrawal may produce delirium tremens.
V. Uses:
    A. Obsolete sedative/hypnotic, currently limited to institutional use; toxic cases are thus rare.
    B. Most often used now only for occasional alcohol withdrawal syndromes.

VI. Toxic mechanism:
   A. Hallmark of toxicity is increased anion gap–type metabolic acidosis, probably resulting from breakdown of paraldehyde to acetaldehyde and acetic acid.
   B. CNS depression.
   C. Direct corrosive damage to tissues at sites of administration.
   D. Toxic hepatitis may occur with fatty changes in the liver.
   E. Pulmonary edema and hemorrhage may occur related to corrosive effect of alveolar excretion of the drug. Liver disease will increase tendency for pulmonary damage because more drug must be excreted via lung.
   F. Toxic nephrosis may result from metabolic acidosis or direct effect of metabolites on the kidney.
   G. Hepatic disease will prolong elimination and greatly increase toxicity. Note that it is precisely in those most prone to severe liver disease, the alcoholic population, who are most likely to receive this drug.
VII. Range of toxicity:
   A. Therapeutic dose:
      1. Oral: 5–10 ml.
      2. Rectal: 30 ml maximum dose.
      3. Intravenous: 2–3 ml.
      4. Narrow therapeutic index and margin of safety.
   B. Fatal dose:
      1. Difficult to establish lethal dose because of wide individual variance in therapeutic and toxic range.
      2. Deaths have occurred after administration of 25 ml by mouth and 12 ml by rectum.
VIII. Clinical features:
   A. CNS depression:
      1. Not always dose related.
      2. Ranges from stupor to coma.
      3. Associated with **respiratory depression** and **hypotension.**
      4. Level of toxicity is graded using Reed's classification of coma (see Chapter 55).
   B. Metabolic acidosis: Increased anion gap acidosis is hallmark of toxicity.
   C. GI:
      1. Esophagitis, hemorrhagic gastritis, proctitis.
      2. Toxic hepatitis.
   D. Local: Sterile abscess, muscle necrosis, neuropathic damage, thrombosis at sites of administration.
   E. Intravenous use may cause several minutes of **paroxysmal coughing** and may precipitate **laryngeal spasm.**
   F. **Pulmonary edema** and hemorrhage.
IX. Laboratory findings and evaluation:
   A. Serum levels: Minimal lethal blood level is about 50 mg/dl. However, levels may be misleading because resultant toxicity and rate of elimination vary enormously from person to person.
   B. Arterial blood gas, electrolytes, stat Na/K$^+$, ECG: Metabolic acidosis.
   C. Chest x-ray examination: Pulmonary edema.

   D. Baseline liver function tests: SGOT, SGPT, bilirubin.

   E. Renal studies: BUN, creatinine, urinalysis.

   F. Monitor coagulation studies, particularly prothrombin time, if severe liver dysfunction.

   G. Hematocrit, type and cross match: Hemorrhagic gastritis.

X. General treatment:

   A. Follow APTLS (see Chapter 8).

   B. General management: Table 57–1 (see Chapter 12 for details).

XI. Specific treatment:

   A. Support vital functions.

   B. Hypotension (see Chapter 10).

      1. Avoid overhydration. Central venous pressure or Swan-Ganz monitoring may be necessary.

   C. Positive end-expiratory pressure (PEEP) ventilation may be necessary.

   D. Metabolic acidosis; $NaHCO_3$, keep pH >7.25.

   E. Dialysis should be used for acidosis unresponsive to bicarbonate administration or in presence of acute renal failure.

XII. Prognosis:

   A. Survival for 48 hours after acute poisoning is associated with good long-term prognosis.

   B. In severe toxicity, however, serious complications are common despite timely and appropriate therapy because of direct toxic effects on organs and degree of metabolic acidosis.

   C. Complete recovery after chronic paraldehyde toxicity is uncommon.

XIII. Disposition considerations:

   A. Admission considerations:

      1. See General Admission Considerations (Chapter 18).

      2. Presence of metabolic acidosis, no matter how minimal.

TABLE 57–1.

General Treatment

Treatment	Indicated	Of No Value	Contraindicated
O₂	+		
IV	+		
ECG monitor	+		
Forced diuresis*		X	
Acidification			X
Alkalinization†	±		
Emesis‡/lavage‡	±/±		
Charcoal	+		
Cathartic	+		
Dialysis§	±		

*Not effective and pulmonary edema a possible complication.
†Depends on severity of acidosis.
‡Emesis and lavage are probably of no value because drug is extremely rapidly absorbed
§In intractable acidosis.

    3. Any symptoms.

    4. ICU: Need for respiratory or cardiovascular support or presence of serious complications such as pulmonary edema.

B. Consultation considerations: Consultation with nephrologist if hemodialysis indicated.

C. Observation period: None. All patients with toxic exposure should be admitted.

D. Discharge considerations: None. All patients with toxic exposure should be admitted.

BIBLIOGRAPHY

Giacoia G, Gessner P, et al: Pharmacokinetics of paraldehyde disposition in the neonate. *J Pediatr.* 1984; 104:291–296.

Gilman AG, Goodman LS, Rall TW, et al: *The Pharmacological Basis of Therapeutics,* ed 7. New York, Macmillan Publishing Co, 1985, pp 366–367.

Goldfrank LR, Flomenbaum NE, Lewin NA: *Toxicologic Emergencies,* ed 3. Norwalk, Conn, Appleton-Century-Crofts, 1986, pp 427–428.

Haddad EM, Winchester JF: *Clinical Management of Poisoning and Drug Overdose.* Philadelphia, WB Saunders Co, 1983, pp 410–413.

Paraldehyde. *Poisindex,* vol 52. Micromedex, Inc, 1987.

58

Ethchlorvynol

V. Gail Ray, M.D., F.A.C.E.P.

I. Route of exposure: Oral intravenous.
II. Common trade name: Placidyl.
III. Pharmacokinetics:
    A. Absorption: Rapidly and completely absorbed from GI tract in therapeutic doses.
    B. Onset of action: 15–30 minutes.
    C. Plasma half-life:
        1. 25 hours with therapeutic dose.
        2. >100 hours with toxic levels.
    D. Peak levels: Peak serum levels at 1–1.5 hours.
    E. Duration of action: Clinical effects last 5 hours.
    F. Elimination: 90% metabolized by liver but not affected by liver disease; 10% excreted unchanged by kidney.
IV. Actions:
    A. CNS depression.
    B. Respiratory depression.
V. Uses: Sedative/hypnotic similar to barbiturate, anticonvulsant, muscle relaxant.
VI. Range of toxicity:
    A. Therapeutic (hypnotic) dose: 500 mg.
    B. Toxic dose: Doses 10 to 25 times therapeutic dose can produce severe intoxication.
    C. Fatal dose: Variable. Lethal ingestions of 10–50 gm have been reported; however, as little as 2.5 gm has produced death. On the other hand, survival has been reported for ingestions ranging from 25–50 gm.

VII. Clinical features:
   A. CNS:
      1. Generalized CNS depression in progressive grades of coma. Coma can be extremely prolonged in severe overdoses (up to 288 hours has been reported).
      2. Flexor-extensor posturing possible.
      3. Flat EEG possible.
      4. Seizures.
   B. Cardiovascular:
      1. Hypotension and bradycardia.
      2. Noncardiac pulmonary edema. More commonly associated with IV use.
   C. Pulmonary: Respiratory depression, adult respiratory distress syndrome.
   D. Hypothermia.
   E. Skin bullae.
   F. Pungent or aromatic breath odor.
   G. Withdrawal: In chronic users abrupt discontinuance of ethchlorvynol may precipitate convulsions and syndrome similar to delirium tremens, with acute psychosis.
VIII. Laboratory findings and evaluation:
   A. Serum levels: May be misleading. Toxicity and rate of elimination vary enormously from person to person.
   B. Toxicology screen: May be helpful in identifying drug.
   C. Chest x-ray examination and arterial blood gas: Indicated for baseline and evaluation of respiratory depression and pulmonary edema.
IX. Treatment:
   A. Follow APTLS (see Chapter 8).
   B. General management: Table 58–1 (see Chapter 12 for details).

TABLE 58–1.

General Treatment

Treatment	Indicated	Of No Value	Contraindicated
O₂	±		
IV	±		
ECG monitor	±		
Forced diuresis		X	
Acidification		X	
Alkalinization		X	
Emesis*/lavage*	+/+		
Charcoal	Repeated doses		
Cathartic	+		
Dialysis		×	
Hemoperfusion	±†		

*Substantial amounts of drug can be removed many hours (8 or more) after ingestion.
†See indications below.

X. Specific treatment:
  A. Hypotension (see Chapter 10).
  B. Seizures:
    1. Avoid treating with barbiturates.
    2. See Chapter 22.
  C. Hemoperfusion
    1. Charcoal hemoperfusion reportedly successful. Should be repeated 4–8 hours after initial treatment, because drug redistributes from lipids to plasma.
    2. Indications:
      a. Ingestion of a potentially fatal dose (>10 gm).
      b. Ingestion of >100 mg/kg body weight.
      c. Serum levels >10 mg/dl in first 12 hours or >7 mg/dl later.
      d. Prolonged coma with life-threatening complications despite intensive supportive therapy.
    3. Amberlite XAD-4 resin hemoperfusion reported to remove 100% of drug in single pass.
    4. Hemodialysis and peritoneal dialysis not effective because of high lipid solubility and redistribution of drug to brain and adipose tissues.
XI. Prognosis:
  A. Expected response to treatment:
    1. If patient can be roused, full recovery is expected.
    2. If patient is comatose with normal vital signs, no evidence of cyanosis, and no pulmonary complications (aspiration, pulmonary edema), recovery should occur in 24–48 hours with good supportive care.
    3. With grade III or IV coma (Reed classification; see Chapter 55), mortality reported to be less than 5%, with recovery of consciousness within 3–5 days.
  B. Expected complications and long-term effects:
    1. Most patients will do well with only supportive therapy, although prolonged coma is common.
    2. Pulmonary aspiration and pneumonia.
    3. Pulmonary edema.
    4. Long-term complications extremely rare.
XII. Special considerations:
  A. Tolerance develops with chronic use.
  B. Ethchlorvynol abusers using up to 4 gm/day may develop a high degree of physical dependence. This is of significant clinical importance because abrupt discontinuance of ethchlorvynol in chronic abusers may precipitate convulsions and a syndrome similar to delirium tremens with acute psychosis.
XIII. Disposition considerations:
  A. Admission considerations:
    1. See General Admission Considerations (Chapter 18).
    2. Development of significant clinical toxicity within 2 hours of ingestion.
    3. ICU: Depression of vital reflexes (e.g., respiration, gag reflex), need for respiratory or cardiovascular support, or presence of serious compli-

cations such as prolonged coma, severe hypotension, pulmonary edema.
B. Consultation considerations:
   1. A nephrologist should be consulted for consideration of hemoperfusion for patients unresponsive to normal supportive care.
C. Observation period: Difficult to make specific recommendations because of variable individual metabolism of ethychlorvynol.
D. Discharge considerations:
   1. General discharge considerations are met (see Chapter 18).
   2. Generally, patients who are easily roused after several hours of emergency department observation may ultimately be safely discharged home if no evidence of serious toxicity or complications have developed.
   3. Suicide risk and psychiatric status have been appropriately assessed.

BIBLIOGRAPHY

Ethchlorvynol. *Poisindex,* vol 47. Micromedex, Inc., 1987.

Gilman AG, Goodman LS, Rall TW, et al: *The Pharmacological Basis of Therapeutics,* ed 7.: New York, Macmillan Publishing Co, 1985, pp 362–363.

Goldfrank LR, Flomenbaum NE, Lewin NA: *Toxicologic Emergencies,* ed 3. Norwalk, Conn, Appleton-Century-Crofts, 1986, p 430.

Haddad EM, Winchester JF: *Clinical Management of Poisoning and Drug Overdose.* Philadelphia, WB Saunders Co, 1983, pp 516–520.

Kathpalia S, Hasbitt J, et al: Charcoal hemoperfusion for treatment of ethchlorvynol overdose. *Artif Organs* 1983; 7:246–248.

Kilner M, Bailey D: Ethchlorvynol ingestion: Interpretation of blood concentrations and clinical findings. *Clin Toxicol* 1983–84; 21(3):399–408.

59

Methaqualone

V. Gail Ray, M.D., F.A.C.E.P.

I. Route of exposure: Usually **oral,** but may be **smoked.**
II. Common names:
  A. Trade names:
    1. **Quaalude, Sopor** (75, 150, 300 mg tablets).
    2. **Mequin, Optimal, Parest, Somnafac** (175, 350 mg tablets).
  B. Street names: **Quaaludes, ludes, sopors, sopes.**
III. Pharmacokinetics:
  A. Onset of action: Rapidly absorbed within 2 hours.
  B. Peak levels: 1–2 hours.
  C. Half-life: Elimination half-life **10–40 hours.**
  D. Duration of action: Depends on half-life.
  E. Elimination: Hydroxylated in **liver** to inactive metabolites, then excreted by kidney. Hepatic microsomal enzyme system is induced. Biliary excretion is 1% to 4%. Renal elimination is less than 1% unchanged.
IV. Action:
  A. Euphoria. Abusers claim a rapid "high" with minimal sedation and falsely attribute aphrodisiac qualities to methaqualone.
  B. Cardiovascular depression usually exceeds that of respiratory depression; both are less severe than in barbiturate poisoning.
  C. CNS depression similar to that with barbiturates develops and potentiates effects of alcohol and other CNS depressants.
V. Uses:
  A. Formerly a major drug of abuse in Europe and the United States until recently withdrawn from the market. Still available through Mexico and Canada (*Med Lett,* 1987; 29:83).
  B. Sedative/hypnotic, anticonvulsant, antispasmodic, local anesthetic, antitussive, weakly antihistaminic.

VI. Toxic mechanism:
   A. Exact mechanism unknown. In high doses, drug appears to selectively depress polysynaptic spinal cord pathways.
   B. Most deaths result from injury related to impaired judgment and reflexes rather than as a direct toxic effect.
VII. Range of toxicity:
   A. Adult: Death has been reported following an 8 gm ingestion. Chronic abusers tolerate up to three times the dose in inexperienced users.
   B. Child: One tablet should be considered toxic.
VIII. Clinical features (also see Action):
   A. CNS depression.
   B. Pyramidal signs of hypertonicity, hyperreflexia, myoclonus, and seizures. Extensor-flexor posturing is possible.
   C. Cardiovascular depression; usually only mild hypotension results. Tachycardia is rare, but myocardial damage possible.
   D. Other:
      1. Bullous skin lesions.
      2. Bleeding diathesis from impaired platelet function.
      3. Increased vascular permeability may manifest as noncardiogenic pulmonary edema, effusions, and increased secretions.
      4. Pyrexia possible.
   E. Physiologic dependence develops rapidly.
      1. In chronic users (e.g., 2 gm/day for 3–4 weeks) abrupt discontinuance of methaqualone may precipitate withdrawal 16–24 hours after last dose, with peak clinical effect in 48–72 hours.
      2. Withdrawal characterized by headache, anorexia, nausea, abdominal cramps, tremor, nervousness, and insomnia. Seizures usually appear after 3–5 days.
IX. Laboratory findings and evaluation:
   A. Toxicology screen:
      1. Serum levels: May be misleading. Degree of intoxication with given level and rate of elimination vary enormously.
      2. 2–3 mg/dl considered lethal blood level.
   B. Blood:
      1. Complete blood cell count, platelets, prothrombin time, partial thromboplastin time, baseline liver function studies, electrolytes.
      2. Arterial blood gas analyses with respiratory symptoms.
   C. ECG: Reversible right bundle branch block, T-wave changes.
   D. Chest x-ray studies to monitor development of pulmonary edema.
X. General treatment:
   A. Follow APTLS (see Chapter 8).
   B. General management: See Table 59–1 (see Chapter 12 for details).
XI. Specific treatment:
   A. Supportive care is usually all that is necessary for most patients.
   B. Hypotension: see Chapter 10.
   C. Dialysis:
      1. Reserved for patients with deterioration despite supportive treatment. Peritoneal and hemodialysis are only minimally effective.

TABLE 59–1.

General Treatment

Treatment	Indicated	Of No Value	Contraindicated
O$_2$	±		
IV	±		
ECG monitor	±		
Forced diuresis			X*
Acidification			X
Alkalinization		X	
Emesis/lavage	+/+		
Charcoal	+		
Cathartic	+		
Dialysis		Minimally effective	
Hemoperfusion	Effective†		

*Tendency for pulmonary edema. Probably not an effective therapeutic method.
†See indications below.

    2. Hemoperfusion with activated charcoal or cation-exchange resins may be effective and should be considered **when plasma levels exceed 40 μg/ml.**

  D. Seizures: Diazepam IV and load with phenytoin (see Chapter 22).

XII. Prognosis:

  A. Expected response to treatment:

    1. Mild intoxication: Patient can be roused at all times in clinical course. No complications expected.

    2. Moderate intoxication: Coma but no cardiopulmonary compromise: Recovery expected in 24–48 hours.

    3. Severe intoxication: Coma, cardiac or pulmonary compromise, areflexia, mild hypothermia: Mortality rate should be less than 5%. Recovery of consciousness, however, may take 3–5 days.

  B. Expected complications and long-term effects:

    1. Severe overdoses are often complicated by **aspiration** pneumonitis and pneumonia.

    2. Long-term complications may include **neuropathy** with weakness and numbness in stocking-glove distribution to distal extremities. These usually resolve spontaneously during convalescence but may persist for years.

XIII. Special considerations:

  A. Street "ludes" may also contain other drugs in varying quantities, including **benzodiazepines, meprobamate, phencyclidine, barbiturates, ephedrine, diphenhydramine.**

XIV. Disposition considerations:

  A. Admission considerations:

    1. See General Admission Considerations (Chapter 18).

2. Altered or depressed level of consciousness decreasing or persistent after 2 hours.
3. Symptomatic within 2 hours after ingestion.
4. Drug levels do not always correlate with toxicity, but 1 mg/dl 2 hours after ingestion is an indication for admission.
5. Suicide risk.

B. Consultation considerations: Nephrology consultation if dialysis or hemoperfusion indicated.

C. Observation period: Significant toxicity should be clinically apparent by 2 hours after ingestion.

D. Discharge considerations:
1. General discharge considerations are met (see Chapter 18).
2. Patient asymptomatic after sufficient observation (at least 2 hours).
3. Suicide risk has been appropriately assessed.

BIBLIOGRAPHY

Bryson PD: *Comprehensive Review in Toxicology.* Rockville, Md, Aspen Systems Corp, 1986, pp 207–209.

Gilman AG, Goodman LS, Rall TW, et al: *The Pharmacological Basis of Therapeutics,* ed 7. New York, Macmillan Publishing Co, 1985, pp 365–366.

Goldfrank LR, Flomenbaum NE, Lewin NA: *Toxicologic Emergencies,* ed 3. Norwalk, Conn, Appleton-Century-Crofts, 1986, p 430.

Haddad LM, Winchester JF: *Clinical Management of Poisoning and Drug Overdose.* Philadelphia, WB Saunders Co, 1983, pp 466–469.

Methaqualone. *Poisindex,* Vol 53. Micromedex, Inc, 1987.

60

Meprobamate

V. Gail Ray, M.D., F.A.C.E.P.

I. Route of exposure: Oral
II. Common trade names:

Bamate	Miltown
Equagesic	Neuromate
Equanil	Pathibamate
Mepripam	SK-Bamate
Meprotabs	Suronil
Milpath	

III. Pharmacokinetics:
  A. Onset of action: Rapid absorption and onset of action.
  B. Half-life: 10 hours, but is dose dependent (range 6–17 hours).
  C. Peak effect: 2–3 hours.
  D. Duration of action: Dependent on half-life; however, most patients should metabolize and clear the drug in 36 hours.
  E. Elimination:
    1. 90% renal elimination of mostly hydroxylated and glucuronide conjugates from the liver, with some unchanged drug.
    2. 10% Fecal.
  F. Active metabolites: None.
IV. Action:
  A. Mild muscle relaxant (related to sedation).
  B. Hyperalgesic.
  C. Poor anticonvulsant except in petit mal seizure disorders.
  D. Hypnotic at doses greater than therapeutic dose.
  E. Euphoric with great abuse potential.

289

V. Uses:
   A. A carbamate derivative that acts like an intermediate barbiturate; approved only as an anxiolytic.
VI. Toxic mechanism:
   A. Site and mode of action not well understood; however, part of its depressant activity appears to involve polysynaptic reflexes leading to CNS depression, respiratory depression, and hypotension.
   B. Possible direct myocardial depressant.
VII. Range of toxicity:
   A. Toxic dose: Serious ingestions roughly correlate with doses >12 gm.
   B. Fatal dose: 12 gm lowest reported; usually >40 gm.
VIII. Clinical features:
   A. Barbiturate-like **CNS depression,** leading to **respiratory depression.**
   B. Cardiac:
      1. **Hypotension:** may occur **suddenly,** even in mild overdoses.
      2. **Arrhythmias.**
      3. **Pulmonary edema** may develop readily, especially after aggressive fluid administration.
   C. Synergistic effect when used with **ethanol** or other depressants.
   D. **Extrapyramidal** symptoms may occur with tonic-clonic reflexes, nystagmus, and ataxia.
   E. Excessive oronasal **secretions.**
   F. Muscle relaxation.
IX. Laboratory findings and evaluation:
   A. Blood:
      1. Quantitative meprobamate level:
         a. Therapeutic level 1 mg/dl.
         b. CNS depression results at 5 mg/dl, coma at 10 mg/dl.
         c. Fatalities reported at levels 5–20 mg/dl; lower with alcohol.
      2. Arterial blood gas on presence of respiratory symptoms.
   B. ECG.
   C. Chest x-ray study with respiratory symptoms.
X. General treatment:
   A. Follow APTLS (see Chapter 8).
   B. General management: Table 60–1 (see Chapter 12 for details).
XI. Specific management:
   A. **Supportive care** usually all that is necessary, but with close monitoring of cardiac status and blood pressure; beware sudden onset of hypotension.
   B. Gastric lavage in combination with endoscopy may be necessary to remove large meprobamate **concretions.** Presence of concretions may prolong clinical effects of drug.
   C. Hypotension: Early use of **vasopressors** indicated because shock is not always responsive to volume expansion and heart failure may be precipitated by fluid loading.
   D. Hemoperfusion:
      1. **Hemoperfusion** with activated charcoal or amberlite XAD-4 resin has been reported to be effective.

TABLE 60–1.

General Treatment

Treatment	Indicated	Of No Value	Contraindicated
O_2	±		
IV	+		
ECG monitor	+		
Forced diuresis*			X
Acidification			X
Alkalinization		X	
Emesis/lavage†	+/+		
Charcoal	Repeated doses		
Cathartic	+		
Suction and cardiopulmonary toilet‡	+		
Dialysis		±	
Hemoperfusion	Effective§		

*Risk of pulmonary edema.
†May need to perform in combination with endoscopy (see below).
‡See Special Considerations.
§See indications below.

2. Indications:
   a. Patient's condition deteriorates despite supportive treatment
   b. Patient has ingested >30 gm and has depression of brainstem functions.
3. Peritoneal dialysis is considered poorly effective; only slightly better results have been obtained with hemodialysis.

XII. Prognosis:
   A. Expected response to treatment:
      1. Supportive care alone has been associated with low incidence of morbidity and mortality. Complications increase in proportion to duration of coma.
      2. Most deaths result from irreversible shock and pulmonary edema.
   B. Expected complications and long-term effects:
      1. Formation of gastric concretions with continued absorption of drug.
      2. CNS depression with secondary aspiration, respiratory depression, pulmonary edema, hypotension.
      3. No direct long-term effects expected.

XIII. Special considerations:
   A. Excessive oronasal secretions may necessitate frequent suctioning and compulsive attention to pulmonary toilet.
   B. Forced diuresis is contraindicated because of increased risk of pulmonary edema.
   C. Withdrawal:
      1. Tolerance develops because of induction of hepatic microsomal enzymes, with physical dependence resulting after daily intake of 1.2 gm.

2. In patients with physical dependence, abrupt discontinuance of methaqualone may precipitate withdrawal 12–48 hours after last dose.
3. Withdrawal is characterized by anxiety, insomnia, tremors, gastrointestinal disturbances, and hallucinations. In severe cases generalized seizures may occur, and at least one death has been reported related to withdrawal.

XIV. Disposition considerations:
   A. Admission considerations:
      1. See General Admission Considerations (Chapter 18).
      2. Symptomatic within 3 hours of ingestion.
      3. Development of cardiac or respiratory symptoms at any time.
      4. Drug levels do not always correlate with toxicity, but 3 mg/dl 3 hours after ingestion is an indication for admission.
      5. Suicide risk.
   B. Consultation considerations:
      1. Nephrology consultation if dialysis or hemoperfusion indicated.
      2. General surgical and GI consultation for removal of large gastric concretions.
   C. Observation period:
      1. Most patients are symptomatic within 3 hours of ingestion.
      2. Concretions may alter this, as may other conditions delaying absorption.
   D. Discharge considerations:
      1. General disposition considerations are met (see Chapter 18).
      2. Asymptomatic.
      3. Suicide risk and psychiatric state have been appropriately addressed.

XV. Related drugs:
   A. **Carisoprodal (Soma, Reia), phenaglycodol,** and **emylcamate** are similar in toxicity to meprobamate. Treatment of overdose is the same.
   B. **Benactyzine** seems to exert toxic effects related to its anticholinergic action.
   C. **Phenprobamate** has not been reported to have severe toxic effects.

BIBLIOGRAPHY

Bryson PD: *Comprehensive Review in Toxicology.* Rockville, Md, Aspen Systems Corp, 1986, pp 210–211.
Gilman AG, Goodman LS, Rall TW, et al: *The Pharmacological Basis of Therapeutics,* ed 7. New York, Macmillan Publishing Co, 1985, pp 364–365.
Haddad LM, Winchester JF: *Clinical Management of Poisoning and Drug Overdose.* Philadelphia, WB Saunders Co, 1983, pp 520–524.
Hassan E: Treatment of meprobamate overdose with repeated oral doses of activated charcoal. *Ann Emerg Med* 1986; 15:73–76.
Meprobamate. *Poisindex,* vol 52. Micromedex, Inc, 1987.

61

Chloral Hydrate

V. Gail Ray, M.D., F.A.C.E.P.

I. Route of exposure: Oral, rectal.
II. Common names:
   A. Most common trade name, "Noctec."
   B. Preparations include 250, 500, and 1,000 mg capsules; elixir, pediatric elixir, mixtures; enema and suppository.
   C. Combination of **chloral hydrate** and **ethanol** referred to as **"Mickey Finn"** or "knockout drops."
III. Pharmacokinetics:
   A. Absorption: Rapidly absorbed from GI tract within minutes.
   B. Onset of action: Within 30 minutes.
   C. Half-life:
      1. Chloral hydrate, minutes.
      2. Active metabolite **trichloroethanol,** 4–12 hours.
   D. Peak effect: Strong hypnotic effect within 1 hour.
   E. Duration of action: Dependent on amount taken and patient's tolerance (see Half-life for rough guidelines).
   F. Elimination: Chloral hydrate is metabolized to trichloroethanol and trichloroacetic acid by alcohol dehydrogenase in the liver and in red blood cells. Further metabolism to inactive metabolites (trichloroethyl glucuronide, urochloralic acid) occurs by conjugation in liver and kidney. All products of chloral hydrate metabolism are then excreted in the urine.
   G. Active metabolites:
      1. Trichloroethanol: Drug rapidly and completely reduced to this active metabolite (as well as an inactive metabolite trichloroacetic acid).
      2. All chloral derivatives are converted to trichloroethanol.

IV. Action:
    A. Rapid development of CNS depression similar to barbiturate toxicity, also resulting in respiratory depression.
    B. Depression of myocardial contractility.
    C. Very little anticonvulsant effect.
    D. May potentiate pain.
    E. Alters sleep cycles similarly to barbiturates, but less potential for "hangover" signs and symptoms.

V. Uses:
    A. One of the first sedative/hypnotics used.

VI. Toxic mechanism:
    A. Active metabolite primarily responsible for symptoms.
    B. Strong direct corrosive effect on GI tract and skin, ranging from minor irritation to necrosis and perforation.
    C. Chloral hydrate is concentrated in the cerebral hemispheres, where it produces global depression of cerebral function.
    D. Hypotension related to vasodilation.
    E. Depression of myocardial contractility and shortening of refractory period.
    F. Hepatotoxicity.
    G. Renal tubular necrosis.
    H. Increased toxicity occurs when taken in combination with ethanol, because ethanol enhances production of the active metabolite trichloroethanol.

VII. Range of toxicity:
    A. Therapeutic dose: 500 mg–1 gm.
    B. Toxic dose:
        1. Doses >2 gm produce toxic symptoms.
        2. Severe intoxication may occur with ingestion of 10 times hypnotic dose.
    C. Fatal dose:
        1. Variable reports: 5–10 gm generally considered adult lethal dose when untreated. However, as little as 1.25–4 gm (approximately 30 mg/kg) have been reported to cause fatalities. On the other hand, recovery has been reported after ingestion of as much as 36 gm in a treated patient.

VIII. Clinical features:
    A. Toxicity develops rapidly within 3 hours of ingestion.
    B. GI tract and skin symptoms, ranging from minor irritation to necrosis and perforation.
    C. Minor CNS effects of ataxia, dizziness, malaise, and nightmares.
    D. Rapid development of CNS depression to grades 3 and 4 coma similar to barbiturate toxicity (see Reed's classification of coma, Chapter 55).
    E. Respiratory depression.
    F. Up to 30% of patients with grades 3 and 4 coma develop cardiac arrhythmias, ranging from AV blocks to supraventricular or ventricular tachycardias and ectopy.
    G. Hypothermia.
    H. Hypotension.

    I. Usually pinpoint pupils; in grade 4 coma pupils may be dilated.

    J. Hepatotoxicity and jaundice may develop after several days.

    K. Albuminuria and renal tubular necrosis may develop after several days. If renal insufficiency develops, electrolyte abnormalities may result.

    L. Delayed GI problems (secondary to caustic effect), with hemorrhage, perforation, and strictures possible.

    M. Delayed skin exfoliation may occur.

 IX. Laboratory findings and evaluation:

    A. Blood:

        1. Serum levels:

            a. Chloral hydrate not detected in blood because of rapid metabolism.

            b. Quantitative levels of metabolite trichloroethanol may be useful in estimating quantity of chloral hydrate ingested.

        2. Complete blood cell count, electrolytes, BUN, creatinine, liver function.

        3. Arterial blood gas: the presence of respiratory depression.

        4. Type and cross match: GI bleed possible.

    B. ECG, urinalysis, chest x-ray examination.

  X. General treatment:

    A. Follow APTLS (Chapter 8).

    B. General management: Table 61–1 (see Chapter 12 for details).

 XI. Specific treatment:

    A. Support of cardiovascular and ventilatory status, as in barbiturate poisoning.

    B. Close cardiac monitoring.

    C. Treat cardiac arrhythmias with appropriate therapy.

TABLE 61–1.

General Treatment

Treatment	Indicated	Of No Value	Contraindicated
O_2	±		
IV	+		
ECG monitor	+		
Forced diuresis*			X
Acidification			X
Alkalinization		X	
Emesis/lavage†	+/+		
Charcoal	+		
Cathartic	+		
Hemoperfusion	Effective		
Dialysis		X	

*Pulmonary edema is a possible complication.
†Gastric lavage probably not necessary in obtunded patient because of rapid and complete absorption of known single-drug ingestion. However, single-drug ingestion can rarely be trusted in such patients, and thus lavage is still advocated.

D. Hemoperfusion:
1. **Charcoal hemoperfusion** indicated in severe toxicity.
2. Hemodialysis and peritoneal dialysis of limited effectiveness because of high lipid solubility and storage of active metabolite in adipose tissue and red blood cells.
E. Hypothermia: Warming blankets, intravenous fluids warmed to room temperature, warm humidified oxygen.
F. Antacids until gastrointestinal tissues heal. Some suggest prophylactic demulcent agents (e.g., eggs, milk).
G. Consider endoscopy with GI symptoms (caustic effect).

XII. Prognosis:
A. Expected response to treatment:
1. If patient can be roused throughout course, full recovery is to be expected.
2. If patient is comatose with normal vital signs, no evidence of cyanosis, and no pulmonary complications (aspiration, pulmonary edema), recovery should occur in 24–48 hours with good supportive care.
3. Grade III or IV coma (Reed classification): Mortality less than 5%, with recovery of consciousness within 3–5 days.
B. Expected complications and long-term effects:
1. Pulmonary edema, aspiration.
2. Hepatotoxicity may develop after several days.
3. Renal tubular necrosis may develop after several days.
4. Delayed GI problems, with hemorrhage, perforation, and strictures.
5. Delayed skin exfoliation.
6. Physiologic and psychologic dependence occur when drugs are used in excess of the sedative dose over 1–2 months.

XIII. Special considerations:
A. Trichloroethanol reported to displace coumadin from albumin, thus potentiating the anticoagulant effects of this drug.
B. Sudden withdrawal of chloral hydrate may precipitate delirium and seizures, with a high mortality rate if untreated.

XIV. Disposition considerations:
A. Admission considerations:
1. See General Admission Considerations (Chapter 18).
2. Development of significant toxicity within 3 hours of emergency department observation.
3. Suicide risk.
B. Consultation considerations:
1. Nephrologist must be consulted for consideration of hemoperfusion (or hemodialysis if hemoperfusion not available) for patients unresponsive to normal supportive care or in whom acid-base or electrolyte problems are uncontrollable.
2. Endoscopist for GI complications.
C. Observation period: Asymptomatic patients must be observed for a minimum of 3 hours in the emergency department.
D. Discharge considerations:
1. General Discharge Considerations are met (see Chapter 18).

2. Generally, patients who can be roused after 3 hours of observation may eventually be discharged home if no evidence of serious toxicity or complications have developed during this period.

3. Suicide potential and psychiatric status have been appropriately evaluated.

XV. Similar drugs:

A. Meparfynol (methypentynol):

1. Similar in structure to chloral hydrate.

2. Sedative/hypnotic that is rapidly and completely metabolized by glucuronidase system and therefore has short duration of action.

3. Toxicity similar to that of chloral hydrate.

4. Other specific toxic effects are exfoliative dermatitis and toxic psychosis.

5. Treatment and disposition same as for chloral hydrate.

BIBLIOGRAPHY

Bowyer K, Glasser S: Chloral hydrate overdose and cardiac arrhythmias. *Chest* 1980; 77(2):232–235.

Brown A, Cade J: Cardiac arrhythmias after chloral hydrate overdose. *Med J Aust* 1980; 1:28–29.

Chloral hydrate. *Poisindex,* vol 47. Micromedex, Inc, 1987.

Gilman AG, Goodman LS, Rall TW, et al: *The Pharmacological Basis of Therapeutics,* ed 7. New York, Macmillan Publishing Co, 1985, pp 360–362.

Goldfrank LR, Flomenbaum NE, Lewin NA: *Toxicologic Emergencies,* ed 3. Norwalk, Conn, Appleton-Century-Crofts, 1986, pp 427–428.

Haddad LM, Winchester JF: *Clinical Management of Poisoning and Drug Overdose.* Philadelphia, WB Saunders Co, 1983, pp 527–531.

Heath A, Krister D, et al: Hemoperfusion with amberlite resin in the treatment of self-poisoning. *Acta Med Scand* 1980; 207:455–460.

62

Glutethimide

V. Gail Ray, M.D., F.A.C.E.P.

Glutethimide is more potent and associated with higher toxicity than barbiturates are.

I. Route of exposure: Oral.

II. Common trade name: Doriden.

III. Pharmacokinetics:
   A. Onset of action: 20–30 minutes.
   B. Duration of action: 48 hours.
   C. Peak effect: 16 hours.
   D. Half-life:
      1. Elimination half-life 5–22 hours.
      2. In overdose plasma half-life is prolonged from 10 to 40 hours.
   E. Elimination:
      1. Biphasic distribution pattern, being highly lipid soluble, sequestered in body fat, and 50% bound to plasma proteins.
      2. 95% metabolized in liver, 50% to the active metabolite. Induction of hepatic microsomal enzymes occurs. Enterohepatic circulation.
      3. Only 2% eliminated unchanged by the kidney.
   F. Active metabolite: Hydroxyglutethimide. Has twice half-life of the parent, with peak level 24 hours after ingestion.

IV. Action: Barbiturate-like CNS depression.

V. Uses:
   A. Sedative/hypnotic.
   B. Drug of abuse.

VI. Toxic mechanism:
   A. Barbiturate-like CNS depression.
   B. Pronounced anticholinergic activity.

VII. Range of toxicity:
    A. Toxic dose: >3 gm.
    B. Fatal dose: 10–20 gm.
VIII. Clinical features:
    A. Clinical effects are unpredictable and **complications may appear suddenly,** even after the patient seems to have recovered from major toxicity.
    B. CNS: **Glutethimide overdose is characterized by profound and prolonged coma.**
        1. Barbiturate-like CNS depression but with more profound and prolonged coma. Coma may be cyclical related to kinetics of redistribution.
        2. Cerebral edema.
        3. Focal and changing neurologic deficits.
        4. Seizures.
    C. Pulmonary:
        1. Respiratory depression (less than barbiturates).
        2. Thick bronchial secretions requiring constant pulmonary toilet and predisposing to pneumonitis.
    D. Cardiovascular:
        1. Hypotension.
        2. Pulmonary edema.
    E. Anticholinergic symptom complex may persist beyond clearance of CNS depression:
        1. See Chapter 91.
        2. Anticholinergic actions of glutethimide may cause dilated pupils with light reactivity or fixed and dilated unilateral or bilateral pupils. Characteristically described as moderate sized and fixed.
    F. Bullous skin lesions may appear.
IX. Laboratory findings and evaluation:
    A. Serum drug level:
        1. Serum levels not indicated. May be misleading, because levels of intoxication and rate of elimination vary enormously.
        2. Low levels are unreliable prognostic indicators.
        3. Repeated levels are also of no value because they may fluctuate considerably and do not correlate with clinical condition.
        4. Toxicologic screen recommended if multiple-drug ingestion suspected.
    B. Arterial blood gas if respiratory symptoms.
    C. ECG if pulse or blood pressure abnormal.
    D. Chest x-ray study with respiratory symptoms.
    E. Abdominal (KUB) x-ray examination; pills may be radiopaque.
    F. Head CT if neurologic symptoms present. Note that unilateral fixed and dilated pupils may be seen in glutethimide-poisoned patients without head injury.
X. General treatment:
    A. Follow APTLS (see Chapter 8).
    B. General management: Table 62–1 (see Chapter 12 for details).

TABLE 62–1.

General Treatment

Treatment	Indicated	Of No Value	Contraindicated
O_2	±		
IV	+		
ECG monitor	+		
Forced diuresis		×	
Acidification			×
Alkalinization		×	
Emesis/lavage*	+/+		
Charcoal	+		
Cathartic	+		
Dialysis		×	
Hemoperfusion	Effective		

*Concretions may require removal under endoscopy.

XI. Specific management:
  A. Pulmonary:
    1. Careful attention to airway.
    2. Pulmonary toilet.
  B. Hypotension: See Chapter 10 for treatment recommendations.
  C. Presence of cerebral edema may require hyperventilation and treatment with mannitol or furosemide.
  D. Seizure activity: See Chapter 22 for treatment recommendations.
  E. Hemoperfusion: See Controversies.
    1. Charcoal or resin hemoperfusion is treatment of choice. Although hemoperfusion will clear large amounts of glutethimide, it is not known if the active metabolite is cleared.
    2. Peritoneal dialysis and hemodialysis are largely ineffective because of large volume of distribution and high lipid solubility of drug (primarily stored in adipose tissue).
XII. Prognosis:
  A. Expected response to treatment:
    1. Moderate symptoms. Coma but no cardiopulmonary compromise: recovery expected in 24–48 hours.
    2. Severe symptoms: Coma, cardiac or pulmonary compromise, areflexia, mild hypothermia: mortality rate should be less than 5%; recovery of consciousness may take 3–5 days.
    3. Mortality with appropriate intensive support is estimated to be 1%. Complications increase in proportion to duration of coma.
    4. Greater than half of mortality is related to pulmonary complications.
    5. Advanced age is a poor prognostic indicator.
  B. Expected complications:
    1. CNS: cerebral edema, convulsions.
    2. Pulmonary:
      a. Sudden apnea.

       b. Pulmonary edema.

       c. Pneumonitis.

       d. Aspiration pneumonia.

    3. Cardiac arrest.

    4. Persistent lactic acidosis.

    5. Acute tubular necrosis.

  C. Long-term effects:

    1. Long-term use may cause osteomalacia.

XIII. Special considerations:

  A. Formation of gastric concretions may thwart gastric emptying procedures, with continued prolonged absorption. Consider endoscopic removal.

  B. Coingestion of alcohol or other CNS depressants will potentiate effects and toxicity of glutethimide.

  C. Euphoria similar to that with heroin when taken with codeine; commonly referred to as "loads," "hits," "setups," or "4s and doors." Usual dose is 1 gm glutethimide taken with 240 mg codeine on empty stomach. Intoxication occurs within 20 minutes; peaks at 40 minutes but may last 3–12 hours.

  D. Withdrawal: In patients taking at least 2.5 gm glutethimide per day, abrupt abstinence may lead to withdrawal symptoms (e.g., tremors, tachycardia, fever, muscle spasms, convulsions).

XIV. Controversies:

  A. Hemoperfusion:

    1. Utility is hotly debated. Clinical outcome and duration of coma do not seem to be affected by active removal of drug. Repeated hemoperfusion is required because drug continues to move from adipose tissue to plasma.

    2. Possible indications for hemoperfusion:

       a. Grade 3 or 4 coma (see Chapter 55 for description of Reed coma classification) with hypotension unresponsive to standard therapeutic measures (see Chapter 10).

       b. Progressive deterioration despite intensive supportive care.

       c. Flat EEG.

XV. Disposition considerations:

  A. Admission considerations:

    1. See General Admission Considerations (Chapter 18).

    2. Any symptomatic patient, even if symptoms only mild.

    3. Any patient with history of ingesting toxic dose, even if presently asymptomatic:

       a. ≥10 gm ingested.

       b. ≥30 µg/ml serum level: NOTE: Low amounts ingested or low plasma levels do not negate possibility of serious toxicity.

    4. ICU: Seizures, hypotension, cerebral edema, pulmonary symptoms, and particularly coma.

  B. Consultation considerations:

    1. Neurology consultation for suspected cerebral edema.

    2. Nephrology if hemoperfusion indicated.

  C. Observation period: None. All patients should be admitted.

   D. Discharge considerations: No patient with a potentially toxic ingestion
      should be discharged.
XVI. Similar drugs:
   A. Methyprylon (Noludar): Ingestion of 2–3 gm considered serious.

BIBLIOGRAPHY

Bailey D, Shaw R: Interpretation of blood glutethimide, meprobamate, and methyprylon
   concentrations in nonfatal and fatal intoxications involving a single drug. *J Toxicol Clin
   Toxicol* 1983; 20:133–145.
Bryson PD: *Comprehensive Review in Toxicology.* Rockville, Md, Aspen Systems Corp,
   1986, pp 205–207.
Gilman AG, Goodman LS, Rall TW, et al: *The Pharmacological Basis of Therapeutics,* ed 7.
   New York, Macmillan Publishing Co, 1985, pp 363–364.
Glutethimide. *Poisindex,* vol 53. Micromedex, Inc, 1987.
Greenblatt D, Allen M, Harmatz J, et al: Correlates of outcome following acute glutethimide
   overdosage. *J Forensic Sci* 1979; 24:76–86.
Haddad LM, Winchester JF: *Clinical Management of Poisoning and Drug Overdose.* Phila-
   delphia, WB Saunders Co, 1983, pp 531–542.
Rotschafer J, Foley C, Zaske D: Glutethimide and a metabolite. *Minn Med* 1980; 63:145–
   147.

Psychotropic Medications

63

Antipsychotic Agents

E. Jackson Allison, Jr., M.D., M.P.H.

I. Route of exposure: Oral, intravenous, intramuscular, rectal.
II. Common generic and trade names: See Table 63–1.
III. Pharmacokinetics: See Table 63–2.
IV. Action: See Table 63–3:
   A. General CNS depression.
   B. Decreases psychotic thinking and delusions.
   C. Decreases anxiety.
   D. NOTE: Butyrophenones less sedating, less anticholinergic effects, more extrapyramidal reactions than phenothiazines.
V. Uses:
   A. Treatment of schizophrenia, psychotic episodes.
   B. Rapid sedation.
VI. Toxic mechanism:
   A. Specific site of toxic action of phenothiazines has not been completely elucidated.
   B. Phenothiazines accumulate in the brain at four to five times plasma concentration, resulting in adverse effects on temperature-regulating centers, extrapyramidal system, and reticular activating system.
VII. Range of toxicity:
   A. Toxic dose:
      1. Antipsychotic drugs in general:
         a. Incidence of toxic reactions: 1% to 5% of patients receiving these drugs for more than 1 month.
      2. Chlorpromazine:
         a. Extremely variable: severe symptoms have occurred with doses <1 mg/kg.
         b. Dystonic reactions may occur with any dose.

305

TABLE 63–1.

Antipsychotic Agents

Generic Name	Trade Name	Available Forms
Chlorpromazine	Thorazine	Oral, slow-release, liquid, injectable, suppository
Trifluoperazine	Stelazine	Oral, liquid, injectable
Prochlorperazine	Compazine	Oral, injectable, suppository
Fluphenazine	Prolixin	Oral, liquid, injectable
Perphenazine	Trilafon	Oral, liquid, injectable
Thioridazine	Mellaril	Oral, liquid
Haloperidol	Haldol	Oral, liquid, injectable
Thiothixene	Navane	Oral, liquid, injectable
Chlorprothixene	Taractan	Oral, liquid, injectable
Loxapine	Loxitane	Oral, liquid, injectable
Molindone	Moban	Oral, liquid

   B. Fatal dose:
      1. Reported fatal doses (see also Table 63–2):
         a. Chlorpromazine: Few deaths reported; 350 mg in 4-year-old child and 26 gm in adult.
         b. Haloperidol: None reported.
         c. Thiothixene: 2.5–4 gm.
VIII. Clinical presentation:
   A. General symptoms: Drowsiness, malaise, anorexia, fever, abdominal pain, nausea, vomiting, pruritis, dry mouth, ataxia, nasal congestion, visual blurring, urinary retention, coma, seizures, hyperthermia or hypothermia.
   B. Extrapyramidal effects: Akathisia, akinesia, pseudoparkinsonism, tardive dyskinesias, acute dystonic reaction.
   C. Anticholinergic effects: See Chapter 91 for details of clinical features.
   D. Cardiovascular effects:
      1. Orthostatic hypotension with reflex tachycardia.
      2. Quinidine effect: Prolongation of Q-T interval.
      3. Dysrhythmias and conduction disturbances (frequent premature ventricular contractions, ventricular tachycardia, ventricular fibrillation).
   E. Photosensitivity: exaggerated sunburn, hyperpigmentation, urticaria.
   F. Hepatic injury (chronic effect):
      1. Probable hypersensitivity reaction.
      2. Intrahepatic cholestasis with clinical jaundice.
   G. Hematologic effect (chronic effect): Leukopenia, agranulocytosis.
   H. Other effects:
      1. Dimethylamines: Hiccoughs, pruritis.
      2. Piperazines: Antiemetic, migraine headaches.
      3. Butyrophenone: Withdrawal syndrome.
IX. Laboratory findings and evaluation:
   A. Phenistix:
      1. Rapid qualitative test for presence of salicylates or phenothiazines; can easily be performed in the emergency department (see Chapter 15).

TABLE 63–2.
Pharmacodynamics of Major Tranquilizers*

	Absorption	Peak Plasma Concentration (hr)	Plasma Half-Life (hr)	Elimination	Lowest Reported Fatal Dose (Humans)
Chlorpromazine (Thorazine)	Varies with dosage and form	2–3	6 (varies markedly among patients)	Renal and fecal	350 mg (about 20 mg/kg) in 4-year-old, 26 gm in adult
Thioridazine (Mellaril)	Rapid	1¼–4	7–42	Similar to chlorpromazine; 12% unchanged in urine	1.5–2.5 gm in adult
Chlorprothixene (Taractan)	Rapid			Renal 29%, fecal 41%	2.5 gm in adult
Haloperidol (Haldol)	Rapid	2–6	21	Bile 15% renal 40% (slow)	None reported

*Adapted from Rosen P: *Emergency Medicine: Concepts and Clinical Practice.* St Louis, The CV Mosby Co, 1988, pp 2102–2103.

TABLE 63–3.

Characteristics of Phenothiazines

Class	Trade Name	Sedative Effects	Extrapyramidal Symptoms	Anticholinergic	Orthostatic Hypotension
Phenothiazines					
Dimethylamine	Thorazine, Vesprin, Sparine, Tentone	+ +	+ +	+ + +	+ + +
Piperazine	Stelazine Compazine Prolixin Trilafon Dartal	+ + + +	+ + + +	+ +	+ +
Piperadine	Mellaril, Pacatal, Mornidine	–	+	+ +	+
Butyrophenones	Haldol	+ +	+ + +	+	+
Thioxanthines	Navane Taractan	+ +	+ +	+ + +	+
Loxapines	Loxitane	+ +	+ +	+ + +	+ +
Heterocyclics	Moban	+ +	+	+ +	–

2. Phenistix turns brown when either salicylates or phenothiazines are present in urine or serum.
3. To differentiate salicylates from phenothiazines, add a drop of 20N H_2SO_4 to the strip. Color will bleach if only phenothiazines are present. (See Chapter 15 for details of performance and interpretation.)
B. Toxicology screen including serum levels of suspected phenothiazines.
C. Blood:
   1. Electrolytes, glucose, BUN, creatinine, liver function.
   2. Complete blood cell count (in presence of fever or suspected leukopenia).
   3. Arterial blood gas with respiratory symptoms.
D. Other laboratory tests:
   1. ECG.
   2. Abdominal (KUB) x-ray examination; phenothiazine pills may be radiopaque.
X. General treatment:
   A. Follow APTLS (Chapter 8).
   B. General management: Table 63–4 (see Chapter 12 for details).
XI. Specific treatment:
   A. Cardiovascular toxic effects:
      1. Malignant cardiac dysrhythmias (e.g., premature ventricular contractions, ventricular tachycardia, ventricular fibrillation):
         a. Treatment: Lidocaine, phenytoin, bretylium, synchronized cardioversion, defibrillation.

TABLE 63–4.

General Treatment

Treatment	Indicated	Of No Value	Contraindicated
O₂	±		
IV	+		
ECG monitor*	+		
Forced diuresis		X	
Acidification			X
Alkalinization		X	
Emesis†/lavage†	±/+		
Charcoal	+		
Cathartic	+		

*If cardiac symptoms or arrhythmias, must monitor until dysrhythmia free for 24 hours.
†May not be effective because of antiemetic properties of several of these drugs; lavage preferred.

    b. Follow most recent Advanced Cardiac Life Support (ACLS) guidelines (*JAMA* 1986; 255:2841–3044).
  2. Hypotension:
    a. See Chapter 10, for treatment recommendations.
  3. Contraindicated drugs (because of myocardial depressant effects): **procainamide, quinidine.**
B. Central nervous system toxic effects:
  1. Extrapyramidal symptoms: Not prevented by anticholinergic drugs.
  2. Acute dystonic reactions:
    a. Benztropine mesylate (Cogentin) 1–2 mg IV.
    b. Diphenhydramine HCl (Benadryl) 25–50 mg IV or IM.
  3. Coma: See Chapter 21, for treatment recommendations.
  4. Seizures: See Chapter 22, for treatment recommendations.
  5. Hypothermia:
    a. Mild (>35° C): Passive techniques usually suffice.
    b. Body temperature <35° C: Acute core rewarming (warmed humidified O₂, warmed IV fluids).
    c. Unstable: Acute core rewarming as above and:
      (1) Administer glucose.
      (2) Intubation.
      (3) GI irrigation.
      (4) Consider:
        a Peritoneal dialysis.
        b Hemodialysis.
        c Extracorporeal rewarming.
  6. Hyperthermia:
    a. Mild <40° C: Cooling blanket, application of wet towels.
    b. >41° C: Rapid cooling to 39° C. Consider:
      (1) Ice wrapped in towels in axilla, neck, and groin.
      (2) Lavage stomach, bladder, rectum with iced saline solution.
      (3) Peritoneal lavage with iced saline solution.

C. Photosensitivity: Withhold drug.

D. Hepatic hypersensitivity: Withhold drug.

XII. Prognosis:

A. Expected response to treatment:

1. Recovery is the rule on cessation of phenothiazines and prompt institution of good supportive and symptomatic care.

2. Several reports of deaths in literature; however, fatalities from phenothiazines and other antipsychotics are not common.

3. Majority of deaths have occurred in children.

4. There are no reported fatalities from ingestions of phenothiazines in the piperazine group, and all reported cases of haloperidol overdoses have been successfully treated with only supportive and symptomatic care.

B. Expected complications and long-term effects:

1. Agranulocytosis: Good prognosis if patient survives 2 weeks.

2. Hepatotoxicity: Good prognosis if drug discontinued.

3. Tardive dyskinesia: Poor prognosis for complete recovery.

XIII. Special considerations:

A. Administration of phenothiazines may exacerbate toxic effects of other drugs, such as opioids, alcohol, certain sedative/hypnotics, and antihistamines.

B. Delayed toxicity may be seen after ingestions with thioridazine.

XIV. Disposition considerations:

A. Admission considerations:

1. See General admission considerations (Chapter 8).

2. Large number of pill fragments found in stomach or intestines by means of lavage, emesis, or abdominal plain film.

3. Unconsciousness at any time after phenothiazine overdose; hospitalize until asymptomatic for at least 24 hours.

4. Any patient who remains symptomatic after treatment and 2–4 hours of observation in the emergency department.

5. Any patient who has ingested a drug that can potentially show delayed toxicity, such as **thioridazine.**

6. Suicide risk.

B. Consultation considerations:

1. Psychiatry consultation for information on various phenothiazine preparations.

2. Cardiologist or internist for management of severe complications.

C. Observation period: At least 4 hours.

D. Discharge considerations:

1. General Discharge Considerations are met (Chapter 18).

2. Must be asymptomatic after 4 hours of observation and treatment. (Does not apply to thioridazine. See Admission considerations.)

3. Suicide risk and psychiatric state have been appropriately evaluated.

E. Patient transfer:

1. Care must be taken to ensure that patients with phenothiazine overdoses are not transferred to a psychiatric facility before they are medically stable.

2. See Chapter 19.

BIBLIOGRAPHY

Ayd FJ: Haloperidol: 20 years of clinical experience. *J Clin Psychiatry* 1978; 39:807.

Davis JM, Bartlett E, Termini BA: Overdosage of psychotropic drugs: A review. *Dis Nerv Syst* 1968; 29:157–164.

Granato JE, Stern BJ, Ringel A, et al: Neuroleptic malignant syndrome: Successful treatment with dantrolene and bromocriptine. *Ann Neurol* 1983; 14:89–90.

Hollister LE: Overdosages of psychotherapeutic drugs. *Clin Pharmacol Ther* 1966; 7:142–146.

Kemper AJ, et al: Thioridazine-induced torsade de pointes. *JAMA* 1983; 249:293A.

Lumpkin J, et al: Phenothiazine-induced ventricular tachycardia following acute overdose. *JACEP* 1979; 8:476.

May DC, Morris SW, Stewart RM, et al: Neuroleptic malignant syndrome: Response to dantrolene sodium. *Ann Intern Med* 1983; 98:183–184.

Niemann JT, Stapczynski JS, Rothstein RJ, et al: Cardiac conduction and rhythm disturbances following suicidal ingestion of mesoridazine. *Ann Emerg Med* 1981; 10:585–588.

Rivera-Calimlin L: The pharmacology and therapeutic application of the phenothiazines. *Ration Drug Ther* 1977; 11(4):1–6.

64

Lithium

E. Jackson Allison, Jr., M.D., M.P.H.

I. Route of exposure: Oral.
II. Common trade names: See Table 64–1.
III. Pharmacokinetics:
    A. Absorption: GI, rapid and complete.
    B. Half-life:
        1. Young person, 18 hours.
        2. Older person, 36 hours.
    C. Peak serum levels in 1–2 hours (except sustained-release preparations).
    D. Duration of action: Depends on half-life and peak effect.
    E. Elimination: Excreted unchanged in urine:
        1. 80% reabsorbed, proximal renal tubule.
        2. 20% excretion in urine.
    F. Active metabolites: None.
IV. Action:
    A. Lithium alters sodium transport in nerve and muscle cells and effects a shift toward intraneuronal metabolism of catecholamines, but the specific biochemical mechanism of lithium action in manic-depressive illness is unknown.
    B. Lithium competes with sodium, potassium, magnesium, and calcium for renal tubular absorption.
    C. Cyclic adenosine monophosphate (cAMP) inhibited, resulting in nephrogenic diabetes insipidus and changes in thyroid function.
    D. Release of endogenous serotonin.
V. Uses:
    A. Manic-depressive psychosis, unipolar depression, LSD psychosis, levodopa-induced mania, aplastic anemia, leukopenias, cluster headache prophylaxis.

TABLE 64–1.

Lithium Preparations*

Trade Name	Dosage
United States	
Lithane (Dome)	300 mg tablets
Pfi-lith (Pfizer)	300 mg capsules
Lithium carbonate USP	300 mg tablets and capsules
Lithium citrate syrup USP	8 mEq/5 ml (300 mg)
Lithonate-S (Rowell)	8 mEq/5 ml (300 mg)
Lithonate (Rowell)	300 mg capsules
Lithotabs (Rowell)	300 mg tablets
Lithoid (Rowell)	300 mg tablets
Eskalith (SmithKline)	300 mg tablets and capsules
Canada	
Carbolith (ICN)	300 mg
Lithane (Pfizer)	300 mg
Lithizine (Maney)	300 mg

*Adapted from Haddad LM, Winchester JF: *Clinical Management of Poisoning and Overdose.* Philadelphia, WB Saunders Co, 1983, p. 373.

VI. Toxic mechanism:
  A. Increase in serum lithium level leads to reduction of renal clearance, which may result in potentiation of lithium's toxic effects (see Action):
    1. Factors leading to decreased renal lithium clearance include:
      a. Volume depletion from any cause.
      b. Renal disease.
      c. Hyponatremia, hypokalemia.
VII. Range of toxicity:
  A. Toxicity determined by serum levels, not by dose (see Laboratory findings and evaluation).
  B. 9% incidence of intoxication with maintenance doses.
VIII. Clinical features:
  A. Prodromal phase: several days to weeks:
    1. Vomiting, diarrhea (often profuse), drowsiness, coarse muscle tremor, muscle twitching, lethargy, coma, ataxia, tinnitus, nystagmus, slurred speech, polyuria, polydipsia, and seizures.
    2. **Caution:** Symptoms may be confused with those of primary depression.
  B. Systemic manifestations of lithium intoxication:
    1. CNS: Fine hand tremor, muscular or reflex hyperirritability, spastic/choreiform movements, parkinsonism, confusion, lateralizing signs, cutaneous hyperalgesia, anxiety, delirium, hyperpyrexia, stupor or coma, abnormal EEG.
    2. GI: Severe gastroenteritis.
    3. Cardiovascular: Dysrhythmias, hypotension, circulatory collapse, interstitial myocarditis.

  4. Renal: Hyponatremia, nephrogenic diabetes insipidus (polyuria, poly-
dipsia, dehydration, sodium depletion, water imbalance).

  5. Other:

   a. Leukocytosis (neutrophilia, lymphocytopenia).

   b. Hypercalcemia, hypermagnesemia.

 C. Serum lithium and toxic manifestations: See Table 64–2:

  1. Lithium toxicity may become manifest even at therapeutic levels, especially in the elderly, when the therapeutic level may be 0.2 mEq/L.

  2. Early signs of toxicity (thirst, fine tremor, irritation, diarrhea) can develop at levels of 0.5–1.5 mEq/L.

  3. Stages 1 and 2: Apathy, tremor, weakness, ataxia, motor agitation, rigidity, fascicular twitching, nausea, vomiting, and diarrhea.

  4. Stage 3: Latent convulsive movements, stupor, and coma.

 D. Chronic toxicity:

  1. Nausea, vomiting, abdominal pain, diarrhea, sedation, and fine tremor.

IX. Laboratory findings and evaluation:

 A. Serum lithium level:

  1. Toxic and fatal levels:

   a. In chronic ingestions, levels >3–4 mEq/L are often fatal.

   b. In acute ingestions, higher levels are tolerated (a patient with a
level of 10.0 mEq/L has been reported to survive).

 B. Electrolytes, calcium, magnesium, BUN, creatinine, complete blood cell
count.

 C. ECG.

 D. Urinalysis.

X. General treatment:

 A. Follow APTLS (see Chapter 8).

 B. General management: See Table 64–3 (see Chapter 12 for details).

XI. Specific management:

 A. Thiazide and loop diuretics should be discontinued because they lead to
increased lithium retention by the kidney.

TABLE 64–2.

Serum Lithium and Toxic Manifestations*

Severity of Symptoms	Toxic Stage	Serum Lithium Concentration (mEq/L)
No toxicity (therapeutic)	0	0.4–1.3
Mild toxicity	1	1.5–2.5
Serious toxicity	2	2.5–3.5
Life-threatening toxicity	3	>3.5

*From Haddad LM, Winchester JF: *Clinical Manage-
ment of Poisoning and Drug Overdose.* Philadelphia, WB Saunders Co, 1983, p 374.

TABLE 64–3.

General Treatment

Treatment	Indicated	Of No Value	Contraindicated
O₂	+		
IV	+		
ECG monitor	+		
Forced diuresis*	+		
Acidification			X
Alkalinization†	+		
Emesis/lavage	+/+		
Charcoal‡	+	X	
Cathartic	+		
Dialysis†	Effective		

*Not with thiazide or loop diuretics (see below).
†See Indications below.
‡Charcoal does not effectively adsorb lithium. It is still recommended because many psychiatric patients have access to several dangerous medications.

   B. Monitor electrolytes closely and correct any sodium-water imbalance.
   C. Urinary alkalinization (see Chapter 13, p. 49 for description of technique or urinary alkalinization):
      1. Indications: Mild to moderate CNS manifestations (adequate cardiac and renal functions are required).
      2. Forced diuresis is reserved for decreased glomerular filtration rate secondary to hypovolemia. Diuresis may be initiated with mannitol or aminophylline. Do not use loop diuretics, such as furosemide, or ethacrynic acid or thiazide diuretics because further sodium loss potentiates lithium absorption.
   D. Hemodialysis:
      1. Indications:
         a. Initial lithium level exceeding 6–8 mEq/L after acute overdose.
         b. Severe CNS manifestations (seizures, coma).
         c. Renal impairment.
 XII. Prognosis:
   A. Expected response to treatment: 25% mortality in acute overdose.
   B. Expected complications and long-term effects: Persistent neurologic deficits, impaired renal function in 10% of lithium-intoxicated patients.
XIII. Special considerations:
   A. Pregnancy: Bottle-feeding recommended because lithium intoxication can occur in infants from breast milk.
   B. Known drug interactions with lithium:

Benzodiazepines	Neuromuscular blockers
Diuretics	Phenytoin
Haloperidol	Potassium supplements
Indomethacin	Sodium bicarbonate
Methyldopa	Tricyclic antidepressants

XIV. Disposition considerations:
  A. Admission considerations:
    1. See General admission considerations (Chapter 18).
    2. Serum lithium levels >2–3 mEq/L.
    3. All symptomatic patients.
    4. If serum lithium levels not readily available, all patients suspected of significant ingestion should be admitted. Indications of significant poisoning include evidence from history or large number of pill fragments found in stomach or intestines by means of lavage or emesis.
    5. Suicide risk.
  B. Consultation considerations:
    1. Nephrology consultation if hemodialysis indicated.
    2. Neurology consultation advised for evaluation of persistent neurological deficits.
  C. Observation period: An observation period of 2 hours in asymptomatic patients with acute ingestion may be sufficient to rule out significant toxicity (sustained-release preparations excepted).
  D. Discharge considerations:
    1. General disposition considerations are met (see Chapter 18).
    2. Asymptomatic.
    3. Suicide potential and psychiatric state have been appropriately evaluated.

BIBLIOGRAPHY

Amdisen A: Lithium and drug interactions. *Drugs* 1982; 24:133.

Clendenin NJ, Pond SM, Kaysen G, et al: Potential pitfalls in the evaluation of the usefulness of hemodialysis for the removal of lithium. *J Toxicol Clin Toxicol* 1982; 19:341.

El-Mallakh RS: Treatment of acute lithium toxicity. *Vet Hum Toxicol* 1984; 26:31.

Fenvez AZ: Lithium intoxication associated with acute renal failure. *South Med J* 1984; 77:1472.

Hansen HE: Renal toxicity of lithium. *Drugs* 1981; 22:461.

Lewis DA: Unrecognized chronic lithium neurotoxic reactions. *JAMA* 1983; 250:2029–2030.

Lydiard RB, Gelenberg AJ: Hazards and adverse effects of lithium. *Annu Rev Med* 1982; 33:327–344.

Parfrey PS: Severe lithium intoxication treated by forced diuresis. *Can Med Assoc J* 1983; 129:979.

Schou M: Pharmacology and toxicology of lithium. *Annu Rev Pharmacol Toxicol* 1976; 16:231.

65

Tricyclic Antidepressants

E. Jackson Allison, Jr., M.D., M.P.H.

I. Route of exposure: Oral.
II. Common generic and trade names: See Table 65–1.
III. Pharmacokinetics:
   A. Absorption: GI absorption rapid but delayed considerably in overdose. Systemic bioavailability 30% to 70%.
   B. Onset of action:
      1. Three weeks of antidepressant effects.
      2. Toxic effects occur within 1–2 hours in acute overdose.
   C. Plasma half-life: 10–76 hours but usually longer in overdose. Note that long half-lives imply that large amounts will be present in tissues even days after overdose.
   D. Peak effect: 4–9 hours.
   E. Duration of action: See Plasma half-life for rough guidelines. Lethal arrhythmias have occurred days after overdose.
   F. Elimination: Demethylation, hydroxylation, glucuronidation in liver, with 35% of metabolites secreted into bile, some secreted into stomach, and the rest excreted by the kidney.
   G. Active metabolites:
      1. Active metabolite of amitriptyline is nortriptyline.
      2. Active metabolite of imipramine is desipramine.
IV. Action:
   A. Mechanism of depression alleviation uncertain but may be related to inhibition of synaptic reuptake of brain norepinephrine and 5-hydroxytryptamine, with increased concentrations of these neurotransmitters at the receptor site.

TABLE 65–1.

Tricyclic Antidepressants*

Amitriptyline	Imipramine
Amid	Imavate
Amitril	Janimine
Elavil	SK-Pramine
Endep	Tofranil
Antipress	Desipramine
Etrafon	Norpramin
Limibitrol	Pertofrane
Perphenyline	Trimipramine
Triavil	Surmontil
Nortriptyline	Maprotilline
Aventyl	Ludiomil
Pamelor	Doxepin
Protriptyline	Adapin
Vivactil	Sinequan
Trazodone	Amoxapine
Desyrel	Asendin

*From Bryson PD: *Comprehensive Review in Toxicology.* Rockville Md, Aspen Publications Corp, 1986, p 46. Used by permission.

   B. Sedative effects related to anticholinergic properties:
      1. Most sedating: Amitriptyline, doxepin, imipramine.
      2. Least sedating: Protriptyline.
   C. Anticholinergic effects:
      1. Predominate in low doses.
      2. Strongest effect: amitriptyline.
      3. Least effect: desipramine.
   D. Sympathomimetic effects: predominate in high doses.
   E. Class I antiarrhythmic properties.
   F. Antihistamine properties (H_1 and H_2 antagonist).
 V. Uses:
   A. Treatment of choice in endogenous depression.
   B. Tricyclics are involved in 10% to 25% of all suicidal ingestions and account for 20% to 25% of all drug-related deaths.
 VI. Toxic mechanism:
   A. Secondary to anticholinergic effects.
   B. Blocking of reuptake of norepinephrine leading to sympathomimetic effects.
   C. Secondary to membrane-stabilizing effects (quinidine-like effect).
   D. Cardiotoxicity from direct effect secondary to preferential uptake by myocardial cells, and anticholinergic and sympathomimetic effects leading to disturbance of both impulse formation and conduction, cardiac dysrhythmias, hypotension, and pulmonary edema.

 E. Direct CNS toxicity.
VII. Range of toxicity:
  A. Toxic dose:
    1. Toxic symptoms can be seen with ingestions of 5 mg/kg, with severe toxicity at 10–20 mg/kg.
  B. Fatal dose:
    1. Adults: 10–30 mg/kg.
    2. Doses as small as 200 mg have produced fatalities in children.
VIII. Clinical features:
  A. Clinical course may progress rapidly from relatively asymptomatic to intractable cardiac arrest.
  B. Vital Signs:
    1. Blood pressure: Hypotension or hypertension.
    2. Pulse: Tachycardia.
    3. Respirations:
      a. Tachypnea if hypoxic (e.g., aspiration).
      b. Bradypnea (respiratory depression).
    4. Temperature: Hypothermia or hyperthermia.
  C. Central nervous system:
    1. Respiratory depression.
    2. Altered mental status: Confusion, agitation, hallucinations, coma.
    3. Seizures common.
    4. Clonus, choreoathetosis, hyperactive reflexes, myoclonic jerks, positive Babinski's sign, extrapyramidal signs, abnormal cerebellar test results.
  D. Anticholinergic effects (see Chapter 91).
  E. Cardiotoxicity:
    1. Conduction delay, quinidine-like effects.
    2. Ventricular arrhythmias (premature ventricular contractions, ventricular bigeminy, ventricular tachycardia, fibrillation).
    3. Sinus tachycardia.
    4. Pulmonary edema:
      a. Results from decreased myocardial contractility.
      b. Worsened considerably by fluid overload.
      c. Increased mortality.
IX. Laboratory findings and evaluation:
  A. Blood:
    1. Plasma levels: Limited or no value:
      a. Unlikely to be available for several hours.
      b. Levels correlate poorly with degree of clinical toxicity.
    2. Arterial blood gas:
      a. Indications: Hypoxia, acidosis.
      b. Necessary if therapy includes blood alkalinization.
    3. Electrolytes.
    4. Complete blood cell count: Rule out infection in presence of hyperthermia.
    5. Blood glucose: Rule out hypoglycemia in presence of coma, altered mental status.

B. ECG: QRS duration >100 msec is a sign of severe toxicity and is associated with the presence of pulmonary insufficiency and adult respiratory distress syndrome (ARDS).

C. Chest x-ray studies: respiratory distress, ARDS, pulmonary edema.

X. General treatment:

A. Follow APTLS (see Chapter 8).

B. General management: See Table 65–2 (see Chapter 12 for details).

XI. Specific treatment:

A. **Supportive care** is of paramount importance (see Chapters 8–10).

B. Respiratory depression: See Chapter 9.

C. Cardiovascular:

1. Hypotension:

a. Sodium bicarbonate (see below for dosage and administration).

b. **Careful fluid administration** with normal saline or Ringer's lactate solution (may precipitate pulmonary edema related to myocardial depressant action of tricyclic antidepressants). Must be managed with strict maintenance IV fluid replacement. May need Swan-Ganz catheter placement to guide therapy.

c. **Dopamine infusion:** 2–50 μg/kg/min, titrating to desired response if necessary.

d. Norepinephrine (Levophed): titrate starting with 0.1 μg/kg/min.

2. Ventricular dysrhythmias:

a. Sodium bicarbonate (see below).

b. If arrhythmias persist after sodium bicarbonate, administer phenytoin sodium (Dilantin) 100 mg IV (adult dose) over 3 minutes.

c. Consider propranolol in children: .01–0.1 mg/kg IV, up to 0.25 mg IV bolus.

d. Consider physostigmine if phenytoin fails. Drug of very last resort (see below).

TABLE 65–2.

General Treatment

Treatment	Indicated	Of No Value	Contraindicated
O_2	+		
IV	+		
ECG monitor	+		
Forced diuresis*	±		
Acidification			X
Alkalinization*	±		
Emesis†/lavage	±/+		
Charcoal	Repeated doses		
Cathartic	+		
Dialysis		X	
Hemoperfusion		X	

*Controversial
†**Caution:** Rapid decrease in level of consciousness is possible; may be ineffective because of antiemetic effect. Lavage is preferred.

    e. **Contraindicated drugs: Quinidine, procainamide, disopyramide.**

    f. Ineffective drugs: Magnesium, calcium, potassium, ?lidocaine.

  3. Prolonged QRS ($\geq$100 msec):

    a. Sodium bicarbonate (see below).

    b. Consider phenytoin 15 mg/kg IV over 30 minutes.

    c. **Avoid: Digoxin, propranolol, physostigmine.**

  4. Bradyarrhythmia or heart block:

    a. Isoproterenol.

    b. Pacemaker.

    c. **Contraindications:** Should avoid **atropine** because of anticholinergic properties.

  5. Pulmonary edema: Fluid restriction and use of positive end-expiratory pressure (PEEP) as necessary.

  6. Cardiac arrest: Follow most recent Advanced Cardiac Life Support (ACLS) guidelines from American Heart Association (*JAMA* 1986; 255:2841–3044).

D. **Metabolic acidosis:** Sodium bicarbonate should be administered IV as needed to reverse severe metabolic acidosis (i.e., pH <7.2).

E. **Seizures:**

  1. Administer bicarbonate to pH 7.5–7.55 (see below).

  2. See Chapter 22.

F. **Sodium bicarbonate** administration:

  1. Indications:

    a. Coma.

    b. QRS >100 msec.

    c. Ventricular dysrhythmias.

    d. Seizures.

    e. Hypotension.

  2. Procedure:

    a. Infuse 44–50 mEq (1 ampule) bicarbonate over 1–5 minutes.

    b. Start drip 0.5 mEq/kg/hr, adjusting rate to maintain blood pH 7.5–7.55.

    c. If condition critical, infuse sodium bicarbonate drip for 24 hours after stabilized.

G. Physostigmine:

  1. Indications:

    a. Treatment of anticholinergic effects only in most severe life-threatening circumstances unresponsive to other therapy:

      (1) Seizures.

      (2) Severe hallucinations.

      (3) Hypertension.

      (4) Arrhythmias (e.g., supraventricular tachycardia, ventricular tachycardia, and any other arrhythmia accompanied by hemodynamic compromise).

  2. Dosage:

    a. Adult: 1–2 mg slow IV (not more than 1 mg/min), repeated in 20 minutes if symptoms persist.

      b. Pediatric: .02 mg/kg (maximum, 0.5 mg/min) slow IV, repeated at 5-minute intervals until maximum dose of 2 mg has been given.

      c. Administer with constant cardiac monitoring and close supervision.

    3. **Contraindications:**

      a. Asthma, gangrene, underlying cardiovascular disease, gastrointestinal or genitourinary tract obstruction.

      b. Cardiac conduction abnormalities, particularly delayed conduction (QRS >100 msec).

    4. Complications: Asystole, heart block, seizures.

  H. Ineffective therapy:

    1. Forced diuresis.

    2. Hemodialysis or peritoneal dialysis.

    3. Hemoperfusion.

XII. Prognosis:

  A. Expected response to treatment:

    1. Factors predictive of severe clinical course:

      a. Anticholinergic symptoms.

      b. QRS >100 msec.

      c. Sinus tachycardia.

      d. Depressed level of consciousness.

    2. Overall mortality 1.7%.

    3. Reported deaths as late as 3 days after ingestion.

    4. Arrhythmias reported to occur several days after ingestion.

  B. Expected complications and long-term effects:

    1. Aspiration pneumonitis, ARDS, pulmonary edema, seizures.

    2. Death.

XIII. Special considerations:

  A. Cautious administration of fluid because of possible precipitation of pulmonary edema.

  B. Monoamine oxidase inhibitors, alpha methyl dopamine, sympathomimetic, and anticholinergic medications should be avoided by patients taking tricyclic antidepressants.

XIV. Disposition considerations:

  A. Admission considerations (see Controversies below):

    1. See General Admission Considerations (Chapter 18).

    2. All patients developing even minor symptoms including noncardiac signs or symptoms such as depressed consciousness or decreased bowel sounds (suggesting the possibility of delayed tricyclic antidepressant absorption) within 6 hours of ingestion should be admitted, with ECG monitoring.

    3. Any history of ingestion in a child.

    4. Suicide potential.

  B. ICU admission considerations:

    1. Any ECG changes, including sinus tachycardia, intraventricular conduction defects of ≥100 msec, complete AV block, severe sinus bradycardia.

    2. Metabolic acidosis.

    3. Pulmonary edema.

    4. Seizures.

    5. Persistent hypotension.

    6. Need for Swan-Ganz catheter.

  C. Consultation considerations:

    1. Cardiology consultation may be helpful in management of severe cardiac arrhythmias resistent to standard therapy.

    2. Psychiatry consultation may be helpful to evaluate suicide potential.

  D. Observation period:

    1. No symptomatic patients should be observed.

    2. If the **treated** patient remains symptom free and there are no anticholinergic signs present, including tachycardia, the patient may be discharged after 6-hour observation.

    3. **Note:** Patients with decreased bowel sounds may have delayed absorption and should not be considered symptom free.

  E. Discharge considerations:

    1. General discharge considerations have been met (see Chapter 18).

    2. Asymptomatic with active bowel sounds.

    3. No acute ECG changes, including sinus tachycardia, after at least 6 hours of observation.

    4. Some authors suggest final dose of charcoal before discharge.

    5. Suicide potential and psychiatric status have been appropriately evaluated.

    6. Appropriate psychiatric follow-up has been arranged.

    7. Patient released in the care of a responsible adult.

  F. Patient transfer considerations: Care must be taken to ensure that patients with tricyclic antidepressant overdose are not transferred to a psychiatric facility before they are medically stable.

XV. Controversies:

  A. The disposition of patients with tricyclic antidepressant overdose is controversial. Recommendations in the literature range from admission of all with confirmed and even suspected overdoses to admission of only unstable patients. Justification for admitting all patients relies on early literature describing deaths as late as several days after ingestion. More recent work, however, provides a more narrow and well-defined population at high risk for serious morbidity and mortality. It appears that **treated** patients who remain completely asymptomatic for 6 hours after ingestion are at virtually no risk for serious sequelae. Others continue to admit all such patients regardless of their clinical condition.

  B. The duration that patients should be monitored is also controversial. Some authors suggest 72 hours of ICU monitoring. Recent studies, however, show that major adverse cardiac symptoms are unlikely to occur if the patient remains free of such symptoms for 24 hours.

BIBLIOGRAPHY

Boehnert MT, Lovejoy FH Jr: Value of the QRS duration versus the serum drug level in predicting seizures and ventricular arrhythmias after an acute overdose of tricyclic antidepressants. *N Engl J Med* 1985; 313:474–479.

Callaham M: Tricyclic antidepressant overdose. *JACEP* 1979; 8:413–425.

Callaham M, Kassel D: Epidemiology of fatal tricyclic antidepressant ingestion: Implications for management. *Ann Emerg Med* 1985; 15:1–9.

Emerman CL, et al: Level of consciousness as a predictor of complications following tricyclic overdose. *Ann Emerg Med* 1987; 16:326–330.

Foulke GE, Albertson TE: QRS interval in TCA overdosage: Inaccuracy as a toxicity indicator in emergency settings. *Ann Emerg Med* 1987; 16:160–163.

Frommer DA, et al: Tricyclic antidepressant overdose: A review. *JAMA* 1987; 257:521–526.

Goldberg RJ, Capone RJ, Hunt JD: Cardiac complications following tricyclic antidepressant overdose. *JAMA* 1985; 254:1772–1775.

Hagerman GA, Hanshiro PK: Reversal of tricyclic antidepressant induced cardiac conduction abnormalities by phenytoin. *Ann Emerg Med* 1981; 10:82–86.

Hoffman JR, McElroy CR: Bicarbonate therapy for dysrhythmia and hypotension in tricyclic antidepressant overdose. *West J Med* 1981; 134:60–64.

Inaccuracy of QRS interval as TCA toxicity indicator (letter). *Ann Emerg Med* 1987; 16:1312–1313.

Kulig K: Management of poisoning associated with "newer" antidepressant agents. *Ann Emerg Med* 1986; 15:1039–1045.

Levitt MA, Sullivan JB Jr, Owens SM, et al: Amitriptyline plasma protein binding: Effect of plasma pH and relevance to clinical overdose. *Am J Emerg Med* 1986:4:121–125.

Mayron R, Ruiz E: Phenytoin: Does it reverse tricyclic-antidepressant-induced cardiac conduction abnormalities? *Ann Emerg Med* 1986; 15:876–880.

McAlpine SB, et al: Late death in tricyclic antidepressant overdose revisited. *Ann Emerg Med* 1986; 15:1349–1352.

Pentel P, Peterson CD: Asystole complicating physostigmine treatment of tricyclic antidepressant overdose. *Ann Emerg Med* 1980; 9:588–590.

Sasyniuk BI, Jhamanda V, Valois M: Experimental amitriptyline intoxication: Treatment of cardiac toxicity with sodium bicarbonate. *Ann Emerg Med* 1986; 15:1052–1059.

Wedin GP, Oderda GM, Klien-Schwartz W, et al: Relative toxicity of cyclic antidepressants. *Ann Emerg Med* 1986; 15:795–804.

66

Monoamine Oxidase Inhibitors

Betty S. Riggs, M.D.

I. Route of exposure: Oral.
II. Common generic and trade names:
   Tranylcypromine (Parnate).
   Phenelzine (Nardil).
   Pargyline (Eutonyl).
   Isocarboxazid (Marplan).
   Iproniazid, pheniprazine, and nialamide (Niamid) no longer marketed in the United States because of toxicity.
III. Pharmacokinetics:
   A. Absorption: Rapid and complete.
   B. Onset of action: With **tranylcypromine** overdose, symptoms usually occur 6–24 hours after ingestion.
   C. Plasma half-life: For **tranylcypromine,** elimination half-life is 1.5–3 hours.
   D. Peak effect:
      1. Therapeutic doses of **tranylcypromine** have produced peak plasma levels 40 minutes–3.5 hours after ingestion.
      2. Peak inhibition of MAO activity does not occur for 5–10 days, however.
   E. Duration of action: With **tranylcypromine** overdose, symptoms usually resolve 48–96 hours after ingestion.
   F. Elimination: Monoamine oxidase inhibitors (MAOIs) undergo hepatic metabolism mainly to an inactive metabolite, which is then excreted in the urine. After the drug is discontinued, effects may persist for days after elimination because of irreversible inhibition of the enzyme.
   G. Active metabolites: Little known.

IV. Action:
  A. MAOIs bind to monoamine oxidase irreversibly; enzyme inhibition persists until new enzyme stores are synthesized (up to 2 weeks after the drugs are discontinued).
  B. MAOIs inhibit the deamination of biogenic amines, such as classical neurotransmitter amines or their precursors (e.g., dopamine, serotonin, norepinephrine, epinephrine, 5-hydroxytryptophan).
  C. These drugs also decrease stores of norepinephrine in postganglionic sympathetic neurons and inhibit enzymes other than MAO, such as dopamine-β-oxidase, diamine oxidase, amino acid decarboxylase, and choline dehydrogenase.
 V. Uses:
  A. Psychiatric: Atypical depression, hysterical depression, phobic disorder, panic attacks.
  B. Neurologic: Parkinson's disease, narcolepsy.
  C. Other: Moderate to severe hypertension resistant to other therapy.
 VI. Toxic mechanism:
  A. Excessive sympathetic stimulation resulting from inhibition of monoamine oxidase and accumulation of neurotransmitters such as norepinephrine in the synaptic cleft. MAOIs also decrease norepinephrine stores in postganglionic sympathetic neurons and inhibit enzymes such as dopamine-β-oxidase.
 VII. Range of toxicity:
  A. Toxic dose: 2–3 mg/kg should be considered life threatening; lesser amounts can cause mild to moderate toxicity.
  B. Fatal dose:
    1. Ingestions of ≥4–6 mg/kg have produced fatalities.
    2. The concept of a "fatal" dose should be considered misleading because with early appropriate therapy no MAOI overdose should be fatal.
VIII. Clinical features:
  A. Mild to moderate toxicity:
    1. Cardiovascular: Hypertension, tachycardia, palpitations.
    2. CNS: Drowsiness, restlessness, irritability, headache, hallucinations, myoclonus, hyperreflexia, opisthotonos.
    3. GI: Nausea, abdominal pain, diarrhea.
    4. Other: Flushing, tremors.
  B. Severe toxicity:
    1. Cardiovascular: Hypotension, bradycardia, shock, asystolic arrest, pulmonary edema.
    2. CNS: Convulsions, coma, respiratory depression.
    3. Hyperpyrexia.
    4. Acute renal failure, hemolysis, rhabdomyolysis.
    5. Coagulopathy.
 IX. Laboratory findings and evaluation:
  A. Serum MAOI levels: No help, because assay procedures and toxic levels of MAOI have not been well defined. Diagnosis of MAOI toxicity is made clinically.

B. Blood:
  1. Liver function studies (SGOT, SGPT, alkaline phosphatase, bilirubin).
  2. Complete blood cell count; rule out infection in face of hyperpyrexia.
  3. Electrolytes, calcium, BUN, creatinine (baseline renal function studies; rule out electrolyte effects for neuromuscular symptoms.
  4. Coagulation studies: prothrombin time, partial thromboplastin time.
  5. Glucose: altered mental status.
  6. Arterial blood gas: with respiratory depression or hypotension.
  7. Serum creatine phosphokinase if suspect rhabdomyolysis.
C. Urinalysis: check for myoglobinuria if rhabdomyolysis suspected.
D. ECG.

X. General treatment:
  A. Follow APTLS (see Chapter 8).
  B. General management: See Table 66–1 (see Chapter 12 for details).

XI. Specific treatment:
  A. Seizures: See Chapter 22.
  B. Hypotension:
    1. See Chapter 10.
    2. Norepinephrine (Levophed) may be useful in treatment of hemodynamically significant hypotension.
  C. Hypertension:
    1. Phentolamine: Dose 2–5 mg over 20 minutes, then titrate up to desired response (maximum dose 10 mg).
    2. See Chapter 68.
    3. **Contraindicated:** Administration of methyldopa and guanethidine may precipitate hypertensive crisis.
  D. Hyperthermia:
    1. See Chapter 63, p. 309.

TABLE 66–1.

General Treatment

Treatment	Indicated	Of No Value	Contraindicated
O$_2$	±		
IV	+		
ECG monitor	+		
Forced diuresis		X	
Acidification			X
Alkalinization		X	
Emesis*/lavage	+/+		
Charcoal	Repeated doses		
Cathartic	+		
Hemodialysis	Effective†		
Hemoperfusion	Effective†		

*Lavage preferred over ipecac in substantial overdose.
†Possibly effective if performed early.

    2. Acetaminophen.

    3. Dantrolene sodium 2.5 mg/kg/dose IV every 6 hours; paralysis with pancuronium may be indicated for malignant hyperthermia.

    4. **Contraindicated:** Phenothiazines may cause irreversible shock.

  E. Rhabdomyolysis with or without renal insufficiency (see Chapter 70).

  F. Hemodialysis or hemoperfusion: May be of benefit if performed early, before distribution phase of the drug. However, patient is likely to be asymptomatic at the time these procedures may be of benefit.

XII. Prognosis:

  A. Expected response to treatment:

    1. Prognosis excellent for those patients who receive early, aggressive, appropriate treatment:

    2. General fatality rate 1%.

  B. Expected complications and long-term effects:

    1. Secondary complications: Acute renal failure, coagulopathy, hemolysis, rhabdomyolysis.

XIII. Special considerations:

  A. Drugs that cause catecholamine release from storage sites of adrenergic neurons may produce sympathetic storm characterized by throbbing headache, sweating, tachycardia, and hyperpyrexia. Such drugs include amphetamines, LSD, ephedrine, metaraminol, phenylephrine, and phenylpropanolamine.

  B. Differential diagnosis: Pheochromocytoma, carcinoid syndrome, stimulant drug toxicity, drug interaction.

  C. Through other mechanisms, such as blocking enzymes other than MAO, MAOIs can prolong and intensify effects of other drugs, such as **meperidine, aspirin, atropine, barbiturates, methyldopa,** and **tricyclic antidepressants.**

  D. Food and drug interactions:

    1. When foods containing tyramine are ingested during treatment with MAOI, tyramine displaces the increased stores of norepinephrine from the presynaptic granules, resulting in increased effect on the alpha receptors and potential precipitation of hypertensive crisis.

    2. Foods to be avoided include hard cheese, smoked or pickled fish, beer, red wine, sherry, liqueurs, beef or chicken liver, broad bean pods, yeast supplements, canned or overripe figs, and fermented sausage (pepperoni, salami, summer sausage).

    3. Foods that may cause a reaction if consumed in large quantities include alcoholic beverages, ripe avocado, ripe fresh banana, yogurt or sour cream, soy sauce, and New Zealand spinach.

XIV. Disposition considerations:

  A. Admission considerations: All patients with acute significant MAOI ingestions must be observed in an ICU for a minimum of 24 hours, even if asymptomatic in the emergency department.

  B. Consultation considerations: Nephrology consultation if hemodialysis or hemoperfusion indicated.

  C. Observation period: There is no role for emergency department observation in a patient in whom a diagnosis of MAOI toxicity is being entertained, regardless of whether the patient is symptomatic.

D. Discharge considerations: No patient with acute MAOI ingestion should be discharged from the emergency department under any circumstances.

BIBLIOGRAPHY

Kaplan RF, Feinglass NG, Webster W, et al: Phenelzine overdose treated with dantrolene sodium. *JAMA* 1986; 255:642–644.

Lindon CH, Rumack BH, Strehlke C: Monoamine oxidase inhibitor overdose. *Ann Emerg Med* 1984; 13:1137–1144.

McDaniel KD: Clinical pharmacology of monoamine oxidase inhibitors. *Clin Neuropharmacol* 1986; 9:207–234.

Drugs of Abuse

67

Narcotics/Opioids

Celeste Madden, M.D.

I. Route of exposure: Oral, parenteral, mucosal, inhalation.
II. Common names: See Tables 67–1 and 67–2.
III. Pharmacokinetics:
   A. Absorption: Well absorbed from all sites.
   B. Onset of action: Time of onset of action varies with different products (see Table 67–4).
   C. Plasma half-life: Most opiates have half-life of 3–6 hours, except methadone (up to 50 hours) and propoxyphene (up to 15 hours) (see Table 67–2).
   D. Peak effect:
      1. 15 minutes IV
      2. 30 minutes IM
      3. 90 minutes SC or oral.
   E. Duration of action: See half-life, Table 67–2.
   F. Elimination: Hepatic metabolism primarily responsible for detoxification. About 90% excreted in the urine, mainly in the form of conjugated metabolites.
   G. Active metabolites:
      a. Codeine: Active metabolite, morphine.
      b. Meperidine: Active metabolite, normeperidine
IV. Action: See Table 67–3.
V. Uses:
   A. Pharmacologic uses: Sedation, analgesia, antitussive, antidiarrheals.
   B. Abuse: Mood alteration.

TABLE 67–1.

Street Opioid Vocabulary

Proper Name or Term	Street Term
Heroin	Skag, dope, shill, horse, H, white stuff, lady Jane, white lady
Intra-arterial injection	Pinkie
Intradermal injection	Skin popping
Intravenous injection	Mainlining
Inhalation	Snorting
Inhalation of pyrolysate	Chinese bowling
Addict	Junkie
Withdrawal	Jones
Needing a dose because of addiction	Strung out
Syringe	Works (syringe, tab, spike fix, cooker)
Occasional use	Chipping
Scars from needle	Tracks
Onset of a high	Rush
Somnolence	Nod
Overdosage	OD, nod out, fall out
Drawing blood in and out of needle	Booting
Attempt at internal jugular injection	Pocket shot
Fentanyl	China white
Postinjection fever	Cotton fever
Heroin-cocaine mixture	Speedball
Site to buy and inject drugs	Shooting gallery
Paregoric and tripelennamine or pyribenzamine	Blue velvet
Cyanide, strychnine, battery acid	Death hit
Codeine and glutethimide	Loads
Acetaminophen with codeine (Phenaphen #4) and glutethimide	4s and doors
Pentazocine and tripelennamine	Ts & Bs, Ts & blues

VI. Toxic mechanism:
   A. Primarily CNS related respiratory depression.
   B. See Actions.
VII. Range of toxicity:
   A. Toxic dose: See Table 67–4.
   B. Fatal dose:
      1. Codeine: 7–14 mg/kg.
      2. Hydrocodone: 2.5 mg in infants, 100 mg in adults.

TABLE 67–2.

Classification, Potency, Pharmacokinetics of Narcotics/Opioids

Opiate	Trade Name	Half-Life	Potency (Equianalgesic Dose, mg IM/IV)
Opium derivatives			
Codeine		2 hr	120
Morphine		2–3 hr	10
Semisynthetic opiates			
Heroin		3 min	3–5
. Hydromorphone	Dilaudid	2–4 hr	1.5
Oxycodone	Percodan/Percocet	1–5 hr*	15
Oxymorphone	Numorphan	1–3 hr	1.5
Synthetic opiates			
Alphaprodine	Nisentil	2 hr	40–60
Butorphanol	Stadol	2.5–3.5 hr	2
Dextromethorphan		2–4 hr*	
Diphenoxylate	Lomotil	14 hr*	
Fentanyl	Sublimaze	1–6 hr	0.1–0.2
Levorphanol	Levo Dromoran	12–16 hr	2
Meperidine	Demerol	2–4 hr	75–100
Methadone	Dolophine	52 hr	8–10
Nalbuphine	Nubain	5 hr	10
Pentazocine†	Talwin	2–6 hr	30–60
Propoxyphene	Darvon/Darvocet	3.5–15 hr	

*Parent compound.
†The combination of pentazocine hydrochloride and tripelennamine hydrochloride (Ts and blues) has been abused as a heroin substitute. In response to this abuse, formulation of pentazocine has been changed to include naloxone hydrochloride, however, abuse of the new pentazocine-naloxone formulation along with tripelennamine has been reported.

  3. Methadone: 10 mg in children.
  4. Etorphine: 0.03–0.12 mg.
VIII. Clinical features:
 A. CNS:
  1. CNS depression: Ranges from stupor to coma.
  2. Seizures: Anoxic, particularly associated with: meperidine, fentanyl, propoxyphene. Common in children.
  3. Respiratory depression. May progress to respiratory arrest. Most common cause of death.
  4. Miosis: Pinpoint pupils.
   a. Mydriasis may be seen with:
    (1) Severe hypoxia, hypotension, acidemia.
    (2) Mixed ingestions.
    (3) Meperidine, propoxyphene, codeine, pentazocine, diphenoxylate.

TABLE 67–3.

Opiate Physiologic Effect

Central Nervous System	Cardiovascular System	Gastrointestinal Tract
Pain tolerance	Peripheral vasodilation	Decreased gastric motility
Anxiety	Orthostatic hypotension	Increased muscle tone
Sedation	Syncope	Antrum
Mood changes		Proximal duodenum
Euphoria		Ileocecal valve
Dysphoria		Anus
Cough reflex		Increased segmental tone
Nausea, vomiting		with decreased
Respiratory depression		peristaltic contractions,
Convulsions		cramping
		Constipation

    B. Cardiovascular:
        1. Orthostatic hypotension, shock secondary to hypoxia or other cause.
        2. Pulmonary edema (noncardiac):
          a. Present in nearly all fatalities.
          b. Presence of pulmonary edema independent of route of administration.
          c. Most common in IV heroin, oral propoxyphene and oral methadone overdoses.
          d. Mechanism probably related to capillary damage.
          e. Onset ranges from immediate to several hours with delay up to 24 hours if narcotic antagonist used.
        3. Arrhythmias: Rare; most likely to be bradyarrhythmias.
    C. Gastrointestinal:
        1. Decreased peristalsis, vomiting.
    D. Genitourinary:
        1. Urinary retention.
 IX. Laboratory findings and evaluation:
    A. Toxicology screen:
        1. Metabolites of some opiates can be detected in urine.
        2. Quantitative blood concentration determinations are difficult and usually not helpful.
        3. It may be helpful to notify the toxicology laboratory when a narcotic antagonist such as naloxone has been given before collection of specimens.
        4. Street additives or adulterants may be detected (see Special considerations).
        5. Many overdoses are the result of multidrug ingestions.
    B. Other laboratory tests:
        1. Arterial blood gas analyses (ABGs): With respiratory depression.
        2. Glucose (Dextrostix): Rule out hypoglycemia.
        3. CBC: Infection can be an important complication.
        4. Chest x-ray: Pulmonary edema, or baseline study in aspiration.

TABLE 67–4.

Relative Toxicity of Narcotics*

Drug (Trade Name)	Dose Causing Respiratory Depression (mg)**		Time of Onset of Respiratory Depression†	Observation Period‡ (hr)
	PO	IM		
Morphine-like drugs				
Alphaprodine (Nisentil)	—	30	Very fast	12
Anileridine (Ieritine)	75	25	Fast	12
Apomorphine	—	10	Fast	12
Brompton's mixture (contains morphine or heroin)	—	—	Fast	Depends on ingredients§
Codeine	200	120	Fast	12
Dextromoramide (Palfium)	10	5	Slow	24
Dihydrocodeine (Paracodin)	150	60	Fast	12
Diphenoxylate (Lomotil)¶	300	—	Delayed	24
Diphenoxylic acid (Difenoxin)¶	400	—	Delayed	24
Dipipanone (Dicanol, Pipadone)	—	20	Slow	24
Etorphine (Immobilon: veterinary use)	—	0.025	Very fast	12
Fentanyl (Sublimaze)	—	0.125	Very fast	12
Heroin	15	3	Fast	12
Hydrocodone (Hycodan, Dicodid)	100	—	Fast	12
Hydromorphone (Dilaudid)	6	—	Fast	12
Levorphanol (Levo-Dromoran)	6	—	Fast	12
Loperamide (Imodium)¶	350	—	Delayed	24
Meperidine (Demerol)	250	100	Fast	12
Methadone (Dolophine, Westadone, Amidone)	20	10	Slow	24
Metopon	8	3	Fast	12
Morphine	70	10	Fast	12
Opium powder USP (Pantopon)	700	—	Fast	12
Opium tincture USP	7 ml	—	Fast	12
Oxycodone (Percodan)	15	10	Fast	12
Oxymorphone (Numorphan)	—	1	Fast	12
Paregoric	175	—	Fast	12
Pethidine	250	100	Fast	12
Phanadoxone (Hepatalgin)	—	15	Fast	12
Propoxyphene HCl (Darvon, Doloxene, Depronal, Dolene)	600	—	Fast	24

(Continued.)

TABLE 67–4 (cont.).

Drug (Trade Name)	Dose Causing Respiratory Depression (mg)**		Time of Onset of Respiratory Depression†	Observation Period‡ (hr)
	PO	IM		
Propoxyphene naphsylate	900	—	Fast	24
Agonists/antagonists‖				
Buprenorphine (Temgesic)	0.8	0.4	Slow	24
Butorphanol (Stadol)	—	2	Fast	12
Levallorphan (Lorfan)	—	3	Fast	12
Nalbuphine (Nubain)	—	10	Fast	12
Nalorphine (Nalline)	—	15	Fast	12
Naloxone (Narcan)	—	—	No respiratory depression	0
Pentazocine (Talwin, Fortral)	120	20	Fast	12
Phenazocine (Primadol, Narphen)	—	3	Fast	12
Antitussives#				
Dextromethorphan				4
Levopropoxyphene (Novrad)				4
Noscapine				4
Pholcodine (Ethnine, Pholdine)				4

*From Rosen P, et al: *Emergency Medicine: Concepts and Clinical Practice.* St Louis: CV Mosby, 1988 pp 2126–2127. Used with permission.

**Equivalent to 10 mg of morphine IM. These dose equivalents are approximate and should be used only as guides. The effects of these doses on any particular patient depend on many factors, such as age, weight, associated drugs, and associated illnesses.

†Onset of respiratory depression varies with the product and the route of administration: (1) With IM: Very fast = 5–30 min; fast = 15–60 min; slow = 1–4 hr. (2) With PO times are approximately double those of IM. (3) IV: Rapid onset, 2–30 min. (4) Delayed onset, in 2–14 hr. Slow or delayed onset produces cumulative effects after several doses.

‡Minimum period of time without any signs of toxicity and without narcotic antagonists for which patient should be observed after overdose.

§Brompton's mixture may contain cocaine, alcohol, and a phenothiazine. Relative amounts of each, and amounts of narcotic, not fixed.

¶Serious poisonings have been reported with diphenoxylate only in young children. Until further evidence is accumulated, diphenoxylic acid and loperamide overdoses should be treated as diphenoxylate overdose.

‖Most agonists-antagonists exhibit a ceiling effect as respiratory depressants. An increased overdose does not cause a proportional increase in respiratory depression, as with morphine.

#These opioid-related products do not depress respirations even in large doses.

X. General treatment:
    A. Follow APTLS (see Chapter 8), particularly important in the unconscious patient with possible narcotic overdose (also see Chapter 21).
    B. General management: Table 67–5. (See Chapter 12 for details.)
XI. Specific treatment:
    A. Airway: See Chapter 9.

TABLE 67–5.

General Treatment

Treatment	Indicated	Of No Value	Contraindicated
O$_2$	+		
IV	+		
ECG Monitor	+		
Forced diuresis*			X
Acidification			X
Alkalinization		X	
Emesis‡/lavage†	± / +		X
Charcoal	+		
Cathartic	+		
Offer counseling	+		

*Noncardiogenic pulmonary edema may be a problem.
†Unstable airway; pentazocine or propoxyphene may cause rapid decrease in level of consciousness.
‡For oral ingestions.

B. Hypotension: See Chapter 10.
C. Pulmonary edema:
   1. Positive-pressure ventilation.
   2. Diuretics and cardiac glycosides not indicated.
   3. Naloxone.
D. Tetanus prophylaxis for parenteral abusers.
E. Narcotic antagonist: Titrate dosage according to reversal of opiate effect. Naloxone (Narcan) is agent of choice.
   1. Naloxone has a half-life of 12–20 minutes, and very little effect is detectable 45 minutes after single intravenous dose of 0.4 mg in an adult.
   2. Most narcotics have a longer half-life, and signs of narcotic overdose may recur after 30–60 minutes, and repeated doses or continuous infusion of naloxone are necessary. Continuous infusion is particularly effective with long-acting narcotics such as methadone, propoxyphene and diphenoxylate.
   3. Dose (bolus):
      a. Route: IV preferred. If an IV line cannot be secured then SC, IM or sublingual.
      b. Adult: 2 mg IV, IM, SC, SL.
      c. Child: 0.01 mg/kg.
      d. Repeat up to a total dose of **10–20 mg** in adults if a single dose fails to reverse the symptoms. Drugs that may require large doses of naloxone to reverse their effects include **propoxyphene, pentazocine, methadone, codeine** and **buphenorphine.**
   4. Continuous intravenous infusion:
      a. Indications: For ongoing reversal of the effects of long-acting opiates (e.g., methadone, pentazocine, propoxyphene, codeine, diphenoxylate, nalbuphine, butorphanol, and the new, potent designer drugs). Provides a convenient alternative to repeated bolus therapy of overdoses with these drugs.

b. Dose:
(1) Two thirds of initial effective naloxone bolus is infused as drip over 1 hour with subsequent infusion rate titrated to desired antagonist effect. Mix with fluid of choice.
(2) 15 minutes after initiation of continuous infusion, administer half initial effective naloxone dose as a bolus.
5. Side effects of naloxone:
a. No known direct side effects of naloxone.
b. May precipitate immediate and severe narcotic withdrawal symptoms.
6. If unconscious patient fails to respond to naloxone, diagnostic possibilities include massive narcotic overdose, drugs relatively resistant to naloxone, overdose of nonnarcotic drug, multiple-drug overdose (e.g., heroin and ethanol), nontoxic etiology.

XII. Prognosis:
A. Expected response to treatment:
1. If good respiratory support has been provided, prognosis is excellent in the uncomplicated case with full recovery expected within 3–4 hours.
2. Pulmonary edema: Recovery within 2–5 days with supportive care, positive-pressure ventilation, and naloxone (Narcan).
B. Expected complications and long-term effects:
1. **Infection:** Bacterial or fungal endocarditis, soft tissue infection or abscess, cellulitis, phlebitis, tetanus, bacteremia, hepatitis, pneumonia, osteomyelitis, AIDS.
2. **Pulmonary:** Aspiration, pulmonary edema, embolism, coma/respiratory depression, lung abscess, atelectasis, pulmonary fibrosis/pulmonary vascular granulomatosis, tetanus-induced respiratory muscle dysfunction.
3. **Neurologic:** Cerebral edema, transverse myelitis, postanoxic encephalopathy.
4. **Hepatic:** Cirrhosis, hepatitis.
5. **Renal:** Immune-complex nephritis, acute tubular necrosis, rhabdomyolysis.
6. **Hematologic:** Thrombocytopenia, neutropenia, anemia.
7. **Skin:** Tracks.
8. **Immunologic:** False positive syphilis serology test results.
9. Also see Chapter 32.

XIII. Special considerations:
A. Narcotic preparations may be combined with other substances and drugs:
1. Local anesthetics: Procaine, lidocaine, tetracaine, benzocaine, butacaine.
2. Stimulants: Amphetamine, caffeine, ergotamine, aminophylline, strychnine, phencyclidine, nicotine, phenylpropanolamine.
3. Hallucinogens: LSD, hashish, marijuana, PCP.
4. Depressants: Alcohol, methapyrilene.
5. Inert substances: Talc, flour, corn starch, sugars (lactose, inositol, sucrose, maltose, mannitol).

6. Other: Quinine, thiamine, $NaHCO_3$ (baking soda), magnesium silicate, $MgSO_4$, salicylamide, cotton fibers, thallium.
B. Many oral and prescribed narcotics are combination preparations, particularly with acetaminophen (APAP) and salicylates (ASA). Therefore one should always have a high index of suspicion for concomitant ASA and APAP toxicity in patients with oral narcotic overdoses.
C. Methadone HCl overdose:
   1. Long duration of action: 72 hours.
   2. May require naloxone drip for as long as 24–48 hours.
D. Withdrawal syndrome: See Chapter 33.
XIV. Special categories of narcotic opioids:
A. **Propoxyphene:**
   1. Fatal overdose occurs much more commonly than with other oral analgesics. Time course is very rapid, with sudden death seen within 15 minutes of ingestion and nearly always within 2 hours.
   2. Toxic symptoms appear with doses of 11 mg/kg with respiratory depression in adults caused by 180 mg and psychotic reactions after 390 mg. Lethal dose reported as 35 mg/kg.
   3. Severe toxicity characterized by convulsions and pulmonary edema.
   4. Treatment:
      a. Emesis should be performed with care because of rapid onset of symptoms.
      b. Patient should be observed for a minimum of 24 hours.
B. **Diphenoxylate:**
   1. Diphenoxylate is a meperidine derivative used in combination with atropine in the antidiarrheal preparation Lomotil.
   2. Extremely toxic in young children younger than 2 years, with reports of just 3 tablets (7.5 mg) resulting in respiratory arrest. No serious toxicity reported for adults.
   3. Anticholinergic symptoms due to presence of atropine in Lomotil.
   4. Late symptoms related to delayed gastric emptying (up to 14 hours after ingestion). May have recurrence of respiratory depression up to 3 days after ingestion.
   5. All patients with overdose must be admitted. Severe overdoses may require continuous naloxone infusion and repeated gastric lavage.
   6. Fluid restriction recommended because of possibility of cerebral edema.
C. **Pentazocine:**
   1. Symptoms of pentazocine overdoses are similar to those of morphine, except more dysphoric symptoms.
   2. Patients who remain asymptomatic after a mild overdose may be discharged after about 6 hours observation. Patients with more severe toxic signs should be observed for at least 12 hours.
D. **Dextromethorphan:**
   1. Dextromethorphan is a narcotic derivative with specific antitussive activity.
   2. Commonly part of combination medication with antihistamines, de-

congestants, or alcohol, which may necessitate modification of treatment.

3. 3–4 hours of observation sufficient to rule out serious toxicity.

E. Narcotic analogues or "designer drugs":

    1. **Fentanyl** analogues:

        a. Fentanyl citrate (Sublimaze, Innovar).

        b. Extremely potent: Fentanyl 20 to 40 times as strong as heroin. Onset of action extremely rapid and lasts 30–60 minutes. Users may become addicted after one injection. 3–Methyl fentanyl is 2,000 times as potent as morphine. Minuscule amounts can have life-threatening effects.

        c. Because of minuscule amounts necessary for effect standard laboratory tests may fail to detect their presence.

    2. Meperidine analogues:

        a. MPPP (1-methyl-4-phenyl-propionoxypiperidine).

        b. PEPAP (1{2-phenylethyl}-4-acetyloxypiperidine).

        c. MPTP (1-methyl-4-phenyl-1,2,3,6-tetrahydropyridine).

            (1) Mistakenly produced during the attempted manufacture of MPPP.

            (2) A neurotoxin that causes syndrome closely resembling Parkinson's disease.

            (3) MPTP also used in chemical manufacturing. May pose risk to chemists unprotected with fume exhaust hoods.

XV. Disposition considerations:

A. Admission considerations:

    1. See General Admission Considerations (Chapter 18).

    2. Social considerations particularly important.

    3. Parenteral overdose: Admit if patient still symptomatic after 4 hours of appropriate treatment.

    4. Oral narcotic considerations:

        a. Patients who are known or suspected to have ingested a toxic amount of narcotics should be hospitalized for 12–24 hours or longer.

        b. Patients with mild symptoms that resolve after 6 hours of observation in the emergency department may be discharged. **Exception:** Patients ingesting any long-acting oral narcotic such as methadone, propoxyphene, or diphenoxylate, regardless of mildness of symptoms, should be admitted, with no observation period.

    5. Suicide risk.

B. Consultation considerations:

    1. Drug counseling should be offered all patients.

C. Observation period:

    1. Asymptomatic patients should be observed for a minimum of 3–4 hours after parenteral opioid overdose.

    2. Difficult to make recommendations for oral narcotics because of great variety of preparations with different half-lives, variable individual metabolism and unpredictable response to treatment.

        a. The patient who is completely asymptomatic after oral ingestion should be observed for a minimum of 6 hours. Observation not appropriate for long- or delayed-action narcotics.

D. Discharge considerations:
1. General discharge considerations are met (see Chapter 18).
2. Asymptomatic.
3. Counseling has been offered.
4. Home environment has been assessed.
5. Suicide potential has been appropriately addressed.

REFERENCES

Bianchine JR: MPTP and parkinsonism. *Ration Drug Ther* 1985; 19:5–7.

Brittain JL: China white: The bogus drug. *J Toxicol Clin Toxicol* 1982; 19:1123–1126.

Goldfrank LR, Weisman RS, Errick JK, et al: A dosing nomogram for continuous infusion intravenous naloxone. *Ann Emerg Med* 1986; 15:566–570.

Handal KA, et al: Naloxone. *Ann Emerg Med* 1983; 12:438–445.

Inturrist CE: Narcotic drugs. *Med Clin North Am* 1982; 66:1061–1071.

Mofenson IIC, Caraccio TR: Continuous infusion of intravenous naloxone (letter to editor). *Ann Emerg Med* 1987; 16:374–375.

Moore RA, Rumack BH, Conner CS, et al: Naloxone: Underdosage after narcotic poisoning. *Am J Dis Child* 1980; 134:156–158.

Reed DA, Schnoll SH: Abuse of pentazocine-naloxone combination. *JAMA* 1986; 256:2562–2564.

Schwartz JA, Koenigsberg MD: Naloxone-induced pulmonary edema. *Ann Emerg Med* 1987; 16:1294–1296.

Ziporyn T: A growing industry and menace: Makeshift laboratory's designer drugs. *JAMA* 1986; 256:3061–3063.

68

Amphetamines/Stimulants

J. Stephen Huff, M.D.

Amphetamines

I. Route of exposure: Oral, IV.
II. Common generic and trade names: See Tables 68–1 and 68–2.
   A. Nomenclature and classification:
      1. Amphetamine is a specific compound, α-methylphenylethylamine (DL-amphetamine, Benzedrine).
      2. The term "amphetamines" can also refer to structural analogues of DL-amphetamine or to some of the other noncatecholamine sympathomimetic drugs with CNS activity. Classification is sometimes arbitrary (see Table 68–1).
      3. Many other compounds have been marketed. Some products also contain barbiturates or phenothiazines.
   B. Amphetamine analogues or "designer drugs":
      1. A number of other newer compounds structurally related to amphetamines have recently been manufactured. CNS effects predominate.
         a. MDA (phenylisopropylamine methylenedioxyamphetamine).
         b. MDA analogue: 3,4-methylenedioxymethamphetamine (MDMA, "Ecstacy," "XTC").
         c. 3,4-Methylenedioxyethamphetamine (MDEA, "Eve").
III. Pharmacokinetics:
   A. Absorption: Oral, rapid.
   B. Onset of action:
      1. Oral: Within 30 minutes.
      2. IV: Immediate.

TABLE 68–1.

Amphetamines/Stimulants

Generic Name	Trade Name
Amphetamines	
DL-Amphetamine (racemic mixture)	Benzedrine
Dextroamphetamine	Dexedrine
Methamphetamine	Desoxyn, Methedrine, Fetamine
Other CNS stimulants	
Ephedrine	See Chapter 94
Diethylpropion HCl	Tenuate, Tepanil
3,4-Methylenedioxyethamphetamine	Eve (street name)
3,4-Methylenedioxymethamphetamine	Ecstacy (street name)
Methylphenidate	Ritalin
Pemolin	Cylert
Phendimetrazine tartrate	Trimtabs, Limit, Wehless
Phenmetrazine	Preludin
Phenylephrine	See Chapter 94
Phenylpropanolamine	See Chapter 94
Phentermine	Ionamin, Fastin

C. Plasma half-life:
  1. Elimination half-life of amphetamine is dependent on urinary pH and urine volume, with more unchanged amphetamine excreted in acidic urine.
    a. Half-life with urine pH of <5.6 is 7–8 hours.
    b. Up to 30 hours or longer with alkaline urine.

TABLE 68–2.

Street Names for Amphetamines*

A's	Crank	Meth	Spliven
BAM	Crosses	Mini-Bennies	Rhythms
Beans	Crossroads	Mollies	Road aspirin
Bennies	Crystal	Nuggets	Roses
Benny bombs	Dexies	Oranges	Tens
Benz	Double cross	Pacific turnabouts	Thrusters
Black beauties	Eye-openers	Peaches	Truck drivers
Blackbirds	Fives	Pen pills	Turnabouts
Black Mollies	Footballs	Purple Hearts	Uppers
Bumblebees	Forwards	St. Louis	Ups
Cartwheels	Hearts	Sparkle Plenties	Wake-ups
Chalk	Jelly beans	Speed	Water
Chicken powder	Leapers	Splash	West Coast turnabouts
Christmas trees	Lid poppers		Whites
Co-pilots	Lightning		

*From Haddad EM, Winchester JF. *Clinical Management of Poisoning and Drug Overdose.* Philadelphia, WB Saunders Co, 1983, p 472. Used by permission.

    D. Peak effect: Within 2–4 hours of oral ingestion.

    E. Duration of action: Dependent on half-life.

    F. Elimination: Metabolism is hepatic by deamination and hydroxylation. Amphetamine and closely related compounds are weak bases; urinary excretion of nonmetabolized compound is pH influenced.

    G. Active metabolites:

        1. Hydroxylated compounds may continue to be significantly active by functioning as "false neurotransmitters."

        2. Amphetamine is a pharmacologically active metabolite of methamphetamine.

IV. Action:

    A. Activity of these compounds thought to involve catecholamine release from adrenergic nerve terminals, inhibition of reuptake of the neurotransmitters, or direct stimulation of alpha and beta adrenergic receptors.

    B. Precise mechanism of action unclear. Some compounds act primarily on central receptors; others have predominantly peripheral effects or combination of the two. CNS activity is reflected in feeling of energy and euphoria that may accompany use. Peripheral nervous system activity is manifest as tachycardia, hypertension, tremors.

V. Uses:

    A. Only current recommended use for amphetamines are treatment of attention deficit disorders in children, and narcolepsy.

    B. Use of phentermine, diethylproprion, and phenylpropanolamine (PPA) as anorectic agents continues.

    C. Ephedrine, PPA, and other agents are used widely as cold remedies in common over-the-counter medications (see Chapter 94).

    D. Abuse:

        1. Both oral and IV abuse.

        2. Alertness, euphoria, and feeling of energy that accompany use are responsible for the abuse problem.

        3. Users seek the "rush" that is intensified with IV use.

VI. Toxic mechanism:

    A. Excessive sympathetic stimulation (sympathetic overdrive) resulting in complications (see Clinical features).

    B. Direct brain damage occurs as a result of both hypertensive cerebral bleeding and direct neurotoxic action in various areas of the brain.

    C. Effects of anorexia, hyperthermia, hypermotility, and typical behavior are believed to be moderated by central dopaminergic stimulation.

    D. Direct toxicity has also been reported from disaggregation of ribosomes with subsequent inhibition of protein synthesis.

    E. Toxicity from adulterants in IV preparations may be present.

VII. Toxic dose: See Table 68–3.

VIII. Clinical features:

    A. Acute toxicity of these compounds seen within hours after oral ingestion.

    B. Sympathetic overdrive:

        1. Restlessness, irritability, agitation.

        2. Pupils may be widely dilated.

        3. Cardiovascular: Hypertension, tachycardia, supraventricular and ventricular dysrhythmias.

TABLE 68–3.

Toxic Dose of Amphetamines/stimulants

	Median Lethal Dose* (mg)
Amphetamines	
DL-Amphetamine (racemic mixture)	10
Dextroamphetamine	20
Methamphetamine	100
Other CNS stimulants	
Ephedrine	200
Methylphenidate	200
Phenmetrazine	200
Phenylephrine	100
Phenylpropanolamine	200
Phentermine	200

*For children. Adult toxic doses may be much higher.

    4. Hyperthermia.

    5. Seizures.

  C. Coma:

    1. Direct toxic effect.

    2. Intracranial hemorrhage secondary to hypertension.

    3. Hypertensive encephalopathy.

    4. Systemic vasculitis.

  D. Behavior:

    1. Agitation, euphoria, hallucinations, psychosis.

    2. Paranoid psychosis is more common in chronic abusers.

  E. Tolerance develops, and regular user may tolerate massive doses of amphetamines.

IX. Laboratory findings and evaluation:

  A. Standard toxicologic screening will reveal presence of amphetamines.

  B. Blood:

    1. Complete blood cell count; search for infection with hyperthermia.

    2. Glucose (Dextrostix): with altered mental status.

    3. Consider electrolytes, BUN, creatinine, calcium, arterial blood gas, urinalysis.

  C. ECG if indicated by clinical findings (e.g., dysrhythmias).

X. Treatment:

  A. Follow APTLS (see Chapter 8).

  B. General management: See Table 68–4 (see Chapter 12 for details).

XI. Specific management:

  A. Anxiety and agitation:

    1. Quiet and calm environment.

    2. If needed, diazepam 15–20 mg PO.

    3. Avoid haloperidol or chlorpromazine; these lower seizure threshold. For severe agitation, violence, or psychosis, major tranquilizers may be necessary.

TABLE 68–4.

General Treatment

Treatment	Indicated	Of No Value	Contraindicated
O$_2$	±		
IV	±		
ECG monitor	+		
Forced diuresis	+		
Acidification*	±		
Alkalinization			X
Emesis/lavage	± / +		
Charcoal	+		
Cathartic	+		
Dialysis		X	

*Controversial.

B. Hypertension (also see Controversies).
  1. Mild hypertension: Frequent blood pressure monitoring, careful observation of vital signs and neurologic symptoms.
  2. Any of several antihypertensives can be used to treat moderate or severe hypertension:
     a. Nifedipine 10 mg SL.
     b. Labetalol 10–80 mg IV.
     c. Propranolol 1 mg IV every minute, up to 6 mg.
     d. If blood pressure rises even further related to unopposed alpha adrenergic effects, may need to add phentolamine.
     e. If diastolic pressure rises above 120 mm Hg, give hydralazine HCl (Apresoline), 25 mg IM or IV. Monitor blood pressure, and repeat initial dose every hour if necessary.
     f. If hypertension is uncontrolled or hypertensive encephalopathy is present, administer sodium nitroprusside initially at 0.5 μg/kg/min by infusion pump or other device that permits precise measurement of rate of flow. Adjust infusion rate upward as necessary, but do not exceed 10 μg/kg/min.
C. Ventricular arrhythmias:
  1. Propranolol has been reported effective in slowing supraventricular tachyarrhythmias associated with PPA overdose.
  2. Lidocaine (1.5 mg/kg bolus followed by IV infusion) is recommended by some for frequent or symptomatic ventricular ectopy. Use is controversial because of potential for seizures.
  3. Experience with other antiarrhythmic agents is limited.
D. Seizures: See Chapter 22.
E. Hyperthermia: See Chapter 63, p. 309.
F. IV fluids should be administered to promote diuresis.
  1. Urinary acidification has been recommended for life-threatening toxic symptoms, but use remains **controversial.** Theoretically will enhance elimination; however, risks appear to outweigh benefits.

XII. Prognosis:
    A. Expected response to treatment:
        1. Toxic symptoms are usually self-limited, lasting generally less than 6 hours.
        2. Prognosis is good with appropriate respiratory support and aggressive control of arrhythmias, seizures, hypertension, and hyperthermia.
    B. Expected complications and long-term effects:
        1. Prolonged use may result in frank psychosis, with recovery requiring weeks or months.
        2. Complications of intravenous drug abuse (see Chapters 32 and 67).
XIII. Special considerations:
    A. Abrupt cessation of amphetamines by the regular user may precipitate a withdrawal syndrome with prominent depressive and suicidal ideation, which should ideally be managed in a hospital setting.
    B. Numerous "look-alike" capsules that resemble the manufactured amphetamines but in fact contain PCP, LSD, cocaine, atropine, strychnine, caffeine, ephedrine, phenylpropanolamine, and other nonrestricted sympathomimetics have wide distribution and are commonly used.
    C. Abusers may take sedatives in combination with amphetamines.
XIV. Controversies:
    A. Urinary acidification has been recommended with life-threatening toxic symptoms but use remains controversial. Efficacy not documented, and acidification may accelerate myoglobinuric renal failure.
    B. The management of hypertension produced by amphetamines is controversial. Some experts recommend treating hypertension prophylactically; others do not treat unless hypertension becomes life threatening. We advocate observation of patients with mild hypertension; antihypertensive agents may be necessary for moderate or severe hypertension.
XV. Disposition considerations:
    A. Admission considerations:
        1. See General Admission Considerations (Chapter 18).
        2. Symptoms persisting after 4–6 hours of appropriate management and observation in the emergency department.
        3. Agitation, paranoid ideation or threatening behavior unresponsive to anxiolytic therapy.
        4. Presence of any major symptoms at any time (coma, seizures, symptomatic hypertension, arrhythmias).
        5. Abrupt cessation of amphetamines by the regular user.
        6. Consideration for admission to ICU:
            a. Hypertensive crisis.
            b. Ventricular arrhythmias.
            c. Seizures.
            d. Hyperthermia.
    B. Consultation considerations:
        1. Consider anesthesiology consultation if patient has intractable seizures, as may occur with massive overdoses of amphetamines.
        2. Psychiatric consultation may be required to treat the depression and suicidal ideation associated with abrupt cessation of amphetamines.

C. Observation period: If no signs of toxicity are seen within 6 hours of ingestion, further medical observation usually is not necessary.
D. Discharge considerations:
1. General disposition considerations are met (see Chapter 18).
2. Patients with mild to moderate symptoms can be discharged if all symptoms are resolved after 6 hours of observation.
3. Suicide potential and psychiatric status have been evaluated.
4. Drug counseling has been offered.

Caffeine

I. Route of exposure: Oral.
II. Compounds containing caffeine: Caffeine is ubiquitous in colas, coffee, tea, chocolate, over-the-counter medications, and in "look-alike" capsules (Table 68–5).
III. Pharmacokinetics:
A. Absorption: Rapidly absorbed after oral ingestion.
B. Onset of action: 10 minutes.
C. Plasma half-life: 3–4 hours in adults.
D. Peak levels: Within 1 hour.
E. Duration of action: Dependent on half-life.
F. Elimination: Hepatic metabolism results in inactive compounds, which are then excreted in the urine.
G. Active metabolites: None known.
IV. Action:
A. Caffeine is a plant-derived xanthine, similar in structure to theophylline.
B. Mechanism of action is not clear but is thought to involve several possibilities:
1. Catecholamine release from nerve terminals.
2. Calcium release.

TABLE 68–5.

Compounds Containing Caffeine

Source	Caffeine* (mg)
Coffee (cup)	100–150
Tea	30–70
Cola	40–60
Chocolate bar	25
Cold preparations	30–75
Stimulants	75–200
Darvon compound	32
Fiorinal	40
Cafergot	100

*Values represent average.

3. Inhibition of phosphodiesterase responsible for degradation of cyclic AMP. As levels of cyclic AMP accumulate intracellularly, the effect is smooth muscle relaxation (with resultant bronchodilation), myocardial stimulation, CNS excitation, and diuresis.
  C. Gastric acid and pepsin secretion stimulant.
V. Uses:
  A. Caffeine has a variety of recreational and medicinal uses.
  B. It is used in cold remedies, as a stimulant, and as an anorectant.
  C. A few cases of severe poisoning have been reported, involving deliberate ingestion of caffeine in tablet form.
VI. Toxic mechanism:
  A. Toxic mechanism not entirely clear.
  B. Excessive sympathetic stimulation resulting from catecholamine release from nerve terminals may cause some toxic symptoms.
  C. The mechanism for CNS toxicity (e.g., seizures) has not been defined but may be the result of cerebral vasoconstriction and hypoxia.
  D. Sinus tachycardia, ventricular tachycardia, and premature ventricular contractions are probably secondary to direct chronotropic action on the myocardium, release of local norepinephrine, and transient decrease in peripheral vagal control.
  E. Direct gastrointestinal irritant.
VII. Range of toxicity:
  A. Toxic dose: 500–1,000 mg.
  B. Fatal dose: 10 gm.
VIII. Clinical features:
  A. Toxic signs and symptoms:
    1. Insomnia, palpitations, tremors, agitation, and tachycardia are common.
    2. Emesis and abdominal pain may occur.
    3. Sympathetic overdrive in some cases (see Chapter 68).
    4. Ventricular dysrhythmias and seizures are rare terminal events.
IX. Laboratory findings and evaluation:
  A. Toxicology screen: Will reveal caffeine in the patient with unknown symptomatic ingestion.
  B. Blood:
    1. Must follow electrolyte status carefully if cathartics used.
    2. Determination of complete blood cell count, BUN, creatinine, and arterial blood gas values potentially useful.
  C. ECG (see Clinical features).
  D. Urinalysis.
X. Treatment:
  A. Follow APTLS (see Chapter 8).
  B. General management: Table 68–6 (see Chapter 12 for details).
XI. Specific treatment:
  A. Arrhythmias:
    1. Follow most recent Advanced Cardiac Life Support (ACLS) guidelines from the American Heart Association (*JAMA* 1986; 255:2841–3044).
    2. **Charcoal hemoperfusion** has been reported to be of benefit in patients with refractory dysrhythmias.

TABLE 68–6.

General Treatment

Treatment	Indicated	Of No Value	Contraindicated
O₂	±		
IV	±		
ECG monitor	±		
Forced diuresis	±		
Acidification			X
Alkalinization		X	
Emesis/lavage*	±/±		
Charcoal†	+		
Cathartic‡	±		
Hemoperfusion‡	±		

*Standard gastrointestinal decontamination, cathartic and charcoal adminis-
tration are recommended with recent ingestions of caffeine in tablet form.
With the unusual massive ingestion, aggressive gastrointestinal decontamination should be initiated.
†Repetitive charcoal administration has not been studied in caffeine ingestions but would be expected to be effective based on reports with theophylline toxicity.
‡See Specific Treatment, below, for indications.

    B. Seizures (see Chapter 22).
    C. Gastritis can be treated with antacids, cimetidine, or ranitidine.
XII. Prognosis:
    A. Expected response to treatment:
        1. Only observation and supportive care are required in the majority of
           cases.
        2. Seizures after theophylline administration result in 50% mortality; sei-
           zures after caffeine are thought less likely to be fatal.
    B. Expected complications and long-term effects:
        1. Complications include psychotic behavior, hypertension, and hyper-
           thermia.
XIII. Disposition considerations:
    A. Admission considerations:
        1. See General Admission Considerations (Chapter 18).
        2. Patients with complications such as psychotic behavior, hypertension,
           hyperthermia or those with prolonged symptoms should be admitted.
        3. Adults who have ingested a potentially fatal dose (>10 gm) should be
           admitted.
        4. Suicide risk.
    B. Consultation considerations: Nephrology consultation if hemoperfusion
       indicated.
    C. Observation period: 3–4 hours.
    D. Discharge considerations:
        1. General Discharge Considerations are met (see Chapter 18).
        2. Asymptomatic after observation period.
        3. Suicide risk and psychiatric status have been evaluated.

Nicotine

I. Route of exposure:
   A. Acute toxicity is generally limited to **oral ingestion** of cigars or cigarette butts. Rarely, inadvertent administration will occur with animal handling or insecticide exposure.
   B. **Green tobacco sickness,** an occupational illness of tobacco handlers, has similar signs and symptoms and is thought to result from **cutaneous absorption** of nicotine.
   C. Cigarette smoking does not cause acute nicotine toxicity.
II. Common trade names and doses:
   A. Cigarettes (thousands of brands worldwide): equivalent to 1–2 mg dose.
   B. Nicotine gum (nicotine polyacrilex, Nicorette): 2 mg/dose.
III. Pharmacokinetics:
   A. Absorption:
      1. Immediately absorbed on inhalation.
      2. Gum must be chewed for nicotine release. If intact gum is swallowed without chewing, little absorption follows.
      3. With oral ingestions, gastric emptying may be delayed, resulting in slower absorption.
      4. A cigarette contains 20–30 mg nicotine, of which only 1–2 mg is absorbed; the majority is burned in the smoking process.
   B. Onset of action:
      1. After inhalation: within 2–3 minutes.
      2. After oral ingestion: within 20–30 minutes.
   C. Plasma half-life: 30 minutes after inhalation or parenteral administration.
   D. Duration of action: Elimination complete in 16 hours.
   E. Elimination: Degradation is primarily hepatic.
   F. Active metabolites: Metabolic breakdown products (e.g., cotinine) have very low toxicity.
IV. Action:
   A. Nicotine derived from tobacco leaves has an acetylcholine-like action on autonomic ganglia and postsynaptic autonomic neurons, resulting first in stimulation and then depolarizing blockage. Both cholinergic and adrenergic postganglionic autonomic neurons are stimulated.
V. Uses:
   A. Toxicity is most commonly seen secondary to oral ingestion of cigarette and other tobacco products.
   B. Nicotine was used widely in the past as an insecticide. Currently only some powdered insecticides contain nicotine.
   C. Used in darts as an animal tranquilizer.
VI. Toxic mechanism:
   A. Accumulation of acetylcholine transiently stimulates but soon paralyzes conduction through cholinergic synapses in the CNS, parasympathetic terminals and some sympathetic terminals (muscarinic effects), and somatic nerves and autonomic ganglionic synapses (nicotinic effects).
   B. Cholinergic crisis results, with usual cause of death being respiratory muscular weakness and increased pulmonary secretions (see Chapters 47 and 106).

      C. Chewing tobacco is strongly associated with oral cancer, although the role that nicotine plays in this process is not clear.

VII. Range of toxicity:

      A. Fatal dose: Estimated at 10 mg/kg (one cigarette generally contains 20–30 mg nicotine).

VIII. Clinical features:

      A. Toxic signs and symptoms:

          1. Diaphoresis, salivation, tachycardias, hypertension, diarrhea (see Cholinergic syndrome, Chapter 47).

          2. Pronounced nausea and vomiting common.

          3. Respiratory failure and cardiovascular collapse have been reported with extreme poisonings.

IX. Laboratory findings and evaluation:

      A. Blood:

          1. Electrolytes (nausea, vomiting).

          2. Arterial blood gas (respiratory symptoms).

      B. ECG.

      C. Chest radiograph if patient has respiratory distress.

X. Treatment:

      A. Follow APTLS (see Chapter 8).

      B. General management: Table 68–7 (see Chapter 12 for details).

XI. Specific management:

      A. For symptoms of cholinergic excess administer atropine (see Chapter 106).

      B. Paralysis: Cardiac monitoring and ventilatory support.

      C. With cutaneous exposure of nicotine-containing insecticides, skin decontamination should be performed (see Chapter 29).

XII. Prognosis:

      A. Expected response to treatment:

          1. Observation until symptoms resolve is frequently the only action necessary.

TABLE 68–7.

General Treatment

Treatment	Indicated	Of No Value	Contraindicated
O_2	±		
IV	±		
ECG monitor	±		
Forced diuresis		X	
Acidification			X
Alkalinization		X	
Emesis/lavage*	± / ±		
Charcoal	±		
Cathartic	±		

*Potassium permanganate has been reported to be an effective neutralizing agent and should be considered for use during lavage; 1:10,000 solution prepared by dissolving 100 mg tablet in 1 L water.

2. The rare fatality usually results from respiratory paralysis, with death occurring in the first 4 hours.

3. With good supportive care, paralysis will resolve as the nicotine is metabolized.

B. Expected complications and long-term effects:

1. Temporary paralysis (see above).

XIII. Special considerations:

A. Green tobacco sickness, an occupational illness of tobacco handlers, has similar signs and symptoms as with oral ingestion and is thought to result from cutaneous absorption of nicotine. With rare cutaneous exposure, skin decontamination should be performed.

XIV. Disposition considerations:

A. Admission considerations:

1. See General Admission Considerations (Chapter 18).

2. Extraordinary case with signs of severe toxicity, such as tachycardia and hypertension.

3. Any patient requiring use of atropine or respiratory support should be admitted for further care and observation.

4. Suicide risk.

B. Observation period: In the patient with mild toxicity, observation for 3–4 hours, until symptoms resolve, is frequently the only action necessary before discharge.

C. Discharge considerations:

1. General disposition considerations are met (see Chapter 18).

2. Asymptomatic after 3–4 hours of observation and treatment.

3. Suicide potential and psychiatric status have been appropriately evaluated.

BIBLIOGRAPHY

Bryson PD: Drugs of abuse: Stimulants, in Bryson PD (ed): *Comprehensive Review in Toxicology.* Rockville, Md, Aspen Systems Corp, 1986, pp 219–237.

Dowling GP, et al: "Eve" and "Ecstasy," a report of five deaths associated with the use of MDEA and MDMA. *JAMA* 1987; 257:1615.

Dreisbach RH, Robertson WO: *Handbook of Poisoning.* Norwalk, Conn, Appleton-Century-Crofts, 1987.

Matick H, et al: Cerebral vasculitis associated with oral amphetamine overdose. *Arch Neurol* 1983; 40:253.

Pentel P: Toxicity of over-the-counter stimulants. *JAMA* 1984; 252:1898.

Treffert DA, Joranson D: Restricting amphetamines: Wisconsin's success story. *JAMA* 1981; 245:1336.

Zimmerman PM, et al: Caffeine intoxication: A near fatality. *Ann Emerg Med* 1985; 14:1227.

Ziporyn T: A growing industry and menace: Makeshift laboratory's designer drugs. *JAMA* 1986; 256:3061–3063.

69

Cocaine

Kevin S. Merigian, M.D.

I. Route of exposure:
   A. Nasal insufflation (snorting).
   B. Smoking (freebase or crack).
   C. Oral.
   D. Mucosal.
   E. Intravenous injection (mainlining, speedballing).
II. Common names:
   A. Cocaine hydrochloride: Topical solution.
   B. Street names: See Table 69–1.
   C. Street measures: Hit (2–200 mg), snort, line, dose, spoon (approximately 1 gm).
   D. Freebase: Cocaine that has been converted to a more volatile base state. Method: add strong alkali to an aqueous solution of cocaine HCl, thereby extracting the cocaine base in a residue or precipitate.
   E. Crack: Potent, purified, smokable form of cocaine; produces effects similar to those with IV injection (Med Lett, 1986; 28:69).
III. Pharmacokinetics:
   A. Absorption: Through mucosal membranes; rapid and complete (e.g., 20 minutes when topically applied to nasal mucosa).
   B. Onset of action:
      1. Oral: 2–5 minutes.
      2. Nasal: 2–5 minutes.
      3. IV: <30 seconds.
      4. Smoked: <30 seconds.

TABLE 69–1.

Street Names for Cocaine*

Bernice	Charlie	Girl	Powder
Bernies	Cholly	Gold dust	Smoke
Blow	Coke	Green gold	Snort
Burese	Corine	Happy dust	Snow
C	Crack	Heaven dust	Snowflake
Cadillac of	Dama Blanca	Jet	Stardust
drugs	Dust	Joy powder	Sugar
Carrie	Dynamite	Leaf	Toot
Cecil	Flake	Paradise	White dust
Champagne	Gin	Pimp's drug	White girl
of drugs			

Combinations: Liquid lady (alcohol and cocaine), Speedball
(heroin and cocaine)

*Adapted from Migliore MJ, Alexander C: *Handbook of Slang Names for Abused Substances.* Jamaica, NY, St Johns University Press 1983.

C. Half-life: 40–90 minutes.
D. Peak effect:
   1. Oral: 20–40 minutes.
   2. Nasal: 20–40 minutes.
   3. IV: 3–5 minutes.
   4. Smoked: 3–5 minutes.
E. Duration of action:
   1. IV: 30–60 minutes.
   2. Nasal insufflation: 20–40 minutes to peak, with gradual decrease over next 60 minutes.
F. Elimination:
   1. Metabolized within 2 hours by liver to major metabolites, benzoylecgonine and ecgonine methyl ester, which are then excreted in urine.
   2. Metabolites can be identified within 5 minutes of IV use, and up to 48 hours after oral ingestion in urine.
IV. Action:
   A. Mechanism of action unclear. Postulated block of reuptake of catecholamines at adrenergic nerve endings.
   B. Possibly increases sensitivity of neuroreceptors and promotes release of norepinephrine.
   C. Intense CNS stimulation.
V. Uses:
   A. Topical anesthetic and vasoconstrictor.
   B. Recreational abuse.
VI. Toxic mechanism: Excessive sympathetic stimulation resulting from blockage of reuptake of neurotransmitters such as norepinephrine, and increased release of epinephrine and norepinephrine from nerve terminals. Concentration in the synaptic cleft leads to hypersensitivity of receptors.

VII. Range of toxicity:
  A. Oral lethal dose: 1,200 mg.
  B. Nasal insufflation:
    1. As little as 30 mg has resulted in death.
    2. Highly publicized reports of fatalities resulting from a single dose.
  C. Parenteral lethal dose: 20 mg.
VIII. Clinical features:
  A. Phase 1:
    1. CNS: Euphoria, agitation, headache, vertigo, twitching, bruxism, non-intentional tremor.
    2. Nausea, vomiting, fever, hypertension, tachycardia.
  B. Phase 2:
    1. CNS: Lethargy, hyperreactive deep tendon reflexes, seizures (status epilepticus).
    2. Sympathetic overdrive: Tachycardia, hypertension, hyperthermia.
    3. Incontinence.
  C. Phase 3:
    1. CNS: Flaccid paralysis, coma, fixed dilated pupils, loss of reflexes.
    2. Pulmonary edema.
    3. Cardiopulmonary arrest.
  D. Psychological presentation: Habituation, paranoia, hallucination (e.g., cocaine "bugs").
IX. Laboratory findings and evaluation:
  A. Toxicology screen (urine) if diagnosis in doubt.
  B. Blood:
    1. Complete blood cell count, electrolytes, glucose, BUN, creatinine, calcium may be indicated.
    2. Arterial blood gas analyses (cardiac or pulmonary findings).
  C. ECG.
  D. Urinalysis.
X. General treatment:
  A. Follow APTLS (see Chapter 8).
  B. General management: See Table 69–2 (see Chapter 12 for details).

TABLE 69–2.

General Treatment

Treatment	Indicated	Of No Value	Contraindicated
O$_2$	±		
IV	+		
ECG monitor	+		
Forced diuresis		X	
Acidification			X
Alkalinization		X	
Emesis/lavage	±/±		
Charcoal	±		
Cathartic	±		

XI. Specific treatment:
   A. Inhalation: Wash nasal passages.
   B. Anxiety:
      1. Diazepam 15–20 mg PO or 5 mg IV for severe agitation.
      2. Avoid haloperidol or chlorpromazine; these lower the seizure threshold.
   C. Seizures: See Chapter 22.
   D. Hypertension: See Chapter 68.
   E. Ventricular arrhythmias:
      1. Propranolol 1 mg/min for up to 6 mg.
      2. Lidocaine 1.5 mg/kg bolus followed by IV infusion. Use is controversial because of potential for causing seizures. Termination of ventricular arrhythmias may be resistant to lidocaine and even to cardioversion.

XII. Prognosis:
   A. Expected response to treatment:
      1. Although prognosis in cocaine overdose is unpredictable and inconsistent, patients who survive for 3 hours after cocaine intoxication generally recover.
   B. Expected complications and long-term effects:
      1. Cardiovascular: Myocardial ischemia or infarction, cardiac arrhythmias, myocarditis.
      2. Ingested cocaine may cause bowel ischemia or infarction.
   C. Bronchiolitis obliterans, organized pneumonia secondary to smoking free-base cocaine.

XIII. Special considerations:
   A. Adulterants, contaminants, and drugs admixed with street cocaine:

Alcohol	Mannitol
Aminophylline	Marijuana
Amphetamines	Meperidine
Benzocaine	Methapyrilene
Butacaine	$MgSO_4$
Caffeine	Morphine
Codeine	$NaHCO_3$ (baking soda)
Corn starch	Nicotine
Cotton fibers	Phencyclidine (PCP)
Ergotamine	Phenylpropanolamine
Flour	Procaine
Hashish	Quinine
Heroin	Salicylamide
Inositol	Strychnine
Lactose	Sucrose
Lidocaine	Talc
LSD	Tetracaine
Magnesium silicate	Thallium
Maltose	Thiamine

   B. Body packing: Ingestion of packets of cocaine. Packets may burst in intestines, causing severe overdose. Packets should be removed with cathartics or surgically.

   C. Multiple-drug ingestion: Frequently patients have used a mixture of cocaine and heroin (speedball) or simultaneously ingested amphetamines, PCP, hallucinogens, or alcohol.
   D. Severe depression may be seen after the effects of cocaine wear off, which **may result in suicide potential.**
XIV. Disposition considerations:
   A. Admission considerations:
      1. See General Admission Considerations (Chapter 18).
      2. Phase 1 toxicity unresponsive to anxiolytic therapy.
      3. Phase 2 or 3 symptoms.
      4. Body stuffer.
      5. Psychosis, agitation.
      6. Suicide risk.
      7. ICU admission considerations:
         a. Chest pain, regardless of age.
         b. ECG changes suggestive of ischemia.
         c. Ventricular arrhythmias.
         d. Uncontrolled sympathetic overdrive.
         e. Recurrent seizures or status epilepticus.
         f. Need for respiratory or cardiovascular support.
   B. Consultation considerations:
      1. Gastroenterology (for endoscopy) or general surgical consultation for body stuffing.
      2. Psychiatric consultation for evaluation of depressive symptoms secondary to withdrawal.
      3. Anesthesiology consultation for seizures unresponsive to emergency treatment.
      4. Cardiology consultation for ventricular arrhythmias unresponsive to standard therapy.
   C. Observation period: Patients with mild toxicity can be discharged if asymptomatic after at least 4 hours of observation in the emergency department.
   D. Discharge considerations:
      1. General discharge considerations are met (see Chapter 18).
      2. Patients with phase 1 symptoms can be discharged if all symptoms are resolved within a 4-hour observation period (with the exception of those who have ingested packets).
      3. Drug counseling has been offered.
      4. Suicide potential and psychiatric status have been appropriately evaluated.
      5. Follow-up has been arranged.

BIBLIOGRAPHY

Caruana DS, Weinbach B, Goerg D, et al: Cocaine-packet ingestion: Diagnosis, management and natural history. *Ann Intern Med* 1984; 100:73–74.
Cregler LL, Mark H: Medical complications of cocaine abuse. *N Engl J Med* 1986; 315:1495–1500.

Gay GR: Clinical management of acute and chronic cocaine poisoning. *Ann Emerg Med* 1982; 11:562.

Hueter DC: Cardiovascular effects of cocaine. *JAMA* 1987; 257:979–980.

Isner JM, et al: Acute cardiac events temporally related to cocaine abuse. *N Engl J Med* 1986; 315:1438–1443.

Kaye BR, Fainstat M: Cerebral vasculitis associated with cocaine abuse. *JAMA* 1987; 258:2104–2106.

Smith HWB, Liberman HA, Brody SL, et al: Acute myocardial infarction temporally related to cocaine use. *Ann Intern Med* 1987; 107:13–18.

Wiener MD, Putnam CE: Pain in the chest of a user of cocaine. *JAMA* 1987; 258:2087–2088.

70

Phencyclidine (PCP)

William P. Fabbri, M.D., F.A.C.E.P.

I. Route of exposure:
   A. Smoked (in treated tobacco or cannabis).
   B. Nasal insufflation (snorted).
   C. IV.
   D. Oral.
II. Common street names: See Table 70–1.
III. Pharmacokinetics:
   A. Absorption: Poorly absorbed in acid media of stomach.
   B. Onset of action: Varies with mode of exposure:
      1. IV: Minutes.
      2. Smoked: Gradually over several minutes.
      3. Oral: No reliable data.
   C. Half-life: 11–89 hours (estimate).
   D. Elimination: 90% by liver enzymes; 10% renal.
   E. Active metabolites: None known.
IV. Action:
   A. Some anticholinergic properties.
   B. Dissociative effects: Altered perception of environmental stimuli.
V. Uses:
   A. Originally developed as an intravenous anesthetic/analgesic. Abandoned because of side effects.
   B. Mind-altering effects and ease of manufacture at low cost have made it a popular drug of abuse.
VI. Toxic mechanism:
   A. Incompletely understood. Proposed mechanism of action: appears to influence several neurotransmitters, may act as a false transmitter.

TABLE 70–1.

Common Street Names for PCP*

Angle dust	KJ
Angel's mist	Magic mist
Cadillac	Mist
CJs	Monkey tranquilizer
Crystal	PCP (Peace)
Crystal joints	Peace pill (San Francisco)
Cyclones	Peace weed (East Coast)
DOA	Rocket fuel
Dust	Scaffle
Elephant embalmer	Sheets
Elephant tranquilizer	Snorts
Flake	Soma
Goon	Super grass
Hog (East Coast)	Super weed
Hog dust	Surfer
Horse tracks	THC
Killer weed	Wobble weed

*Total PCP: Angel dust, 88%–100% pure; crystal, 50%–100%; others, 10%–30%.

    B. Poorly absorbed in the stomach's acid milieu and readily absorbed in the basic pH of the small bowel. After absorption in the small bowel PCP is resecreted into stomach. It is thought that this sequestration within the gastric lumen and subsequent reabsorption in the small intestine may explain the characteristic fluctuating symptomatology after ingestion of a single dose.

    C. The relative low pH of cerebrospinal fluid relative to brain tissue may also produce a similar sequestration phenomenon in the CSF space.

  VII. Range of toxicity:

    A. Toxic dose:

      1. Mild intoxication: 5 mg.

      2. Moderate intoxication: 5–10 mg.

      3. Severe intoxication: >10 mg.

    B. Fatal dose: 1 mg/kg.

    C. Some authors believe published fatal and toxic doses for PCP are not important information, because the ingested amount is seldom known and at least 40% of PCP overdoses involve more than one drug.

  VIII. Clinical features:

    A. Three stages of intoxication:

      1. Stage I: Mild intoxication:

        a. Patient may be hallucinating, disoriented, confused, or violent. Violence and agitation particularly associated with IV or PO exposure.

        b. May observe anxiety or depression.

        c. Sensory dissociation: Patients may ignore pain, manifest detachment from surroundings (blank stare, automatic behavior).

      d. Tachycardia, tachypnea, hypertension.

      e. Nystagmus (in fewer than 50% of patients).

  2. Stage II: Moderate intoxication:

      a. Stupor or coma lasting 0.5 to 1 hour.

      b. May observe generalized spasticity, myoclonus, decreased or absent laryngeal and pharyngeal reflexes, and seizures.

      c. Hyporeflexia, muscular rigidity.

  3. Stage III: Severe intoxication:

      a. Coma lasting longer than 2 hours.

      b. May exhibit status epilepticus, opisthotonos.

      c. Respiratory failure, apnea.

      d. Hypertensive crisis.

      e. Rhabdomyolysis.

      f. Acute renal failure.

      g. Unresponsive to deep pain.

      h. Fatal arrhythmias.

B. Other signs and symptoms:

  1. Trauma: Patients with PCP intoxication may have trauma secondary to violence and agitation (e.g., fractures, lacerations). Unless the clinician has a high index of suspicion for concomitant PCP use, the toxicologic cause of trauma may be missed.

  2. CNS:

      a. Sudden changes in neurological status.

      b. Seizures.

      c. Sudden loss of consciousness.

      e. Sudden apnea.

  3. Adrenergic crises:

  4. Difficult to determine level of intoxication because of waxing and waning nature of symptoms, with alternating periods of alertness and coma.

IX. Laboratory findings and evaluation:

A. Toxicological screen:

  1. Serum levels not of value in the emergency department:

      a. Serum levels do not correlate well with symptoms.

      b. Depending on the assay method used, approximately 15% of patients admitted with PCP intoxication have negative laboratory results. Also, patients subjected to serial urine testing while inpatients have displayed resolution and then reappearance of positive test results.

  2. Routine screen recommended to rule out multiple-drug ingestion.

B. Blood:

  1. Complete blood cell count:

      a. Leukocytosis common.

      b. Differential diagnosis of altered mental status includes sepsis.

  2. Chemistry:

      a. Creatine phosphokinase.

      b. BUN, creatinine to assess renal function, especially if evidence of rhabdomyolysis.

      c. Uric acid: Early finding in rhabdomyolysis.

      d. Hypoglycemia: 20% incidence.

      e. Serum ammonia: Rule out Reye's syndrome.

      f. Electrolytes: Hyperkalemia may be seen, particularly in the presence of rhabdomyolysis, and serial serum potassium levels may be indicated.

      g. Liver function studies: SGOT, SGPT, alkaline phosphatase.

    3. Arterial blood gas analysis: Monitor acid/base status, respiratory depression.

  C. Urinalysis: Myoglobinuria.

X. General treatment:

  A. Follow APTLS (see Chapter 8).

  B. General management: See Table 70–2 (see Chapter 12 for details).

XI. Specific management:

  A. Continuous gastric suction may be indicated in severe toxicity (stupor or coma). The rationale for this therapy is based on the observation that PCP is resecreted into the stomach after absorption in the small intestine (see Toxic mechanism). Continuous gastric suction, however, cannot be routinely recommended.

  B. Agitation:

    1. Place patient in quiet area.

    2. Restraint:

      a. Frequent monitoring of vital signs, neurologic examination, and serial physical examinations are necessary components of safe restraint.

TABLE 70–2.

General Treatment

Treatment	Indicated	Of No Value	Contraindicated
O_2	+		
IV (D_5NSS)	+		
ECG monitor*	+		
Forced diuresis	+		
Acidification†			X
Alkalinization†	±		
Emesis‡/			X
lavage	+		
Charcoal§	Repeated		
Cathartic	+		
D_{50}¶	±		
Dialysis**	±		

*Continuous cardiac monitoring for cardiac arrhythmias.
†See Controversies.
‡Risk of sudden seizure or apnea.
§Dose: 1 gm/kg every 2–4 hours.
¶Incidence of hypoglycemia 20%.
**See Indications below.

     b. Proper restraint requires trained personnel. "Choke holds" have resulted in sudden bradycardia and cardiovascular collapse. Metal restraints such as handcuffs are contraindicated because they have resulted in severe orthopedic and neurological injury when applied to disoriented patients. Plastic or leather restraints are preferred, although not without risks to the wildly agitated patient. On the other hand, gauze restraints may be totally ineffective in restraining out-of-control patients. See Chapter 27 for suggestions.

     c. In cases of severe violent behavior or prolonged agitation, the patient may develop exhaustion, severe hypertension, or self-injury.

     d. Diazepam 2–5 mg IV initially, titrated upward to desired sedative response. Generally 10 mg or less is adequate; however, up to 20 mg or more may be required.

  3. Dangerous or **contraindicated** therapy:

     a. Phenothiazines: Prolonged hypotension, lowered seizure threshold.

     b. Haloperidol: Associated with neuroleptic malignant syndrome in one study.

C. Adrenergic crisis:

  1. Mild hypertension:

     a. Observation only.

     b. Propranolol HCl (Inderal), up to 40 mg PO. Repeat if necessary in doses of 20–40 mg every 4–6 hours.

  2. Moderate or severe hypertension: See Controversies:

     a. Also see Chapter 68.

  3. Tachycardia associated with hemodynamic compromise not responsive to sedation may be cautiously treated with IV propranolol.

D. Seizures: See Chapter 22 for treatment suggestions.

E. Rhabdomyolysis:

  1. Treatment of PCP-induced myoglobinuria:

     a. Correct volume depletion with IV fluids.

     b. Alkalinization for rhabdomyolysis is controversial and some authors recommend that it definitely **should not** be performed in the setting of phencyclidine toxicity.

  2. Hemodialysis:

     a. Indications:

       (1) If urine flow does not increase in response to forced diuresis.

       (2) Renal failure.

XII. Prognosis:

A. Expected response to treatment:

  1. Mild toxicity:

     a. Most patients are communicative within 1–2 hours and alert and oriented within 6–8 hours.

     b. No medical sequelae expected.

     c. Psychiatric sequelae (toxic psychosis and major depression) increase with repeated abuse, regardless of level of intoxication in the acute event. With mild intoxication, symptoms may resolve in 6–24 hours; however, there are reports of persistent and recurrent behavioral abnormalities for several weeks or months.

2. Moderate to severe toxicity:
    a. High rate of medical complications.
    b. Patients usually recover consciousness in 24–48 hours, but complete recovery may take a week or longer.
B. Expected complications and long-term effects:

Apnea	Intracerebral hemorrhage
Cardiac arrest	Laryngospasm
Hypertensive encephalopathy	Psychosis
Hyperthermia	Rhabdomyolysis
	Seizures

XIII. Controversies:
  A. Urine acidification is often suggested in texts. It is of questionable value, difficult to achieve, and may be inappropriate in patients at risk for rhabdomyolysis.
  B. Hypertension: Some experts recommend treating hypertension prophylactically; others do not treat unless hypertension becomes life threatening.
  C. Use of physostigmine, haloperidol, chlorpromazine, and meperidine has been recommended by some for treatment of PCP toxicity. **Phenothiazines** and **butyrophenones** may lower seizure threshold and cause acute dystonic reactions. **Physostigmine** has been associated with significant side effects, including seizures and cardiac arrhythmias. **Meperidine** has not been completely evaluated in large-scale studies.
  D. Urinary alkalinization for PCP-induced rhabdomyolis is controversial.
XIV. Special considerations:
  A. Treatment of hypertension: Hypertension associated with PCP overdose is produced by peripheral vasoconstriction and increased cardiac output and heart rate. Although propranolol is effective in treatment of PCP-induced hypertensive crisis, it has been observed on occasion to actually worsen the hypertension. The reason for this idiosyncratic reaction is related to the fact that beta blockers may result in unopposed alpha receptor stimulation, leading to increased vasoconstriction, causing the blood pressure to rise even higher.
  B. Similar drugs: Phencyclidine-like analogs:
    1. PCC: Peperidinocyclohexane carbonitrile.
    2. PHP: Phenylcyclohexylpyrrolidine.
    3. TCP: Thienylcyclohexylpiperidine.
    4. PCE: Cyclohexamine.
    5. Ketamine.
XV. Disposition considerations:
  A. Admission considerations:
    1. See General Admission Considerations (Chapter 18).
    2. Mild intoxication: Consider admission:
      a. Anxiety or depression if patient has no social supports.
      b. Question whether patient will follow up with drug or psychiatric counseling.
      c. If admitted, patients with mild intoxication may be admitted to a psychiatric unit until symptoms clear, usually in 6–24 hours.

   3. Moderate intoxication: consider admission:
      a. Sustained hypertension.
      b. Myoglobinuria.
      c. Renal failure (secondary to myoglobinuria).
      d. Aspiration or apneic episodes.
   4. Severe intoxication: All patients should be admitted to an ICU for at least 24 hours.
B. Consultation considerations:
   1. Acute psychiatric evaluation indicated for all patients exhibiting initial self-destructive behavior. Follow-up psychiatric evaluation indicated for all cases of PCP intoxication, regardless of severity, because of potential for delayed sequelae (e.g., subtle thought disorders, depression).
C. Observation period:
   1. Mild toxicity: If mentally and neurologically stable, 4 hours. If patient then asymptomatic, may be discharged in company of responsible adult.
D. Discharge considerations:
   1. General discharge considerations have been met (see Chapter 18).
   2. Transient episodes of serious symptoms in the prehospital phase (e.g., transient apnea, catatonia) have been definitely excluded.
   3. Patients with mild intoxication without complicating factors may be discharged if they are asymptomatic after 4 hours of observation.
   4. Rhabdomyolysis has been ruled out.
   5. Multiple-drug ingestion has been ruled out (value of toxicology screening).
   6. **All patients must be assessed for suicide risk before discharge.**
   7. Drug counseling has been offered. Psychiatric follow-up arranged.
   8. Patient warned that episodes of disorientation and depression may continue for up to 4 weeks.
   9. Patient released in the care of a responsible adult.
E. Transfer considerations:
   1. Interhospital transfer of patients with PCP intoxication should be avoided because of potential for sudden changes in status. Transfer only if initial treating center does not have resources to care for the patient. Transfer with physician in attendance if possible, and with ability to cope with agitation or violence.
   2. See Chapter 19.

BIBLIOGRAPHY

Bryson PD: *Comprehensive Review in Toxicology.* Rockville, Md, Aspen Systems Corp, 1986.

Budd RD, Lindstrom DM: Characteristics of victims of PCP-related deaths in Los Angeles County. *J Toxicol Clin Toxicol* 1982; 9:997–1004.

Castellani S, Adams PM, Giannini AJ: Physostigmine treatment of acute phencyclidine intoxication. *J Clin Psychiatry* 1982; 43:10–12.

Castellani S, Giannini AJ: Phencyclidine intoxication: Assessment of possible antidotes. *J Clin Toxicol* 1982; 19:313–319.

Giannini AJ, Eighan MS, Loiselle RH: Comparison of chlorpromazine and haloperidol in phencyclidine psychosis: Role of the DA-2 receptor. *J Clin Pharmacol* 1984; 24:202–204.

Giannini AJ, Loiselle RH, Price WA, et al: Comparison of chlorpromazine and meperidine in the treatment of phencyclidine psychosis: Role of the opiate receptor. *J Clin Psychiatry* 1985; 46:52–54.

Lahmayer HW, Stock PG: Phencyclidine intoxication, physical restraint, and acute renal failure: Case report. *J Clin Psychiatry* 1983; 5:184–185.

McCarron MM: Phencyclidine intoxication, in *Phencyclidine: An Update.* Bethesda, Md, National Institute on Drug Abuse, NIDA Monograph 64, 1986, pp 209–217.

Pradhan SN: Phencyclidine (PCP): Some newer studies. *Neurosci Biobehav Rev* 1984; 8:493–501.

Rosen P, Baker FJ, Barkin RM, et al: *Emergency Medicine: Concepts and Clinical Practice.* St Louis, CV Mosby Co, 1988.

71

Marijuana (Tetrahydrocannabinol)

Jeanne C. Rubenstone, M.D.

I. Route of exposure: Inhalation, oral (e.g., baked in brownies), IV (hashish oil).
II. Common names:
    A. Synthetic tetrahydrocannabinol (THC) is available in the United States (FDA approved) as dronabinol (trade name Marinol). Used as an antiemetic for patients receiving chemotherapy.
    B. Street names:

Acapulco gold	Kif
Brick	Mary
Bull	Mohasky
Bush	Mooters
Butter	Mu
Grass	Mud
Griffo	Mutah
Hash	Panama
Hashish	Pot
Hemp	Red stick
Indiana hay	Smoke
J	Splim
Jane	Straw
Jive	Weed
Joint	

III. Pharmacokinetics:
    A. Absorption: When smoked, immediate.

B. Onset of action:
   1. Inhalation: 6–12 minutes.
   2. Oral: 30–120 minutes.
C. Plasma half-life:
   1. Accurate determinations are difficult because plasma concentrations generally cannot be detected below 1–5 ng/ml.
   2. In humans, plasma half-life estimated at 56 hours for inexperienced users and 28 hours for chronic users.
D. Peak effect: Peak blood level of THC is reached within minutes of inhalation, then declines rapidly. Blood levels do not correlate well with symptoms; patients may remain intoxicated for 2–3 hours after smoking.
E. Duration of action:
   1. Inhalation: Clinical effects may last 3–4 hours.
   2. Oral: Clinical effects may last 4–6 hours.
F. Elimination:
   1. Rapidly metabolized by the liver and lungs, with metabolites slowly eliminated by release from various body compartments.
   2. Biliary excretion predominates. Metabolites are detectable in both feces and urine.
G. Active metabolite: 11-hydroxy-THC.

IV. Action:
A. Active ingredients:
   1. The hemp plant *Cannabis sativa* contains up to 2%–6% THC.
   2. More potent forms include sensimilla (seedless marijuana, containing approximately 8% THC), hashish (often more than 10%), and hash oil (may contain more than 20% THC).
   3. A standard U.S. joint contains 500–1,000 mg marijuana. THC concentrations typically range from 1%–2%, equivalent to 5–20 mg THC.
B. Mechanism of action:
   1. Postulated mechanism of action involves an unknown interaction with serotonin release and GABA actions.
   2. Increased sympathetic activity and parasympathetic inhibition.
   3. Bronchodilation.
   4. Antiemetic effect.
   5. Ocular hypotensive effect.
   6. Anticonvulsant effect. No present clinical application.

V. Uses:
A. Illegal recreational abuse.
B. Therapeutic applications:
   1. Antiemetic for patients receiving chemotherapy. Use limited by CNS effects.
   2. Decreases intraocular pressure; under investigation for open-angle glaucoma.
   3. Bronchodilator:
      a. Oral dose required for bronchodilation produces adverse effects (see Clinical features).
      b. Unable to formulate aerosol preparation because of low water solubility.

      c. No present clinical application.
VI. Toxic mechanism:
  A. Autonomic effects:
    1. Orthostatic hypotension, dry mouth, decreased GI motility, urinary retention.
    2. At high doses: Tachycardia, bradycardia, congestive heart failure.
  B. Direct irritant effects (e.g., bronchitis).
  C. May potentiate seizures in toxic doses.
  D. Anaphylactoid reactions.
VII. Range of toxicity:
  A. Toxic dose: 15 mg/kg absorbed THC.
  B. Fatal dose: No lethal overdose in humans has been clearly documented.
VIII. Clinical features:
  A. Acute effects:
    1. Cardiovascular:
      a. Sinus tachycardia:
        (1) Dose related.
        (2) Maximal within 15–30 minutes of inhalation, then slow decline over 4 hours.
        (3) Can be inhibited by beta blockade.
      b. ECG changes:
        (1) Premature ventricular contractions.
        (2) Nonspecific ST-T changes generally rate related.
      c. Orthostatic hypotension thought to be related to decreased peripheral vascular resistance secondary to $beta_2$ stimulation. This also can be inhibited by beta blockade.
    2. Central nervous system:
      a. Relaxation; altered time/space/sensory perception; dose-related drowsiness; impaired short-term memory, cognition, speech, and complex motor skills.
      b. With high doses or in some inexperienced users or in certain predisposed individuals, may be dysphoric symptoms, such as anxiety, paranoia, psychosis.
      c. Reports of muscle weakness, fine tremor, marked lateral gaze nystagmus.
      d. Alterations in rapid eye movement (REM) sleep and sleeplike EEG patterns while awake have been observed.
    3. Behavioral: Persons with underlying psychiatric disorders or inexperienced users may be at higher risk for severe reactions to marijuana, including psychosis, paranoid ideation, panic, and visual hallucinations.
    4. Miscellaneous:
      a. Conjunctival hyperemia.
      b. THC may potentiate seizures in patients with seizure disorders.
      c. Increased appetite, thirst, dry mucous membranes.
      d. Urinary frequency or retention.
  B. Chronic effects:
    1. Respiratory:
      a. Chronic pharyngitis, rhinitis, hoarseness, bronchitis, sinusitis, wheezing.

  b. No evidence of carcinogenesis in humans; however, malignant changes observed in tissue culture and animal studies.

 2. Pregnancy: Increased incidence of protracted labor, meconium staining, infants with low birth weight and developmental features resembling those of fetal alcohol syndrome.

 3. Behavioral: May cause apathy and loss of energy, commonly referred to as amotivational syndrome.

IX. Laboratory findings and evaluation:

 A. Serum levels:

  1. Not helpful in acute intoxication, because of poor correlation between blood level and clinical effect.

  2. Standard assays of urinary metabolites may detect presence of THC up to 10 days after use in inexperienced users and up to 4 weeks in chronic users.

   a. False positive test results rare. Experimental evidence suggests that passive inhalation from nearby marijuana smokers can produce urinary metabolite levels detectable by highly sensitive assays; detection by standard screening methods highly unlikely.

   b. False negative test results are possible by adulteration of urine specimen with sodium chloride, acidic substances such as lemon juice, alkaline substances such as chlorine bleach, or dilution with water. This is known to some drug abusers, who surreptitiously add these substances to their urine samples to produce false negative results. Thus both pH and specific gravity of the urine should be measured before performing the assay.

 B. Toxicologic screen: If diagnosis is in doubt or multiple-drug ingestion cannot be definitely ruled out.

 C. Consider glucose test (Dextrostix) in patients with altered mental status or decreased level of consciousness.

 D. Other tests dictated by clinical situation.

X. General treatment:

 A. Follow APTLS (see Chapter 8).

 B. General management: Table 71–1 (see Chapter 12 for details).

XI. Specific treatment:

 A. Reassurance and quiet environment for mood-altering or psychoactive effects.

 B. For severe, refractory behavioral effects (e.g., extreme agitation), may consider administering benzodiazepine (e.g., diazepam 5–10 mg PO or IV).

XII. Prognosis: Physical and behavioral effects generally resolve within 6 hours of THC use.

XIII. Special considerations:

 A. Acute multiple-drug toxicity:

  1. Marijuana and alcohol: Frequent combination. May augment usual autonomic and CNS effects (synergism of perceptual, cognitive, and motor impairment).

  2. Marijuana and amphetamines: One report of additive increase in systolic blood pressure, with synergistic increase in duration and intensity of the "high."

TABLE 71–1.

General Treatment

Treatment	Indicated	Of No Value	Contraindicated
O₂	±		
IV	±		
ECG monitor	±		
Forced diuresis		X	
Acidification			X
Alkalinization		X	
Emesis*/lavage*	±/±		
Charcoal*	±		
Cathartic*	±		

*For oral intoxication, may lavage or induce emesis with ipecac. This should be followed by activated charcoal, which is most effective when given within 30 minutes of ingestion.

---

   3. Marijuana and phencyclidine (PCP): Smoked together as "super grass." Produces marked sympathomimetic symptoms (hypertension, tachycardia, salivation, flushing, sweating, agitation).

   4. Marijuana and opiates, barbiturates, sedatives: marked CNS depression.

B. Intravenous intoxication:

   1. Syndrome produced by intravenous injection of marijuana has been reported:

     a. Abdominal pain, nausea, vomiting, diarrhea, fever, and chills occur within 1 hour of injection.

     b. Patients come to emergency department about 12 hours after injection and may be cyanotic, febrile, and hypotensive, with renal insufficiency (azotemia), leukocytosis (or leukopenia), bleeding disorder (thrombocytopenia), and rhabdomyolysis, with elevated creatinine phosphokinase level and myoglobinuria.

   2. Given good supportive care, patients ordinarily recover without any permanent sequelae. Cause of syndrome unknown at present.

C. Contaminants:

   1. Pesticide contamination of marijuana leaves: Prime example is paraquat-contaminated marijuana from Mexico (see Chapter 107). No documented cases of paraquat poisoning in marijuana users, despite potential for severe pulmonary toxicity; the paraquat may be destroyed by the burning joint prior to inhalation.

   2. Bacterial gastroenteritis: One documented epidemic of *Salmonella muenchen* gastroenteritis traced to contaminated marijuana. Cause of contamination unclear. May have been related to fertilization of marijuana plants with contaminated manure or adulteration with dried manure to increase weight.

D. Tolerance and dependence:

   1. Tolerance develops to both psychological and physiological effects.

   2. Cross tolerance with alcohol has been reported. Chronic marijuana

users have shown less impairment than expected after alcohol consumption.

3. Physical dependence remains controversial. No solid experimental evidence exists that addiction occurs, but several investigators report restlessness and irritability after cessation of chronic use.

XIV. Disposition considerations:

A. Admission considerations:
  1. See General Admission Considerations (Chapter 18).
  2. Symptomatic after 6 hours of observation.
  3. Severe psychotic episodes with paranoid ideation, agitation, and hallucinations not responding to therapy.
  4. All patients who have injected marijuana IV.

B. Consultation considerations: Patients with severe psychiatric symptoms, including psychosis, paranoid ideation, panic, and visual hallucinations, should be evaluated by a psychiatrist.

C. Observation period: Symptoms usually dissipate within 6 hours. Even toxic psychosis usually requires no treatment other than protecting the patient from consequences of behavioral toxicity as a result of disorientation. Patient can be observed if quiet area exists and personnel are adequate.

D. Discharge considerations:
  1. All General discharge considerations have been met (see Chapter 18).
  2. Symptoms have abated.
  3. Follow-up visit with a psychiatrist should be scheduled within 1 week for all patients discharged from the emergency department after an episode of marijuana-induced psychosis, to determine any underlying psychopathologic condition.
  4. Suicide potential and psychiatric state have been appropriately evaluated.

BIBLIOGRAPHY

Brandenberg D, Wernick R: Intravenous marijuana syndrome. *West J Med* 1986; 145:94–96.

Huber G, O'Connell D, McCarthy C, et al: Toxicologic pharmacology of tetrahydrocannabinol (THC) and marijuana (MJ) smoke components. *Clin Res* 1976; 24:A255.

Kolansky H, Moore WT: Toxic effects of chronic marijuana use. *JAMA* 1972; 222:35–41.

Landrigan PJ, Powell PE, James LM, et al: Paraquat and marijuana: Epidemiologic risk assessment. *Am J Public Health* 1983; 73:784–788.

Payne RJ, Brand SN: The toxicity of intravenously used marijuana. *JAMA* 1975; 223:351–354.

Peterson RC (ed): *Marijuana Research Findings: 1980.* Bethesda, Md, National Institute on Drug Abuse, Research Monograph 31, 1980.

Tashkin DP, Soares JR, Hepler RS, et al: Cannabis, 1977. *Ann Intern Med* 1978; 135:1213–1215.

Vachon K, et al: Single-dose effect of marijuana smoke. *N Engl J Med* 1973; 288:985–989.

72

Lysergic Acid Diethylamide and Other Hallucinogens

Donna L. Seger, M.D., F.A.C.E.P.

Lysergic Acid Diethylamide (LSD)

LSD is a colorless, odorless, tasteless solution prepared as crystal-clear solution or sold in bright-colored tablets. Synthetic psychedelic related to the psychoactive alkaloids found in morning glory seeds.

I. Route of exposure:
   A. Oral: Placed on crackers, blotting paper, gelatin, or sugar cubes. Often adulterated with other drugs.
   B. Rarely SC, IV, or insufflation.
II. Common street names:

Acid	Lysergide
The beast	LSD-25
Blotter acid	Pink dots
Blue caps	Sunshine
The chief	Window panes
Crackers	25+

III. Pharmacokinetics:
   A. Onset of action: 0.5 to 2 hours after ingestion.
   B. Duration of action:
      1. Hallucinogenic effects: 2–4 hours.
      2. Physiologic effects: Usually absent by 6 hours.
      3. Psychic effects persist for 8–12 hours.
      4. Possible flashbacks long after ingestion.

C. Peak effect: 1–2 hours.

D. Elimination: Rapidly metabolized to 2-oxy-lysergic acid diethylamide and eliminated in bile.

E. Active metabolites: None.

IV. Action:

A. Psychotropic effects.

B. Sympathomimetic and parasympathomimetic effects.

V. Uses: Illegal in all states since 1969. Originally used in psychiatry but abandoned because of disturbing psychotropic effects. Estimated 5% of adult Americans have tried LSD or similar hallucinogen at least once.

VI. Toxic mechanism:

A. Unknown. Postulated to reduce activity of serotonin-containing neurons. These neurons inhibit a variety of sensorimotor processes and modulate an organism's perception and behavior; therefore LSD inhibits inhibitory neurons.

B. Recent evidence that LSD causes cerebral arterial vasospasm.

VII. Range of toxicity:

A. Toxic dose: Depends on potency and purity; 1 mg/kg gives short encounter ("trip"), 4 mg/kg longer "trip."

B. Lethal dose: Unknown.

VIII. Clinical features:

A. Mind altering:

1. Altered perception of time and space. Sensory perception becomes unusually brilliant and intense.

2. Mood changes abruptly. Emotions are intense.

3. Thinking: Early memories may be recalled. Depersonalization or separation of self from body may occur.

4. Visual illusions frequently occur, but patient remains lucid.

B. Sympathomimetic and parasympathomimetic effects:

1. Pupillary dilation, tachycardia, piloerection, hyperglycemia, salivation, and lacrimation may occur.

2. Hyperthermia has been reported but is uncommon.

C. Acute adverse reactions:

1. May last minutes, days, or infrequently years (toxic psychosis).

2. Acute panic reaction: Most frequent emergency department presentation. Patient thinks he or she is going crazy; exhibits anxiety, paranoid illusions, depression. **May become suicidal.** Sweating and tachycardia add to anxiety.

3. 20% of trips unpleasant.

4. Usual duration of adverse reactions: 8–12 hours.

D. Chronic adverse reaction:

1. Flashback: Episode of spontaneous recurrences of LSD experience after immediate effects of drug have dissipated:

a. Usually lasts only minutes.

b. Rarely occurs more than a year after last LSD experience.

c. Most common precipitant is smoking marijuana. Also occurs during periods of stress and fatigue.

2. Toxic psychosis: usually acute but may become chronic.

    3. Depression.

    4. Exacerbation of preexisting psychiatric illness.

IX. Laboratory findings and evaluation:

  A. Serum LSD levels: Of no value in treating LSD intoxication.

  B. Toxicology screen: If diagnosis in doubt or multidrug ingestion suspected.

  C. Glucose test (Dextrostix): Any patient with altered mental status.

X. General treatment:

  A. Follow APTLS (see Chapter 8).

  B. General treatment: Table 72–1 (see Chapter 12 for details).

XI. Specific management:

  A. Agitation:

    1. Protect patient from self.

    2. May need to "talk down."

    3. Sedation:

      a. **Diazepam** 5–10 mg PO or titrate to effect IV. May be repeated three or four times over next 24 hours. Higher doses occasionally indicated.

      b. Alternative: **Haloperidol.**

    4. **Contraindicated: Phenothiazines** (lower seizure threshold).

  B. Adverse reactions:

    1. Prolonged reactions should be treated in hospital by a psychiatrist.

    2. Tranquilizers or antipsychotics may be needed.

XII. Prognosis:

  A. Expected response to treatment: Very good.

  B. Expected complications and long-term effects:

    1. Chronic adverse reaction (see above).

    2. Personality dissociation may lead to traumatic behavior and death.

    3. Panic reactions may result in suicide.

XIII. Special considerations:

  A. LSD does not cause physical addiction, organic brain syndrome, withdrawal syndrome, or drug-seeking behavior.

  B. Teratogenicity of LSD unknown.

TABLE 72–1.

General Treatment

Treatment	Indicated	Of No Value	Contraindicated
O$_2$	±		
IV	±		
ECG monitor	±		
Forced diuresis		X	
Acidification		X	
Alkalinization		X	
Emesis/lavage		X	
Charcoal		X	
Cathartic		X	

XIV. Disposition considerations:
  A. Admission considerations:
    1. See General Admission Considerations (Chapter 18).
    2. Persistent confused or paranoid behavior.
    3. Prolonged adverse reactions should be treated in hospital by a psychiatrist.
    4. Suicide potential.
  B. Consultation considerations: Psychiatrist for adverse reactions.
  C. Observation period: If doubt exists as to the diagnosis, patient should be observed for up to 12 hours to see if significant changes in condition occur. If no improvement, patient should be admitted.
  D. Discharge considerations:
    1. General discharge considerations have been met (see Chapter 18).
    2. Most patients with LSD intoxication may be observed in the emergency department and ultimately sent home in the company of a responsible adult after "coming down."
    3. Warn patients regarding possible long-term effects.
    4. Suicide potential and psychiatric state have been appropriately evaluated.

Other Hallucinogens

I. Common names:

Bufotenine (dimethyl serotonin; also from *Piptadenia peregrina, Amanita muscaria,* and skin of a toad *(Bufo marinus)*

Cannabinols (like marijuana)

DET (diethyltryptamine)

Ditran

DMT (dimethyltryptamine)

DOM (see STP)

Harmine and **harmaline** (from plants, *Peganum harmala* and *Banisteria caapi*)

Ibogaine (from plant, *Tabernanthe iboga*)

Jimsonweed seeds

Psilocybin, psilocin (derivatives of 4-hydroxytryptamine; also from a mushroom, *Psilocybe mexicana*)

Mescaline

MDA (3,4-methylene dioxamphetamine)

MDMA (Ecstacy, 3,4-methylene dioxymethamphetamine)

Muscal (peyote; from plant, *Lophophora williams:* Contains mescaline)

Nutmeg

Peyote (see muscal)

STP (dimethoxy-4-methyl amphetamine)

Wood rose

II. Discharge considerations: Most patients who have taken a hallucinogen other than PCP may be observed in the emergency department and ultimately sent home in the company of a responsible adult after "coming down."

BIBLIOGRAPHY

Altura B, Altura BM: Phencyclidine, lysergic acid diethylamide and mescaline: Cerebral artery spasms and hallucinogenic activity. *Science* 1981; 212:1051–1052.

Davis W: LSD and DOB? *Am J Psychiatry* 1982; 139:1649.

Litovitz T: Hallucinogens, in Haddad LM, Winchester JF: *Clinical Management of Poisoning and Drug Overdose*. Philadelphia, WB Saunders Co, 1983, p 455–461.

Livingstone M: LSD—A generation later. *Hawaii Med J* 1982; 41:462–471.

Mace S: LSD. *Clin Toxicol* 1979; 15:219–224.

Smith D, Seymour R: Dream becomes nightmare: Adverse reactions to LSD. *J Psychoactive Drugs* 1985; 17:297–303.

Caustics and Corrosives

73

Alkalis and Acids

Robert F. Shesser, M.D., F.A.C.E.P.

Alkalis

I. Route of exposure: Oral, cutaneous, ocular, inhalation.
II. Common trade names: See Table 73–1.
III. Action (see Toxic mechanism).
IV. Uses:
    A. "Lye"-like compounds:
        1. Home products: Drain cleaners, oven cleaners, urinary glucose test tablets, phosphate detergents, concrete floor cleaner, button batteries.
        2. Industrial products: Quick-lime, slaked lime, Portland cement, lithium hydride, calcium carbide.
    B. Ammonia and amines that form strongly alkaline solutions:
        1. Household products: Household ammonia, metal polish, hair dye, jewelry cleaner.
        2. Industrial products: Fertilizer, industrial refrigerant, emulsifier in polishes and hair wave solution.
    C. Bleaching agents.
    D. Borates: Denture cleaners, ketone test tablets.
V. Toxic mechanism:
    A. Esophagus main target organ after ingestion.
    B. Time course of injury:
        1. 0–4 days: Deep, rapid liquefaction necrosis; heat damage to cells; vascular necrosis, bacterial infiltration, fatty saponification.
        2. 4–7 days: Mucosal sloughing, enhanced fibroblast activity.
        3. 7–21 days: Esophageal wall weakest.
        4. 3 weeks–years: Symptomatic strictures.

TABLE 73–1.

Alkalis

Product	Contents
Red Devil Drain Opener	Sodium hydroxide (96%–100%)
Crystalline Drano	Sodium hydroxide (50%)
Clinitest reagent tablets	Sodium hydroxide (50%)
Liquid Drano	Sodium hydroxide (2%–10%)
Mr. Clean liquid	Sodium carbonate
Purex	Sodium carbonate (15%–25%)
Top Job	Sodium carbonate/ammonia
Liquid Clorox	Sodium hypochlorite (5.25%)
Lysol Deodorizing Cleaner	Ammonium chloride (2.7%)
Swish Toilet Bowl Cleaner	Ammonium chloride (1.25%)
Tide	Sodium silicate (4%)
Polident	Potassium monopersulfate
Efferdent	Potassium monoperborate
Acetest tablets	Sodium borate (37%)

C. Factors influencing extent of injury:
  1. High pH, concentration, amount ingested, duration of contact, absence of other fluid or food in stomach, increased pyloric sphincter tone.
  2. Solid lye more painful initially, more oral burns, less likely to pass through esophagus.
  3. Liquid lye less painful initially, more likely to cause gastroesophageal injury.
  4. Bleaches less injurious than lye.
VI. Range of toxicity:
  A. Estimated lethal dose (gm)
    Calcium hydroxide: 30
    Calcium oxide: 10
    Cement (Portland): 60
    Diethanolamine: 20
    Potassium carbonate: 20
    Potassium hydroxide: 5
    Sodium carbonate: 30
    Sodium hydroxide: 5
    Sodium silicate: 50
VII. Clinical features:
  A. History:
    1. Suspect mixed ingestion in adult suicide attempts.
    2. May not be clear in children because they are rarely observed actually drinking substance; may see children near open container.
    3. Child may smell like alkaline product.
    4. Suspect ingestion if child drooling, has stridor, complains of dysphagia, refuses to eat.

B. Physical examination:
1. Signs of systemic toxicity (e.g., hypotension, tachycardia, altered mental status).
2. Check oropharynx carefully:
   a. Burns indicate possible ingestion.
   b. Glottic and subglottic edema.
3. Check eyes carefully for evidence of inflammation, ulceration.
4. Check for fever (41% of patients with significant esophageal burns have fever).
5. Examine for signs of esophageal rupture and gastric perforation:
   a. Severe abdominal pain, decreased or absent bowel sounds.
   b. Subcutaneous emphysema at thoracic outlet.
   c. Hamman's crunch on cardiac auscultation.
6. Gastrointestinal bleeding.
7. Pulmonary aspiration and adult respiratory distress syndrome.

VIII. Laboratory findings and evaluation:
A. Upright chest x-ray examination.
B. Blood:
1. Complete blood cell count, electrolytes, BUN, creatinine.
2. Arterial blood gas (with pulmonary findings).
3. Methemoglobin level if strong oxidizing agent suspected.
4. Type and cross match.
C. Stool Hemoccult.

IX. General treatment:
A. Follow APTLS (see Chapter 8).
B. General management: Table 73–2 (see Chapter 12 for details).

TABLE 73–2.

General Treatment

Treatment	Indicated	Of No Value	Contraindicated
O_2	+		
IV	+		
ECG monitor	±		
Forced diuresis		X	
Acidification		X	
Alkalinization		X	
Emesis/			X
lavage			X
Charcoal		X	X
Cathartic			X
Dilution*	±		
Nasogastric tube			X
Cross match†	+		

*Controversial (see Dilution, below).
†Type and cross match for 4 units packed red blood cells.

C. Dilution (controversial):
   1. Reasons for:
      a. Irrigation of residual caustic from oropharynx and esophagus.
      b. Lower concentration of caustic at mucosal surface.
   2. Reasons against:
      a. Potential for inducing emesis, leading to aspiration pneumonitis and esophageal injury.
      b. May make esophagoscopy more difficult.
   3. Milk or water is preferred diluent in solid lye ingestion.
   4. Diluents are of **no value in liquid lye ingestion.** By the time the patient reaches the emergency department, tissue injury is probably complete.
   5. Contraindications:
      a. Severe ingestions with signs of:
         (1) Gastric or esophageal perforation.
         (2) Shock.
      b. Ingestion of liquid lye.
D. Contraindicated therapeutic procedures:
   1. Do not neutralize base with acid because of potential for exothermic reaction releasing significant amounts of heat.
X. Specific management:
   A. Supportive care is of paramount importance.
      1. Respiratory support:
         a. Respiratory distress uncommon; if present, suspect upper airway obstruction.
         b. Avoid blind nasotracheal intubation. Endotracheal intubation and assisted ventilation may be unavoidable if airway compromised, inadequate ventilation.
      2. Cardiovascular support:
         a. Hypotension (see Chapter 10 for treatment recommendations).
      3. Copiously irrigate any obvious skin or mucosal contamination.
      4. Begin eye irrigation as soon as possible (see Chapter 28).
   B. Endoscopy:
      1. Indications:
         a. Consider nature of alkali. Lye ingestions mandate endoscopy regardless of symptoms; endoscopy may not be necessary for bleach.
         b. Patients with obvious signs or symptoms of serious alkali ingestion. Usually performed within 12–24 hours of injury.
         c. Small children or unreliable adults with normal findings on physical examination.
      2. Findings from endoscopy will help guide subsequent therapy.
      3. Esophagus should not be examined beyond first visualized burn, to minimize risk of perforation.
      4. Gastric injury is often present but not detected.
   C. Surgery:
      1. Indications for immediate operative intervention:
         a. Signs of perforation.

D. Antibiotics: Administer if perforation suspected (e.g., triple antibiotic coverage with clindamycin (or metronidazole), ampicillin, and gentamicin).

E. Therapy for strictures:
1. Medical: Esophageal bougienage.
2. Surgical: Colonic interposition, gastrostomy.

XI. Prognosis:
A. Expected response to treatment:
1. Fatality rate from strong alkali 25%.
2. Injury to esophagus and stomach may occur despite optimal therapy.
3. Alkaline button batteries that pass the esophagus usually travel through the gastrointestinal tract with little or no damage.
4. Corneal damage usually permanent despite immediate irrigation.
B. Expected complications and long-term effects:
1. Late death from peritonitis.
2. Incidence of esophageal stricture 95%.
3. Tracheoesophageal and aortoenteric fistula.
4. Esophageal carcinoma.
5. Gastric outlet obstruction.
6. Heavy metal toxicity.
7. Tracheotomy frequently required.

XII. Special considerations:
A. Ocular exposures (see Chapter 28).
B. Common vehicle for suicide attempt by adults in second and third decades.
C. Button battery ingestion:
1. Button or disk batteries may contain sodium or potassium hydroxide. Ingestion may result in necrosis of esophagus and trachea, with massive mediastinitis.
2. Ascertain if battery is in esophagus:
   a. Radiographs of nasopharynx, chest, abdomen.
   b. If in esophagus for less than 24 hours, most authorities suggest removal with Foley catheter.
   c. If in esophagus for longer than 24 hours, remove with aid of endoscopy.
3. If battery has passed beyond esophagus, observe patient for symptoms.
4. Once past the pylorus, cathartic administration may speed passage of battery.
5. Obtain x-ray studies at 8-hour intervals (for progression and evidence of perforation). Surgical intervention considered if battery impeded for 8 hours at specific site. Impaction at site for more than 8 hours associated with high risk of tissue damage.
6. Most button batteries will pass spontaneously in the feces within 1 week (particularly if smaller than 18 mm (size of dime); all stools during this period should be collected and examined carefully.
7. If symptoms suggestive of tissue injury are noted, remove battery surgically.

XIII. Controversies:
A. Administration of prophylactic antibiotics.

    B. Corticosteroids to prevent stricture formation:
1. Recommended by some for all circumferential burns or when burns are suspected but esophagoscopy not available.
2. Others do not recommend steroids, because of lack of evidence of efficacy, suppression of immune system, and masking of infection.
3. It is recommended that antibiotics (e.g., penicillin or ampicillin) be given concurrently if steroids are used.

XIV. Disposition considerations:
    A. Admission considerations:
1. See General Admission Considerations (Chapter 18). Low threshold for admission in these patients.
2. All patients with known or suspected strong alkali exposure (e.g., lye).
3. Symptomatic with any ingestion (including low or moderate toxicity alkalis).
4. All small children.
5. All button battery ingestions.
6. Suicide risk.
    B. Consultation considerations:
1. Early GI consultation for endoscopy in all ingestions.
2. Immediate ophthalmology consultation for ocular exposures.
3. Surgeon for evidence of perforation or serious ingestion.
4. Burn specialist or plastic surgeon for severe skin burns.
    C. Observation period:
1. Applies only to ingestion of alkali with low toxicity.
2. Difficult to make recommendations because symptoms often do not correlate with extent of injury.
3. Asymptomatic adults and older children who have been exposed to alkalis with low potential for tissue damage (e.g., bleaches) may be considered for release after several hours of observation.
    D. Discharge considerations:
1. General discharge considerations have been met (see Chapter 18).
2. Only asymptomatic adults and older children with ingestions of alkalis with low toxicity should be considered for discharge.
    E. Patient transfer:
1. Transfer to burn center may be indicated in severe caustic exposure (see Chapter 29).
2. See Chapter 19.

Acids

  I. Route of exposure: Oral, cutaneous, ocular, inhalation.
 II. Common trade names: See Table 73–3.
III. Action: See Toxic mechanism.
IV. Uses: See Table 73–3.
 V. Toxic mechanism:
    A. Stomach is the main target organ (usually antrum, pylorus) because squamous epithelium of esophagus is relatively resistant to acids.

TABLE 73–3.

Acids

Primary Use	Chemical Name	Brand Name
Inorganic:		
Aluminum cleaner	Hydrofluoric acid	Al-Brite
Metal etching	Hydrofluoric acid	
Toilet bowl cleaners	Hydrochloric acid	Vanish, Ajax,
	Sulfuric acid	Sani-Flush
Swimming pool cleaner	Hydrochloric acid	
Brick cleaner	Hydrochloric acid	
	Muriatic acid	
Automobile battery fluid	Sulfuric acid	
Organic:		
Detergents	Formic Acid	
	Lactic acid	
Boiler cleaner	Oxalic acid	

    B. Produces early injury through heat release and tissue desiccation.

    C. Does not penetrate as deeply as alkalis.

    D. Same general factors influencing severity of tissue damage as for alkalis.

  VI. Range of toxicity:

    A. Hydrochloric, peracetic, perchloric, phosphoric, and trichloracetic acids: Reported fatal dose 1 ml.

    B. Acetic acid: Reported fatal dose 5 ml.

    C. Formic acid: Reported fatal dose 30 ml.

 VII. Clinical features:

    A. History (see Alkalis).

    B. Physical examination (see Alkalis):

      1. Acids more likely to produce skin burns.

      2. May see immediate complications (gastric perforation, edema leading to gastric outlet obstruction, peritonitis, shock).

VIII. Laboratory findings and evaluation: See Alkalis.

  IX. General treatment:

    A. Follow APTLS (see Chapter 8).

    B. General management: See Table 73–4 (see Chapter 12 for details).

   X. Specific management:

    A. Supportive care: See Alkalis; Chapters 8–10.

    B. If evidence of inhalation injury, see Table 108–1.

    C. Contraindicated: Do not neutralize acid with base because of potential for exothermic reaction releasing significant amounts of heat, producing thermal injury and increased tissue damage.

    D. Endoscopy: See Alkalis for indications.

    E. Surgery: See Alkalis.

    F. Steroids: See Controversies, under Alkalis (usually not considered for acids).

TABLE 73–4.

General Treatment

Treatment	Indicated	Of No Value	Contraindicated
O₂	±		
IV	+		
ECG monitor	±		
Forced diuresis		X	
Acidification		X	
Alkalinization		X	
Emesis/			X
lavage			X
Charcoal		X	X
Cathartic			X
Dilution*		X	
Nasogastric			X
tube			

*Tissue injury occurs rapidly.

    G. Antibiotics: See Alkalis.

    H. Therapy for strictures: See Alkalis.

  XI. Prognosis:

    A. Expected response to treatment:

      1. Fatality rate from one series 30%.

    B. Expected complications and long-term effects:

      1. Incidence of esophageal strictures 16%. Most severe scarring to gastric antrum and pylorus, the latter leading to outlet obstruction.

      2. Late death from peritonitis and exposure to corrosive fumes.

      3. Bowel perforation.

      4. Sepsis.

      5. Severe scarring from skin burns.

  XII. Special considerations:

    A. Hydrofluoric acid burns:

      1. Produces deep burns because fluoride penetrates epidermal barrier.

      2. Can produce systemic fluoride toxicity after extensive skin exposure (profound hypocalcemia, hyperkalemia, hypomagnesemia, circulatory collapse; see Fluoride intoxication, Chapter 110).

      3. Pain from skin burns may be disproportionate to degree of obvious damage.

    B. Ocular exposure: See Chapter 28.

  XIII. Controversies: See Alkalis.

  XIV. Disposition: See Alkalis.

BIBLIOGRAPHY

Crain EF, Gershel JC, Mezey AP, et al: Caustic ingestions. *Am J Dis Child* 1984; 138:863.

DiConstanzo J, Noirclerc M, Jouglard J, et al: New therapeutic approach to corrosive burns of the upper gastrointestinal tract. *Gut* 1980; 21:370–375.

Dreisbach RH, Robertson WO: *Handbook of Poisoning.* Norwalk, Conn, Appleton-Century-Crofts, 1987.

Gaudreault P, Parent M, McGuigan M, et al: Predictability of esophageal injury from signs and symptoms: A study of caustic ingestion in 378 children. *Pediatrics* 1983; 71:767–770.

Goodman L, Weigert J: Corrosive substance ingestion: A review. *Am J Gastroenterol* 1984; 79:85–90.

Haller JA, Andrews JG, White JJ, et al: Pathophysiology and management of acute corrosive burns of the esophagus. *J Pediatr Surg* 1971; 6:578–583.

Harris J, Rumack BH, Bregman DJ: Comparative efficacy of injectable calcium and magnesium salts in the therapy of hydrofluoric acid burns. *Clin Toxicol* 1981; 18:1027–1032.

Howell JM: Alkaline ingestions. *Ann Emerg Med* 1986; 15:820–825.

Litovitz TL: Battery ingestions: Product accessibility and clinical course. *Pediatrics* 1985; 75:469.

Litovitz TL, Butterfield D, Holloway B, et al: Button battery ingestion: Assessment of therapeutic modalities and battery discharge state. *J Pediatr* 1984; 105:868–873.

McIvor ME: Delayed fatal hyperkalemia in a patient with acute fluoride intoxication. *Ann Emerg Med* 1987; 16:1165–1167.

Maull KI, Osmand AP, Maull CD: Liquid caustic ingestions: An in vitro study of the effects of buffer, neutralization, and dilution. *Ann Emerg Med* 1985; 14:1160–1162.

Maull KI, Scher LA, Greenfield LJ: Surgical implications of acid ingestion. *Surg Gynecol Obstet* 1979; 148:895.

Oakes D, Sherck J, Mark J: Lye ingestion: Clinical patterns and therapeutic implications. *J Thorac Cardiovasc Surg* 1982; 83:194–204.

Penner GE: Acid ingestion: Toxicology and treatment. *Ann Emerg Med* 1980; 9:374.

Range DR, Hirokawa RH, Bryarly RC: Caustic ingestion. *Ear Nose Throat J* 1983; 62:46–63.

Sugawa C, Mullins R, Lucas C, et al: The value of early endoscopy following caustic ingestion. *Surg Gynecol Obstet* 1981; 153:553.

Tepperman PB: Fatality due to acute systemic fluoride poisoning following a hydrofluoric acid skin burn. *J Occup Med* 1980; 22:691–692.

Trevino MA, Herrmann GH, Sprout WL, et al: Treatment of severe hydrofluoric acid exposures. *J Occup Med* 1983; 25:861.

Votteler TP, Nash JC, Rutledge JC: The hazard of ingested alkaline disk batteries in children. *JAMA* 1983; 249:2504–2506.

74

Formaldehyde

Robert F. Shesser, M.D., F.A.C.E.P.

I. Route of exposure: Inhalation, dermal, ocular, oral, parenteral.
II. Formaldehyde preparations:
   A. Formaldehyde (HCHO) is a gas.
   B. Formalin: Aqueous solution containing formaldehyde, ethanol, or methanol.
III. Pharmacokinetics:
   A. Absorption: Rapid.
   B. Onset of action: Irritation and coagulation necrosis may occur immediately on contact.
   C. Elimination: Excreted by kidneys as formate.
   D. Active metabolites: Metabolized to toxic formic acid and formate.
IV. Actions: See Toxic mechanism.
V. Uses:
   A. Formalin used as disinfectant, antiseptic, deodorant, tissue fixative, embalming fluid.
   B. Manufacture of plastics and resins.
   C. Major constituent of foam insulation.
   D. Can be a component of smoke from fires involving structures built with wood containing urea formaldehyde resins.
VI. Toxic mechanism:
   A. Toxic metabolic products, formic acid, and formate rapidly necrose cells. Mucous membranes shrink and become necrotic, and degenerative changes are found in the liver, kidneys, heart, and brain.
   B. Normal metabolite that can react chemically with cellular proteins, leading to depression of cellular function.

C. Converted metabolically to formic acid, leading to severe metabolic acidosis.

VII. Range of toxicity:
   A. 60–90 ml often fatal. In one case 30 ml concentrated (37%) solution caused death in an adult.
   B. Few drops of 100% solution has been reported to cause death in a child.

VIII. Clinical features:
   A. Exposure to fumes:
      1. Eye, skin, respiratory tract irritation.
      2. Can cause asthma-like syndrome, pneumonitis, pulmonary edema.
   B. Dermal exposure:
      1. Skin and conjunctival irritation.
      2. Potent experimental allergen.
   C. GI exposure: Severe nausea, vomiting, diarrhea, abdominal pain from corrosive esophagitis, gastritis, ulceration, potential perforation.
   D. Parenteral exposure: Reports of hemolytic anemia in dialysis patients given high doses parenterally.
   E. Severe exposures: Metabolic acidosis, hypotension, anuria, CNS depression, coma.

IX. Laboratory evaluation:
   A. Blood:
      1. Complete cell count, electrolytes, BUN, creatinine, glucose.
      2. Arterial blood gas (especially with exposure to fumes, or to monitor acidosis in severe toxicity).
   B. Urinalysis (may see protein, casts, red blood cells).
   C. Radiographs:
      1. Chest x-ray studies (including upright film to look for free air under diaphragm).
      2. Abdominal x-ray studies (possible obstruction).

X. General treatment:
   A. Follow APTLS (see Chapter 8).
   B. General management: Table 74–1 (see Chapter 12 for details).

XI. Specific management:
   A. For inhalation injury, see Table 108–1.
   B. Tap water, milk, and ammonium salts (which change formaldehyde into methenamine) should be administered orally.
   C. Hypotension (see Chapter 10 for treatment recommendations).
   D. Acidosis:
      1. Bicarbonate (if pH <7.15).
      2. Hemodialysis if acidosis uncorrectable with sodium bicarbonate or if patient anuric.

XII. Prognosis:
   A. Expected response to treatment:
      1. Prognosis excellent for patients surviving first 48 hours after exposure.
   B. Expected complications and long-term effects:
      1. Esophageal stricture.
      2. Aspiration of stomach contents containing formalin may result in pulmonary edema, aspiration pneumonitis.

TABLE 74–1.

General Treatment

Treatment	Indicated	Of No Value	Contraindicated
O$_2$	±		
IV	+		
ECG monitor	±		
Forced diuresis		X	
Acidification			X
Alkalinization		X	
Emesis/			X
lavage			X
Charcoal			X
Cathartic			X
Diluent	+		
Cross match*	+		

*Type and cross match for four units.

XIII. Disposition considerations:
   A. Admission considerations: All patients with known or suspected exposure (inhaled or ingested).
   B. Consultation considerations:
      1. Nephrology consultation if hemodialysis indicated (severe metabolic acidosis).
      2. See Consultation considerations (Alkalis), Chapter 73.
   C. Observation period: None; all patients should be admitted.
   D. Discharge considerations: None; all patients should be admitted.

BIBLIOGRAPHY

Eells JT, McMartin KE, Black K, et al: Formaldehyde poisoning: Rapid metabolism to formic acid. *JAMA* 1981; 246:1237.

Hanrahan LP, et al: Formaldehyde vapor in mobile homes: A cross-sectional survey of concentrations and irritant effects. *Am J Public Health* 1984; 74:1026.

Starr TB, Gibson JE: The mechanistic toxicology of formaldehyde and its implications for quantitative risk estimation. *Ann Rev Pharmacol Toxicol* 1985; 25:745.

Yodaiken RE: Formaldehyde toxicity. *JAMA* 1981; 246:1677.

75

Phenols

James L. Baker, M.D., F.A.C.E.P.

I. Route of exposure: Oral, transdermal, mucous membranes, inhalation of toxic fumes.

II. Common names:
   A. Campho-Phenique contains 2%–5% phenol.
   B. Phenol derivatives in:
      1. Creosote (a wood preservative).
      2. Guiacol and hexachlorophene (antiseptics).
      3. Resorcinol (bactericidal ointment).
      4. Low concentrations in shampoos.
   C. Medicinal products containing phenol:
      1. Castellani's paint (carbol-fuchsin solution).
      2. Chloraseptic Liquid and Lozenges.
      3. Oraderm.
      4. Osti-Derm lotion.

III. Pharmacokinetics:
   A. Onset of action: Rapid absorption from all body surfaces. Coma has been reported to occur within 30 minutes in some cases.
   B. Elimination:
      1. Portion of absorbed phenol oxidized to hydroquinone and pyrocatechol; another portion oxidized more completely.
      2. 80% excreted by kidneys, either unchanged or conjugated with glycuronic acid and sulfuric acids.
      3. Lesser amount may be excreted through pulmonary circulation, causing aromatic odor.

IV. Action:
   1. Phenol denatures proteins and is therefore directly poisonous to cells.
   2. Bacteriostatic in 0.2% solution; bactericidal at 1%. Fungicidal in 1.3% solution.
   3. Becomes relatively inactivated when incorporated into soaps.
 V. Uses:
   1. Nonsubstituted phenol is carbolic acid, originally used as a disinfectant.
   2. Currently used as an ingredient in many types of disinfectants and medicinals.
   3. Dinitro derivatives of phenol and cresol used as insecticides and herbicides.
VI. Toxic mechanism:
   1. Phenol denatures proteins and is a general protoplasmic poison; thus acts as a local corrosive.
   2. Dinitrophenols uncouple oxidative phosphorylation within cellular mitochondria.
   3. Action on central nervous system through an unknown mechanism, first causing stimulation, followed by respiratory depression.
   4. May cause cardiovascular collapse by direct toxic effect.
   5. Has potent antipyretic effect through mechanism similar to that of salicylates.
   6. Hepatic and renal failure have been reported; mechanism unknown.
   7. Methemoglobinemia may be seen following systemic absorption of dinitrophenol and hydroquinone.
VII. Range of toxicity:
   1. Although accepted lethal dose is 2 gm, death has been reported from as little as 1 gm pure phenol taken orally.
VIII. Clinical features:
   A. Dermal exposure:
      1. When phenol is applied directly to skin, a white pellicle of precipitated protein is formed. This soon turns red and is eventually sloughed, leaving the surface stained lightly brown. If phenol remains on skin for a long period, it penetrates deeply and may cause extensive gangrene.
      2. A 5% solution applied to intact skin will produce local anesthesia; in this concentration phenol is irritating to exposed tissue and may cause necrosis. May cause partial-thickness chemical burn.
      3. Contact with **mucus membranes** following oral exposure produces protein denaturation and white discoloration of involved tissue, with a border of erythema.
   B. Mucous membrane exposure:
      1. Necrosis of mucous membranes (see Chapter 73).
   C. Systemic absorption:
      1. Cardiovascular: Hypotension and tachycardia.
      2. Pulmonary: Tachypnea followed by respiratory depression, cyanosis resistant to oxygen therapy (with dinitrophenol).
      3. CNS: Fleeting excitation followed by seizures and coma.
      4. GI: Nausea, vomiting, abdominal pain, diarrhea.

5. Other:
   a. Intense diaphoresis common.
   b. Methemoglobinemia may follow absorption of dinitrophenol, hydroquinone.
   c. Deep venous thrombosis has been reported following injections of dilute phenol solutions to produce chemical neurolysis or motor point blocks.
   d. Renal failure.
IX. Laboratory findings and evaluation:
   A. Toxicologic screen:
      1. Phenol can be detected in urine and serum.
      2. 10% ferric chloride reagent may be positive (violet or blue color) but is nonspecific (see Chapter 15, p. 58).
   B. Blood:
      1. Arterial blood gas (in presence of respiratory symptoms).
      2. Electrolytes, BUN, creatinine, glucose (with nausea and vomiting or seizures).
      3. Methemoglobin levels (with dinitrophenol, hydroquinone).
   C. Urine:
      1. Urinalysis may reveal albumin, red blood cells, casts.
      2. Myoglobin.
X. General treatment:
   A. Follow APTLS (see Chapter 8).
   B. General management: See Table 75–1 (see Chapter 12 for details).
   C. Gastric emptying:
      1. Dilution with 100–300 ml milk or water (15 ml/kg in child) should precede emesis or lavage.
      2. Emesis is preferred in awake patients for ingestion of dilute solutions (<5% phenol).

TABLE 75–1.

General Treatment (Ingestions)

Treatment	Indicated	Of No Value	Contraindicated
O$_2$	+		
IV	+		
ECG monitor	+		
Forced diuresis		X	
Acidification			X
Alkalinization		X	
Emesis*/lavage*	+/+		
Charcoal†	+		
Cathartic	±		
Hemodialysis		X	

*Should be preceded by dilution with milk (see Gastric emptying, below).
†Withhold if endoscopy likely.

3. Lavage is preferred for solutions >5% or in patients in whom emesis is contraindicated.

XI. Specific management:
   A. Dermal exposure:
      1. Copious quantities of water should be used to cleanse involved areas, followed by repeated gentle soap-and-water washes.
      2. Some recommend use of undiluted polyethylene glycol as a solvent, but this may be no more effective than water.
      3. Olive oil has also been recommended.
   B. Ocular exposure: See Chapter 28.
   C. Systemic toxicity:
      1. Support respiratory and cardiovascular function.
      2. Esophagoscopy within 24 hours to rule out esophageal injury.
   D. Systemic exposure:
      1. It has been reported that 30–60 ml castor oil may slow gastric absorption.
      2. Seizures: See Chapter 22 for treatment recommendations.
      3. Methemoglobinemia: See Management of methemoglobinemia, Chapter 102.
      4. Dialysis: Neither peritoneal dialysis nor hemodialysis has been shown effective.

XII. Prognosis:
   A. Expected response to treatment:
      1. Prior to use of lavage, mortality 65%; with lavage, mortality has dropped to 15%.
      2. In patients who have died from severe poisonings, death usually occurred within the first 24 hours.
      3. Renal and hepatic failure may lead to delayed death in isolated cases.
   B. Expected complications and long-term effects:
      1. Liver failure.
      2. Anuria.
      3. Esophageal strictures.

XIII. Special considerations:
   A. Dinitrophenol and hydroquinone may cause methemoglobinemia (see Management of methemoglobinemia, Chapter 102).
   B. Concentrated phenol is highly toxic. Medical staff should use appropriate precautions to prevent potential injury to themselves.
   C. Chemical spills involving phenol may produce toxic vapors and must be managed by trained personnel to prevent inhalation exposure (see Chapter 111).

XIV. Disposition considerations:
   A. Admission considerations:
      1. See General Admission Considerations (Chapter 18).
      2. Any evidence of systemic toxicity from any form of exposure.
      3. Dermal exposure: See Admission considerations, Chapter 29.
      4. Exposure to toxic fumes.
   B. Consultation considerations:
      1. If indicated, endoscopy should be performed within 24 hours.

2. Ophthalmologist for ocular exposures.
3. Nephrologist if renal failure develops.
C. Observation period:
1. Symptomatic: Not appropriate to observe.
2. Initially asymptomatic: 6 to 8 hours.
D. Discharge considerations:
1. No initially symptomatic patient should be discharged.
2. Asymptomatic patients may be discharged if still no symptoms after 6 hours of observation and General discharge considerations have been met (see Chapter 18).
3. Suicide potential and psychiatric status have been evaluated.

BIBLIOGRAPHY

Brown VKH, Box VL, Simpson BJ: Decontamination procedures for skin exposed to phenolic substances. *Arch Environ Health* 1975; 30:1–6.

Conning DM, Hayes MJ: The dermal toxicity of phenol: An investigation of the most effective first-aid measures. *Br J Ind Med* 1970; 27:155.

Deichman WB, Gerarde HW: *Toxicology of Drugs and Chemicals.* Orlando, Fla, Academic Press, 1969.

Gilman AG, Goodman LS, Gilman A: *The Pharmacological Basis of Therapeutics,* ed 6. New York, Macmillan Publishing Co, 1980.

Gosselin RE, Hodge HC, Gleason MN, et al: *Clinical Toxicology of Commercial Products,* ed 4. Baltimore, Williams & Wilkins Co, 1976.

Haddad LM, Diamond KA, Schweistris JE: Phenol poisoning. *JACEP* 1979; 8:267.

Macek C: Venous thrombosis results from some phenol injections. *JAMA* 1983; 249:1807.

Soares ER, Tift JP: Phenol poisoning: Three fatal cases. *J Forensic Sci* 1982; 27:729–731.

Common Therapeutic Medications

76

Salicylates

Betty S. Riggs, M.D.

I. Route of exposure: Oral, rectal, transdermal (rub and liniment)
II. Common trade names: See Table 76–1.
III. Pharmacokinetics:
    A. Absorption:
        1. Primarily in small bowel.
        2. Absorption of orally administered soluble aspirin (ASA) is rapid and complete, particularly in solutions.
        3. Absorption may be slower after large doses, in part because of the inhibitory effect of aspirin on gastric emptying.
        4. Acute overdose with enteric-coated or sustained-release preparations may also result in prolonged absorption.
        5. Oil of wintergreen (methyl salicylate) is rapidly absorbed from the GI tract and may produce symptoms sooner than salicylates in tablet form.
    B. Onset of action: Serum levels are detectable in 15–30 minutes under normal conditions.
    C. Plasma half-life:
        1. ASA in therapeutic doses: 20 minutes.
        2. Salicylic acid:
            a. In therapeutic range: 3–6 hours.
            b. In overdose: Can be as long as 15–30 hours because of acidosis interfering with clearance and dose-dependent elimination kinetics.
    D. Peak effect:
        1. Peak plasma concentration reached within 25 minutes after ingestion of standard formulations but not until 4–6 hours after enteric coated or sustained-release preparations.

TABLE 76–1.

Common Products Containing Salicylates

Alka-Seltzer	Excedrin
Anacin	4-Way Cold Tablets
Ascriptin	Goody's Headache
Bayer Aspirin	Powders
Bayer Children's Cold	Midol
Tablets	Norwich Aspirin
Bufferin	St. Joseph Cold Tablets
Coricidin D	for Children
Ecotrin Tablets	Sine-Off Tablets–Aspirin
	formula

2. Levels after large overdoses may continue to rise for 12 hours related to inhibition of gastric emptying.
3. Acute overdose with enteric-coated or sustained-release preparations may result in persistently elevated levels, with peak plasma concentrations not occurring until 12 hours after ingestion.

E. Metabolism and elimination:
1. Rapid hydrolysis of ASA to salicylic acid is by esterases in the GI mucosa, liver, plasma, red blood cells, and synovial fluid.
2. Elimination includes renal excretion of unchanged salicylic acid and hepatic metabolism to salicyl phenolic glucuronide, salicyl acyl glucuronide, salicyluric acid, and gentisic acid.
3. Elimination kinetics are nonlinear; thus elimination half-life increases with increasing dose.
4. In the kidneys salicylates undergo glomerular filtration, active secretion in the proximal tubules, and passive reabsorption in the distal tubules; renal excretion is greatly enhanced by alkaline urine (pKa of salicylic acid is 3).

F. Active metabolites: Aspirin is rapidly hyrolyzed to salicylic acid.

IV. Action and uses:
A. Salicylates are used for their properties as antipyretics, anti-inflammatories, and analgesics and for their antiplatelet activities.

V. Toxic mechanism:
A. Metabolic effects:
1. Stimulation of the CNS respiratory center:
a. Effect: Respiratory alkalosis with compensatory renal excretion of bicarbonate; occurs early in intoxications. May not be seen in children.
2. Uncoupling of oxidative phosphorylation:
a. Effect:
(1) Increased catabolism leading to increased CO_2 production and respiratory acidosis, although respiratory alkalosis predominates early.

   (2) Increased heat production.

   (3) Increased glycolysis and peripheral demand for glucose.

   (4) Increased production of metabolic intermediates, which contribute to metabolic acidosis seen later in intoxications.

3. Inhibition of Krebs cycle enzymes:

   a. Effect: Increased anion gap metabolic acidosis (from production of high concentration of organic anions and decreased HCO_3).

4. Stimulation of gluconeogenesis, increased tissue glycolysis, stimulation of lipid metabolism, inhibition of amino acid metabolism:

   a. Effect: Impaired glucose metabolism (tendency for hyperglycemia in adults, hypoglycemia in children).

5. Bleeding diathesis secondary to impaired platelet aggregation, and decreased thrombin, decreased factor VII production, and increased capillary fragility.

6. Fluid and electrolyte imbalance:

   a. Metabolic alkalosis secondary to vomiting.

   b. Hypokalemia secondary to renal tubule stimulation to excrete $K+$, and inhibition of active transport, resulting in flux of Na^+ and H_2O into cells and K^+ out (increasing loss).

   c. Hypovolemia secondary to increased renal losses, vomiting, and increased cutaneous and pulmonary insensible losses.

VI. Range of toxicity:

   A. Acute ingestion:

      1. Mild toxicity: <150 mg/kg.

      2. Moderate toxicity: 150–300 mg/kg.

      3. Severe toxicity: 300–500 mg/kg.

      NOTE: **If untreated or inappropriately treated, toxic doses may result in death.**

   B. Chronic ingestion:

      1. As a result of nonlinear, saturable kinetics, repeated doses of >100 mg/kg/day for 2 or more days may result in chronic salicylism.

      2. Chronic salicylism is associated with a higher degree of morbidity and mortality in both pediatric and adult patients than is acute ingestion.

VII. Clinical features:

   A. Head, ears, eyes, nose, and throat: Tinnitus often associated with levels >30 mg/dl.

   B. Respiratory:

      1. Hyperpnea and tachypnea.

      2. Noncardiogenic pulmonary edema may be seen in severe cases.

   C. GI: Vomiting usually occurs 3–8 hours after acute overdose.

   D. Hyperthermia may be seen in severely poisoned patients.

   E. Neurologic: Lethargy may be present in mild to moderate cases; convulsion and coma may occur with severe toxicity.

   F. Acid-base abnormalities:

      1. Respiratory alkalosis (early).

      2. Increased anion gap metabolic acidosis (late, severe).

      3. Concomitant metabolic alkalosis (volume loss secondary to vomiting, increased renal losses).

4. Respiratory acidosis (secondary to increased CO_2 production); respiratory alkalosis predominates except in very high doses.
G. Bleeding diathesis secondary to impaired platelet aggregation and decreased thrombin (increased prothrombin time).
H. Death: Either brain death or acute respiratory or cardiac arrest.
VIII. Laboratory findings and evaluation:
  A. Screening tests for suspected toxicity are qualitative only; results are positive even with therapeutic levels. Cannot be used to identify toxin in gastric contents.
    1. Because serum salicylate levels are easily obtained, neither Phenistix Reagent Strips nor the ferric chloride test should be accepted as a substitute. An unacceptably high number of false positive results occur with these tests. Ketone bodies can give a false-positive reaction but can be removed by acidifying and boiling the urine before adding ferric chloride. False-positive results can also be produced by coal tar dyes and some phenothiazines, although the latter tend to give a more pinkish color. (For more detailed discussion, see Chapter 15, p. 58.)
      a. Ferric chloride test (see also Chapter 15):
        (1) Few drops of 10% ferric chloride may be added to 1–5 ml boiled, acidified urine. (Urine can be acidified by adding a couple drops H_2SO_4).
        (2) If salicylates are present, sample will turn purple within minutes.
      b. Phenistix test:
        (1) Dip Phenistix Reagent Strip into urine.
        (2) Color gives a rough indication of the degree of toxicity.
          a Tan: Mild poisoning.
          b Brown: Moderate toxicity.
          c Maroon: Severe poisoning.
  B. Serum levels:
    1. Acute ingestion:
      a. Blood for plasma salicylate level determination should be drawn at 6 hours after ingestion and plotted on the Done nomogram (Fig 76–1). In symptomatic patients blood may be drawn prior to 6 hours to document exposure, and again at 6 hours after ingestion. **Do not wait for the 6-hour blood level to confirm suspicion prior to initiating treatment in clinically toxic patients.**
    2. Chronic ingestion:
      a. Diagnosis of chronic salicylism is based on clinical findings.
      b. Although a plasma salicylate level documents the presence of salicylate, it cannot be plotted on the Done nomogram and levels do not correlate with clinical findings.
    3. Serum salicylate level may not always correspond to the clinical condition, which may warrant more aggressive therapy than the blood level suggests.
  C. Blood:
    1. Electrolytes (hypokalemia, anion gap, volume loss, aid in diagnosing acid-base abnormalities).
    2. Blood glucose (hypoglycemia or hyperglycemia).

DONE NOMOGRAM FOR SALICYLATE POISONING

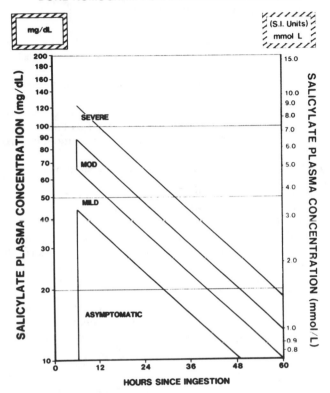

FIG 76–1.
Done nomogram for salicylate poisoning. (From Done AK: Salicylate intoxication: Significance of measurements of salicylate in blood in cases of acute ingestion. *Pediatrics* 1960; 26:800. Used with permission.)

3. Arterial blood gases (acidemia, respiratory function).
4. BUN, creatinine.
5. Liver function tests, prothrombin time, partial thromboplastin time (bleeding diathesis).
6. Complete blood cell count, spun hematocrit, platelets (bleeding diathesis).
D. Chest x-ray (pulmonary edema).

E. ECG.

F. Urinalysis (urine pH).

IX. General treatment:

A. Follow APTLS (see Chapter 8).

B. General management: Table 76–2 (see Chapter 12 for details).

C. Accidental childhood ingestion:

1. Ingestions definitely <150 mg/kg considered nontoxic and can be treated at home with fluids and close observation.

2. Ingestions definitely 150–300 mg/kg can be treated with ipecac-induced emesis at home and close follow-up for 24 hours. **If any doubt as to amount taken, or health status, patient must be brought to a hospital.**

3. Ingestions of >300 mg/kg must be treated at a hospital.

X. Specific management:

A. Fluid management and alkalinization:

1. Goals of IV therapy include:

a. Rehydration.

b. Alkalinization of urine to pH 7–8 to enhance excretion of salicylates. pKa of salicylates is 3.0. It is the nonionized form that penetrates cell membranes. Alkalinization traps salicylate in the intravascular compartment, enhancing renal excretion and decreasing resorption.

c. Replacement of potassium to prevent paradoxical aciduria (acid urine in the face of alkalemia, which occurs when the kidneys excrete acid in exchange for potassium, related to intracellular hypokalemia).

TABLE 76–2.

General Treatment

Treatment	Indicated	Of No Value	Contraindicated
O_2	+		
IV	+		
ECG monitor	+		
Forced diuresis*			X
Acidification			X
Alkalinization of urine	+		
Emesis/lavage†	+/+		
Charcoal‡	+		
Cathartic§	+		
Dialysis¶	±		

*Not recommended due to risk of pulmonary edema.
†Lavage preferred.
‡Repeat every 4 hours until charcoal stool.
§Give with first dose of charcoal and thereafter as indicated. Serum magnesium levels should be monitored if magnesium-containing cathartics are given in repeated doses.
¶See specific indications.

2. If patient is volume depleted, prepare an IV solution of:
   a. Two ampules sodium bicarbonate in 1 L 5% dextrose in one-half normal saline solution (D_5 0.45% NS + 88 mEq/L HCO_3). Administer as required to correct volume loss. Monitor serum and urine pH.
   b. NOTE: **Hypokalemia must be corrected before effective urinary alkalinization can take place. Shift in pH will cause K+ to go into cells and lower serum K+ further.**
3. Once adequate hydration is established (with demonstrated urine output), IV fluids should be changed to D_5W with 2 ampules sodium bicarbonate per liter plus 40 mEq KCl/L at a rate of 2–3 ml/kg/hr.
4. Insert Swan-Ganz catheter if patient at high risk for developing pulmonary edema (underlying cardiac disease, history of congestive heart failure).
5. Forced alkaline diuresis is not recommended because pulmonary edema is a real danger during diuresis.

B. Monitor:
1. Serum salicylate level: In significant ingestions, monitor every 2 hours until a peak has been reached; thereafter, every 4–6 hours to confirm that it is falling toward the nontoxic range.
2. Urinary pH should be 7 or greater.
3. Serum K+ frequently. For each increase in H+ concentration of 10 (pH decrease of 0.10) serum K+ is increased by 0.5 related to shift from intracellular to extracellular space. Sudden or rapid correction of acidemia without consideration of K+ status may result in further hypokalemia, leading to ventricular tachycardia or cardiac arrest.

C. Acidemia: Correct as needed with additional sodium bicarbonate (keep pH >7.25).

D. Bleeding diathesis:
1. For severe salicylate poisoning, administer single 25 mg dose of vitamin K_1 (AquaMEPHYTON, Konakion); do not give more than 1 mg/min. If prothrombin time has not decreased within 6–8 hours, repeat dose.

E. Hemodialysis: Although hemodialysis is preferred, charcoal hemoperfusion is also effective. Peritoneal dialysis is not recommended.
1. Indications:
   a. CNS symptoms.
   b. Noncardiogenic pulmonary edema.
   c. Acidosis refractory to conservative therapy.
   d. Renal failure.
   e. Clinical deterioration despite aggressive conservative therapy.
   f. High salicylate level alone is not an indication for extracorporeal elimination, although some authorities recommend hemodialysis for levels >100 mg/dl.

F. Contraindicated therapy:
    1. Acetazolamide: alkalinizes urine but concomitantly acidifies blood, causing increased distribution of salicylate to tissues, such as the CNS, and a resultant increase in symptoms.
    2. Forced diuresis (see Controversies).
    3. Alkalinization without consideration of effect on serum $K+$.

XI. Prognosis:
  A. Expected response to treatment:
    1. Prognosis excellent when appropriate treatment is initiated early.
    2. In chronic toxicity, prognosis dependent on many factors, including underlying medical problems, phase of salicylate toxicity on presentation, and delay in diagnosis and treatment.
    3. Mortality among young persons about 2%; however, among older patients not diagnosed early, mortality may approach 25%.
    4. Serum salicylate level is poor predictor of outcome.
    5. Prolonged acidemia carries a grave prognosis.
  B. Expected complications and long-term effects:
    1. Noncardiogenic pulmonary edema.
    2. Hyperthermia.
    3. Rhabdomyolysis.
    4. Gastric perforations.
    5. GI hemorrhage from hypoprothrombinemia.

XII. Special considerations:
  A. Elderly patients with chronic salicylate use have atypical presentation of toxicity. May not have acidosis and may have therapeutic serum salicylate levels.
  B. Infants with severe, life-threatening cumulative intoxication may have low serum salicylate levels.
  C. 1 ml 98% oil of wintergreen equals 1.4 gm aspirin (ASA).
  D. Aspirin is often found in fixed combination preparations with drugs such as oxycodone and codeine and may be overlooked in the patient with presumed "pure" narcotic overdose.

XIII. Controversies:
  A. Many texts recommend forced alkaline diuresis. Although alkalinization may be beneficial, forced diuresis may lead to potential complications such as pulmonary edema and thus we do not recommend it.
  B. Traditionally, enteric-coated salicylates were considered radiopaque; however in a recent study (Savitt DL, Hawkins HH, Roberts JR: *Ann Emerg Med* 1987; 16:331) salicylates (including enteric-coated ones) were not radiopaque.

XIV. Disposition considerations:
  A. Admission considerations:
    1. See General Admission Considerations (Chapter 18).
    2. Salicylate level >45 mg/dl 6 hours after ingestion.
    3. All patients with a toxic serum level (into the moderate or severe toxicity area of the nomogram) 6 hours or more after an acute ingestion.

4. Signs and symptoms of salicylism in a patient taking salicylates chronically, regardless of serum level.
5. All patients suspected of or with a history of ingestion of enteric-coated or sustained-release preparations.
6. Patients with symptoms of serious toxicity (tachypnea secondary to acidosis, dehydration, seizures, CNS changes) should be admitted for observation and aggressive therapy.
7. Any abnormal arterial blood gas level, no matter how minor, because acid-base status may rapidly worsen without immediately obvious change in the patient's clinical appearance.
8. Any infant or child with symptoms.
9. Any signs and symptoms of salicylism in a patient with a history of oil of wintergreen ingestion, regardless of serum level.
10. Suicide risk.
11. ICU:
   a. Respiratory or cardiovascular support, seizures, arrhythmias, or persistent hypotension.
   b. Patients with metabolic acidosis are probably best treated in intensive care.
B. Consultation considerations:
   1. Consultation with a nephrologist is usually warranted for any patient whose salicylate level is >80 mg/dl, regardless of whether hemodialysis is to be undertaken.
   2. Cardiology consultation for any patient with evidence of cardiac dysfunction (e.g., congestive heart failure, arrhythmias) and development of pulmonary edema.
   3. Pediatric consultation for any child with seizures or significant hypotension.
   4. Psychiatric consultation for any patient who attempted suicide.
C. Observation period:
   1. Symptomatic: None; all patients should be admitted.
   2. Asymptomatic: Until 6-hour and repeat blood level confirms nontoxic ingestion.
D. Discharge considerations:
   1. General discharge considerations are met (Chapter 18).
   2. Initial (at least 6 hours after ingestion) and repeat salicylate levels in nontoxic range.
   3. Asymptomatic.
   4. Psychiatric considerations including suicide risk have been appropriately assessed.
   5. For older patients who chronically abuse salicylates and unintentionally overdose, family members or other responsible persons have been educated and are able to monitor salicylate use.
E. Patient transfer issues:
   1. Failure of the patient to respond to conservative therapy may necessitate transfer to a higher level facility if hemodialysis or charcoal hemoperfusion are not readily available (see Chapter 19).

BIBLIOGRAPHY

Aderson RJ, Potts DE, Gabow PA, et al: Unrecognized adult salicylate intoxication. *Ann Intern Med* 1976; 85:745–748.

Barone JA, Raia JJ, Huang YC: Evaluation of the effects of multiple-dose activated charcoal on the absorption of orally administered salicylate in a simulated toxic ingestion model. *Ann Emerg Med* 1988; 17:34–37.

Broder JN: The ferric chloride screening test (letter). *Ann Emerg Med* 1987; 16:1188.

Done AK: Salicylate intoxication: Significance of measurements of salicylate in blood in cases of acute ingestion. *Pediatrics* 1960; 26:800–807.

Gabow PA: How to avoid overlooking salicylate intoxication. *J Crit Illness* Oct 1986; 77–85.

Hillman RJ, Prescott LF: Treatment of salicylate poisoning with repeated oral charcoal. *Br Med J* 1985; 291:1472.

Levy G: Gastrointestinal clearance of drugs with activated charcoal. *N Engl J Med* 1982; 307:676–678.

McGuigan MA: A two-year review of salicylate deaths in Ontario. *Arch Intern Med* 1987; 147:510–512.

Needs CJ, Brooks PM: Clinical pharmacokinetics of the salicylates. *Clin Pharmacokinet* 1985; 10:164–177.

Savitt DL, Hawkins HH, Roberts JR: The radiopacity of ingested medications. *Ann Emerg Med* 1987; 16:331.

Temple AR: Acute and chronic effects of aspirin toxicity and their treatment. *Arch Intern Med* 1981; 141:364–369.

77

Acetaminophen

Betty S. Riggs, M.D.

I. Route of exposure: Oral, rectal

II. Common trade names: See Table 77–1.

III. Pharmacokinetics:
   A. Absorption: Rapid and usually complete by 1 hour in therapeutic dosages; faster with liquid preparations. In overdoses, absorption is complete in 4 hours.
   B. Onset of action: Within 1 hour.
   C. Half-life: After therapeutic doses 1–3 hours; extended in overdose.
   D. Peak effect: After therapeutic doses peak plasma levels occur between 1–2 hours after ingestion; after overdose peak may not be reached for 4 hours.
   E. Duration of action: 4 hours (PO).
   F. Elimination: Liver metabolism accounts for 98% of acetaminophen elimination.
   G. Metabolites:
      1. After therapeutic doses approximately 94% of acetaminophen (APAP) is conjugated to sulfate and glucuronide; neither APAP nor these metabolites are toxic.
      2. Approximately 4% of **therapeutic** dose metabolized by P-450 mixed-function oxidase system to a reactive metabolite, which is detoxified by glutathione and excreted as cysteine and mercapturate conjugates.

IV. Action and uses:
   A. Acetaminophen is an antipyretic and analgesic with only weak anti-inflammatory properties:
      1. Fever reduction is mediated by the hypothalamus, involves brain prostaglandin synthetase, and is accomplished by cutaneous vasodilation.

TABLE 77–1.

Common Products Containing Acetaminophen

Anacin-3	Excedrin P.M.
Comtrex	Liquiprin
Congespirin Liquid Cold Medicine	Sinarest Tablets
	Sine-Aid Sinus
CoTylenol Cold Formula Liquid and Tablets	Headache Tablets
	Sinutab Extra Strength
Datril	Capsule Formula
Dristan AF Decongestant Tablets	Tempra
	Tylenol
Excedrin	Vanquish

    2. The mechanism of analgesia is also thought to be a centrally mediated effect on prostaglandins.

V. Toxic mechanism:

  A. Mechanism of hepatotoxicity:

    1. In APAP overdose, increased amount of available drug quickly overwhelms normal metabolism because the sulfate and glucuronide pathways are saturable. Consequently, more drug undergoes metabolism by the P-450 pathway, depleting glutathione. When glutathione is depleted by 70% or more, the reactive intermediate metabolite, which cannot be detoxified, becomes covalently bound to hepatocellular proteins, causing hepatocellular necrosis.

  B. Renal toxicity:

    1. Acute renal failure has been reported both with and without associated hepatocellular injury after APAP ingestion; because P-450 enzyme is present in the renal cortex, the same mechanism may explain renal injury resulting directly from APAP.

VI. Range of toxicity:

  A. Toxic dose:

    1. Adults: 7.5 gm (140 mg/kg).

    2. Children: 140 mg/kg.

  B. Fatal dose:

    1. Concept of a fatal dose is misleading because history of amount of APAP is frequently erroneous. If properly treated early after ingestion, no patient can be claimed to have ingested a "fatal" dose.

VII. Clinical features:

  A. The clinical course generally follows four stages:

    1. Stage 1:

      a. Patients with toxic levels develop nausea, vomiting, anorexia, and diaphoresis during the first 24 hours after ingestion.

      b. Patients in the probable-risk category on the Rumack-Matthew nomogram (Fig 77–1) had a mean time of 6 hours to onset of symptoms; 100% had symptoms by 14 hours after ingestion.

      c. Children younger than 6 years generally have vomiting after acetaminophen overdose even with nontoxic levels; they develop vom-

SEMI-LOGARITHMIC PLOT OF
PLASMA ACETAMINOPHEN LEVELS VS. TIME

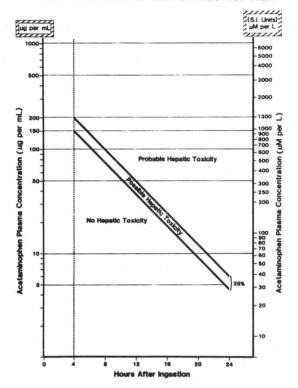

RUMACK – MATTHEW NOMOGRAM
FOR ACETAMINOPHEN POISONING

CAUTIONS FOR USE OF THIS CHART:
1) The time coordinates refer to time of ingestion.
2) Serum levels drawn before 4 hours may not represent peak levels.
3) The graph should be used only in relation to a single acute ingestion.
4) The lower solid line 25% below the standard nomogram is included to allow for possible errors in acetaminophen plasma assays and estimated time from ingestion of an overdose.

FIG 77–1.
Rumack-Matthew nomogram shows plasma acetaminophen levels plotted against time after ingestion. The area above the lines corresponds with possible or probable hepatotoxicity; below the lower line, hepatotoxicity is unlikely. Even one reading that falls above the lower line mandates a complete course of treatment with *N*-acetylcysteine (Mucomyst). (From Rumack BH, et al: Acetaminophen overdose: 662 cases with evaluation of oral acetylcysteine treatment. *Arch Intern Med* 1981; 141:380. Used with permission.)

iting earlier than adults and do not develop diaphoresis.
    2. Stage 2: Symptoms decrease during 24–48 hours after ingestion, but transaminase levels, prothrombin time, and bilirubin begin to rise. (PT and bilirubin are best prognosticators of outcome.)

3. Stage 3: Peak hepatotoxicity occurs at 72–96 hours after ingestion.
4. Stage 4: Recovery occurs at 7–8 days.
B. Specific problems:
   1. Hepatotoxicity: Although liver function test values may be elevated at 24 hours after ingestion, peak values do not occur until 72–96 hours.
   2. Both hypoglycemia and hyperglycemia have been reported.
   3. Acute renal failure.
   4. Pancreatitis.
   5. Myocardial necrosis.
VIII. Laboratory findings and evaluation:
   A. Serum level:
      1. All patients should have blood for serum acetaminophen level drawn 4 or more hours after ingestion.
      2. Rumack-Matthew nomogram (Fig 77–1):
         a. If the level falls on or above the lower line in the Rumack-Matthew nomogram, treatment with *N*-acetylcysteine (NAC) is indicated.
         b. If it is unclear precisely how long since overdose, err on the side of exaggerating time lapse when you read the nomogram. For example, if the overdose might have taken place anytime in the last 4–8 hours, assume 8 hours.
   B. If level is toxic (see Fig 77–1) the following laboratory studies should be performed:
      1. Baseline liver function tests (transaminases, bilirubin, PT), electrolytes, glucose, renal function tests, complete blood cell count, platelet count, urinalysis, amylase, and ECG.
      2. Toxicology screen (many ingestions are combination preparations and multiple-drug poisonings).
IX. General treatment:
   A. Follow APTLS (see Chapter 8).
   B. General management: Table 77–2 (see Chapter 12 for details).
X. Specific management:
   A. Indications for *N*-acetylcysteine:
      1. APAP level determined 4 or more hours after ingestion within toxic range.
      2. If APAP levels cannot be obtained before 10 hours after ingestion. Treatment should be started if the history indicates a significant ingestion (140 mg/kg in a child or 7.5 gm in an adult) but may be discontinued if the level is found later to be nontoxic.
   B. Protocol for oral NAC:
      1. Optimally started before 16–24 hours after ingestion.
      2. Loading dose 140 mg/kg.
      3. Maintenance doses: 70 mg/kg every 4 hours for 17 doses.
      4. NAC available as 10% or 20% solution and should be diluted to 5% solution with a soft drink or fruit juice to make it more palatable.
      5. Any dose vomited within 1 hour should be repeated; administration of an antiemetic such as droperidol (0.5 ml IV in an adult) or prochlorperazine 30 minutes prior to dose of NAC may be effective.

TABLE 77–2.

General Treatment

Treatment	Indicated	Of No Value	Contraindicated
O$_2$	±		
IV	+		
ECG monitor	±		
Forced diuresis		X	
Acidification		X	
Alkalinization		X	
Emesis/lavage	+/+		
Charcoal*	+		
Cathartic	+		
Dialysis†		X	

*Repeated doses. Activated charcoal is indicated if patients present early after a pure APAP overdose or in patients who ingest multiple drugs. Use of N-acetylcyteine (NAC) should not be delayed by use of activated charcoal. Use of charcoal with oral NAC is controversial. Some authorities suggest using it simultaneously; others suggest adjustment of dosage; still others suggest administering activated charcoal and NAC alternately every 2 hours. We advocate using charcoal even when oral NAC is called for, using the latter technique (see Controversies).
†APAP is dialyzable, but hemodialysis has not been shown to change clinical course.

6. With persistent vomiting unresponsive to antiemetics, NAC can be given by nasogastric or duodenal tube, as slow drip.
7. Intravenous NAC is being tested under an investigational new drug number by the Rocky Mountain Poison Center (1-800-525-6115); a separate protocol is being studied by the National Capital Poison Center (1-202-625-3333).

XI. Prognosis:
   A. Expected response to treatment:
      1. Prognosis correlates more closely with time after ingestion that treatment is begun than with APAP levels. Patients whose treatment is begun more than 16 hours after ingestion have a worse prognosis than patients whose treatment is begun early.
      2. Deaths are infrequent (less than 3%–4% of untreated cases).
      3. In a series of 1,559 cases treated with NAC less than 16 hours after ingestion only two deaths (0.13%) were reported. In a series of 479 patients with treatment begun 16–24 hours after ingestion, eight deaths were reported (1.67%).
   B. Expected complications and long-term effects:
      1. Major acute complication is fulminant hepatic necrosis.
      2. If patient survives to stage 4, complete recovery without long-term sequelae is the rule.
XII. Special considerations:
   A. Potentially significant hepatic toxicity may not be apparent for up to 3 days, during which time patient may feel well.

B. Chronic exposure to drugs that stimulate the P-450 enzyme system may enhance APAP toxicity. Examples of such "inducer" drugs include:

Antihistamines	Haloperidol
Barbiturates	Meprobamate
Ethchlorvynol	Phenylbutazone
Glutethimide	Phenytoin
Griseofulvin	Tolbutamide

C. Pediatric overdose: Children younger than 6 years who ingest a toxic amount of APAP seem to be at less risk for serious hepatotoxicity than older children and adults do, possibly because of differences in acetaminophen metabolism. Nevertheless, treatment with NAC is indicated for children with toxic acetaminophen levels.

D. Acetaminophen is often found in fixed combination preparations with drugs such as propoxyphene, oxycodone, and codeine and may be overlooked in the patient with a presumed "pure" narcotic overdose.

E. Cimetidine, which interferes with the metabolism of many drugs, has been shown in a study of human volunteers to have no effect on the formation of toxic APAP metabolites.

XIII. Controversies:

A. Concurrent use of activated charcoal and NAC remains controversial. Some experts claim that activated charcoal may reduce the absorption and hence the effectiveness of oral NAC, related to presumed adsorption and inactivation. However, evidence for this is primarily from in vitro studies, and NAC may not in fact be significantly adsorbed by activated charcoal.

XIV. Disposition considerations:

A. Admission considerations:

1. See General Admission Considerations (Chapter 18).
2. Patients with toxic serum levels.
3. Suspected potential for acetaminophen toxicity, based on history of amount ingested (>140 mg/kg).
4. Admission threshold should be low with ingestion of drugs such as acetaminophen, which have potential delayed lethal effects.

B. Consultation considerations:

1. Dialysis service for correction of metabolic abnormalities in the setting of renal failure.
2. Hepatic failure should be managed with standard therapy in consultation with a gastroenterologist.

C. Observation period:

1. Observe until APAP levels are available to decide disposition.
2. Treatment should begin before return of laboratory results (e.g., serum APAP level) in emergency department, including administration of NAC if significant toxicity is suspected.

D. Discharge considerations:

1. General discharge considerations are met (Chapter 18).
2. Asymptomatic with a nontoxic level obtained at least 4 hours after ingestion.
3. Suicide potential and psychiatric status have been appropriately evaluated.

BIBLIOGRAPHY

Linden CH, Rumack BH: Acetaminophen overdose. *Emerg Med Clin North Am* 1984; 2:103–119.

Rumack BH, Peterson RC, Koch GG, et al: Acetaminophen overdose: 662 cases with evaluation of oral acetylcysteine treatment. *Arch Intern Med* 1981; 141:380–385.

Rumack BH: Acetaminophen overdose in children and adolescents. *Pediatr Clin North Am* 1986; 33:691–701.

Jeffery WH, Lafferty WE: Acute renal failure after acetaminophen overdose: Report of two cases. *Am J Hosp Pharm* 1981; 38:1355–1358.

Curry RW, Robinson JD, Sughrue MJ: Acute renal failure after acetaminophen ingestion. *JAMA* 1982; 247:1012–1014.

Pillans P, Hall C: Paracetamol-induced acute renal failure in the absence of severe liver damage. *South Afr Med J* 1985; 67:791–792.

Sato C, Lieber CS: Mechanism of the preventive effect of ethanol on acetaminophen-induced hepatotoxicity. *J Pharmacol Exp Ther* 1981; 218:811–815.

Barker JD, deCarle DJ, ANuras S: Chronic excessive acetaminophen use and liver damage. *Ann Intern Med* 1977; 87:299–301.

Critchley JAJH, Scott AW, Dyson EH, et al: Is there a place for cimetidine or ethanol in the treatment of paracetamol poisoning? *Lancet* 1983; 1:1375–1376.

Renzi FP, et al: Concomitant use of activated charcoal and *N*-Acetylcysteine. *Ann Emerg Med* 1985; 14:568–572.

Kaysen GA, Pond SM, Roper MH, et al: Combined hepatic and renal injury in alcoholics during therapeutic use of acetaminophen. *Arch Intern Med* 1985; 145:2019–2023.

Acetaminophen levels (letter). *Ann Emerg Med* 1987; 16:1096.

78

Theophyllines

Samuel S. Spicer, M.D., F.A.C.E.P.

I. Route of exposure:
   A. Oral, intravenous, rectal.
   B. Iatrogenic and intentional overdoses are the most common causes of theophylline toxicity. Iatrogenic causes of toxicity include intravenous therapy, especially in those on maintenance therapy, and decreased clearance secondary to medications (erythromycin, cimetidine).

II. Common generic and trade names: See Table 78–1.
   B. Other sustained-release theophylline products:

Aerolate	Slo-Bid
Aminodur	Somophyllin CRT
Bronkodyl SR	Sustaire
Choledyl SA	Theo-24
Constant-T	Theobid
Duracap	Theobid Jr
Dura-Tab	Theobron SR
Gyrocaps	Theoclear L.A.
LaBid	Theophyl-SR
Lodane	Theospan SR
Phyllocontin	Theovent
Respbid	Uniphyl

III. Pharmacokinetics:
   A. Absorption: See Table 78–1.
   B. Onset of action: Rapid and complete absorption within 2 hours of ingestion in non-sustained-release products.

TABLE 78-1.

Theophylline Compounds*

Generic Name	Trade Name	Percent Anhydrous Theophylline	Percent Absorption	Peak Action (hr)
Aminophylline	Aminophylline	85	100	1–2
	Elixophylline	100	100	
	Somophylline	86	100	1
Oxtriphylline	Choledyl	64	100	3
	Brondecon			
Dyphylline	Lufyline	70†	100	0.5–1
Slow-release theophylline	Slo-Phyllin Gyrocaps	100	100	3–5
	Theo-Dur	100	100	6–10
	Elixophylline SR	100		
	Quibron	100		
	Theolair SR	100		
Slow-release aminophylline	Aminodur Duratabs	79	65	5

*From Haddad LM, Winchester JF: *Clinical Management of Poisoning and Drug Overdose.* Philadelphia, WB Saunders Co, 1983, p 921. Used by permission.
†Equivalent to 70% anhydrous theophylline.

C. Half-life:
1. 3.5 hours in children, 8–9 hours in adults.
2. Shorter in:
   a. Chronic smokers.
   b. Patients taking phenytoin.
3. Longer in:
   a. Liver impairment.
   b. Congestive heart failure.
   c. Patients taking cimetidine or erythromycin.
   d. Influenza vaccine.
   e. Some viral illnesses.
4. In acute toxicity, may be markedly prolonged up to 50 hours.
D. Peak effect: See Table 78–1.
E. Duration of action: Sustained-release products will provide constant levels for 8–12 hours, with one product (Theo-24) claiming sustained levels for up to 24 hours.
F. Elimination: Major route is by liver; 10% excreted unchanged in the urine.
G. Active metabolites:
1. 3-Methyl xanthine is the only active metabolite in both children and adults. Rate of formation of the active metabolite is slower than rate of excretion. Serum levels are <1 µg/ml for theophylline level of 10 µg/ml.
2. Caffeine as an active metabolite may be responsible for adverse effects

in premature neonates who otherwise have therapeutic theophylline levels (5–12 µg/ml).

IV. Action: Inhibits action of phosphodiesterase; responsible for degradation of cyclic AMP (cAMP). As levels of cAMP increase intracellularly, effect is smooth muscle relaxation (with resultant bronchodilation), myocardial stimulation, and CNS excitation. Also has mild diuretic effect.

V. Uses: Because of its bronchodilator effect, theophylline is used in treatment of asthma, pulmonary edema, and chronic obstructive pulmonary disease with reversible airway disease.

VI. Toxic mechanism:
   A. Mechanism for CNS toxicity (e.g., seizures) has not been defined but may be the result of cerebral vasoconstriction and hypoxia.
   B. Sinus tachycardia, ventricular tachycardia, and premature ventricular contractions are probably secondary to the direct chronotropic action on the myocardium, release of local norepinephrine, and a transient decrease in peripheral vagal control.
   C. Drug levels measure both protein bound and unbound theophylline. Sixty percent of the drug is protein bound, but the remaining unbound portion is responsible for physiological and toxic effects. Patients with low albumin such as the elderly or those with liver disease have less protein binding and are more likely to become toxic, at therapeutic drug levels.
   D. Liver capacity to metabolize theophylline is saturated at the drug level of 20 µg/ml or more. Small changes in dosages may then cause a large change in serum levels and prolong the half-life up to 50 hours.
   E. Factors that increase likelihood of theophylline toxicity include:
      1. Maintenance theophylline therapy, especially delayed-release preparations.
      2. Cor pulmonale.
      3. Drugs (cimetidine, erythromycin, noncardioselective beta blockers).
      4. Age over 60 years.
      5. Congestive heart failure.
      6. Chronic obstructive lung disease and acute exacerbation.
      7. Influenza vaccine.
      8. Liver disease (cirrhosis, hepatitis, cholestasis).
      9. Viral illnesses, influenza.
      10. Febrile illnesses.

VII. Range of toxicity:
   A. Toxic dose: Over 10 mg/kg or 700 mg in average adult.
   B. Fatal dose:
      1. Report of death resulting from 100 mg aminophylline administered IV push.
      2. 25–100 mg/kg by rectal suppository.
      3. Reports of deaths from 8.4 mg/kg orally in a child.

VIII. Clinical features:
   A. Mild toxicity: Theophylline level 20–35 µg/ml.
      1. Signs and symptoms:
         a. Nausea and vomiting are often first clues to toxicity.
         b. Tremors, irritability, tachycardia, tachypnea, headache, polyuria.

B. Severe toxicity:
   1. Signs and symptoms:
      a. Arrhythmias (ventricular and supraventricular).
      b. Seizures (usually generalized tonic-clonic).
      c. Hypotension and cardiac arrest.
   2. Acute overdoses in otherwise healthy individual: Little risk of seizures or ventricular arrhythmias until theophylline levels >60 μg/ml, and often will not see these until level >90 μg/ml. May see hypokalemia, metabolic acidosis, hyperglycemia, hypocalcemia, hypomagnesemia, and hypophosphatemia in acute intoxication.
   3. Patients receiving long-term maintenance therapy may develop seizures and ventricular arrhythmias when theophylline levels are >40–50 μg/ml. When seizures occur in patients in the 25–40 year age range, there is usually coexisting congestive heart failure, cirrhosis, viral illnesses, fever, or prior history of seizure disorder.

IX. Laboratory findings and evaluation:
   A. Theophylline serum levels: Should be obtained every 2 hours until a peak level is obtained; continue to obtain levels until values begin to decrease.
   B. ECG.
   C. Calcium, magnesium, blood glucose.
   D. Must follow electrolyte status carefully if cathartics used. Although hypokalemia is seen in acute toxicity, observe closely for hyperkalemia, which may develop as theophylline is cleared from the serum and if patient is receiving potassium replacement therapy.
   E. May see elevated leukocyte count.

X. General treatment:
   A. Follow APTLS (see Chapter 8).
   B. General management: Table 78–2 (see Chapter 12 for details).

Table 78–2.

General Treatment

Treatment	Indicated	Of No Value	Contraindicated
O$_2$	±		
IV	+		
ECG monitor	+		
Forced diuresis		X	
Acidification			X
Alkalinization		X	
Emesis*/lavage*	+/+		
Charcoal†	+		
Cathartic†	+		

*Patients will often have protracted vomiting from toxicity. Use gastric emptying procedures only if such spontaneous vomiting has not taken place. Gastric emptying may be successful up to 10 hours after massive ingestions because of clumping of tablets into large concretions.
†May need repeated doses (see below).

C. Multiple doses of activated charcoal:
   1. Indications:
      a. Serum theophylline concentrations >30 μg/ml in all patients who are able to tolerate oral activated charcoal therapy.
      b. Sustained-released products may not have peak effect for 12–24 hours.
   2. Dosing schedule: 25 gm every 2–4 hours. Administer cathartic every 12 hours to facilitate passage of toxin-charcoal complex through GI tract.
D. Charcoal hemoperfusion:
   1. Indications:
      a. Seizures.
      b. Hypotension, ventricular arrhythmias, intractable vomiting, not responding to supportive or corrective measures.
      c. Adults: Serum theophylline concentration:
         (1) >60 μg/ml after single acute ingestion.
         (2) >40 μg/ml in patients receiving prolonged theophylline therapy or with:
            a High-risk factors for developing toxicity (see Toxic mechanism).
            b Inability to tolerate oral activated charcoal therapy.
            c Known seizure disorder or focal CNS lesion.
      d. Children: Serum theophylline concentration >80 μg/ml.
E. Seizures:
   1. See Chapter 22 for treatment recommendations.
   2. Intractable seizure is an indication for hemoperfusion.
F. Arrhythmias:
   1. Supraventricular tachycardia:
      a. Verapamil 5–10 mg IV.
      b. Propranolol 1 mg IV. CAUTION: May worsen bronchoconstriction.
      c. In the future, esmolol, a short-acting more cardioselective beta blocker may become useful in treatment of hemodynamic abnormalities of acute theophylline poisoning without risk of bronchospasm.
   2. Ventricular arrhythmias:
      a. Lidocaine 1 mg/kg IV bolus.
      b. Bretylium 5–10 mg/kg IV bolus.
      c. Hemoperfusion for refractory arrhythmias.
XI. Prognosis:
   A. Expected response to treatment:
      1. Variable response to treatment may be noted, related to clumping of tablets, prolonged half-life with sustained-release preparations, or persistent vomiting, which may interfere with use of activated charcoal.
      2. Fatality rate is about 50% if patient has seizures secondary to theophylline toxicity.
   B. Expected complications and long-term effects:

1. Seizures may be intractable, resulting in prolonged hypoxia and permanent neurological damage.
2. Survival with neurological deficits has been noted at toxic levels of 190 μg/ml.

XII. Special considerations: Sustained-release products may not have peak effect for 12–24 hours. Therefore, early theophylline levels may be misleadingly low and patient only minimally symptomatic despite significant overdose.

XIII. Controversies:
  A. Theophylline toxicity appears to be a catecholamine excess syndrome in which short-acting beta blockers, such as esmolol, may play a role.
  B. Phenobarbital in animal studies was superior to phenytoin (Dilantin) in prevention of seizures.
  C. Hemoperfusion is effective in reducing theophylline levels, but controlled studies documenting decrease in morbidity or mortality have not been conducted.

XIV. Disposition considerations:
  A. Admission considerations:
    1. See General Admission Considerations (Chapter 18).
    2. Any patient with serum levels >30 μg/ml must be admitted to a monitored bed, with seizure precautions.
    3. Any patient who has had a significant ingestion of sustained-release products (by history or large number of pill fragments found by means of lavage or emesis), regardless of symptoms or initial theophylline level, requires admission, monitoring, and repeated oral charcoal every 2–4 hours until theophylline level is <20 μg/ml.
    4. Suicide risk.
  B. Consultation considerations:
    1. Referral to hemoperfusion specialist if indicated (see Treatment).
    2. Anesthesiology consultation for prolonged seizures unresponsive to treatment.
  C. Observation period:
    1. Difficult to make specific recommendation. Not appropriate with sustained-release ingestions; all patients should be admitted.
    2. If emergency department observation is attempted, it should be done only in those patients with levels <30 μg/ml. Levels must be determined every 2 hours until values begin to decline. Patients with theophylline levels <30 μg/ml may be considered for discharge when a repeat theophylline level is <20 μg/ml and they are asymptomatic.
  D. Discharge considerations:
    1. General discharge considerations have been met (see Chapter 18).
    2. Significant ingestion of sustained-release products absolutely ruled out.
    3. Asymptomatic.
    4. Level prior to discharge <20 μg/ml.
    5. Long-term theophylline regimen has been reevaluated and adjusted if necessary.
    6. Suicide potential and psychiatric status have been appropriately evaluated.

BIBLIOGRAPHY

Aitken ML, Martin TR: Life-threatening theophylline toxicity is not predictable by serum levels. *Chest* 1987; 91:10.

Bertino JS, Walker JW: Reassessment of theophylline toxicity: Serum concentrations, clinical course and treatment. *Arch Intern Med* 1987; 147:757–760.

D'Angio R, Sabatelli F: Management considerations in treating metabolic abnormalities associated with theophylline overdose. *Arch Intern Med* 1987; 147:1837–1838.

Gaar GG, Banner W, Laddu AR: The effects of esmolol on the hemodynamics of acute theophylline toxicity. *Ann Emerg Med* 1987; 16:1334–1339.

Gal P, Miller A, McCue JD: Oral activated charcoal to enhance theophylline elimination in acute overdosage. *JAMA* 1984; 251:3130–3131.

Hendles L, Weinberger M: Theophylline: A "state-of-the-art" review. *Pharmacology* 1983; 3:2–44.

Kulig KW, et al: Intravenous theophylline poisoning and multiple-dose charcoal in an animal model. *Ann Emerg Med* 1987; 16:842–846.

Lim DT, Singh P, Nourtsis S: Absorption inhibition and enhancement of sustained-release theophylline tablets by oral activated charcoal. *Ann Emerg Med* 1986; 15:1303–1307.

Olson KR, Benowitz NL, Woo OL: Theophylline overdosage: Acute single ingestion versus chronic repeated overmedication. *Am J Emerg Med* 1985; 3:386.

Paloucek FP, Rodvold KA: Evaluation of theophylline overdoses and toxicities. *Ann Emerg Med* 1988; 17:135–144.

Park GD, Spector R, Roberts RJ, et al: Use of hemoperfusion for treatment of theophylline intoxication. *Am J Med* 1983; 74:961.

79

Hypoglycemic Agents

Donna L. Seger, M.D., F.A.C.E.P.

Insulin

I. Route of exposure: Intramuscular, intravenous, subcutaneous, intraperitoneal.
II. Common generic and trade names: See Table 79–1.
III. Pharmacokinetics:
  A. See Table 79–1.
  B. Elimination: Largely metabolized in the liver (>50%), via glutathione insulin transhydrogenase.
IV. Action:
  A. Beta cells of pancreas synthesize and store insulin.
  B. Insulin stimulates hepatic glycogen synthesis, inhibits glycogenolysis, gluconeogenesis, and lipolysis.
V. Uses:
  A. Treatment of hyperglycemic disorders (diabetes mellitus, diabetic ketoacidosis, nonketotic hyperosmolar hyperglycemia).
  B. Acute hyperkalemia (in conjunction with glucose).
  C. Maple syrup urine disease.
VI. Toxic mechanism:
  A. Deleterious effects of hypoglycemia are felt in all organ systems; however, CNS derives all its energy from glucose metabolism (except in starvation states, when it can utilize ketones), and it is here that the effects of hypoglycemia are most profoundly felt. If insulin causes the level of blood glucose to fall to low values, CNS metabolism is depressed.
  B. As blood glucose falls, CNS neurons become hyperexcitable, leading to nervousness, trembling, diaphoresis, hallucinations, seizures, and finally coma.

TABLE 79–1.

Insulin Preparations

Insulin	Preparation	Onset (hr)	Peak (hr)	Duration of Action (hr)
Fast acting	Regular	0.5–1	1–2	5–7
	Insulin Zinc Prompt (Semi-lente)	0.5–1	1–2	12–16
Intermediate acting	Isophane (NPH)	1.5–2	8–12	20–28
	Insulin Zinc (Lente)	1.5–2	8–12	20–28
Long acting	Protamine Zinc (PZI)	3–4	8–12	36
	Insulin Zinc Extended (Ultralente)	3–4	8–14	36

VII. Range of toxicity:
   A. Toxic dose:
      1. Dependant on multiple factors including metabolic state, level of activity, glycogen stores.
      2. There is no reported minimum toxic dose, but as low as 20 units has been reported to produce death. It is safe to assume the minumum toxic dose is at least this low, and probably lower.
   B. Fatal dose:
      1. Minimum lethal dose recorded is 20 units.
      2. Maximum dose survived is reported as 1,200 units.
VIII. Clinical features:
   A. Individual response to decreasing serum glucose is variable. Hypoglycemic symptoms depend on rate at which serum glucose falls rather than specific blood glucose levels.
   B. Signs and symptoms of hypoglycemia secondary to insulin:
      1. Excess adrenergic discharge (diaphoresis, anxiety, palpitations, flushed skin, tachycardia, weakness).
      2. Neurogenic:
         a. Confusion, headache, drowsiness, incoordination, uncontrollable yawning, tremor, seizures, coma.
         b. Focal neurologic signs (particularly in elderly) may mimic cerebrovascular accident.
IX. Laboratory findings and evaluation:
   A. Immediate Dextrostix, Chemstrip, or stat serum glucose if rapidly available.
   B. Frequent repeat serum glucose.
   C. If patient has seizures or is comatose, check electrolytes, especially potassium, calcium, magnesium, phosphorus.
   D. Renal function studies (BUN, creatinine).

    E. Complete blood cell count if infectious cause suspected for changed mental status.

X. Treatment:

    A. Follow APTLS, particularly approach to altered mental status and coma (see Chapter 8).

    B. Specific management:

        1. Administer 50 ml D_{50} (50% glucose in water) IV, 1 mg/kg $D_{25}W$ in children. If patient potentially nutritionally deficient (e.g., severely debilitated alcoholic), also administer thiamine 100 mg IV.

        2. If no or variable effect, repeat above.

        3. If unsure of cause of altered level of consciousness, also administer naloxone.

        4. If 50% glucose successful in reviving patient, start $D_{10}W$ infusion to maintain blood sugar 100–200 mg/dl. Severely hypoglycemic patients may even require $D_{20}W$, with intermittent boluses of D_{50}.

        5. Once patient able to tolerate oral intake, can change IV to D_5W.

XI. Prognosis:

    A. Expected response to treatment: Intravenous administration of concentrated glucose solution usually reverses mental status changes of hypoglycemia within about 1 minute.

    B. Expected complications and long-term effects: If recognition and treatment are not immediate in comatose, severely hypoglycemic patients, permanent damage to neuronal cells of CNS may occur.

XII. Special considerations:

    A. Anaphylaxis to nonhuman forms of insulin.

    B. Intentional overdose (suicide or homicide attempt) may be misinterpreted as accidental hypoglycemia.

    C. Hypoglycemia in a child may be the result of child abuse.

    D. Factitious hypoglycemia: Patients who surreptitiously administer insulin or oral hypoglycemic agents to themselves to simulate organic disease.

    E. Effect of insulin increased by ethanol, propranolol, levodopa, and monoamine oxidase inhibitors.

XIII. Controversies:

    A. Some authorities suggest administering glucagon 1–2 mg IM if IV access a problem; others believe glucagon should never be administered, because of ketogenic properties.

    B. Some authorities consider diazoxide, epinephrine, and glucocortocoids for refractory hypoglycemia, but there are no data to substantiate administration.

XIV. Disposition considerations:

    A. Admission considerations:

        1. See General Admission Considerations (Chapter 18).

        2. All **intentional** insulin overdoses. Hypoglycemia may occur far longer than predicted by insulin's duration of action.

        3. All patients who have taken a massive insulin overdose, even if euglycemic. Therre is limited predictability of time of onset and extent of hypoglycemia.

        4. All patients with reactions from long-acting insulin, regardless of intent.

5. Patients with severe overdoses (coma resistent to administration of glucose, persistent seizures) should be admitted to the intensive care unit until intravenous glucose is no longer necessary.
6. All patients with a second episode following a recent presentation with insulin-induced hypoglycemia, regardless of form of insulin or intent, should be admitted for metabolic reevaluation and possible readjustment of their insulin doses.
7. Suicide risk.

B. Consultation considerations:
1. Psychiatry consultation may be indicated for suicide attempt or for evaluation of factitious hypoglycemia.
2. Social worker should be involved in cases of child abuse.
3. Visiting nurse arrangements may be necessary for patients with difficulty with self-administration of insulin (e.g., elderly, vision impaired).

C. Observation period: Difficult to make recommendations, because of limited predictability of time of onset and extent of hypoglycemia and the fact that hypoglycemia may last far longer than predicted by insulin's duration of action.

D. Discharge considerations:
1. General discharge considerations have been met (see Chapter 18).
2. Asymptomatic and physical examination is unremarkable.
3. Patient has not taken a long-acting insulin preparation such as UltraLente or Protamine Zinc.
4. Patient has acceptable blood glucose level at time of discharge.
5. If patient is receiving maintenance insulin, regimen has been reviewed and adjusted if necessary.
6. Patient has been instructed to take sugar orally if symptoms of hypoglycemia occur.
7. Patient is compliant and will return if symptoms of hypoglycemia appear.
8. Suicide potential and psychiatric status have been appropriately evaluated.

Sulfonylurea Hypoglycemic Agents

I. Route of exposure: Oral.
II. Common generic and trade names: See Table 79–2.
III. Pharmacokinetics:
   A. Absorption: All readily absorbed.
   B. Onset of action:
      1. Tolbutamide: Within 20 minutes.
      2. Glyburide: Within 60 minutes.
      3. Chlorpropamide: Within 60 minutes.
   C. Plasma half-life: See Table 79–2.
   D. Peak effect: See Table 79–2.
   E. Duration of action: See Table 79–2.
   F. Elimination: See Table 79–2.
   G. Active metabolites: See Table 79–2.

TABLE 79–2.

Pharmacokinetic Profile of Sulfonylurea

Generic Name	Trade Name	Plasma Half-Life (hr)	Peak Effect (hr)	Duration of Action (hr)	Metabolism	Metabolites
Tolbutamide	Orinase, Orinade	6	3–4	6–12	Hepatic	Inactive
Acetohexamide	Dymelor	3.5–11	3	12–18	Hepatic	1 Active 1 Inactive
Tolazamide	Tolinase	7	3–4	12–14	Hepatic	3 Active 3 Inactive
Glipizide	Glucotrol	3–7	1–3	<24	Hepatic	Inactive
Glyburide	Diabeta, Micronase	10	4	<24	Hepatic	Inactive
Chlorpropamide	Diabinase	24–28	3–6	60	Hepatic	Active and inactive

IV. Action:
   A. Exact mechanism unknown.
   B. Stimulates insulin release from pancreatic beta cell. Also inhibits hepatic glucose production, enhances uptake of glucose and binding of insulin to insulin receptors.
 V. Uses:
   A. To lower blood glucose level in patients with non-insulin-dependent diabetes mellitus (type II) whose hyperglycemia cannot be controlled by diet alone.
   B. Central diabetes insipidus.
   C. Sulfonylureas are agents that most frequently cause hypoglycemia in patients over the age of 40 years. Chlorpropamide, in particular, is the drug most commonly reported in accidental and suicidal hypoglycemia. Note that chlorpropamide also has the longest serum half-life (up to 38 hours) and consequently the longest duration of action. It has caused refractory hypoglycemia for 6 days after ingestion.
 VI. Toxic mechanism: See Insulin.
VII. Range of toxicity:
   A. Toxic dose:
      1. The following doses have produced coma:
         a. Tolbutamide 500 mg/day for 5 days.
         b. Chlorpropamide 500 mg/day for 2 weeks.
         c. Single dose of acetohexamide in a patient with renal failure.
   B. Fatal dose:
      1. Single dose of glyburide 2.5 gm has been reported to produce death.
VIII. Clinical features: See Insulin.
 IX. Laboratory findings and evaluation: See Insulin.
  X. General treatment:
   A. Follow APTLS, especially if presentation is altered mental status, coma, or seizures (see Chapter 8).
   B. General management: Table 79–3 (see Chapter 12 for details).

Table 79–3.

General Treatment

Treatment	Indicated	Of No Value	Contraindicated
O_2	±		
IV*	+		
ECG monitor	±		
Forced diuresis		X	
Acidification	−		
Alkalinization	−		
Emesis†/lavage‡	+/+		
Charcoal†	+[a]		
Cathartic†	+[a]		
Dialysis		X	

*D_{10} may be necessary.
†Indicated in ingestions. Not indicated in patients who are hypoglycemic secondary to maintenance therapy. If history is unclear, it is best to proceed with gastric decontamination procedures.
‡Lavage is preferred in symptomatic patients (risk of coma, seizures).

XI. Specific treatment:
   A. See Insulin.
   B. Prolonged glucose administration usually required because of long half-life and duration of action.
   C. Dialysis, forced diuresis, charcoal hemoperfusion of no value.
XII. Prognosis:
   A. Expected response to treatment:
      1. Prognosis or expected response to treatment of hypoglycemia secondary to ingestion of oral hypoglycemics is unpredictable.
   B. Expected complications and long-term effects:
      1. All sulfonylureas can cause delayed, recurrent, or refractory hypoglycemia.
      2. If recognition and treatment are not effected immediately in comatose, severely hypoglycemic patients, permanent damage to neuronal cells of the CNS may occur.
XIII. Special considerations:
   A. Hypoglycemic effect of sulfonylureas increased by ethanol, dicumarol, sulfafenazole, oxyphenbutazone, aspirin, phenylbutazone, and chloramphenicol.
   B. Other drugs causing hypoglycemia: Ethanol, aspirin, haloperidol, propoxyphene, organophosphates, propanolol, insulin.
   C. Populations at high-risk of developing drug-induced hypoglycemia:
      1. Elderly with hepatic or renal disease.
      2. Malnourished patients.
      3. Alcoholics.
      4. Salicylate users.

5. Patients using drugs that increase hypoglycemic effect of sulfonylureas and insulin (see above).
6. Young children, particularly those with ethanol intoxication (e.g., young children may drink half-empty glasses of liquor left after their parents' party).

XIV. Controversies: See Insulin, p. 429.

XV. Disposition considerations:
   A. Admission considerations:
      1. **All** hypoglycemic patients, whether from overdose or maintenance therapy. Delayed, prolonged, and refractory hypoglycemia cannot be predicted.
      2. Suicide risk.
   B. Observation period: Not appropriate to observe; **all** patients should be admitted.
   C. Discharge considerations: Not appropriate to discharge.

BIBLIOGRAPHY

Arem R, Zoghbi W: Insulin overdose in eight patients: Insulin pharmakokinetics and review of the literature. *Medicine* 1985; 64;5:323–332.

Bobzien W: Suicidal overdoses with hypoglycemic agents. *JACEP* 1979; 8:467–470.

Forrest J: Chlorpropamide overdosage: Delayed and prolonged hypoglycemia. *Clin Toxicol* 1974; 7:19–24.

Goldfrank L, Kirsten R: Chlorpropamide and other hypoglycemic agents, in Goldfrank LR, Flomenbaum NE, Lewin NA (eds): *Goldfrank's Toxocologic Emergencies,* ed 3. Norwalk, Conn, Appleton-Century-Crofts, 1986, pp 263–269.

Stapczynski J, Haskall R: Duration of hypoglycemia and need for intravenous glucose following intentional overdoses of insulin. *Ann Emerg Med* 1984; 13:505–511.

80

Phenytoin

Samuel S. Spicer, M.D., F.A.C.E.P.

I. Route of exposure: Oral, intravenous, intramuscular.
II. Common generic and trade names: See Table 80–1.
III. Pharmacokinetics:
    A. Onset of action:
        1. Without oral loading dose, 7–10 days until steady state reached.
        2. With oral loading dose (18 mg/kg), therapeutic levels achieved within 8–12 hours.
        3. With IV loading dose (18 mg/kg) onset is immediate.
    B. Peak action:
        1. May be delayed with extended forms up to 7 days.
        2. Peak blood levels from 4–12 hours after ingestion of capsules, with prolonged absorption up to 48 hours.
    C. Half-life:
        1. Elimination half-life varies from 7–40 hours, with average of 24 hours at therapeutic levels.
        2. Plasma drug concentration increases disproportionately as dosage is increased (half-life 8–62 hours).
        3. Half-life increased by:
            a. Hepatic disease.
            b. Toxic blood levels.
            c. Other agents that compete for same metabolic enzyme system: **isoniazid, clofibrate, phenylbutazone, chloramphenicol, dicumarol, cimetidine, disulfiram, some sulfonamides).**
        4. Half-life decreased by **carbamazepine, alcohol, phenobarbital,** related to enhanced microsomal enzyme induction and biotransformation.

TABLE 80–1.

Common Phenytoin Preparations

Generic Name	Trade Name	Strength
Extended Phenytoin Sodium Capsules*	Dilantin Kapseals	30, 100 mg
Prompt Phenytoin Sodium Capsules*	Diphenylan	30, 100 mg
Dilantin		
Diphenylhydantoin		
Phenytoin Oral Suspension	Dilantin-30 Pediatric	30/5 ml
Phenytoin Chewable Tablets	Dilantin 125	125/5 ml
	Dilantin Infatabs	50
Phenytoin Sodium Injection*	Dilantin	50/1 ml

*Generic product available.

D. Elimination:
  1. In acute overdose, liver hydoxylation and conjugation capacity quickly saturated, resulting in fixed rate of metabolism estimated at 3,000 mg/day.
  2. Less than 4% of drug is excreted unchanged in the urine.
E. Active metabolites: Major metabolite (60%–75%) is inactive.
IV. Action: Reduces speed of focal seizures and limits maximal seizure activity through promotion of neuronal sodium outflow.
V. Uses:
  A. First drug of choice for generalized tonic-clonic seizures and partial complex seizures.
  B. Useful for control of digoxin toxicity–induced arrhythmias.
VI. Toxic mechanism:
  A. Alters flow of Na^+, K^+, and Ca^{++} ions at both rest and during action potential.
    1. Stabilizes membranes of cardiac and neuronal Purkinje cells.
      a. In cardiac tissue, phenytoin (like lidocaine) decreases automaticity (type II antiarrhythmic). In particular, decreases secondary depolarizations occurring early in diastole (delayed afterdepolarizations) that are triggered by digitalis.
      b. Similarly, phenytoin limits maximal intensity and generalization of a seizure focus.
  B. Mechanism of phenytoin toxicity is presumably an extension of therapeutic action.
  C. Most common cause of phenytoin toxicity is a large dose increment, which because of nonlinear pharmacokinetics results in a disproportionately large increase in plasma level.
  D. Drug interactions: **Isoniazid, disulfiram** (Antabuse), **cimetidine,** and

chloramphenicol may elevate levels into the toxic range by decreasing hepatic clearance.

E. Free (unbound) phenytoin is responsible for toxicity; 90% is normally protein bound, 80% with uremia.

F. Aside from intentional overdosage, toxicity may occur because of failure to shake oral suspensions, injecting >50 mg/min, or drug interactions.

VII. Range of toxicity:

A. Toxic dose: Variable.

B. Fatal dose: Deaths are rare. Estimates of minimum lethal doses are unreliable.

VIII. Clinical features:

A. Serum (total) drug levels roughly correlate with toxicity (see Table 80–2).

B. Cardiac toxicity

1. Particularly associated with rapid intravenous use (possibly secondary to the diluent, propylene glycol).

2. Bradycardia, asystole, and hypotension less likely if given <40 mg/min or at a concentration <6–7 μg/ml.

C. Hypersensitivity reactions: Hepatitis, erythema multiforme, exfoliative dermatitis, Stevens-Johnson syndrome.

IX. Laboratory findings and evaluation:

A. Blood:

1. Serum phenytoin levels: Repeated every 2–4 hours during treatment, until peak noted. Toxic level considered to be greater than 20 μg/ml.

2. Glucose: Hyperglycemia.

B. ECG: Asystole and bradycardia have been reported.

X. General treatment:

A. Follow APTLS (see Chapter 8).

B. General management: Table 80–3 (see Chapter 12 for details).

XI. Specific treatment:

A. Seizures:

1. **Diazepam** 5–10 mg IV every 10 minutes up to 30 mg in adults; 0.25–0.40 mg/kg up to 10 mg in children.

2. **Phenobarbital** 10 mg/kg every 15 minutes up to 40 mg/kg with close monitoring of respiratory status.

TABLE 80–2.

Serum Phenytoin Levels and Clinical Signs of Toxicity

Level (μg/ml)	Toxicity
<15	Rare
>20	Nystagmus
>30	Ataxia, slurred speech
>40	Drowsiness, verbally unresponsive, seizures

TABLE 80-3.

General Treatment

Treatment	Indicated	Of No Value	Contraindicated
O_2	±		
IV	+		
ECG monitor	+		
Forced diuresis		X	
Acidification			X
Alkalinization		X	
Emesis/lavage	+/+		
Charcoal*	+		
Cathartic	+		

*Repeated doses of charcoal may be particularly effective in enhancing elimination of phenytoin.

    B. Bradycardia, asystole:
       1. Stop any phenytoin infusions.
       2. Atropine 0.5–1.0 mg.
       3. Pacing for refractory arrhythmias.
    C. Hypotension: See Chapter 10 for treatment recommendations.
    D. The efficacy of hemodialysis, charcoal hemoperfusion, exchange transfusion, peritoneal dialysis are questionable.
 XII. Prognosis:
    A. Expected response to treatment: With supportive care, death and morbidity are very uncommon from acute oral ingestion. Toxicity may last up to 7–10 days after ingestion.
    B. Expected complications and long-term effects:
       1. Bradyarrhythmia.
       2. Trauma related to self-injury from ataxia and depressed mental status.
       3. Patients receiving prolonged phenytoin therapy may experience withdrawal seizures if levels are allowed to drop below therapeutic range.
XIII. Disposition considerations:
    A. Admission considerations:
       1. See General Admission Considerations (Chapter 18).
       2. Admission is advisable in **all** acute overdoses because peak levels are frequently delayed 24–48 hours.
       3. Plasma levels >30 µg/ml associated with significant toxicity.
       4. Suicide risk.
    B. Observation period:
       1. Only if admission criteria are in doubt and patient asymptomatic.
       2. Only until peak is established.
       3. If stat phenytoin levels are not available, admit.
    C. Discharge considerations:
       1. General discharge considerations have been met (Chapter 18).
       2. Peak phenytoin serum level <30 µg/ml.

3. Asymptomatic.
4. No potential drug interaction or hepatic disease.
5. Patient can be discharged in care of responsible person.
6. Patient educated regarding medication regimen.
7. Suicide potential and psychiatric status have been appropriately evaluated.

BIBLIOGRAPHY

Atkinson AJ, Shaw JM: Pharmacokinetic study of a patient with diphenylhydantoin toxicity. *Clin Pharmacol Ther* 1973; 14:521–528.

Baehler RW, Work J, Smith W, et al: Charcoal hemoperfusion in the therapy for methsuximide and phenytoin overdose. *Arch Intern Med* 1980, 140: 1466–1468.

Earnest MP, Marx JA, Drury LR: Complications of intravenous phenytoin for acute treatment of seizures. *JAMA* 1983; 249:762–765.

Glaser GH, Penry JK, Woodbury DM (eds): *Antiepileptic Drugs: Mechanism of Action.* New York, Raven Press, 1980.

Mauro LS, Mauro VF, Brown DL, et al: Enhancement of phenytoin elimination by multiple-dose activated charcoal. *Ann Emerg Med* 1987; 16:1132–1135.

Osborn HH, Zisfein J, Sparano R: Single-dose oral phenytoin loading. *Ann Emerg Med* 1987; 16:407–412.

Weichbrodt GD, Elliott DP: Treatment of phenytoin toxicity with repeated doses of activated charcoal. *Ann Emerg Med* 1987; 16:1387–1389.

Wilder BJ, Buchanan RA, Serrano EE: Correlation of acute diphenylhydantoin intoxication with plasma levels and metabolic excretion. *Neurology* 1973; 23:1329–1332.

81

Digitalis

Teri A. Manolio, M.D., M.H.S.

I. Route of exposure:
   A. Oral, intravenous.
   B. Excess ingestion: Accidental or suicidal overdose, errors in preparation (excess amount in tablet), increased bioavailability of preparation.
II. Common generic and trade names:
   A. Digoxin (Lanoxin, Lanoxicaps).
   B. Digitoxin (Crystodigin).
   C. Deslanoside (Cedilanid-D).
III. Pharmacokinetics: See Table 81–1.
IV. Action:
   A. Mechanism of action: Enhances availability of calcium to myocardial contractile elements, probably by inhibition of Mg^{++} and ATP-dependent Na-K-ATPase (sodium pump) in sarcolemma; increases force of myocardial contraction.
   B. Effects on autonomic nervous system: Hypersensitizes carotid sinus baroreceptors; stimulates central vagal nucleus and nodose ganglia; enhances vagal activity and sensitization of cardiac tissues to effects of exogenous acetylcholine.
   C. Other cardiac effects:
      1. Sinus node: Slowing of rate (probably related to cholinergic and antiadrenergic mechanisms).
      2. Atrium: Accelerates repolarization and abbreviates effective refractory period; increases conduction velocity; predisposes to automatic impulse formation.
      3. AV node: Slowing of conduction and prolongation of AV nodal effective refractory period.

TABLE 81–1.

Oral Administration of Digitalis

	Digoxin	Digitoxin
GI absorption (%)	50–80	90–100
Onset of action (hr)	0.5	1–2
Plasma half-life (day)	1.5	4–6
Peak effect (hr)	3–6	4–12
Duration of action	3–6 day	2–3 wk
Elimination (%)	Renal 60–80, hepatic, GI	Hepatic primarily, some renal
Active metabolites	None	Digoxin

V. Uses:
  A. Congestive heart failure: Increases force of cardiac contraction.
  B. Supraventricular tachycardia: Increases refractoriness of AV node, leading to slowing of ventricular rate in atrial fibrillation and flutter.
VI. Toxic mechanism:
  A. Toxic effects are usually extensions of cellular mechanisms that augment inotropic state or slow conduction.
    1. Atrium: Increases automatic impulse formation and depresses conduction.
    2. AV node: Slows and eventually blocks AV nodal conduction.
    3. Purkinje fibers and ventricular muscle: Increases rate of spontaneous (phase 4) diastolic depolarization, leading to rapid spontaneous rhythms. Effect much more common in patients with heart disease.
  B. Factors predisposing to digitalis intoxication:
    1. Decreased volume of distribution: Ventricular failure, shock.
    2. Decreased elimination: Renal disease, decreased renal blood flow, decreased metabolism.
    3. Increased sensitivity to effects of digitalis:
      a. Electrolyte imbalance (hypokalemia, hypernatremia, hypomagnesemia, hypercalcemia).
      b. Excess sympathetic activity.
      c. Acute hypoxia, acid-base abnormalities.
      d. Severe heart disease, myocardial infarction, ischemia or fibrosis, myocarditis, recent heart surgery, cor pulmonale.
      e. Old age, hypothyroidism.
    4. Drug interactions: Diuretics, steroids, reserpine, catecholamines, quinidine, verapamil, amiodarone, lorcainide, propafenone.
VII. Range of toxicity:
  A. Toxic dose:
    1. Digoxin: Toxicity rarely seen with oral ingestions of <5 mg; however, symptoms of digoxin toxicity have been reported in oral ingestions as low as 2–3 mg in healthy adults.
    2. Digitoxin: 3–5 mg.

B. Fatal dose:
    1. Digoxin: Usually more than 10–20 mg in acute digoxin overdoses in healthy adults; less in patients with heart disease or hypokalemia. Deaths reported in patients receiving prolonged oral digoxin therapy after acute ingestion of 6 mg.
    2. Digitoxin: Estimated single lethal dose 3–10 mg.

VIII. Clinical features:
  A. Noncardiac symptoms:

Nausea	Visual disturbances
Fatigue	Color vision disturbances
Dizziness	Diarrhea
Vomiting	Neuropsychiatric disturbances
Headache	

  B. Cardiac manifestations:
    1. **Bradyarrhythmias** (e.g., sinus bradycardia, sinus arrest, AV block) common in toxic patients without heart disease, especially children and young adults. Usually related to increased vagal activity. May progress to **asystole** without ever developing tachyarrhythmias.
    2. **Tachyarrhythmias:** Common in toxic patients with heart disease.
      a. Atrial tachycardia with AV block and nonparoxysmal AV junctional tachycardia.
      b. Nonspecific ventricular tachyarrhythmias, ranging from ventricular extrasystoles (usually multiform) to ventricular bigeminy to ventricular tachycardia (often bidirectional) and fibrillation.
  C. Severe **hyperkalemia:**
    1. Although hypokalemia is found in chronic digitalis toxicity, elevated serum potassium may occur in acute digitalis poisoning.
    2. Can result from poisoning of sodium pump; elevated potassium levels closely correlate with increased mortality.
    3. ECG manifestations of hyperkalemia, such as peaked T waves, should be taken extremely seriously, but may be absent even with life-threatening serum potassium elevations.

IX. Laboratory findings and evaluation:
  A. Serum digitalis levels:
    1. Digoxin or digitoxin level by radioimmunoassay usually not available for several hours; therefore serum levels not usually helpful in emergency situation.
    2. Substantial overlap between toxic and therapeutic ranges, and no precise value clearly separates toxic from nontoxic doses. Much individual variation. Toxic patients usually have levels >2 ng/dl, but may be toxic with lower doses especially in presence of hypokalemia.
  B. ECG essential (see Clinical features).
  C. Other blood tests:
    1. Electrolytes, particularly potassium; magnesium and calcium if available.
    2. BUN, creatinine (assess likelihood of toxicity with "therapeutic" digitalis dosages and time course of clearance).

TABLE 81–2.

General Treatment of Ingested Overdose

Treatment	Indicated	Of No Value	Contraindicated
O$_2$	+		
IV	+		
ECG monitor	+		
Forced diuresis			X
Acidification			X
Alkalinization		X	
Emesis*/	−		
lavage	+		
Charcoal	+		
Cathartic	+		
Dialysis†	±		

*Ipecac administration may increase vagal reflexes and worsen bradyarrhythmias and therefore should be used with caution.
†Dialysis and hemoperfusion not effective in removing digitalis. May be necessary for treatment of refractory hyperkalemia.

3. Consider arterial blood gases to determine if acute hypoxia (which increases toxic effect) is present.
X. General treatment:
   A. Follow APTLS (see Chapter 8).
   B. General management: Table 81–2 (see Chapter 12 for details).
XI. Specific treatment:
   A. Mild toxicity (without arrhythmias):
      1. Admit to hospital, withhold a few doses, restart at lower dose when signs and symptoms have disappeared, replace potassium as necessary.
   B. Large ingestions:
      1. See Table 81–2.
      2. Consider oral administration of nonabsorbable resins (cholestyramine, colestipol) to prevent further absorption of digitalis in GI tract.
   C. Cardiac arrhythmias:
      1. Withhold drug, replace potassium, and observe with appropriate monitoring.
      2. AV block and bradyarrhythmias:
         a. Usually responsive to atropine 0.5 mg IV in adults, 10–30 μg/kg/dose up to 0.4 mg/dose in children.
         b. May require transvenous pacemaker.
         c. Avoid isoproterenol because of arrhythmogenic potential.
      3. Tachyarrhythmias:
         a. Replace potassium when serum K$^+$ low or normal (assess renal function prior to administration of potassium).
         b. Drugs of choice for management of arrhythmias:
            (1) Lidocaine:
               a Loading dose: 1 mg/kg/dose IV; repeat 0.5–1 mg/kg 20 minutes later if needed.

        b Maintenance dose: 10–40 µg/kg/min by continuous IV infusion.

        c Lidocaine does not impair AV nodal conduction.

    (2) Phenytoin:

        a Phenytoin actually improves AV conduction.

        b Loading dose: 15 mg/kg up to 1 gm IV, not to exceed rate of 0.5 mg/kg/min.

        c Maintenance for control of ventricular arrhythmias:

          i. Adults: 2 mg/kg IV every 12 hours as needed.

          ii. Child: 2 mg/kg IV every 8 hours as needed.

        d Maintenance to improve AV conduction:

          i. Adult: 25 mg/dose IV every 1–2 hours.

          ii. Child: 0.5–1 mg/kg/dose IV every 1–2 hours.

    (3) Refractory arrhythmias have been successfully treated with **amiodarone** 300 mg IV, but experience is scant.

D. Hyperkalemia:

  1. Can be managed with bicarbonate therapy and glucose with insulin (to shift potassium into intracellular space) or with potassium-binding resins (kayexalate) or hemodialysis or hemoperfusion to remove excess serum potassium.

  2. Hemoperfusion and hemodialysis are not effective in removing digoxin because of substantial protein and tissue binding of drug and large volume of distribution.

  3. Aggressive measures to lower elevated potassium levels will lead to total body depletion and may cause life-threatening hypokalemia once digitalis effect wears off.

  4. Administering calcium in digitalis-related hyperkalemia may be dangerous.

E. Digoxin-specific antibody fragments (Digibind) for treatment of life-threatening digoxin or digitoxin overdose.

  1. Indicated for patients in shock or cardiac arrest, ventricular tachycardia or fibrillation, or with progressive bradyarrhythmias such as severe sinus bradyarrhythmias or second- or third-degree AV block unresponsive to atropine. Severe hyperkalemia may also be an indication.

  2. Action: Binds digoxin in serum, causing shift of tissue-bound drug to intravascular compartment, where it is bound and can be excreted by kidneys. Free digoxin or digitoxin levels drop to unmeasurable levels less than 1 minute after IV injection. **Therefore digoxin-specific antibody fragments may interfere with immunoassay techniques to detect digoxin.**

  3. Adverse effects: Mild exacerbation of congestive heart failure or ventricular rate in patients with atrial fibrillation related to withdrawal of therapeutic effect of digitalis. No hypersensitivity reactions reported to date, but effect of repeated exposures unknown. Should be avoided in mild overdoses.

  4. Dosage:

    a. IV infusion over 30 minutes or bolus if cardiac arrest imminent; may require a second dose several hours later.

b. Packaged in 40 mg vials; each will bind 0.6 mg digoxin or digitoxin.

c. Reconstitute vials with 4 ml sterile water or sterile isotonic saline solution.

d. Number of vials = body load (mg)/[0.6 mg/vial]. Body load for digoxin (mg) = dose ingested × 0.8; for digitoxin (mg) = dose ingested.

5. Availability: Soon to be commercially available throughout United States. Call manufacturer 24 hours a day (1-800-334-4828; in North Carolina 1-800-672-7223) for further information on local supplies.

F. Hemofiltration therapy: Reported to successfully lower digoxin and potassium levels in a patient with refractory hyperkalemia, congestive heart failure, and complete AV block (Lai KN, Swaminathan R, Pun CO, et al: *Arch Intern Med* 1986; 146:1219–1220). More experience with this technique, however, is required before hemofiltration can be recommended as a therapeutic alternative.

XII. Prognosis:

A. Expected response to treatment:

1. Mortality in up to 50% in patients with hyperkalemia without digitalis antibody therapy.

2. With adequate and timely treatment, recovery should be rapid and complete, especially if patient survives for 24 hours after ingestion.

B. Expected complications and long-term effects:

1. Even after removal of digitalis and correction of hyperkalemia, patients may die of cerebral or myocardial hypoperfusion after prolonged hypotension and low cardiac output. No other reported long-term effects.

XIII. Disposition considerations:

A. Admission Considerations:

1. See General Admission Considerations (Chapter 18).

2. Healthy adults with **acute ingestions** of >3 mg should be admitted to monitored setting for detection of arrhythmias. If no arrhythmias in 12–24 hours after ingestion, discontinuation of monitoring may be considered.

3. Any child who has ingested >0.07 mg/kg digitalis preparation should be considered at high risk for serious toxicity and should be admitted to a monitored setting.

4. All symptomatic patients following **acute overdose,** including those with mild nonspecific symptoms (see Clinical features).

5. ICU monitoring for patients with ECG findings.

6. Suicide risk.

B. Consultation Considerations: Cardiology consultation for any patient for whom therapy with digoxin-specific antibody fragments is being considered.

C. Observation period:

1. Symptomatic patients with evidence of **acute digitalis toxicity** should be admitted and not observed in the emergency department.

2. Asymptomatic patients with history of significant **acute** ingestion (>3 mg) should not be observed in the emergency department because of long half-life of digitalis preparations (see Table 81–1).

D. Discharge considerations:
  1. General discharge considerations have been met (Chapter 18).
  2. Patients with **mild chronic toxicity** with noncardiac symptoms only can be discharged with close follow-up after discontinuation of drug. Replace potassium and correct any other metabolic abnormalities predisposing to toxicity before discharge from the emergency department. If any doubt, admit.
  3. Suicide potential and psychiatric status have been appropriately evaluated.

BIBLIOGRAPHY

Antman EM, Smith TW: Digitalis toxicity. *Annu Rev Med* 1986; 36:357.

Baud F, Bismuth CH, Pontal PG, et al: Time course of antidigoxin FAB fragment and plasma digitoxin concentrations in an acute digitalis intoxication. *J Toxicol Clin Toxicol* 1982; 19:857.

Bigger JT: Digitalis toxicity. *J Clin Pharmacol* 1985; 24:514–521.

Cardiac glycosides. *Poisindex,* vol 53. Micromedex Inc, 1987.

Digoxin antibody fragments for digitalis toxicity. *Med Lett Drugs Ther* 1986; 28:87–8.

Lai KN, Swaminathan R, Pun CO, et al: Hemofiltration in digoxin overdose. *Arch Intern Med* 1986; 146:1219–1220.

Standards and guidelines for cardiopulmonary resuscitation and emergency cardiac care: American Heart Association. *JAMA* 1986; 255:2841–3044.

Vincent JL, Dufaye P, Berre J, et al: Bretylium in severe ventricular arrhythmias associated with digitalis intoxication. *Am J Emerg Med* 1984; 2:504.

Warren SE, Fanestil DD: Digoxin overdose: Limitations of hemoperfusion-hemodialysis treatment. *Arch Intern Med* 1979; 242:2100–2101.

82

Calcium-Channel Blockers

Samuel S. Spicer, M.D., F.A.C.E.P.

I. Route of exposure: Oral, sublingual, intravenous.
II. Common generic and trade names: See Table 82–1.
III. Pharmacokinetics: See Table 82–2.
IV. Action:
   A. Calcium-channel blockers interfere with transport of calcium and other ions through the Ca^{++}-dependent slow channels in cardiac muscle, SA and AV nodes, and vascular smooth muscle, resulting in:
      1. Relaxation of arterial smooth muscle, with resultant lowering of peripheral resistance.
      2. Negative inotropic effect on heart.
   B. All three calcium channel-blockers have markedly different chemical structures and preferential site of actions (see Table 82–3).
V. Uses: Treatment of angina, arrhythmias, hypertension, migraine prophylaxis.
VI. Toxic mechanism:
   A. Drugs block reentry of calcium into muscle fibers, which can result in cardiac toxicity, including AV dissociation, sinus arrest, bradycardia, asystole.
   B. Reflex increase in adrenergic tone counteracts negative inotropic and bradycardia side effects at therapeutic drug levels. Such compensating mechanisms may be insufficient at toxic levels.
   C. Inhibits release of insulin.
VII. Range of toxicity:
   A. Toxic dose:
      1. Toxic doses have not been established except by case reports.
         a. Concomitant use of ophthalmic timolol 0.5% twice a day and oral verapamil 160 mg resulted in asymptomatic bradycardia at a rate of 36 in one patient.

TABLE 82–1.

Calcium-Channel Blockers

Generic Name	Trade Name	Strength (mg)
Verapamil	Isoptin	80, 120, 240 (SR)
	Calan	80, 120, 240 (SR)
Nifedipine	Procardia	10, 20
	Adalat	10
Diltiazem	Cardiazem	30, 60

B. Fatal dose:
  1. Like toxic doses, fatal doses have not been established except by case reports.
     a. 9.6 gm verapamil has resulted in death.
     b. An 11-month-old infant ingested 400 mg and survived.
     c. Survival has been noted after 10.8 gm of diltiazem in one patient and 900 mg nifedipine in another.
  2. Overdose with sustained-release forms has resulted in small intestine deposits and death after ingestion of 2.4 gm verapamil.
VIII. Clinical features:
  A. Clinical signs of toxicity are usually an extension of pharmacological properties. However, actions normally not expressed in some calcium channel blockers may be present in the acutely poisoned patient.

TABLE 82–2.

Pharmacokinetics

	Verapamil	Nifedipine	Diltiazem
Absorption*	Rapid	Rapid	Rapid
Onset of action	3 min IV	3 min SL	1 min IV
	60–120 min PO	20 min PO	15 min PO
Half-life (hr)†	1 IV	4–5 PO	4 PO
	5 PO		
Peak effect	5–15 min IV	30 min SL	30–60 min PO
	2–4 hr	60–90 min PO	
Elimination‡	Kidney mostly	Kidney mostly	Liver mostely
Active metabolites§	Yes	No	No

*Except for sustained-release forms, all calcium-channel blockers are rapidly absorbed. Bioavailability is limited by hepatic transformation, resulting in oral doses five to 20 times IV doses.
†Hepatic dysfunction may prolong half-life up to 16 hours.
‡Verapamil and diltiazem are extensively metabolized by the liver, with only 2%–4% excreted unchanged in the urine. Nifedipine is also extensively metabolized to inert products. Eighty percent to 85% of verapamil and nifedipine metabolic products are excreted via the kidney. Diltiazem products are excreted 60% by the liver and 35% by the kidney.
§Verapamil has an active metabolite, norverapamil, which is present only after oral administration.

TABLE 82–3.

Effects and Uses of Calcium-Channel Blockers

Drug	Peripheral Vasodilation	Bradycardia and AV Block	Decreased Contractility	Angina	Essential Hypertension	SVT Atrial Fibrillation Atrial Flutter
Verapamil	+	+ +	+ +	+	+	+
Nifedipine	+ + +	0	0	+		
Diltiazem	+	+	+	+		

B. Excessive vasodilation results in dizziness, peripheral edema, hypotension.

C. Other side effects include: Headaches, digital dysesthesias, flushing, nausea, vomiting, seizures, confusion, constipation.

D. ECG changes: A-V dissociation, sinus arrest, including sinus bradycardia, atrial flutter, PACs, PVCs (fusion beats), heart block, and asystole may be noted in the same patient.

E. Laboratory findings: Hyperglycemia, metabolic (lactic) acidosis.

F. Hepatotoxicity reported after several days to months of nifedipine therapy.

IX. Laboratory findings and evaluation:

A. Serum levels: Correlate with A-V conduction delays, but are not commonly available.

B. Minimum laboratory tests in symptomatic patients include electrolytes, glucose, ECG.

C. In more seriously ill patients: arterial blood gases, creatinine, BUN, calcium, serum lactate, liver function tests (SGOT/bilirubin), and baseline chest x-ray.

X. General treatment:

A. Follow APTLS (see Chapter 8).

B. General management: Table 82–4 (see Chapter 12 for details).

TABLE 82–4.

General Treatment

Treatment	Indicated	Of No Value	Contraindicated
O$_2$	+		
IV	+		
ECG monitor	+		
Forced diuresis		X	
Acidification			X
Alkalinization		X	
Emesis*/ lavage	+		X
Charcoal	+		
Cathartic	+		

*Emesis is relatively contraindicated. Vagal stimulation could possibly exacerbate AV conduction disturbances. During the first hour after ingestion, patients with intact airway may be candidates for emesis.

XI. Specific treatment:
  A. Clinical trials of treatment protocols are not available. Limited experience with treatment protocols dictates caution in interpretation of any recommendations. Supportive therapy, prevention of absorption, and aggressive management of hypotension and conduction abnormalities are major therapies.
  B. Hypotension:
    1. NaCl fluid challenge:
      a. Adult: 500 ml.
      b. Child: 20 ml/kg.
      c. Pulmonary edema because of excessive fluid resuscitation or rapid return of vascular tone usually responds to diuretics and oxygen.
    2. Trendelenburg position or pneumatic antishock garment.
    3. Vasopressors: Dopamine 5–50 μg/kg/min (use cautiously if underlying cardiac disease).
    4. CaCl 10%:
      a. Adult: 1–2 gm every 30 minutes for 8 hours.
      b. Child: 10–25 mg/kg.
    5. Inotropic agents: Dobutamine, epinephrine (use cautiously if underlying cardiac disease).
  C. Symptomatic conduction delay abnormalities including asystole:
    1. Atropine:
      a. Adult: 0.5–1 mg IV.
      b. Child: 0.02 mg/kg (0.15 mg minimum).
    2. CaCl 10%: 1–2 gm every 30 minutes for 8 hours.
    3. Isoproterenol 2 to 20 μg/min. CAUTION: Isoproterenol can accentuate peripheral vasodilation and exacerbate hypotension.
    4. Conduction defects may not respond to atropine, calcium, or isoproterenol and often require transvenous pacing. (Experience with cutaneous pacing has not been reported to date but may be of value).
XII. Prognosis:
  A. Expected response to treatment:
    1. Three of 17 patients with verapamil overdose died and one was left with significant brain damage. Diltiazem and nifedipine overdoses have been reported with no fatalities.
    2. Most ingestions are self-limited, with resolution of cardiovascular compromise in 24–72 hours. Survival for 24 hours has been followed by complete recovery.
  B. Expected complications and long-term effects:
    1. Aspiration pneumonia or cardiac arrest may prolong hospitalization and prevent full recovery.
    2. Severe hepatocellular injury secondary to verapamil.
XIII. Special considerations:
  A. Calcium channel blockers may increase digitalis levels 50%–75%.
  B. Overdose with sustained-release forms may result in toxicity with as little as 2.4 gm verapamil (see Range of toxicity).
  C. Abrupt withdrawal of a calcium-channel blocker may precipitate angina.
  D. In one report, overdose with diltiazem (1.2 gm) and metoprolol (500

mg) was treated with charcoal hemoperfusion, which resulted in rapid clinical improvement.

XIV. Disposition considerations:
  A. Admission considerations:
    1. See General Admission Considerations (Chapter 18).
    2. Any symptomatic patient.
    3. Those with underlying conduction system disease or concomitant use of beta blockers, regardless of mildness of symptoms, warrants hospitalization with cardiac monitoring.
    4. Ingestions of long-acting preparations, regardless of clinical presentation.
    5. ICU: Refractory hypotension, ECG abnormalities.
    6. Suicide risk.
  B. Observation period:
    1. Asymptomatic patients or those with very mild symptoms (e.g., dizziness) with normal examination and vital signs may be considered for discharge if they continue to show no evidence of systemic toxicity from ingestion after 6–8 hours of observation in the emergency department. Symptomatic patients taking beta blockers or who have underlying conduction disease should be admitted regardless of severity of symptoms.
  C. Discharge considerations:
    1. General discharge considerations have been met (Chapter 18).
    2. Asymptomatic patients with normal examination may be considered for discharge if they continue to show no evidence of toxicity after 6–8 hours of observation.
    3. Suicide potential and psychiatric status have been appropriately evaluated.

BIBLIOGRAPHY

Anthony T, Jastremski M, Elliot W, et al: Charcoal hemoperfusion for treatment of a combined diltiazem and metoprolol overdose. *Ann Emerg Med* 1986; 15:1344–1348.

Hariman RJ, Mangiardi LM, McAllister RG, et al: Reversal of the cardiovascular effects of verapamil by calcium and sodium: Differences between electrophysiologic and hemodynamic responses. *Circulation* 1979; 59:797–804.

Herrington DM, Insley BM, Weinmann GC: Nifedipine overdose. *Am J Med* 1986; 81:344–346.

Richter WO, Schwandt P: Serious side effect of nifedipine (letter). *Arch Intern Med* 1987; 147:1850.

Standards and guidelines for cardiopulmonary resuscitation and emergency cardiac care: American Heart Association. *JAMA* 1986; 255:2841–3044.

Young GP: Calcium channel blockers in emergency medicine. *Ann Emerg Med* 1984; 13 (part I):712–722.

83

Lidocaine

John G. Keene, M.D., F.A.C.E.P.

I. Route of exposure:
  A. Parenteral:
    1. Infused IV as antiarrhythmic; can also be given IM and via orotracheal tube.
    2. Infiltrated SC as local anesthetic.
  B. Oral:
    1. Topical preparations (e.g., viscous lidocaine).
II. Common name: Xylocaine.
III. Pharmacokinetics:
  A. Absorption from GI tract: Rapid.
  B. Onset of action:
    1. IV within minutes.
    2. Seizure has been reported 30 minutes after ingestion of lidocaine HCl jelly by a child.
  C. Peak levels: 30–60 minutes after ingestion.
  D. Duration of action: Initial IV bolus for antiarrhythmic action remains in therapeutic range for 8–10 minutes. Effect of 50–100 mg bolus disappears within 10–20 minutes.
  E. Half-life: Elimination half-life after IV bolus 1.5–2 hours.
  F. Elimination:
    1. Deethylation in liver.
    2. Metabolites excreted by kidneys.
    3. Clearance decreased in heart failure and liver disease.
  G. Active metabolites:
    1. Monoethyl glycylxylidine is the first metabolite and has some antiarrhythmic and toxic activity.
    2. Then glyginexylidine is produced, which has little effect.

IV. Actions:
    A. Direct cardiac action:
        1. Decreases automaticity in Purkinje fibers by decreasing slope of normal phase 4 depolarization.
        2. Increases threshold for excitation in Purkinje fibers; increases ventricular fibrillation threshold.
        3. Can abolish reentrant arrhythmias.
    B. Local anesthetic action:
        1. Prevents generation and conduction of nerve impulses.
        2. Stabilizes neuron membrane, preventing ionic movement necessary for impulse generation and conduction.
V. Uses:
    A. Local and topical anesthetic.
    B. Effective agent for ventricular dysrhythmias and tachydysrhythmia of Wolff-Parkinson-White syndrome.
VI. Toxic mechanism:
    A. CNS: Excitatory or depressant effects characterized by drowsiness, respiratory depression, convulsions.
    B. Cardiovascular system:
        1. Effects require large concentrations and usually occur after CNS effects.
        2. Depression of electrical excitability, conduction rate, and force of contraction. These may lead to bradycardia, hypotension, and cardiac arrest.
    C. Hypersensitivity or allergic reactions: Virtually nonexistent with amide class local anesthetics.
    D. Methemoglobinemia.
    E. Patients at risk for toxicity include those with congestive heart failure, shock, liver disease, those receiving cimetidine and propranolol, and the elderly.
VII. Range of toxicity:
    A. Toxic dose:
        1. Toxic reactions occur in 6%–15% of patients with IV infusion of lidocaine at 3 mg/min.
        2. Oral ingestions >5–10 mg/kg may result in seizures. Oral ingestions 10–30 ml 2%–4% viscous lidocaine solutions have resulted in seizures in children.
    B. Fatal dose: Any toxic dose resulting in seizure can result in death secondary to complications (e.g., airway obstruction, aspiration pneumonia).
    C. Maximum recommended dose as local anesthetic:
        1. 60 ml 0.5% solution.
        2. 30 ml 1% solution.
        3. 15 ml 2% solution.
VIII. Clinical features:
    A. CNS: Restlessness, tremor, euphoria, confusion, dizziness, tinnitis, blurred vision, vomiting, slurred speech, clonic convulsions, coma, respiratory arrest.

B. Cardiovascular system: Sinus arrest, AV block, hypotension, ventricular arrhythmias (e.g., ventricular tachycardia, fibrillation), cardiac arrest.

C. Hypersensitivity: Urticaria, edema, anaphylaxis.

D. Methemoglobinemia (see Chapter 102).

IX. Laboratory findings and evaluation:

A. Serum lidocaine levels: Toxic reactions (usually CNS) are commonly first seen with blood levels about 5 µg/ml.

B. ECG.

C. Patients given lidocaine as local anesthesia who develop CNS symptoms should have standard acute altered mental status workup (see Chapter 21).

D. Methemoglobin level if appropriate.

E. Liver function tests.

X. General treatment:

A. Follow APTLS (see Chapter 8).

B. General management: Table 83–1 (see Chapter 12 for details).

XI. Specific management:

A. Stop IV infusion.

B. Seizures: See Chapter 22 for treatment recommendations.

C. Hypotension: See Chapter 10.

D. Bradycardia:

a. Atropine 0.5 mg; repeat every 5 minutes if necessary, to maximum of 2 mg.

b. Temporary pacing may be necessary.

E. Methemoglobinemia: See Chapter 102 for details of treatment.

XII. Prognosis:

A. Expected response to treatment:

1. Symptoms of intravenous toxicity should begin to abate within 10–15 minutes after lidocaine infusion stopped.

2. Survival for 1 hour indicates that patient will recover.

TABLE 83–1.

General Treatment

Treatment	Indicated	Of No Value	Contraindicated
O$_2$	+		
IV	+		
ECG monitor	+		
Forced Diuresis		X	
Acidification			X
Alkalinization		X	
Emesis/	−		
Lavage	−		
Charcoal	−		
Cathartic	−		

XIII. Special considerations: There are two general classes of local anesthetics. Lidocaine is a group II (amide class) local anesthetic, which includes bupivacaine, etidocaine, and prilocaine. Group I (ester class) anesthetics include procaine, tetracaine, benzocaine, and cocaine. Inasmuch as there is less demonstrated cross-reactivity between the amide and ester types of local anesthetics, patients allergic to one of the amide anesthetics, such as lidocaine, may safely be given any of the ester anesthetics.

XIV. Disposition considerations:
  A. Admission considerations:
    1. See General Admission Considerations (Chapter 18).
    2. Patients with severe reactions (convulsions, respiratory depression, loss of consciousness, bradycardia, hypotension).
    3. Persistent mild symptoms (see below) after observation.
  B. Consultation considerations: Hematologist should be consulted for inpatient follow-up if methemoglobinemia develops.
  C. Observation period: Patients with mild symptoms (shakiness or tremors, giddiness or euphoria, slight confusion, slightly slurred speech, vomiting) may be observed with cardiac monitoring for 3–4 hours.
  D. Discharge considerations:
    1. General discharge considerations have been met (Chapter 18).
    2. Asymptomatic and without clinical findings.

BIBLIOGRAPHY

Fruncillo RJ, Gibbens W, Bowman SM: CNS toxicity after ingestion of topical lidocaine. *N Engl J Med* 1982; 306:426.

Pfeifer HJ, Greenblatt DJ, Koch-Weser J: Clinical use and toxicity of intravenous lidocaine: A report from the Boston Collaborative Drug Surveillance Program. *Am Heart J* 1976; 92:168–173.

Rothstein P, Dornbusch J, Shaywitz B: Prolonged seizures associated with the use of viscous lidocaine. *J Pediatr* 1982; 101:461–463.

Saito S, Chen CM, Buchanan JW, et al: The effect of lidocaine. *Circ Res* 1978; 42:246.

Sakai R, Lattin J: Lidocaine ingestion. *Am J Dis Child* 1980; 134:323.

Stein JM, Warfield CA: Local anesthetics: Principles of safe use. *Hosp Prac* 1983; 18:73–78.

84

Quinidine/Procainamide/ Disopyramide: Type I Antiarrhythmic Agents

John G. Keene, M.D., F.A.C.E.P.

Procainamide

    I. Route of exposure: Oral, intravenous, intramuscular.
   II. Common trade names: Procan SR, Pronestyl.
 III. Pharmacokinetics:
      A. Absorption: Oral bioavailability 75%–95%
      B. Plasma half-life:
         1. 3 hours (average).
         2. Markedly prolonged in heart failure or renal insufficiency (half-life 8–10 hours).
         3. *N*-acetyl procainamide (NAPA, an active metabolite) has half-life of 6 hours and up to 36 hours in overdoses.
      C. Peak effect:
         1. Oral: 1 hour.
         2. IM: 30 minutes.
         3. IV: Within several minutes.
      D. Elimination: 40% acetylated by liver to NAPA, 60% excreted unchanged in urine.
      E. Active metabolites: *N*-acetylprocainamide (NAPA).

IV. Action:
  A. Class I antiarrhythmic:
    1. Decreases automaticity.
    2. Slows conduction velocity.
    3. Prolongs refractory period.
  B. Can produce serious toxicity, which is often life threatening (see Toxic mechanism).
V. Uses:
  A. Suppression of ventricular arrhythmias.
  B. Treatment of automatic and reentrant supraventricular tachycardia.
  C. Conversion of atrial fibrillation or flutter.
VI. Toxic mechanism:
  A. Cardiovascular effects:
    1. Depresses automaticity and intracardiac conduction:
      a. Vagolytic effects and reflex sympathetic stimulation.
      b. Usually in severe toxicity depressed automaticity predominates.
      c. Depressed automaticity and conduction may render heart refractory to pacing.
    2. Myocardial depression and hypotension:
      a. Dose-related depression of contractility.
      b. Decreased vascular resistance secondary to direct vasodilation.
      c. Some alpha adrenergic blocking.
  B. CNS depression manifested by lethargy, confusion, respiratory depression.
  C. Anticholinergic effects.
VII. Range of toxicity:
  A. Toxic dose:
    1. Single oral dose of 2 gm may produce symptoms of toxicity. Ingestion of 3 gm may be dangerous, especially if patient is slow acetylator or has renal impairment of underlying heart disease.
  B. Fatal dose:
    1. Death reported from IV administration of 200 mg (2 ml 10% solution). Postulated mechanism of death either hypersensitivity reaction or too rapid injection.
VIII. Clinical features:
  A. Cardiovascular:
    1. Vagolytic effects and reflex sympathetic stimulation may result in sinus or atrial tachycardia.
    2. Ventricular tachyarrhythmias: May present as Adams-Stokes disease.
    3. Myocardial depression and hypotension:
      a. Hypotension, with some patients having warm, pink skin.
      b. Pulmonary edema.
  B. Other toxic manifestations:
    1. Gastrointestinal irritation:
      a. Nausea, vomiting, diarrhea, abdominal pain.
      b. Seen commonly with both therapeutic doses and overdoses.
    2. CNS depression:
      a. Lethargy may progress to coma.
      b. Subject to respiratory arrest.

  c. Onset of CNS symptoms delayed.

  d. Recovery from coma often delayed.

 3. Anticholinergic effects (see Chapter 91).

 4. Mild hypovolemia, hypokalemia, metabolic acidosis possible.

IX. Laboratory findings and evaluation:

 A. Serum concentration:

  1. Plasma levels >10 μg/ml increasingly associated with toxic findings.

  2. Levels of procainamide and NAPA >60 μg/ml suggest severe toxicity.

 B. ECG findings:

  1. Widened QRS complex (characteristic in overdose).

  2. Prolongation of QT interval (characteristic in overdose).

  3. U waves.

  4. Bundle branch block.

  5. Sinoatrial block.

  6. Atrioventricular block.

  7. Sinus arrest.

  8. Junctional or ventricular bradycardia.

  9. Asystole.

  10. Ventricular tachycardia.

  11. Torsade de pointes.

  12. Ventricular fibrillation.

 C. Arterial blood gas (mild metabolic acidosis, respiratory depression, monitor alkalinization treatment [see below]).

 D. Other laboratory tests depending on clinical situation:

  1. Blood sugar (in presence of altered mental status).

  2. Chest radiograph (pulmonary edema).

  3. Electrolytes, BUN, creatinine (fluid and electrolyte status if severe vomiting, diarrhea).

  4. Complete blood cell count (neutropenia, thrombocytopenia, hemolytic anemia have been reported as rare adverse reaction).

X. General treatment:

 A. Follow APTLS (see Chapter 8).

 B. General management: Table 84–1 (see Chapter 12 for details).

XI. Specific treatment:

 A. Cardiovascular support:

  1. **Cardiac arrest:** Follow most recent Advanced Cardiac Life Support guidelines from the American Heart Association (*JAMA* 1986; 255:2841–3044).

  2. Use epinephrine or norepinephrine with caution; they may lead to ventricular arrhythmias.

  3. Bradycardia:

   a. Isoproterenol 2–10 μg/min.

   b. Temporary cardiac pacing; may need higher energies to stimulate refractory myocardium.

  4. Ventricular dysrhythmias (especially premature ventricular contractions [PVCs] and ventricular tachycardia).

   a. Lidocaine, phenytoin, bretylium may be effective.

   b. Overdrive pacing (may be refractory in severe poisoning)

TABLE 84–1.

General Treatment

Treatment	Indicated	Of No Value	Contraindicated
O_2	+		
IV	+		
ECG monitor	+		
Forced diuresis			X
Acidification			X
Alkalinization (see below)	+		
Emesis/lavage	+/+		
Charcoal*	+		
Cathartic	+		
Dialysis	±		

*May be effective hours later because of delayed absorption.

5. Sinus tachycardia usually does not require treatment; however, if hemodynamically unstable and there are no conduction defects, propranolol may be effective.
   6. Sodium bicarbonate:
      a. May reverse toxic electrophysiologic effects.
      b. Dose: 44–50 mEq IV every 5–10 minutes until pH 7.45–7.50.
   B. Hypotension and cardiogenic shock:
      1. See Chapter 10.
      2. Intractable cardiogenic shock may require placement of intraaortic balloon pump or cardiopulmonary bypass.
   C. CNS effects:
      1. Protect airway (see Chapter 9).
   D. Hemodialysis and resin hemoperfusion:
      1. Indications for hemodialysis:
         a. Serum procainamide concentration >20 μg/L.
         b. Severe cardiovascular manifestations.
         c. Inadequte renal function.
   XII. Prognosis:
      A. Expected response to treatment: Presence of PVCs and runs of ventricular tachycardia almost always successfully treated. Prognosis excellent if these rhythms do not progress to ventricular fibrillation or asystole.
      B. Expected complications and long-term effects: Agranulocytosis from hypersensitivity reaction associated with 90% recovery rate.
   XIII. Disposition considerations:
      A. Admission considerations:
         1. All procainamide overdoses should be admitted to a monitored bed for observation and treatment for the following reasons:
            a. Potentially life-threatening nature of toxicity

      b. Possibility of delayed absorption secondary to gastric irritation and anticholinergic effects

      c. Delayed onset of CNS complications

      d. Long half-life of active metabolite

B. Consultation considerations:

    1. Cardiology.

    2. Dialysis service, particularly if patient has renal impairment.

C. Observation period: Not appropriate to observe in emergency department.

D. Discharge considerations: Not appropriate to discharge patients with known or suspected ingestions.

Quinidine

I. Route of exposure: Oral, intravenous.

II. Common trade names:

    Cinn-quin

    Quinora

    SK-Quinidine Sulfate

    Quinidine Extentabs

    Duraquin

    Quinaglute Dura-tabs

    Cardioquin

III. Pharmacokinetics:

A. Absorption:

    1. Rapidly absorbed, with systemic bioavailability 70%–95% for both quinidine sulfate and slow-release preparations.

    2. Anticholinergic or gastric effects delay absorption.

B. Plasma half-life: Average 6–8 hours (range 3–19 hours).

C. Peak effect:

    1. 1–2 hours for quinidine sulfate.

    2. 4–8 hours for quinidine gluconate (slow-release preparation).

D. Elimination: 80% metabolized by liver, 20% excreted unchanged in urine.

E. Active metabolites: Yes.

IV. Action:

A. Class I antiarrhythmic similar to procainamide.

B. Pharmacologic effects similar to those of procainamide (see Procainamide).

C. Can produce serious toxicity, which is often life threatening (see Toxic mechanism).

V. Uses:

A. Suppression of ventricular arrhythmias.

B. Treatment of automatic and reentrant supraventricular tachycardia.

C. Conversion of atrial fibrillation or flutter.

VI. Toxic mechanism:
   A. See Procainamide.
   B. Potentially prolonged toxicity with quinidine:
      a. Gastric irritation slows absorption.
      b. Hypotension delays excretion.
VII. Range of toxicity:
   A. Fatal Dose: May be as low as 0.2 gm as a result of hypersensitivity.
VIII. Clinical features:
   A. See Procainamide.
   B. Cardiovascular
      1. Ventricular tachyarrhythmias may result in Adams-Stokes disease (quinidine syncope).
      2. Depressed automaticity and intracardiac conduction with bradyarrhythmias.
      3. Myocardial depression with hypotension.
   C. Prominent gastrointestinal irritation:
      1. Nausea, vomiting, diarrhea, abdominal pain
      2. Seen commonly with both therapeutic doses and overdoses.
   D. Seizures associated with quinidine toxicity.
   E. Quinidine toxicity may present with symptoms of cinchonism:
      1. Tinnitus.
      2. Vertigo.
      3. Hearing loss.
      4. Blurred vision.
      5. Yellow vision.
      6. Contracted visual fields.
      7. Scotomas.
      8. Diplopia.
      9. Photophobia.
      10. Headache.
      11. Confusion, delirium, excitement.
      12. Fever.
   F. Lethargy, coma, respiratory arrest.
   G. Hypokalemia.
   H. Thrombocytopenic purpura in chronic poisoning.
IX. Laboratory findings and evaluation:
   A. Serum quinidine levels generally not helpful.
   B. Other laboratory tests: See Procainamide.
X. Treatment:
   A. See Procainamide. Check for hypokalemia.
   B. Dialysis generally not effective in quinidine poisoning, but in liver failure resin hemoperfusion may be helpful.
XI. Prognosis:
   A. Expected response to treatment:
      1. Mortality from use of quinidine for treatment of cardiac arrhythmias is 1%.
      2. Survival after acute ingestion for 24 hours associated with good prognosis for complete recovery.

XII. Special considerations: May elevate serum digoxin levels.
XIII. Disposition considerations: See Procainamide.

Disopyramide

I. Route of exposure: Oral.
II. Common trade name: Norpace.
III. Pharmacokinetics:
   A. Absorption: Oral bioavailability 80%–90%, but absorbed slowly because of anticholinergic effects.
   B. Plasma half-life: 8 hours (prolonged renal insufficiency).
   C. Peak effect: 1–3 hours.
   D. Elimination: 45% metabolized in liver with production of active metabolites, 55% excreted unchanged in urine.
   E. Active metabolites: Metabolite has some antiarrhythmic and pronounced anticholinergic activity.
IV. Action: See Procainamide.
V. Uses: Suppression of ventricular and supraventricular arrhythmias.
VI. Toxic dose: Not established.
VII. Clinical features:
   A. See Procainamide.
   B. Myocardial depression may lead to severe pulmonary edema.
   C. Pronounced anticholinergic effects (more than procainamide and quinidine).
VIII. Laboratory findings and evaluation:
   A. Serum disopyramide concentrations difficult to interpret.
   B. Other laboratory tests: See Procainamide.
IX. Treatment:
   A. See Procainamide.
   B. Hemodialysis and resin hemoperfusion should be considered in **All** cases of life-threatening disopyramide overdose.
X. Prognosis: Good with adequate support of vital functions.
XI. Disposition considerations: See Procainamide.

BIBLIOGRAPHY

Atkinson AJ, Krumlovsky FA, Huang CM, et al: Hemodialysis for severe procainamide toxicity: Clinical and pharmacokinetic observations. *Clin Pharmacol Ther* 1976; 20:585.

Conrad KA, Molk BL, Chidsey CA: Pharmacokinetic studies of quinidine in patients with arrhythmias. *Circulation* 1977; 55:1.

Desai JM, Desai JM, Scheinman MM, et al: Cardiovascular collapse associated with disopyramide therapy. *Chest* 1981; 79:545.

Gosselin B, et al: Acute intoxication with disopyramide: Clinical and experimental study by hemoperfusion on Amberlite XAD-4 resin. *Clin Toxicol* 1980; 17:439.

Hayler AM, Hold DW, Volans GN: Fatal overdosage with disopyramide. *Lancet* 1978; 1:968.

Karlsson E: Clinical pharmacokinetics of procainamide. *Clin Pharmacokinet* 1978; 3:97.

Shub C, Gau GT, Sidell PM, et al: The management of acute quinidine intoxication. *Chest* 1978; 73:173–178.

Swerdlow CD, Yu JO, Jacobson E: Safety and efficacy of intravenous quinidine. *Am J Med* 1983; 75:36.

Villalba-Pimental L, Epstein LM, Sellers EM, et al: Survival after massive procainamide ingestion. *Am J Cardiol* 1973; 32:727.

85

Antihypertensive Agents

John G. Keene, M.D., F.A.C.E.P.
Mary L. Dunne, M.D.

Many of the medications covered in this chapter produce adverse effects (side effects) from prolonged use in therapeutic doses. However, given the scope of this book, discussion of these medications is generally limited to toxicity from acute overdose. Adverse effects are noted if they can be produced with acute toxicity, or if presence as an underlying condition from long-term use may influence emergency care.

Captopril

   I. Route of exposure: Oral.
  II. Common trade name: Capoten.
 III. Pharmacokinetics:
   A. Absorption: Food reduces absorption by 30%–40%.
   B. Plasma half-life: 2–3 hours.
   C. Elimination: 95% excreted by kidneys; 40%–50% unchanged in urine.
  IV. Action: Inhibits angiotensin I converting enzyme.
   V. Toxic mechanism:
   A. Mild hypertension secondary to inhibition of angiotensin I converting enzyme.
   B. Theoretically, could result in hyperkalemia, and the patient needs to be monitored for this effect.

VI. Range of toxicity:
   A. Toxic dose: A 5 gm ingestion has been survived with only mild hypotension.
   B. Fatal dose: No deaths reported.
VII. Clinical features:
   A. Acute effects: Hypotension, tachycardia.
   B. Adverse (chronic) effects: Neutropenia, agranulocytosis, proteinuria, rash, Raynaud's phenomenon, angina, myocardial infarction, loss of sense of taste, vertigo.
VIII. Laboratory findings and evaluation (acute toxicity):
   A. Electrolytes (may have hyperkalemia).
   B. Spun hematocrit (if diagnosis in doubt, must rule out hemorrhage as cause of hypotension).
   C. Renal function studies (BUN, creatinine).
   D. Urinalysis (may see proteinuria).
   E. ECG (may have ischemia, myocardial infarction).
IX. Treatment:
   A. Follow APTLS: See Chapter 8.
   B. General management: Table 85–1.
   C. Hypotension: See Chapter 10.
   D. Dialysis effective.
X. Prognosis: Excellent with good supportive care.
XI. Disposition considerations:
   A. Admission considerations:
      1. See General Admission Considerations (Chapter 18).
      2. Symptomatic or clinical findings.
      3. Intractable hypotension (ICU).
      4. Myocardial ischemia (ICU).
      5. Suicide risk.
   B. Observation period: Each patient requires individual evaluation for toxic manifestations. At minimum, all patients with symptoms after ingestion should be treated and observed for several hours in the emergency de-

TABLE 85–1.

General Treatment

Treatment	Indicated	Of No Value	Contraindicated
O$_2$	+		
IV	+		
ECG monitor	+		
Forced diuresis		X	
Acidification			X
Alkalinization		X	
Emesis/lavage	+/+		
Charcoal	+		
Cathartic	+		
Dialysis	±		

partment if discharge is entertained. For most overdoses observation is not appropriate.

   C. Discharge considerations:

     1. General disposition considerations have been met (see Chapter 18).

     2. Asymptomatic without clinical findings after sufficient observation.

     3. If patient is receiving maintenance therapy, dosage has been evaluated and patient has been counseled.

     4. Suicide potential and psychiatric status have been appropriately evaluated.

Methyldopa

    I. Route of exposure: Oral.

   II. Common trade name: Aldomet.

  III. Pharmacokinetics:

    A. Absorption: Oral bioavailability variable.

    B. Plasma half-life: 2 hours.

    C. Peak effect: 4 hours.

    D. Elimination: 25%–60% excreted in urine; remainder metabolized, producing active metabolites.

    E. Active metabolites: Methyldopa-O-sulfate, the major metabolite, probably has little or no antihypertensive activity; however, under conditions of renal failure may be pharmacologically active.

  IV. Action: Stimulates inhibitory alpha adrenergic receptors centrally, decreasing sympathetic outflow from CNS.

   V. Toxic mechanism:

    A. Toxic effects result from CNS actions of methyldopa.

    B. Abnormalities of temperature regulation: Hypothermia.

    C. Cardiovascular regulation: Hypotension, bradycardia, dizziness, weakness.

    D. CNS: Weakness, coma.

  VI. Range of toxicity:

    A. Toxic dose: 7.5 gm.

    B. Fatal dose: 25 gm.

  VI. Clinical features:

    A. Neurologic: Sedation, postural hypotension, dizziness, dry mouth, headache, decreased mental acuity, sleep disturbance, Parkinsonian signs, weakness, coma.

    B. Cardiovascular: Bradycardia, hypotension.

    C. Hematologic: Mostly chronic adverse effects: Hemolytic anemia, lupus-like syndrome (20% of patients have positive Coombs' test results).

    D. Methyldopa may cause confusion in elderly patients who may inadvertently overdose.

 VIII. Laboratory findings and evaluation:

    A. Spun hematocrit (if diagnosis in doubt, must rule out bleeding as source of hypotension).

    B. ECG (may see dysrhythmias, especially bradycardias).

    C. Blood glucose (in presence of sedation, dizziness, or altered mental status).

IX. Treatment:
   A. See Captopril.
   B. Patients with severe poisoning may benefit from hemodialysis.
X. Prognosis: Excellent with good supportive care.
XI. Special considerations:
   A. Oral suspension contains sodium bisulfite; tablets do not. Some patients have bisulfite sensitivity.
   B. Sudden cessation may produce rebound hypertension.
XII. Disposition considerations:
   A. Admission considerations:
      1. See General Admission Considerations (Chapter 18).
      2. Symptomatic.
      3. Bradycardia (ICU).
      4. Refractory hypotension (ICU).
      5. Suicide risk.
   B. Consultation considerations: Dialysis service if symptoms severe.
   C. Observation period: In milder cases of methyldopa poisoning, observation period of 6 hours may be sufficient to rule out significant toxicity.
   D. Discharge considerations: See Captopril.

Calcium-Channel Blockers

I. See Chapter 82.

Diazoxide

I. Route of exposure: Intravenous, oral.
II. Common trade name: Hyperstat.
III. Pharmacokinetics:
   A. Absorption: Oral bioavailability 100%.
   B. Plasma half-life: 28 hours (range 20–60 hours).
   C. Elimination: 70% metabolized in liver to inactive compounds, 30% excreted unchanged by kidneys.
   D. Active metabolites: None known.
IV. Action:
   A. Direct arterial smooth muscle relaxation with peripheral vasodilation.
   B. Marked water retention.
   C. Decreased insulin secretion and utilization of glucose.
V. Toxic mechanism: Related to direct effect on smooth muscle.
VI. Range of toxicity:
   A. Fatal dose and toxic doses have not been well established.
   B. Old dosage of 300 mg IV caused sudden hypotension with attendant complications.
VII. Clinical features:
   A. Acute toxicity: Hypotension, shock (rarely, hypertension), hyperglycemia, nonketotic hyperosmolar coma, hyperglycemic ketoacidosis, myocardial

ischemia, angina myocardial infarction, cerebral infarction, arrhythmias, seizures.
B. Adverse (chronic) affects: Sodium and water retention, rash, hyperuricemia.
VIII. Laboratory findings and evaluation:
    A. Spun hematocrit (if diagnosis in doubt, rule out bleeding as cause of hypotension).
    B. Serum glucose (hyperglycemia).
    C. Renal function tests (BUN, creatinine, urinalysis).
    D. ECG (ischemic changes).
    E. Uric acid (hyperuricemia).
    F. Serum osmolality, ketones, electrolytes, arterial blood gases.
IX. Treatment:
    A. See Captopril.
    B. Hyperglycemia, nonketotic hyperosmolar coma, ketoacidosis:
        1. Insulin.
        2. Restoration of fluid and electrolyte balance.
    C. Peritoneal dialysis and hemodialysis have lowered diazoxide levels in two patients.
X. Prognosis:
    A. Expected response to treatment: Toxicity usually subsides.
    B. Expected complications and long-term effects: Myocardial infarction and cerebrovascular accident are grave complications.
XI. Special considerations:
    A. Drug interactions: Marked potentiation of antihypertensive and hyperuricemic effects if given:
        1. Concomitantly with **thiazides.**
        2. Within 6 hours of **hydralazine, reserpine, methyldopa, beta blockers, prazosin, minoxidil, papaverine**-like compounds.
XII. Disposition considerations:
    A. Admission considerations:
        1. Because of dizoxide's long half-life (approximately 30 hours), symptoms of overdose require prolonged surveillance for up to 7 days until blood glucose level stabilizes within normal range.
        2. ICU admission mandatory for life-threatening signs: Hypotension, shock (rarely, hypertension), nonketotic hyperosmolar coma, hyperglycemic ketoacidosis, myocardial ischemia, angina, myocardial infarction, cerebral infarction, arrhythmias, seizures.

Thiazide Diuretics

    I. Route of exposure: Oral.
    II. Common names: See Table 85–2.
    III. Pharmacokinetics:
        A. Absorption: Oral bioavailability 60%–90%.
        B. Onset of action: 1 hour after oral dose.

TABLE 85–2.

Common Thiazide Diuretics

Generic Name	Trade Name
Bendroflumethiazide	Naturetin
Benzthiazide	Exna
Chlorothiazide	Diuril
Hydrochlorothiazide	Hydrodiuril, Esidrix
Hydroflumethiazide	Diucardin, Saluron
Methyclothiazide	Aquatensin, Enduron
Polythiazide	Renese
Trichloromethiazide	Naqua, Trizdaide, Metahydrin
Related agents:	
Chlorthalidone	Hygroton
Quinethazone	Thalitone, Hydromox

   C. Plasma half-life:
      1. Chlorthiazide: 1.5 hours.
      2. Chlorthalidone: 44 hours.
   D. Peak effect: 3–6 hours.
   E. Duration of action: Most last 6–12 hours, with following exceptions:
      1. Quinethazone: 18–24 hours.
      2. Methyclothiazide: 24 hours.
      3. Polythiazide: 24 hours.
      4. Chlorthalidone: 48 hours.
   F. Elimination: Excreted unchanged in urine.
   G. Active metabolites: None.
IV. Action:
   A. Diuretic action by inhibition of sodium and chloride reabsorption at distal convoluted tubule of the kidneys.
   B. At higher doses, thiazides are carbonic anhydrase inhibitors.
   C. Increased excretion of sodium, potassium, chloride, bicarbonate, water.
   D. Inhibits insulin secretion.
   E. Inhibits synthesis of vitamin D and thus absorption of calcium from gut; also inhibits renal excretion of calcium.
 V. Toxic mechanism: Toxicity related to fluid and electrolyte losses from above actions and associated clinical effects.
VI. Clinical features:
   A. Intravascular volume depletion: Orthostatic hypotension, tachycardia, dry mouth, oliguria.
   B. Neurologic: Drowsiness, restlessness, CNS depression, coma, seizures secondary to hyponatremia.

C. Metabolic: Hypokalemia (muscle cramps, weakness, arrhythmias), hyponatremia, hypochloremic metabolic alkalosis, hyperglycemia, hyperuricemia.

D. GI: Pancreatitis, irritation (nausea, vomiting, diarrhea), jaundice, hepatic cirrhosis.

VII. Laboratory findings and evaluation:

A. Electrolytes, BUN, creatinine.

B. Serum glucose (check for hyperglycemia and for hypoglycemia in presence of weakness, drowsiness).

C. Amylase (check for pancreatitis).

D. Liver function studies.

E. Uric acid.

F. Consider serum calcium (see Action).

G. ECG (hypokalemia-induced arrhythmias).

VIII. Treatment:

A. Follow APTLS: see Chapter 8.

B. General management: See Table 85–1.

C. Hypotension:

1. Fluid challenge and replacement (normal saline solution).

2. If arrhythmia induced, suspect hypokalemia and treat as for specific arrhythmia and replete potassium (see below).

D. Hypokalemia:

1. Replace potassium (KCl 10–40 mEq/hr IV slowly) and monitor for dysrhythmias.

2. Repeat serum K^+ often.

3. Careful K^+ replacement in face of renal failure (acute tubular necrosis).

E. Hyponatremia: Replace sodium with sodium chloride. Hypertonic saline solution rarely required.

F. Hypochloremic alkalosis: Saline-sensitive metabolic acidosis; replace volume with normal saline solution.

G. CNS depression: See Chapter 21.

H. Dialysis ineffective for drug clearance.

IX. Prognosis:

A. Expected response to treatment: Good prognosis with appropriate treatment.

B. Expected complications and long-term effects: With severe volume loss, may see acute tubular necrosis if not treated early.

X. Special considerations:

A. Elderly may accidentally overdose.

B. Precipitation or aggravation of diabetes mellitus.

C. Careful K^+ repletion with renal impairment.

XI. Disposition considerations:

A. Admission considerations:

1. See General Admission Considerations (Chapter 18).

2. Dysrhythmias (ICU).

3. Persistent hypotension (ICU).

4. Severe hypokalemia (ICU).

    5. Pancreatitis.

    6. Suicide risk.

  B. Observation period: For milder cases of thiazide poisoning or for initially asymptomatic patients, observation for 6–8 hours may be sufficient to rule out significant toxicity. Chlorthalidone, which has a very long half-life (44 hours) has very low toxicity.

  C. Discharge considerations:

    1. General discharge considerations have been met (see Chapter 18).

    2. No evidence of toxicity after at least 6 hours of observation and treatment.

    3. Repeat serum potassium just prior to discharge to make sure level is within normal range.

    4. Suicide potential and psychiatric status have been appropriately evaluated.

Potassium-Sparing Diuretics

  I. Route of exposure: Oral.

  II. Common generic and trade names:

    Amiloride (Midamor)

    Triamterene (Dyrenium)

    Spironolactone (Aldactone)

  III. Pharmacokinetics:

  A. Peak serum levels:

    1. Spironolactone: 2–4 hours.

    2. Triamterene: 3 hours.

    3. Amiloride: 3–4 hours.

  B. Plasma half-life: Amiloride: 6–9 hours.

  C. Elimination: Amiloride excreted unchanged. Triamterene metabolized to active compounds with some diuretic action; these are excreted in urine.

  D. Active metabolites: Triamterene has metabolite with active pharmacologic properties.

  IV. Action:

  A. Spironolactone is competitive antagonist of aldosterone, resulting in increased sodium and water secretion and potassium retention.

  B. Triamterene inhibits reabsorption of sodium ions in exchange for potassium by direct effects on renal tubule (independent of effects of aldosterone).

  C. Amiloride exerts its natriuretic and potassium-conserving effects independent of aldosterone.

  V. Toxic mechanism: Insufficient data in the literature to accurately characterize a toxic syndrome related to acute ingestion of large amounts of potassium-sparing diuretics.

  VI. Range of toxicity: Fatal and toxic doses not established.

  VII. Clinical features:

  A. Fluid and electrolytes: Hyperkalemia, hyponatremia, hypochloremia.

  B. Cardiovascular: Arrhythmias secondary to hyperkalemia, hypotension.

C. GI: Nausea, vomiting, diarrhea, abdominal cramps.

D. Headache.

VIII. Laboratory findings and evaluation:

    A. Electrolytes: Prolonged diuretic effect (long half-life). Repeat potassium level every 1–2 hours in emergency department to monitor changes (less frequently after peak).

    B. Renal function studies (BUN, creatinine, urinalysis).

    C. ECG.

IX. Treatment:

    A. Follow APTLS: See Chapter 8.

    B. General management: See Table 85–1.

    C. Hyperkalemia:

        1. Consider dialysis.

X. Disposition considerations:

    A. Admission considerations:

        1. See General Admission Considerations (Chapter 18).

        2. Severe hyperkalemia (ICU).

        3. Dysrhythmias (ICU).

        4. Suicide risk.

    B. Observation period: For milder cases of potassium-sparing diuretic poisoning, observation period of 6 hours may be sufficient to rule out significant toxicity.

    C. Discharge considerations: See Thiazide diuretics.

Loop Diuretics

I. Route of exposure: Oral, intravenous.

II. Common generic and trade names:

    Furosemide (Lasix)

    Bumetamide (Bumex)

    Ethacrynic acid (Edecrin)

III. Pharmacokinetics:

    A. Absorption: Oral bioavailability:

        1. Furosemide: 50%–60%

        2. Bumetamide: 20%–40%

    B. Plasma half-life: 1–1.5 hours.

    C. Peak effect: 1–2 hours.

    D. Duration of action: 4–8 hours.

    E. Elimination: Primarily excreted unchanged by kidneys, with smaller portion metabolized in liver.

IV. Action:

    A. Inhibits reabsorption of electrolytes in ascending limb of loop of Henle.

    B. Increases venous capacitance in patients with pulmonary edema, thus decreasing cardiac filling pressure.

V. Uses:

    A. Management of all types of edema including that related to advanced renal failure, ascites related to cirrhosis, congestive heart failure.

    B. Hypercalcemia.

    C. Short-term treatment of hypertension; however, little place in long-term therapy of uncomplicated hypertension because of tendency to cause clinically significant hypokalemia.

  VI. Toxic mechanism: Fluid and electrolyte losses with associated hypokalemia, hypochloremic alkalosis, volume depletion.

  VII. Range of toxicity: No established toxic or fatal doses, because of variable individual response to wide dosage range of loop diuretics.

 VIII. Clinical features:

    A. Acute overdose: Hypotension volume depletion, hypokalemia (with possible secondary arrhythmias, weakness), hypocalcemia, hypomagnesemia, tetany related to electrolyte imbalance.

    B. Adverse (chronic) effects: Weakness, dizziness, confusion, cramps, skin rash, pruritus, paresthesia, deafness, visual blurring, nausea, vomiting, diarrhea, leukopenia, thrombocytopenia, acute pancreatitis, hyperuricemia (with ethacrynic acid).

  IX. Laboratory findings and evaluation:

    A. Electrolytes (electrolyte imbalance).

    B. Calcium, magnesium levels (check for hypocalcemia, hypomagnesemia).

    C. Renal function studies (BUN, creatinine).

    D. Amylase if GI symptoms.

    E. Blood glucose (rule out hypoglycemia in presence of confusion, visual blurring, weakness).

    F. CBC (look for leukopenia, thrombocytopenia if patient on chronic diuretic regimen).

    G. ECG (hypokalemia-induced dysrhythmias).

  X. Treatment:

    A. Follow APTLS (see Chapter 8.)

    B. General management: See Table 85–1.

    C. Hypotension: See Chapter 10 for treatment recommendations.

    D. Hypokalemia: See Thiazide diuretics.

    E. Dialysis not effective for drug treatment.

  XI. Prognosis: Good prognosis with appropriate fluid, electrolyte replacement, supportive care.

  XII. Disposition considerations: See Thiazide diuretics.

Clonidine

  I. Route of exposure: Oral, transdermal.

  II. Common trade name: Catapres.

  III. Pharmacokinetics:

    A. Absorption: Rapidly absorbed with oral bioavailability 65%–95%.

    B. Onset of action: Within 30–60 minutes.

    C. Plasma half-life: 12–16 hours.

    D. Peak effect: 1–3 hours.

    E. Duration of action: Approximately 8 hours.

F. Elimination: 30%–60% excreted by kidneys; remainder metabolized by liver.

IV. Action:

 A. Specific alpha$_2$ agonist, stimulating central adrenergic receptors that inhibit sympathetic outflow.

 B. At high doses clonidine acts as peripheral partial alpha agonist, resulting in increased blood pressure and heart rate.

V. Uses:

 A. Antihypertensive.

 B. Opiate withdrawal symptoms.

VI. Toxic mechanism:

 A. Central adrenergic inhibition results in miosis, sedation, lethargy, coma, bradycardia, hypotension, respiratory depression, apnea, hypothermia.

 B. Stimulation of peripheral alpha receptors may result in hypertension.

VII. Range of toxicity:

 A. Toxic dose:

 1. Symptoms in children have been reported after doses of 0.025–3 mg.

 2. Maximum adult dose documented (with survival) is 16.8 mg.

 B. Fatal dose: No deaths reported.

VIII. Clinical features:

 A. Cardiovascular:

 1. Sinus bradycardia, hypotension, ischemia, congestive heart failure.

 2. Paradoxical hypertension: Very short-lasting and may rapidly progress to severe hypotension.

 B. Neurological: Dizziness, somnolence, hallucinations, nightmares, agitation, seizures.

 C. GI: Nausea, vomiting, diarrhea.

 D. Chronic adverse reactions: Xerostomia, Raynaud's phenomenon, rash.

IX. Laboratory findings and evaluation:

 A. Clonidine serum level: Peak at 1–3 hours.

 B. ECG (AV heart block, Wenkebach period, trigeminy, bradydysrhythmias).

 C. Other laboratory tests:

 1. Arterial blood gases (with pulmonary symptoms).

 2. Electrolytes, BUN, creatinine (if significant vomiting).

 3. Blood glucose (if altered mental status).

 4. Chest radiograph (pulmonary symptoms).

X. Treatment:

 A. Follow APTLS: See Chapter 8.

 B. General management: See Table 85–1.

 C. Cardiovascular:

 1. Sinus bradycardia:

 a. Treatment needed only if symptoms (e.g., chest pain, dyspnea, lightheadedness, hypotension, ventricular ectopy).

 b. Atropine 0.5 mg IV; may repeat 0.5 mg doses up to maximum of 2.0 mg.

 c. Isoproterenol infusion 2–10 µg/min.

 d. Temporary transvenous pacemaker.

    2. Hypotension:
      a. See Chapter 10.
      b. Refractory hypotension:
        (1) Naloxone 0.4–0.8 mg IV (give cautiously to avoid rebound hypertension).
        (2) Tolazoline (Priscoline):
          a Use only in life-threatening situations.
          b Dose: 10 mg IV at 30-minute intervals.
    3. Paradoxical hypertensive phase: If potential for end organ damage, treat with nitroprusside.
  D. Seizures: see Chapter 22 for treatment recommendations.
  E. Dialysis not effective for drug clearance.
XI. Prognosis: Overdose can be life threatening in both adults and children; however, prognosis good with rapid institution of basic overdose management and good supportive care.
XII. Special considerations:
  A. Hypertensive crisis may be precipitated on sudden discontinuance of clonidine in patients receiving maintenance doses.
  B. At high doses clonidine may stimulate peripheral alpha receptors, resulting in severe hypertension.
XIII. Disposition considerations:
  A. Admission considerations: All patients with known or suspected overdose should be admitted.
  B. Observation period: Not appropriate to observe patients in the emergency department, even if asymptomatic.
  C. Discharge considerations: Not appropriate to discharge patients, even if asymptomatic.

Reserpine

  I. Route of exposure: Oral.
 II. Common trade name: Serpasil.
III. Pharmacokinetics:
  A. Absorption: Fair.
  B. Plasma half-life: 33 hours.
  C. Peak effect: 2 hours.
  D. Elimination: Slow, over 4 days; renal 14%, fecal 60%.
 IV. Action: Reduces stores of norepinephrine, dopamine, and serotonin in many tissues including brain (medulla oblongata).
  V. Toxic mechanism: Reduction of neurotransmitter in CNS results in CNS depression, coma, ataxia, tachycardia followed by bradycardia, initial hypertension followed by hypotension.
 VI. Range of toxicity:
  A. Toxic dose: Ingestions of up to 260 mg have been reported with patient survival.

B. Fatal dose: Unknown.

VII. Clinical features:

    A. Signs and symptoms of acute overdose:

       1. Hypotension, hypothermia, CNS depression, GI hemorrhage, bradycardia, abdominal pain, diarrhea, sedation.

       2. See also Toxic mechanism.

    B. Adverse (chronic) effects: Nightmares: may induce depression so severe as to require hospitalization.

VIII. Laboratory findings and evaluation:

       1. ECG (bradycardia, tachycardia).

       2. Electrolytes, glucose.

       3. Spun hematocrit (GI hemorrhage).

IX. Treatment:

    A. Follow APTLS: See Chapter 8.

    B. General management: See Table 85–1.

    C. Hypotension:

       1. See Chapter 10 for treatment recommendations.

       2. Consider blood loss (GI hemorrhage) as potential etiology.

    D. GI hemorrhage:

       1. Monitor intravascular volume, obtain spun hematocrit, order cross-match.

       2. Antacids (aluminum hydroxide) if bleeding mild.

       3. Replace volume (including PRBCs if indicated)

    E. Dialysis ineffective for drug clearance.

X. Prognosis: No known deaths.

XI. Disposition considerations:

    A. Admission considerations: All patients with reserpine overdose should be admitted because of the long half-life of reserpine.

    B. Observation period: Not appropriate to observe patients in the emergency department.

    C. Discharge considerations: Not appropriate to discharge.

Guanethidine

I. Route of exposure: Oral.

II. Common trade name: Ismelin.

III. Pharmacokinetics:

    A. Absorption: 50%–80% absorbed.

    B. Plasma half-life: 5.2 days.

    C. Peak effect: 3 hours.

    D. Elimination: Metabolized in liver to less active compounds, which are excreted by kidneys.

IV. Action: Inhibits response to stimulation of sympathetic nerves by displacing norepinephrine from nerve endings, producing functional denervation of peripheral sympathetic nervous system.

V. Toxic mechanism:
  A. Toxic effects related to sympathetic blockade (dizziness, weakness, syncope).
  B. Toxic effects related to unopposed parasympathetic activity (bradycardia, diarrhea).
  C. Augments sensitivity of postsynaptic receptors to exogenously administered sympathomimetic agents, resulting in hypertension and cardiac arrhythmias.
VI. Range of toxicity:
  A. Toxic dose: No human data available.
  B. Fatal dose: No deaths reported.
VII. Clinical features:
  A. Reactions related to sympathetic blockade.
    1. Dizziness, weakness, lassitude, syncope resulting from either postural or exertional hypotension.
    2. Hypotension may be present for days.
  B. Reactions related to unopposed parasympathetic activity:
    1. Bradycardia, increase in bowel movements, nausea, vomiting, diarrhea.
  C. Adverse (chronic) effects:
    1. Inhibition of ejaculation.
    2. Tendency toward fluid retention and edema, with occasional development of congestive heart failure.
    3. Nasal congestion, blurred vision, tremor.
VIII. Laboratory findings and evaluation:
  A. Electrolytes (imbalance secondary to diarrhea).
  B. Renal function tests (BUN, creatinine); usually transient elevations
  C. ECG (monitor for bradycardia, ischemic changes).
  D. Arterial blood gases, chest radiograph (with pulmonary symptoms or findings; e.g., congestive heart failure).
  E. Blood sugar (rule out hypoglycemia in presence of dizziness, weakness).
IX. Treatment:
  A. Follow APTLS: See Chapter 8.
  B. General management: See Table 85–1.
  C. Hypotension: See Chapter 10 for treatment recommendations.
  D. Bradycardia: See Clonidine.
  E. Dialysis ineffective for drug clearance.
X. Prognosis: No known deaths.
XI. Special considerations:
  A. Drug interactions:
    1. Concurrent use of guanethidine and *Rauwolfia* derivatives (e.g., reserpine) may cause excessive postural hypotension, bradycardia, mental depression.
    2. Tricyclic antidepressants antagonize effects of guanethidine; withdrawal may precipitate profound hypotension.
  B. Guanethidine may sensitize postsynaptic receptors to effects of sympathomimetic agents, which can lead to hypertensive crises when some cold remedies containing direct-acting sympathomimetics are used.

XII. Disposition considerations:
   A. Admission considerations: All patients with guanethidine overdose should be admitted because of long half-life of guanethidine (5.2 days).
   B. Observation period: Not appropriate to observe even asymptomatic patients in emergency department.
   C. Discharge considerations: Not appropriate to discharge.

Hydralazine

   I. Route of exposure: Oral, intravenous.
   II. Common trade name: Apresoline.
   III. Pharmacokinetics:
   A. Absorption: 80% after oral dose.
   B. Plasma half-life: 3–7 hours.
   C. Peak effect: 2–4 hours.
   D. Elimination: Acetylation in liver with excretion in urine.
   IV. Action: Direct arteriolar smooth muscle relaxation.
   V. Uses: In addition to uses in essential hypertension, hydralazine is frequently used in eclampsia and preeclampsia.
   VI. Toxic mechanism:
   A. Severe hypotension secondary to arteriolar vasodilation.
   B. Toxicity greatest in "slow acetylators."
   VII. Range of toxicity:
   A. Toxic dose:
      1. Incidence of serious reactions following prolonged administration is 10%–20%.
      2. Toxic dose not established; severity of intoxication must be determined based on clinical findings.
   B. Fatal dose: No deaths documented related to acute overdose; deaths from chronic poisoning may result from GI bleeding.
   VIII. Clinical features:
   A. Cardiovascular: Hypotension, tachycardia, palpitations, myocardial ischemia (angina, infarction), ventricular arrhythmias, profound shock.
   B. Neurological: Headache.
   C. Chronic adverse reactions: Anxiety, sleep disturbance, nausea, vomiting, weakness, fatigue, postural hypotension, nasal congestion, lupus-like syndrome (myalgia, arthralgia, joint swelling, fever, ANA positive).
   IX. Laboratory findings and evaluation:
   A. ECG (tachydysrhythmias, ischemia, infarction).
   B. Blood glucose (rule out hypoglycemia in presence of headache, dizziness, weakness).
   C. Electrolytes (if significant vomiting).
   D. Urinalysis (protein, red blood cells).
   X. Treatment:
   A. Follow APTLS: See Chapter 8.
   B. General management: See Table 85–1.

C. Hypotension:
   1. See Chapter 10 for treatment recommendations.
   2. Plasma expanders.
   3. If possible, avoid vasopressors because of increased possibility of dysrhythmias.
D. Symptomatic tachycardia:
   1. Consider beta blocker such as propranolol: Dose: 1 mg IV or 10–30 mg PO three or four times per day.
E. Dialysis not effective for drug clearance.
XI. Prognosis: No known deaths from acute overdose directly attributable to hydralazine.
XII. Disposition considerations:
   A. Admission considerations:
      1. See General Admission Considerations (Chapter 18).
      2. Persistent hypotension, tachycardia.
      3. Suicide risk.
   B. Observation period: For milder cases of hydralazine poisoning that resolve with treatment, observation for 4–6 hours may be sufficient to rule out significant toxicity.
   C. Discharge considerations:
      1. General discharge considerations have been met (see Chapter 18).
      2. Asymptomatic without clinical findings after sufficient observation.
      3. If patient is receiving maintenance therapy, dosage has been evaluated and patient counseled.
      4. Suicide potential and psychiatric status have been appropriately evaluated.

Prazosin

I. Route of exposure: Oral.
II. Common trade name: Minipress.
III. Pharmacokinetics:
   A. Absorption: Oral bioavailability 90%.
   B. Onset of action: 30–60 minutes.
   C. Plasma half-life: 2–3 hours.
   D. Peak effect: 1–3 hours
   E. Elimination: Metabolized in liver, excreted in bile.
IV. Action: Direct smooth muscle relaxation by competitive blockade of postsynaptic alpha adrenergic receptors. Results in decreased peripherial vascular resistance.
V. Uses: Hypertension and resistant congestive heart failure.
VI. Toxic mechanism: Severe hypotension from peripheral vasodilation.
VII. Range of toxicity: Fatal and toxic doses not established.
VIII. Clinical features:
   A. First dose phenomenon: 30–60 minutes after first dose patient becomes hypotensive and may have syncopal episode; may be preceded by tachycardia.

    B. Other signs and symptoms of acute overdose: drowsiness, depressed reflexes.

    C. Adverse (chronic) effects: Dizziness, headache, drowsiness, weakness, palpitations, nausea, vomiting, peripheral edema, syncope, rash, nasal congestion.

IX. Laboratory findings and evaluation:

    A. Spun hematocrit (if diagnosis in doubt, rule out bleeding as cause of hypotension).

    B. Serum glucose (hypoglycemia).

    C. Electrolytes and renal function tests (BUN, creatinine, urinalysis).

    D. ECG (tachydysrhythmias, ischemic changes).

    E. Uric acid (hyperuricemia).

X. Treatment:

    A. Follow APTLS: See Chapter 8.

    B. General management: see Table 85–1.

    C. Hypotension: See Chapter 10 for treatment recommendations.

    D. Tachycardia: Usually resolves with supine position and fluids.

    E. Dialysis not effective for drug clearance.

XI. Prognosis: Good with appropriate supportive treatment.

XII. Disposition considerations:

    A. Admission considerations:

        1. See General Admission Considerations (Chapter 10).

        2. Refractory hypotension or tachycardia.

        3. Suicide risk.

    B. Observation period: For asymptomatic patients or milder cases of prazosin poisoning, observation for 4 hours may be sufficient to rule out significant toxicity.

    C. Discharge considerations:

        1. General discharge considerations have been met (see Chapter 18).

        2. Asymptomatic without clinical findings after sufficient observation.

        3. If patient is receiving maintenance therapy, dosage has been evaluated and patient counseled.

        4. Suicide potential and psychiatric status have been appropriately evaluated.

Minoxidil

    I. Route of exposure: Oral, topical.

   II. Common trade name: Loniten.

  III. Pharmacokinetics:

    A. Absorption: Oral absorption complete.

    B. Plasma half-life: 3–4 hours.

    C. Peak effect: 30–60 minutes.

    D. Duration of action: Antihypertensive effect may last 1–3 days because of tissue sequestration.

    E. Elimination: Conjugated in liver, with metabolites excreted by kidneys; 12% excreted unchanged.

    F. Active metabolites: (Exert much less pharmacologic effect than minoxidil itself).

IV. Action: Direct smooth muscle relaxation resulting in arterial vasodilation.

V. Uses: Hypertension, alopecia, male-pattern baldness.

VI. Toxic mechanism: Severe hypotension form direct arteriolar vasodilation.

VII. Range of toxicity: Fatal and toxic doses not established.

VIII. Clinical features:
    A. Cardiovascular: Hypotension, tachycardia.
    B. Adverse (chronic) effects: Sodium and fluid retention, exacerbation of angina, congestive heart failure, pericardial effusion or tamponade, thrombocytopenia, leukopenia, Stevens-Johnson syndrome.

IX. Laboratory findings and evaluation:
    A. ECG (may see tachydysrhythmias, ischemic changes).
    B. Complete blood cell and platelet count (may see hemodilution from fluid retention, leukopenia, thrombocytopenia.
    C. Renal function studies (BUN, creatinine).
    D. Arterial blood gases (if pulmonry symptoms).
    E. Chest radiograph (congestive heart failure).

X. Treatment:
    A. Follow APTLS: See Chapter 8.
    B. General management: See Table 85–1.
    C. Hypotension:
       1. See Chapter 10 for treatment recommendations.
       2. Avoid epinephrine and norepinephrine because of excess cardiac stimulation.
       3. Dopamine may be used if evidence of severe underperfusion.
    D. Angina: Beta blockers may be effective if accompanied by tachydysrhythmia.
    E. Dialysis ineffective for drug clearance.

XI. Prognosis: Good with appropriate supportive care.

XII. Disposition considertions:
    A. Admission considerations: See Prazosin.
    B. Observation period: For milder cases of minoxidil poisoning, observation for 6–8 hours may be sufficient to rule out significant toxicity.
    C. Discharge considerations: See Prazosin.

Sodium Nitroprusside (Nipride)

I. Route of exposure: Intravenous.

II. Common trade name: Nipride.

III. Pharmacokinetics:
    A. Onset of action: Hypotensive effect extremely rapid, within minutes.
    B. Plasma half-life: 2 minutes.
    C. Duration of action: Few minutes.
    D. Elimination: Metabolized by cyanide, which combines with thiosulfate to form thiocyanate, which is excreted by kidneys.
    E. Active metabolites: Thiocyanate, cyanide.

IV. Action: Direct smooth muscle relaxation resulting in both arteriolar and venous vasodilation.

V. Uses:
  A. Emergency treatment of accelerated hypertension.
  B. Cardiogenic shock.
  C. Ergot poisoning.
  D. Dissecting aneurysm (used in combination with propranolol).

VI. Toxic mechanism:
  A. Severe hypotension results from direct peripheral vasodilation.
  B. Nitroprusside reacts with hemoglobin and is then nonenzymatically converted to cyanide and thiocyanate. Cyanide toxicity rare and may be seen in patients with hepatic dysfunction. Thiocyanate toxicity also rare unless large doses (>8 μg/kg/min) of nitroprusside are given, prolonged infusions (more than 2–3 days) are given, or patient has renal failure.

VII. Range of toxicity: Median lethal dose (LD_{50}) approximately 10 mg/kg.

VIII. Clinical features:
  A. Direct toxic effects of nitroprusside
    1. Hypotension.
    2. Substernal chest pain.
    3. Bradycardia, tachycardia.
    4. Muscular twitching.
    5. Increased intracranial pressure.
    6. Methemoglobinemia (see Chapter 102).
  B. Cyanide toxicity:
    1. Coma, barely palpable pulse, absent reflexes, widely dilated pupils, pink color, respiratory arrest.
    2. See Chapter 101.
  C. Thiocyanate toxicity:
    1. Tinnitus, visual blurring, confusion, mental status changes (e.g., psychotic behavior), nausea, abdominal pain, hyperreflexia, seizures.

IX. Laboratory findings and evaluation:
  A. See Chapter 101.
  B. Methemoglobin level (see Chapter 102).
  C. Thiocyanate level: Should not exceed 10 mg/dl.
  D. Arterial blood gases with measured percent oxygen saturation.
  E. Electrolytes (may be imbalance if vomiting severe).
  F. Renal function studies (elimination of thiocyanate primarily by kidneys).
  G. Blood glucose (rule out hypoglycemia in presence of coma, altered mental status).
  H. ECG.
  I. Chest radiograph if respiratory distress.

X. Treatment:
  A. Follow APTLS: See Chapter 8.
  B. General management:
    1. Stop infusion.
    2. Airway management (see Chapter 9).
    3. Administer oxygen, 100% initially.

    C. Cardiovascular support:
      1. Hypotension:
        a. Continuous blood pressure monitoring via arterial catheter; potent dose-related lowering of blood pressure.
        b. See Chapter 10.
      2. Arrhythmias: If required, antiarrhythmic therapy should be specific for arrhythmia present (follow most recent Advanced Cardiac Life Support guidelines from the American Heart Association (*JAMA* 1986; 255:2841–3044).
    D. Cyanide toxicity:
      1. See Chapter 101 for approach to management.
      2. Signs of cyanide toxicity may recur and therapy should be repeated at half-hour intervals.
    E. Methemoglobinemia: See Chapter 102 for approach to management.
    F. Thiocyanate toxicity:
      1. Stop or decrease infusion rate.
      2. Dialysis may be effective in lowering thiocyanate levels, and may be considered for patients with severe symptoms.
  XI. Prognosis:
    A. Good if hypotension is only sign of toxicity. Direct toxic effects of nitroprusside dissipate quickly when infusion stopped.
    B. Presence of toxic effects such as cyanide or thiocyanate toxicity, methemoglobinemia, ischemic cardiac changes worsen prognosis considerably.
  XII. Disposition: Patients who become toxic from nitroprusside are usually already in an ICU, monitored setting.

86

β-*Blockers*

Samuel S. Spicer, M.D., F.A.C.E.P.

I. Route of exposure: Oral, ophthalmic, parenteral.
II. Common generic and trade names: See Table 86–1.
III. Pharmacokinetics: See Tables 86–2 and 86–3.
   A. Absorption: In general, rapid but incomplete (see Table 86–2). Onset of severe toxic symptoms may occur within 2 hours of ingestion.
   B. Duration of action:
      1. Drugs with short half-lives, such as propranolol (see Table 86–2), should be eliminated entirely within 24–48 hours.
      2. Drugs with long half-lives, such as nadolol, may take several days for complete elimination.
   C. Elimination:
      1. Propranolol and metoprolol eliminated entirely by liver metabolism.
      2. Nadolol and atenolol eliminated by kidney.
   D. Active metabolites:
      1. 4-OH-propranolol, 4-OH-pindolol, 4-OH-alprenolol, and one metabolite of acebutolol.
IV. Action: β-Blockers compete with catecholamines for receptor sites, blocking receptor action (Table 86–4).
V. Uses: Approved clinical indications: Angina pectoris, hypertension, arrhythmias, open-angle glaucoma, idiopathic hypertrophic subaortic stenosis, pheochromocytoma, prophylaxis for sudden death and migraine headache.
VI. Toxic mechanism:
   A. Toxicity is often a combination of underlying medical illness and excessive β-blockade (e.g., bronchospasm in asthmatics or complete heart block in patients with conduction system disease).

TABLE 86–1.

Common β-Blocker Preparations

Generic Name*	Trade Name	Tablets (mg)	Ophthalmic Solution (%)	Injection (mg/ml)
Acebutolol	Sectral	200, 400	—	—
Atenolol	Tenormin	50, 100	—	—
Betaxolol	Betoptic	—	0.5	—
Esmolol	Brevibloc	—	—	250
Labetalol	Normodyne	100, 200, 300	—	5.0
	Trandate	100, 200, 300	—	5.0
Levobunolol	Betagan	—	0.5	—
Metoprolol	Lopressor	50, 100	—	1.0
Nadolol	Corgard	40, 80, 120, 160	—	—
Pindolol	Visken	5, 10	—	—
Propranolol†	Inderal‡ (sustained release)	10, 20, 40, 80, 120, 160‡	—	1.0
	Ipran	10, 20, 40, 60, 80, 90	—	—
Timolol	Blocadren	5, 10, 20	—	—
	Timoptic	—	0.25 0.50	—

*Alprenolol, Pratolol, Sotalol, Oxprenolol not available in United States.
†Generic available.
‡Oral solution available (10 mg/ml).

B. Cardioselective agents in therapeutic doses predominantly block β_1 and not β_2 receptors (Table 86–5). At toxic levels both receptors are affected and cardioselectivity is lost.

VII. Range of toxicity:
  A. Toxic dose:
    1. Because of variable sensitivity and role of underlying disease, degree of β-blockade cannot be estimated from amount of ingested drug.
    2. Minimum toxic dose not established; however, serious symptoms can occur after oral administration of 1 gm propranolol in adults or 10 mg/kg in children.
  B. Fatal dose: Several deaths have been reported in the literature:
    1. Propranolol: Patients have died with doses as little as 1 mg IV; others have survived 2 gm oral ingestion.
    2. Metoprolol: Death has been reported with 7.5 gm; however survival has been documented with 10.0 gm.
    3. Atenolol: Deaths have been reported from 12.8 gm.

VIII. Clinical features:
  A. Most life-threatening toxic findings relate to β_1 blockade (Table 86–4): **bradycardia, hypotension, cardiogenic shock, intraventricular conduction delay, AV block, asystole.**

TABLE 86–2.

Properties of β-Blockers

Drug	Absorption, Bioavailability (%)	Half-Life (hr)	Protein Binding (%)	Renal Excretion (%)	Lipid Solubility*
Acebutolol	50	3–4†	26	30–40	Low
Atenolol	55	6–9‡	3	85–95	Low (0.2)
Betaxolol	70–90	12–22	50–60	3–12	—
Labetolol	50	3–8	50	55–60	Low
Levobunolol	—	6	—	15	—
Metoprolol	50	3–7§	12	3–10	Moderate (2.1)
Nadolol	30	14–24	20–30	70	Low (0.7)
Propranolol	30	3.5–6§	93	0.5	High (3.6)
Timolol	75	3–5	10	20	Moderate (2.1)

*As expressed by log portion coefficient in octanol and water.
†Major metabolite (diacetolol) is active and cardioselective; half-life 8–15 hours.
‡With renal insufficiency, 16 hours or longer.
§With hepatic insufficiency, 30 hours or longer.

B. Propranolol, which possesses moderate solubility (Table 86–2) is more likely to cross the blood-brain barrier and cause **coma, convulsions, respiratory depression.**

C. Beta blockers with intrinsic sympathomimetic activity (Table 86–5) may exhibit non-life-threatening **hypertension** or **tachycardia.** They are also less likely to depress cardiac function.

TABLE 86–3.

Peak Effect Time of Common β-Blockers

Generic Drug	Peak Effect
Acebutol	2.5–3.5 hr
Atenolol	2–4 hr
Betaxolol	—
Esmolol (IV)	<5 min
Labetolol (IV)	5 min
Levobunolol	—
Metoprolol	1–2 min
Nadolol	3–4 min
Pindolol	1.25 hr
Propranolol	1.5 hr
Timolol	1–2 hr

TABLE 86–4.

Physiologic Action of β-Blockers

Beta Receptor	Site	Receptor Action	Toxic Effect
β_1	Heart	SA, AV conduction Contractility	Heart block Asystole Congestive heart failure
β_1	Kidney	Renin	
β_2	Arterioles	Relaxation	
β_2	Bronchus	Smooth muscle relaxation	Bronchospasm
β_2	Pancreas	Insulin	Hypoglycemia

  D. β-Blockers with significant membrane depressant effects (quinidine-like
     effect) depress contractility and intraventricular conduction (see Table
     86–5).
  E. Pulmonary edema and bronchospasm in patients with history of conges-
     tive heart failure or chronic obstructive pulmonary disease.
  F. Hypoglycemia (also reports of hyperglycemia).
IX. Laboratory findings and evaluation:
  A. Use of serum β-blocker levels to predict outcome or guide therapy have
     not been established.
  B. Electrolytes (potential differential cause of arrhythmias or symptoms).
  C. Blood glucose.
  D. ECG, cardiac monitor.
  E. Consider arterial blood gases and chest radiograph (with pulmonary com-
     plications).

TABLE 86–5.

Pharmacologic Properties of Common β-Blockers

Drug	Cardioselectivity*	Membrane Depression†	Partial Agonist Activity‡
Acebutolol	+	+	+
Atenolol	+	0	0
Betaxolol	+	0	0
Labetolol§	0	0	0
Levobunolol	0	0	0
Metoprolol	+	±	0
Nadolol	0	0	0
Pindolol	0	+	+ + +
Propranolol	0	+ +	0
Timolol	0	0	+

*Diminishes with increased dosage.
†Quinidine-like effect.
‡Intrinsic sympathomimetic activity.
§Also has α-adrenergic blocking effect.

TABLE 86–6.

General Treatment

Treatment	Indicated	Of No Value	Contraindicated
O$_2$	+		
IV*	+		
ECG monitor	+		
Forced diuresis†			X
Acidification			X
Alkalinization		X	
Emesis‡			X
Lavage	+		
Charcoal	+		
Cathartic	+		
Dialysis§	±		

*IV D$_5$W, keep vein open.
†Potential for congestive heart failure.
‡Potential for rapid onset of cardiovascular complications.
§See text.

X. General treatment:
   A. Follow APTLS: See Chapter 8.
   B. General management: Table 86–6.
XI. Specific management:
   A. Hypotension with or without severe bradycardia and conduction defects:
     1. Glucagon:
       a. 0.05 mg/kg IV bolus.
       b. Follow with 2–5 mg/hr continuous infusion.
       c. Use D$_5$W, not provided phenol diluent. Also avoid solutions with sodium chloride, potassium chloride, or calcium chloride.
     2. Atropine:
       a. Adult: 0.5 mg IV; may repeat dose up to maximum of 2.0 mg.
       b. Child: 0.01–0.03 mg/kg IV; may repeat dose up to maximum of 0.5 mg.
     3. Isoproterenol:
       a. Adult: 2–10 μg/kg/min.
       b. Child: 1.5 μg/kg/min.
       c. Isoproterenol without dopamine may make some patients more hypotensive; use with caution.
     4. Transvenous pacemaker if heart block or hemodynamically significant bradycardia refractory to drug treatment.
     5. One case report of successful use of intraaortic balloon pump to support a patient in cardiogenic shock from massive propranolol overdose unresponsive to glucagon or high doses of β- and α-agonists.
   B. Hypoglycemia: Treated with administration of 50% glucose solution or glucagon.
   C. Bronchospasm: Treated with adrenergic agents such as metaproterenol, isoetharine, intravenous aminophylline.

D. Seizures: See Chapter 22 for treatment recommendations.

E. **Hemodialysis:** May be of value in drugs with low protein binding and high renal clearance (Table 86–2), such as acebutolol, atenolol, nadolol. **Charcoal hemoperfusion** has been used with clinical improvement in a mixed overdose (verapamil and metoprolol).

XII. Prognosis:

A. Expected response to treatment:

1. Most patients eliminate the drug within 48 hours and recover within 2–3 days when drugs with short half-lives such as propranolol (3.6–6 hours) are ingested. Hypotension, hepatic insufficiency, renal failure will prolong the clinical course.

2. If hypotension in particular can be avoided or controlled, prognosis excellent.

B. Expected complications and long-term effects:

1. Pulmonary edema from excessive fluid resuscitation or ventricular arrhythmias from excessive vasopressors.

2. Refractory hypotension.

XIII. Special considerations: Several reports link rapid withdrawal of propranolol in patients receiving prolonged maintenance regimens with induction of myocardial infarction.

XIV. Controversies: All treatment protocols described are not based on clinical trials. Role of dobutamine, charcoal hemoperfusion, and external pacing not clearly defined.

XV. Disposition considerations:

A. Admission considerations:

1. General admission considerations have been met (see Chapter 18).

2. Minimum toxic dose has not been established. Because of the role of underlying disease, each patient requires individual evaluation for toxic manifestations. If doubt exists as to outcome or development of symptoms, admit.

3. ICU: All patients with significant symptoms (hypotension, congestive heart failure, seizures, bradycardia).

4. Suicide risk.

B. Consultation considerations: Nephrologist in severe overdoses with atenolol, nadolol, or acebutolol; patients may benefit from hemodialysis.

C. Observation period: Difficult to make recommendation because of variable individual sensitivity to β-blockers, role of underlying diseases, and because degree of β-blockade cannot be estimated from amount of ingested drug.

D. Discharge considerations:

1. General discharge considerations have been met (see Chapter 18).

2. See Special Considerations, above.

3. Suicide potential and psychiatric status have been appropriately evaluated.

BIBLIOGRAPHY

Frishman W, Jacob H, Eisenberg E, et al: Clinical pharmacology of the new beta adrenergic blocking drugs. VIII: Self-poisoning with beta adrenoreceptor blocking agents: Recognition and management. *Am Heart J* 1979; 98:798.

Gwinup GR: Propranolol toxicity presenting with early repolarization, ST segment elevation, and peaked T waves on ECG. *Ann Emerg Med* 1988; 17:171–174.

Lane AS, Woodward AC, Goldman MR: Massive propranolol overdose poorly responsive to pharmacologic therapy: Use of the intra-aortic balloon pump. *Ann Emerg Med* 1987; 16:1381–1383.

Peterson CD, et al: Glucagon therapy for β-blocker overdose. *Drug Intell Clin Pharm* 1984; 18:394.

Weinstein RS: Recognition and management of poisoning with beta-adrenergic blocking agents. *Ann Emerg Med* 1984; 13:1123–1131.

87

Vitamins

Richard A. Christoph, M.D., F.A.C.E.P.

Vitamin A

  I. Route of exposure: Oral, parenteral, topical.
 II. Common preparations: See Table 87–1.
    A. Topical agents for acne, such as retinoic acid (Tretinoin).
    B. Other sources of Vitamin A: Liver (polar bear, seal, shark, beef, chicken).
III. Pharmacokinetics:
    A. Absorption: Completely absorbed except in liver failure or extremely high oral doses.
    B. Plasma half-life: 9 hours.
    C. Elimination: Metabolized in liver and excreted in feces and urine.
 IV. Action:
    A. Vitamin A aldehyde or retinol is a constituent of visual pigment in retina.
    B. Maintenance of normal membrane structure and function.
    C. May be necessary for glycoprotein synthesis by mucus-secreting cells.
  V. Uses:
    A. Vitamin therapy; food fads; empirical treatment of learning disorders, cancer, psychiatric illness.
    B. High doses of oral retinoids (e.g., 13-*cis*-retinoic acid [Accutane] and etretinate [Tigason]) for treatment of acne or psoriasis.
 VI. Toxic mechanism:
    A. Signs and symptoms of chronic hypervitaminosis A are usually the result of overzealous vitamin therapy, food fads, or use of high doses of oral retinoids for treatment of acne or psoriasis.
    B. Precise mechanism unknown.

TABLE 87–1.

Products Containing Vitamin A

Trade Name	Product	Vitamin A per Dosage Unit
ACE Tablets	Legree	
Aquasol A	Armour	
Beta Carotene Capsules	Nature's Bounty	5,000 IU/tablet
Bio-AE-Mulsion	Biotics Research	50,000 IU/capsule
Bio-AE-Mulsion Forte	Biotics Research	25,000 IU/capsule
Bugs Bunny Multivitamin Supplement	Miles	2,000 IU/drop
Eldercaps	Mayrand	12,500 IU/drop
Flintstones Multivitamin Supplement	Miles	2,500 IU/tablet
Halibut Liver Oil Capsules	Nature's Bounty	4,000 IU/capsule
Iromin-G	Mission	2,500 IU/tablet
Lobana Derm-Aide Cream	Ulmer	5,000 IU/tablet
Megadose	Arco	4,000 IU/capsule
Natalins	Mead-Johnson	?
One-A-Day Essential Vit	Miles	25,000 IU/capsule
One-A-Day Maximum Formula	Miles	8,000 IU/capsule
Oyster Calcium Tablets	Nature's Bounty	5,000 IU/capsule
Pedivit Cream	Pedinol	5,000 IU/capsule
Prenate	Bock	800 IU/capsule
Slim Plan Meal Replacement	Shaklee	?
Stressgard Stress Formula	Miles	8,000 IU/capsule
Therabid	Mission	1,750 IU/2 oz
Tri-Vi-Sol, Poly-Vi-Sol	Mead-Johnson	5,000 IU/capsule
Ultra "A" Caps	Nature's Bounty	8,000 IU/capsule
Vicon Forte	Glaxo	1,500 IU/1 ml
Vidaylin	Ross	5,000 IU/0.6 ml
Vi-Penta Multivitamin drops	Roche	5,000 IU/4 tablets
Vita-Lea Multivitamins	Shaklee	2,000 IU/2 tablets
Vita-Lea Multivitamins for Children	Miles	25,000 IU/capsule
Vitamin A Capsules, Natural	Mission	5,000 IU/tablet
Vizac	Mead-Johnson	500 IU/tablet

    C. May adversely affect membranes, leading to damaged intracellular organelles and release of proteolytic enzymes. Proteolytic enzymes may be direct agent of tissue toxicity.

VII. Range of toxicity:

    A. Therapeutic dose: Recommended daily allowance 5,000 IU (1.5 mg) for males and 4,000 IU (1.2 mg) for females.

    B. Toxic dose:

        1. Acute intoxication from commercial vitamin A preparations:

            a. Adults: 2 million IU.

            b. Infants: 75,000 IU.

        2. Acute toxicity syndrome from retinol:

            a. Adult: 500 mg

       b. Child: 100 mg.

       c. Infant: 30 mg.

    3. Chronic intoxication from vitamin A (after daily intake of those doses for several months):

       a. Adult: 100,000 IU.

       b. Child: 80,000 IU.

       c. Infant: 18,000 IU.

    4. Acute hypervitaminosis A has been reported following ingestion of polar bear liver.

VIII. Clinical features:

  A. Acute hypervitaminosis A:

    1. Neurological: Irritability or drowsiness, severe headache and papilledema related to increased intracranial pressure, dizziness.

    2. GI: Hepatomegaly, vomiting.

    3. Skin: Generalized peeling after 24 hours.

  B. Chronic hypervitaminosis A:

    1. General: Fatigue, malaise, abdominal pain, nausea, vomiting, hypomenorrhea, leukopenia.

    2. Skin: Dryness, pruritus, desquamation, hair growth disturbance, erythematous dermatitis, lip fissures.

    3. Skeletal: Hyperostosis, increased osteoblastic activity with resultant hypercalcemia, bone tenderness, migratory arthralgias, premature epiphyseal closure with resultant growth retardation.

    4. CNS: Irritability, headache, increased intracranial pressure resulting in papilledema or bulging fontanelles in infants.

    5. GI: Hepatosplenomegaly, jaundice, hepatic fat storage increase, hepatic fibrosis and cirrhosis resulting in portal hypertension and ascites.

IX. Laboratory findings and evaluation:

  A. Serum vitamin A levels:

    1. Normal total vitamin A concentration: 20–60 μg/dl.

    2. Toxic total vitamin A concentrations: >100 μg/dl.

    3. Toxic levels in patients with cirrhosis or low retinol-binding protein: 60 μg/dl.

  B. Other laboratory tests:

    1. Complete blood cell count (rule out leukopenia, evaluation of hepatosplenomegaly).

    2. Blood glucose (rule out hypoglycemia in presence of fatigue, malaise, altered mental status).

    3. Liver function tests, amylase, urinalysis (evaluation of abdominal pain, jaundice).

    4. Electrolytes (assess fluid, electrolyte status in severe vomiting).

    5. Consider skeletal series (for chronic toxicity, calcifications).

    6. Arterial blood gases (to help guide therapy in increased intracranial pressure).

X. General treatment:

  A. Follow APTLS: See Chapter 8.

  B. General management: See Table 87–2 (see Chapters 12 and 13 for details).

TABLE 87–2.

General Treatment

Treatment	Indicated	Of No Value	Contraindicated
O$_2$	±		
IV	+		
ECG monitor	±		
Forced diuresis		X	
Acidification		X	
Alkalinization		X	
Emesis/lavage	+/+		
Charcoal	+		
Cathartic	+		

XI. Specific treatment:
   A. Acute toxicity:
      1. Increased intracranial pressure:
         a. Usually gradually improves over course of several weeks after cessation of vitamin A.
         b. Rarely, severe cases that do not resolve may require daily lumbar punctures, diuretics, steroids, acetazolamide, mannitol.
      2. Other signs and symptoms of acute toxicity resolve after cessation of vitamin A and appropriate supportive care.
   B. Chronic toxicity:
      1. No therapy usually required other than stopping vitamin A.
      2. Hypercalcemia may need to be treated.
XII. Prognosis:
   A. Expected response to treatment: Prospects for full recovery from both acute and chronic hypervitaminosis A excellent, with most signs and symptoms of toxicity resolving within a week.
   B. Expected complications and long-term effects: Rarely, chronic liver disease, skeletal deformities, optic atrophy, and blindness.
XIII. Disposition considerations:
   A. Admission considerations:
      1. See General Admission Considerations (Chapters 17 and 18).
      2. Neurologic symptoms.
      3. Intractable vomiting.
      4. Suicide risk.
   B. Consultation considerations:
      1. Immediate neurosurgical consult if evidence of increased intracranial pressure. Not unreasonable to consult for any patient with neurological finding, including altered mental status.
      2. Dermatology for serious skin reaction.
   C. Observation period: Not enough information in literature to make recommendations; use half-life information as guideline.

D. Discharge considerations:
1. General discharge considerations have been met (see Chapters 17 and 18).
2. No neurological symptoms.
3. Easy access to high level medical care should untoward developments occur.
4. Patients taking vitamin therapy prescribed either by self or physician have been counseled regarding cessation or correct dose.
5. Suicide potential and psychiatric status have been appropriately evaluated.

Hypervitaminosis D

I. Wide variation in amount of vitamin D that results in toxicity. However, in a person with normal parathyroid function and normal responsiveness to vitamin D, doses of >50,000 IU/day may cause poisoning.
II. Signs and symptoms related chiefly to effects of hypercalcemia and hypercalciuria.
III. In children, severe hypercalcemia may arrest bone growth for 6–8 months, and ultimate growth potential may be irreversibly affected. In all age groups, peripheral tissues affected by metastatic calcifications can become so severely damaged as to result in end-organ failure and death.
IV. Treatment:
A. Stop vitamin D.
B. Low calcium diet and possibly calcium disodium edetate orally to increase fecal excretion of calcium.
C. Serious hypercalcemia will require hydration, steroids, calcitonin, mithramycin. Peritoneal or hemodialysis may be required if unable to give large amounts of fluid.

Vitamin C (Ascorbic Acid)

I. Megadoses of ascorbic acid have been controversially proposed for treatment of viral respiratory illnesses and terminal cancer, among many other conditions. Studies attempting to confirm these hypotheses have yielded negative or inconsistent findings.
II. Risks associated with megadoses of ascorbic acid:
A. Nephrolithiasis.
B. Rebound scurvy on sudden cessation of large amounts of vitamin C.
C. Interference with concurrent anticoagulation therapy, enhanced absorption of iron.
D. Calcium oxalate nephrolithiasis associated with ingestions >2 gm/day. Diarrhea may result when >10 gm ascorbic acid are ingested daily.

BIBLIOGRAPHY

Favus MJ: Vitamin D physiology: Some clinical aspects of the vitamin D endocrine system. *Med Clin North Am* 1978; 63:1291.

Haussler MR, McCain TA: Basic and clinical concepts related to vitamin D metabolism and action. *N Engl J Med* 1979; 297:974.

Herbert V: The vitamin craze. *Arch Intern Med* 1980; 140:173–176.

Hodges RE: Megavitamin therapy. *Primary Care* 1982; 9:605–619.

Lawton JM, Conway LT, Crossan JT, et al: Acute oxalate nephropathy after massive ascorbic acid administration. *Arch Intern Med* 1985; 145:950.

Muenter M, Perry H, Ludwig J: Chronic vitamin A intoxication in adults. *Am J Med* 1971; 50:129–136.

Podell RN: Vitamin A overdose. *Postgrad Med* 1983; 74:297.

Smith RF, Goodman DS: Vitamin A transport in human vitamin A toxicity. *N Engl J Med* 1976; 294:805.

88

Iron

M. Douglas Baker, M.D.

I. Route of exposure: Oral.
II. Common Generic and Trade Names:
  A. Variety of different iron salts manufactured, each containing different amounts of elemental iron (see Table 88–1). Because of variability by brand and often deficient labeling practices, consultation with local poison control centers to verify amount of elemental iron ingested is recommended early in management of these cases.
  B. Over 120 iron-containing preparations are listed in the current *Physician's Desk Reference,* many available over-the-counter (Table 88–2).
III. Pharmacokinetics:
  A. Absorption:
    1. Bioavailability poor, approximately 10%, increasing to about 20% in iron deficiency.
    2. Primarily absorbed in duodenum.
    3. Absorption affected by a number of factors:
      a. Fasting state (increased).
      b. Ascorbic acid (increased).
      c. Enteric coatings (decreased).
      d. Antacids (decreased).
    4. Ferric salts much less well absorbed than ferrous salts.
  B. Onset of toxic effect: Vomiting and diarrhea, often bloody, may occur 30 minutes–2 hours after ingestion.
  C. Peak effect: Peak serum iron levels usually occur 3–5 hours after ingestion.
  D. Metabolism: After absorption into duodenal cell, ferrous salt is oxidized to ferric form, which then binds to storage proteins (ferritin). Ferric form

TABLE 88–1.

Elemental Iron Equivalents of Common Iron Preparations

Iron Salt	% Elemental Iron*
Ferrous sulfate (most common)	20
Ferrous gluconate	12
Ferrous fumarate (Flintstones Plus Iron Multivitamin Supplement)	33
*May vary by brand.	

may then be released from ferritin into plasma, where it binds to transport globulins (transferrin) for distribution and utilization.

    E. Elimination: In contrast to absorption, no specific mechanism for excretion of iron exists. Normal daily losses from intestine, skin, and urinary tract total approximately 1 mg.

IV. Action: Essential to the body as part of hemoglobin and several enzymes.

V. Uses:

    A. Iron therapy indicated in treatment of iron-deficiency anemias resulting from poor nutrition, increased demands, or blood loss.

    B. Present in many multivitamins including prenatal and postnatal supplements.

    C. Acute iron poisoning is one of the most common intoxications reported, particularly in the pediatric population.

VI. Toxic mechanism:

    A. During overdose, binding capacity of transferrin is exceeded. A small amount of excess binds to albumin; the remainder circulates in free unbound form, which becomes deposited in various tissues, such as liver, kidney, heart, and lungs, where it functions as a potent mitochondrial poison.

    B. Locally corrosive agent with potential for significant gastrointestinal mucosal damage.

    C. Because of its hepatotoxic effects, iron salts can effect subsequent ferritin release from periportal cells, which results in vasodepressor effect.

    D. Iron salts can cause coagulation defects.

VII. Range of toxicity:

    A. Toxic dose: >30 mg/kg (elemental iron).

    B. Fatal dose:

        1. >250–300 mg/kg.

        2. Doses as low as 60 mg/kg have caused death.

VIII. Clinical features: Four clinical stages of acute iron poisoning have been described (Table 88–3).

    A. Patients have primarily GI symptoms, such as abdominal pain, vomiting, diarrhea (stage 1), which may progress to shock, coma, and seizures in massive ingestions.

TABLE 88–2.

Products Containing Iron*

Name of Product	Iron Component per Dosage Unit (mg)	Total Elemental Iron per Dosage Unit (mg)
Adabee with Minerals Tablets	50	15
A/G-Pro	—	10/6 tablets
Aldol with Minerals		15
Arne Timesules	150	50
A.V.P. Natal	200	60
B-Nutron		6
Calcicaps with Iron	—	8
Cebetinic Tablets	324	37.5
Cefera-Plus Tablets	194	60
Cefera Tablets	200	60
Chel Iron Liquid	417/5 ml	50/5 ml
Chel Iron Pediatric Drops	208/5 ml	25/5 ml
Chel Iron Tablets	330	40
Chenatal	—	20/3 tablets
Chocks Bugs Bunny Plus Iron	55	18
Chocks plus Iron	55	18
Chromagen	200	66
C-Ron	200	66
C-Ron Forte	200	66
C-Ron FA	200	66
C-Ron Freckles	100	33
Dayalets plus Iron Filmtab	90	18
DEQUASine	—	5
Dical-D with Iron Capsules	87	10
Engran	—	9
Fenemaid	—	10
Feminins Tablets	—	18
Feosol Elixir	220/5 ml	44/5 ml
Feosol Plus Capsules	200	65
Feosol Spansule Capsules	167	50
Feosol Tablets	200	65
Ferancee Chewable Tablets	3.1 grains	67
Ferancee-HP	330	110
Fergon Capsules	435	50
Fergon Elixir 6%	300	34
Fergon Tablets	320	36
Fergon with C	450	50
Fer-In-Sol Capsules	190	60
Fer-In-Sol Drops	75/0.6 ml	15/0.6 ml
Fer-In-Sol Syrup	90/5 ml	18/5 ml
Fermalox Tablets	200	40.17
Fero-Folic-500	525	105
Ferro-Grad-500 Tablets	525	105
Fero-Fradument Filmtab	525	105

(Continued.)

Fe-Plus		50
Ferralet	320	37
Ferralet Plus	400	46.33
Ferritrinsic Tablets	187.7	60
Ferrolip Plus	200	24
Ferrolip Syrup	417/5 ml	50/5 ml
Ferrolip Tablets	333	40
Ferro-Mandets	60	20
Ferronord	240	40
Ferro-Sequels	150	50
Ferrous-G	5 grains/5 ml	37.36/5 ml
Ferrous Sulfate Tablets	325	65
Ferrous Sulfate Tablets USP	325	
Filibon Capsules	90	30
Filibon OT Tablets	90	30
Flintstones Plus Iron Multivitamin Supplement	55	18
Folvron	182	57
Fosfree	125	14.5
Gerilets Filmtab	135	27
Geriplex Kapseals	30	6
Geriplex FS Kapseals	30	6
Geriplex FS Liquid		15/30 ml
Geritinic Tablets	195	63
Geritonic Liquid	200/5 ml	35/5 ml
Gerix Elixir	87.60	15
Gerizyme	43.17	5
Gevrabon Liquid	174	20
Gevral T Capsules	45	15
Gevrite	30	10
Glytinic	—	25
Golden Bounty Multivitamin Supplement with Iron	—	18
Hemocyte Plus Tablets	324	106
Hepp-Iron Drops	120/ml	20/ml
Heptuna Plus Capsules	340	100
Hytinic Capsules	—	150
Hytinic Elixir	—	100/5 ml
Iberet Filmtab	525	105
Iberet-500 Filmtab	525	105
Iberet-Folic-500	525	105
Iberet-Liquid	131.25/5 ml	26.25/5 ml
Iberet 500 Liquid	131.25/5 ml	26.25/5 ml
Iberol Filmtab	525	105
Iberol-F Filmtab	525	105
I.L.X.B$_{12}$ Elixir	3 grains/5 ml	36/5 ml
I.L.X.B$_{12}$ Tablets	5 grains	37.56
Imferon	—	50/ml
Incremin with Iron Syrup	250	30
Ironized Yeast	5.25 grains	100

(Continued.)

TABLE 88–2 (cont.).

Name of Product	Iron Component per Dosage Unit (mg)	Total Elemental Iron per Dosage Unit (mg)
Iromin-G	333.3	38.6
Iron with Vitamin C	—	50
Laud-Iron Folic Tablets	320	105
Laud-Iron Forte Tablets	300	100
Laud-Iron Plus Chewing Tablets	100	33
Laud-Iron Tablets	324	108
Laud-Iron Suspension	100/5 ml	33/5 ml
L-Glutavite Capsules	5.3	1.7
Livitamin Capsules	100	33
Livitamin Chewable Tablets	50	16.4
Livitamin Liquid	420/oz	70/oz
Livitamin Prenatal Tablets	152	50
Livitamin Capsules with Intrinsic Factor	100	33
Lofenalac	—	12/150 gm
Lysmins		10
Mevanin-C Capsules	65	14
Mol-Iron Capsules	399	78
Mol-Iron Liquid	195/4 ml	39/4 ml
Mol-Iron Tablets	195	39
Mol-Iron with Vitamin C	195	39
Mol-Iron with Vitamin C Chronosule Capsules	390	78
Mol-Iron Panhemic Chronosule Capsules	390	100
Mission Prenatal	333.3	38.6
Mission Prenatal F.A.	333.3	38.6
Mission Prenatal H.P.	333.3	38.6
Myadec Capsules	—	20
Myadec Tablets	—	20
Natabec Kapseals	150	30
Natabec-FA Kapseals	150	30
Natalins Rx Tablets	—	60
Natalins Tablets	—	45
Niferex Elixir	—	100/5 ml
Niferex Capsules	—	150
Niferex Tablets	—	50
Niferex with Vitamin C Tablets	—	50
Niferex-PN	—	60
Nuclomin	—	10/2 tablets
Nu-Iron 150 Caps	—	150
Nu-Iron Elixir	—	100/5 ml
Nu-Iron-V Tablets	—	60
Norlac	180	60
Norlac RX	180	60

(Continued.)

Oblate-Plus Tablets	90	30
One-A-Day Vitamins Plus Iron	55	18
One-A-Day Vitamins Plus Minerals	55	18
Optilets-M-500	100	20
Ostrex Tonic Tablets	38.33	14.12
Paladac with Minerals	—	5
Perihemin Capsules	168	55
Peritinic Tablets	300	100
Poly-Vi-Flor Vitamin Tablets with Iron	40	12
Poly-Vi-Flor Vitamin Drops with Iron	—	10/ml
Poly-Vi-Sol Vitamin Tablets with Iron	40	12
Poly-Vi-Sol Vitamin Drops with Iron	—	10/ml
Progiatric Tablets	—	10
Pronemia Capsules	350	115
Ragus	—	20/3 tablets
Recoup Hematinic Tablets	150	50
Sclerex	—	110/3 tablets
Simron Capsules	—	10
Simron Plus Capsules	—	10
S.S.S. Tonic	—	220/100 ml
Stuart Formula (tablets)	54	18
Stuart Formula (liquid)	25/5 ml	5/5 ml
Stuart Hematinic Tablets	66	22
Stuart Hematinic Liquid	200/5 ml	22/5 ml
Stuartinic Tablets	330	100
Stuart Prenatal Tablets	182	60
Stuart Prenatal with Folic Acid Tablets	197	65
Stuartnatal 1 + 1 Tablets	182	65
Tabron Filmseal	304.2	100
Theragran-M Tablets	—	12
Therapeutic Vitamins and Minerals	—	12
Theron Tablets	45	15
Toleron Suspension	100/5 ml	33/5 ml
Toleron Tablets	200	66
TriHemic 600 Tablets	350	115
Tri-Vi-Sol Vitamin Drops with Iron	50/ml	10/ml
Troph-Iron Tablets	250	30
Troph-Iron Liquid	250/5 ml	30/5 ml
Unicap M Plus Iron	50	10
Unicap Plus Iron	18	
Unicap Senior Tablets	50	10
Unicap Therapeutic	50	10

(Continued.)

TABLE 88–2 (cont.).

Name of Product	Iron Component per Dosage Unit (mg)	Total Elemental Iron per Dosage Unit (mg)
Vi Aquamin Capsules	100	30
Vi Aquamin Therapeutic Capsules	102	30
Vio-Geric	55	18
Vi-Syneral One Caps	—	18
Vitacrest Capsules	—	10
Vitron-C	200	66
Vitron-C-Plus	400	132
Zymasyrup	130/5 ml	15/5 ml
Zymalixir Drops	65/ml	7.5/ml

*From Krenzelok EP, Hoff JV: Accidental childhood iron poisoning: A problem of marketing and labeling. *Pediatrics* 1979; 63:591–596. Used with permission.

B. Following initial (stage 1) symptoms is a deceptive "latent" phase of clinical improvement (stage 2) from 6–24 hours after ingestion, during which time the patient may be relatively asymptomatic.

C. With large ingestions, symptoms progress to hepatic and renal shutdown, with cardiovascular collapse (stage 3).

D. Patients who survive these events and some who never develop systemic symptoms are at risk for later development of gastrointestinal strictures and obstruction (stage 4).

TABLE 88–3.

Acute Iron Poisoning: Clinical Symptoms

Time Since Ingestion	Mechanism of Toxicity	Symptoms and Toxic Effects
Stage 1: 0.5–6 hr	Direct mucosal irritation	Vomiting, diarrhea (bloody), fever, leukocytosis
	Increased ferritin release	Vasodilation, venous pooling, metabolic acidosis, shock
	?Direct CNS effect	Lethargy, seizures (massive overdose), coma
Stage 2: 6–24 hr	Tissue distribution	Absent or improving: **Latent period**
Stage 3: 12–48 hr	Mitochondrial poisoning via lipid peroxidation or electron transport chain disruption	Hepatic failure Shock, vascular collapse, pulmonary edema Renal shutdown
Stage 4: 3–4 wk	Late effects of mucosal damage	GI stricture formation, small bowel obstruction, pyloric scarring, hepatic cirrhosis

IX. Laboratory findings and evaluation:
  A. Serum iron and total iron binding capacity (TIBC).
    1. Determine blood level 2–4 hours after ingestion (peak level).
    2. Interpretation of serum iron levels:
      a. 100 μg/dl: Normal.
      b. 100–300 μg/dl: Minimal toxicity.
      c. 300–500 μg/dl: Mild to moderate toxicity; less than 6% risk of shock and coma.
      d. 500–1,000 μg/dl: Serious toxicity; 20% risk of shock and coma.
      e. >1,000 μg/dl: Potentially lethal; 60% risk of shock and coma.
      f. >5,000 μg/dl: Usually fatal.
  B. Other laboratory tests:
    1. Complete blood cell count: Leukocytosis (WBC >15,000/mm^3).
    2. Blood glucose: (Hyperglycemia).
    3. Arterial blood gas (with electrolytes): Significant (increased anion gap) metabolic acidosis (lactate).
    4. Abdominal radiograph: Iron medications are opaque. An absence of opaque material on x-ray does not exclude the possibility of iron ingestion, since complete dissolution of many solid iron preparations can occur within 1.5–2 hours after ingestion.
    5. Electrolytes, BUN, creatinine, liver function tests (transaminases, bilirubin).
    6. Urinalysis.
    7. Check stool and gastric aspirate for occult blood.
    8. Chest radiograph if respiratory distress.
    9. Prothrombin time, partial thromboplastin time.
    10. Type and cross match for 4 units blood.
  C. Deferoxamine challenge test:
    1. Deferoxamine is a specific iron-binding agent that can be used to test for or treat significant iron poisoning.
    2. Deferoxamine binds toxic free Fe to form a ferrioxamine complex, which is excreted in urine. Ferrioxamine is a reddish complex that produces characteristic "vin rose"-colored urine.
    3. Challenge test:
      a. Administer 25–50 mg/kg (maximum 1–2 gm) IM or 15 mg/kg IV over 1 hour.
      b. Appearance of reddish (vin rose) urine within 4–6 hours indicates presence of potentially toxic level. However, absence of urine color change does not completely rule out toxic exposure, since only about 10% of patients with toxic iron levels show such a color change.
      c. CAUTION: May lead to hypotension.
X. General treatment:
  A. Follow APTLS: See Chapter 8.
  B. General management: Table 88–4 (See Chapter 12 for details).
  C. Activated charcoal does not bind iron effectively and may accumulate in mucosal ulcerations, interfering with endoscopy. However, should be administered if multiple-drug ingestion is suspected.

TABLE 88–4.

General Treatment

Treatment	Indicated	Of No Value	Contraindicated
O_2	+		
IV	+		
ECG monitor	+		
Forced diuresis		X	
Acidification			X
Alkalinization		X	
Emesis	+		
Lavage*	+		
Charcoal†		X	
Cathartic‡			X
Dialysis		X	

*Examine aspirate for iron or test with deferoxamine. Follow with HCO_3 instillation (see Specific management).
†See General Treatment below.
‡Contraindicated in presence of GI bleed, and usually diarrhea a problem.

   D. Maintain electrolyte and acid-base balances. Monitor urine output closely.
   C. Initial resuscitation and supportive care of paramount importance.
      1. Respiratory support:
         a. Administer oxygen, 100% initially.
         b. Endotracheal intubation if necessary; see Chapter 9 for indications.
      2. Hypotension:
         a. See Chapter 10 for treatment recommendations.
         b. Transfusion if significant GI bleeding present.
      3. Seizures: See Chapter 22 for treatment recommendations.
XI. Specific management:
   A. Gastric lavage should be followed with 50–100 ml 2%–3% bicarbonate solution instilled into stomach. This converts free ferrous salt into poorly absorbed ferrous carbonate.
   B. Correct clotting abnormalities with vitamin K or fresh-frozen plasma.
   C. Early surgical or GI consultation for identification and treatment of bleeding sites.
   D. Chelation therapy with deferoxamine:
      1. Indications:
         a. Ingestion >30 mg/kg elemental iron.
         b. Signs of significant iron toxicity:
            (1) Serum iron greater than total iron-binding capacity.
            (2) Serum iron >300 μg/dl.
            (3) WBC >15,000, serum glucose >150 mg/dl, iron tablets visible on abdominal radiograph.
            (4) Signs and symptoms suggestive of significant ingestion (vomiting, abdominal pain, diarrhea, black or bloody stools).
         c. Positive deferoxamine challenge test.

2. Procedure
   a. If normotensive administer 90 mg/kg/dose (maximum 1–2 gm/dose) IM every 8 hours (maximum 6 gm/24 hr).
   b. If hypotensive administer 1 gm IV no faster than 10–15 mg/kg/hr every 4–6 hours.
   c. Continue until patient asymptomatic, urine no longer vin rose in color, serum iron levels below toxic range.
   d. Observe closely for:
      (1) Hypotension (if IV infusion too rapid).
      (2) Allergic reactions (blushing, urticaria, erythema).
   E. Dialysis:
      1. Not effective.
      2. May be necessary to clear deferoxamine in presence of renal failure.
   F. Total bowel irrigation: Experimental.
   G. Upper GI series needed 6 weeks after ingestion to check for strictures or obstructions.
XII. Prognosis:
   A. Expected response to treatment:
      1. Depends largely on amount ingested. Patients who ingest small amounts and who remain asymptomatic through the first 6 hours after ingestion generally have full recovery.
      2. Patients with systemic symptoms at higher risk for significant morbidity and mortality.
         a. Coma or shock indicative of grave prognosis (mortality 10%).
         b. Patients not in coma or shock should survive with good supportive care.
   B. Expected complications and long-term effects:
      1. Strictures may occur in patients who survive the systemic phase and some who never develop systemic symptoms.
      2. Other complications include increased coagulation time and bowel infarction.
XIII. Special considerations:
   A. Renal failure requiring hemodialysis, especially when deferoxamine used.
   B. Persistent iron concretions requiring endoscopic removal or gastrostomy.
   C. Exchange transfusion in small infants.
   D. Do not be misled by latent period between 6–24 hours, during which time patient may be relatively asymptomatic. Can be followed by fulminant life-threatening conditions such as pulmonary edema, shock, seizures, hepatic and renal failure.
XIV. Controversies: Inconclusive data on safety and efficacy of orally administered deferoxamine.
XV. Disposition considerations:
   A. Admission considerations:
      1. Indications of significant poisoning:
         a. WBC >15,000.
         b. Blood glucose >150 mg/dl.
         c. Opacity on abdominal radiographs.
         d. Four-hour serum Fe level >300 μg/dl.

    e. Serum Fe greater than total iron-binding capacity.

    f. Positive deferoxamine challenge test.

    g. History of lethal ingestion (>300 mg/kg).

  2. Patients with severe early symptoms:

    a. Vomiting, diarrhea.

    b. GI bleeding.

    c. Hemoglobin <10 gm/dl.

    d. Electrolyte imbalance, metabolic acidosis.

    e. Altered sensorium.

    f. Circulatory compromise.

  3. Patients initially symptomatic, then later asymptomatic should be admitted; may be latent phase.

  4. Suicide risk.

 B. Consultation considerations:

  1. Nephrologist if hemodialysis indicated (renal impairment).

  2. GI for endoscopy.

  3. General surgery consultation (early) for severe GI bleeding and persistent gastric concretions.

 C. Observation period: Asymptomatic patients should be observed for a minimum of 6 hours.

 D. Discharge considerations:

  1. General discharge considerations have been met (see Chapters 17 and 18).

  2. Asymptomatic throughout observation period.

  3. Four-hour serum Fe level <300 μg/dl.

  4. Follow-up including 6-week barium upper GI study arranged.

  5. Suicide potential and psychiatric status have been appropriately evaluated.

BIBLIOGRAPHY

Banner WJ, Tong TG: Iron poisoning. *Pediatr Clin North Am* 1986; 33:393–409.

Goldfrank LR, Kulberg AG, Kirstein RM: Iron, in Goldfrank LR, Flomenbaum NE, Lewin NA, et al (eds): *Goldfrank's Toxicologic Emergencies.* Norwalk, Conn, Appleton-Century-Crofts, 1986, pp 619–628.

Henretig FM, Karl SR, Weintraub WH: Severe iron poisoning treated with enteral and intravenous deferoxamine. *Ann Emerg Med* 1983; 12:306–309.

Krenzelok EP, Hoff JV: Accidental childhood iron poisoning: A problem of marketing and labeling. *Pediatrics* 1979; 63:591–596.

Lacouture PG, Watson S, Temple AR, et al: Emergency assessment of severity in iron overdose by clinical and laboratory methods. *J Pediatr* 1981; 99:89–91.

Robotham JL, Lietman PS: Acute iron poisoning, a review. *Am J Dis Child* 1980; 134:875–879.

Rumack BLT (ed): *Poisondex.* Denver, Micromedex, 1985.

Whitten CF, Chen YC, Gibson GW: Studies in acute iron poisoning. III: The phemodynamic alterations in acute experimental iron poisoning. *Pediatr Res* 1968; 2:479–485.

89

Pyridoxine

James L. Baker, M.D., F.A.C.E.P.

I. Route of exposure: Oral.
II. Common generic and trade names:
   A. Pyridoxines: Rodex, Rodex T.D.
   B. Many multivitamins contain pyridoxine, for example:

Alba-Lybe	Glutofac
Al-Vite	Hemo-Vite
B Complex 100	Hexa-betalin
Beelith Tablets	Mega-B
Besta Capsules	Nu-Iron-V
Eldertonic	Vicon-C
	Vicon-Plus Capsules

   C. Herpecin-L Cold Sore Lip Balm contains pyridoxine and other agents.
III. Pharmacokinetics:
   A. Absorption: Pyridoxine is readily absorbed from the gastrointestinal tract.
   B. Elimination: Excreted in the urine as 4-pyridoxic acid following hepatic aldehyde oxidase conversion of free pyridoxal.
   C. Active metabolites: Pyridoxal phosphate, pyridoxamine phosphate.
IV. Action: Pyridoxine serves as a coenzyme in a wide variety of metabolic transformations of amino acids, including transamination, decarboxylation, and racemization, and is also vital in enzymatic steps in the metabolism of tryptophan, sulfur-containing amino acids, and hydroxy amino acids. Symptoms of deficiency in humans include glossitis, stomatitis, hypochromic anemia, and seizures.

V. Uses:
  A. Sources: Pyridoxine is most commonly available as a vitamin supplement and is usually supplied as a component of multivitamins. It is also included as an ingredient in certain emollient lip balms.
  B. Pyridoxine has been identified as potentially useful as an adjunct in the control of refractory seizures in isoniazid (INH) toxicity, or in poisoning by monomethylhydrazine (MMH). MMH is used as a rocket fuel in the aerospace industry, and toxicity results from percutaneous or inhalation exposure. Exposure may also occur from ingestion of raw *Gyromitra esculenta,* a false morel mushroom.
VI. Toxic mechanism:
  A. Pyridoxine is a coenzyme in multiple metabolic transformations and deficiency states are more significant than excess states.
  B. There have been reports of several patients with sensory neuropathy with long-term high-dose ingestion, of seizures associated with high doses, and of a possible dose-related association with ulcer formation.
VII. Range of toxicity:
  A. Toxic dose: Toxic effects have been noted after 2 gm/day for 4 months or 5 gm/day for 2 months. (The United States Recommended Daily Allowance of pyridoxine for adults is 2 mg).
  B. Fatal doses: Although doses of 3–4 gm/kg have resulted in death in experimental animals, no fatal dose has been established in humans.
VIII. Clinical features:
  A. Symptoms of **chronic excess** are uncommon, but may include peripheral sensory neuropathies (sensory ataxia, impaired position and vibration sense), ulcerations, or seizures. No deaths have been reported.
  B. As noted, **symptoms of deficiency** are more common than symptoms of excess, and include seborrhea-like lesions about the eyes, nose, and mouth, glossitis, stomatitis, seizures, and rarely hypochromic anemia.
IX. Laboratory findings and evaluation:
  A. No specific laboratory determination has been established as useful in the diagnosis or treatment of suspected pyridoxine toxicity.
  B. Laboratory evaluation should be guided by clinical presentation.
X. General treatment:
  A. Follow APTLS: (See Chapter 8).
  B. General management: Table 89–1 (see Chapter 12 for details).
XI. Specific treatment:
  A. When specific symptoms are suspected to be related to chronic pyridoxine overdosage, withdrawal of pyridoxine compounds until symptoms resolve should suffice.
  B. If a single ingestion of vitamins is suspected, treat as for other important components of the vitamin preparation, such as iron.
XII. Prognosis: The prognosis for uneventful complete recovery is good following discontinuance of pyridoxine until symptoms resolve.
XIII. Disposition considerations:
  A. Admission considerations:
    1. See General Admission Considerations (Chapters 17 and 18).
    2. Toxicity following even large doses of pyridoxine is quite unusual and

TABLE 89–1.

General Treatment of Acute Ingestion

Treatment	Indicated	Of No Value	Contraindicated
O_2	−		
IV	−		
ECG monitor	−		
Forced diuresis		X	
Acidification		X	
Alkalinization		X	
Emesis/lavage	+/+		
Charcoal	+		
Cathartic	+		

resolution of symptoms is expected following discontinuance. Thus, admission for management is usually unnecessary.

   3. Suicide risk.

B. Observation period:

   1. For pure pyridoxine ingestions, patients usually should be kept in the emergency department until basic poisoning management is complete.

   2. For multivitamin ingestions, observation is dictated by other components in the preparation.

C. Discharge considerations:

   1. General discharge considerations have been met (see Chapters 17 and 18).

   2. Suicide potential and psychiatric status have been appropriately evaluated.

BIBLIOGRAPHY

Dipalma JR, Ritchie DM: Vitamin toxicity. *Ann Rev Pharm Toxicol* 1977; 17:133.

Goodman LS, Gilman A: *The Pharmacological Basis of Therapeutics,* ed 7. New York, Macmillan Publishing Co, 1985.

Holtz P, Palm D: Pharmacological aspects of vitamin B_6. *Pharmacol Rev* 1964; 16:113–178.

Lincoff G, Mitchell DH: *Toxic and Hallucinogenic Mushroom Poisoning.* New York, Van Nostrand Reinhold, 1977.

Schaumberg H, Kaplan J, Windebank A, et al: Sensory neuropathy from pyridoxine abuse. *N Engl J Med* 1983; 309:445–448.

Vitamin B_6 toxicity: A new megavitamin syndrome. *Nutr Rev* 1984; 42:44–46.

Watson S, Lacouture PG, Lovejoy FH: Single high-dose pyridoxine treatment for isoniazid overdose. *JAMA* 1981; 245:1102–1104.

90

Thyroid Replacement Drugs

Donna L. Seger, M.D., F.A.C.E.P.

I. Route of exposure: Oral, intravenous.
II. Common generic and trade names: Triiodothyronine (T_3), thyroxine (T_4); see also Table 90–1.
III. Pharmacokinetics:
    A. Absorption:
        1. Readily absorbed from the GI tract, predominantly from the stomach, within hours.
        2. T_3 is 95% absorbed; T_4 absorption varies from 30%–90%.
    B. Onset of action:
        1. Oral: Within hours.
        2. IV: 6–8 hours.
        3. Patients ingesting T_4 may be well for several days after the ingestion, until peripheral conversion of T_3 is significant and toxicity develops.
    C. Duration of action:
        1. Oral: Clinical effects have been observed for 3–16 hours in massive overdoses and 3–5 days with therapeutic administration.
        2. Approximately one third of extrathyroidal hormone is stored in the liver, and serum thyroid hormone slowly saturates other tissues, reaching equilibrium in several days.
    D. Peak effect: Maximum pharmacologic response after oral ingestion occurs within 2–3 days.
    E. Half-life:
        1. Published estimates of normal half-life of T_3, 1.3–2.5 days.
        2. T_4 turnover is normally 7 days, but this value may be halved in children and in settings of thyroid hormone excess and more than dou-

TABLE 90–1.

Thyroid Preparations

Generic Name	Trade Name	T_3, T_4 Composition
Thyroid tablets	Thyrar, Westhroid, others	T_3 and T_4
Thyroglobulin	Proloid	T_3 and T_4
Levothyroxine sodium (IV)	Synthroid, Levothyroid (IV)	T_4
Liothronine sodium	Cytomel	T_3
Liotrix	Euthroid, Thyrolar	$T_4/T_3 = 4:1$

bled in hypothyroidism. T_4 has a metabolic clearance rate of 0.84–1.37 L per day and fractional turnover rate of 9.7%–14.2% per day.

F. Elimination: After penetration into the cell, T_4 and T_3 undergo a variety of reactions that ultimately lead to excretion and inactivation.

G. Active metabolites: Perhaps the most important intermediate product of T_4 metabolism is formation of T_3, found in appreciable amounts within 3 days of T_4 administration.

IV. Action:

  A. Thyroid physiology:

    1. Iodine trapped by thyroid attaches to tyrosine and is oxidized to form monoiodotyrosine (MIT) and diiodotyrosine (DIT). MIT + DIT = T_3; DIT + DIT = T_4. Thyroid stimulating hormone (TSH) stimulates release of T_3 and T_4 into circulation.

    2. T_4 derived solely from thyroid secretion; 80% of T_3 derived from monodeiodination of T_4, which occurs at 3–7 days.

V. Uses:

  A. Treatment of hypothyroidism.

  B. Factitious thyrotoxicosis; most cases stem from subacute self-medication by patients eager to lose weight.

  C. Massive overdoses are decidedly uncommon, and many mild overdoses result from medication errors by nurses, misplaced decimal points by physicians and pharmacists, or patients continuing to take doses that were once considered to be appropriate but now are believed excessive (e.g., 300 µg thyroxine per day).

VI. Toxic mechanism:

  A. Stimulatory effect on sympathetic nervous system and metabolism result in excessive production of heat, increased motor activity, increased autonomic function.

  B. Reports of sudden death in patients without heart disease thought to be related to thyroid-induced myocarditis or increased myocardial sensitivity to catecholamines.

VII. Range of toxicity:

  A. Toxic dose:

    1. Ingestion of dessicated thyroid 0.3 gm/kg has caused fever, tachycar-

dia, hypertension, hyperactivity, cardiovascular collapse followed by complete recovery.

2. Therapeutic dose, patients without underlying heart disease tolerate intravenous doses of T_4 up to 750 μg.

3. Euthyroid persons appear to have a wide range of tolerance to the effect of acute or chronic overdose.

4. Some cardiologists contend that women tolerate thyroid excess less well than men do.

5. Cardiovascular system in aged or debilitated patients is vulnerable to even modest overdoses.

6. Type of preparation involved: Ingestion of up to 1,600 μg T_3 may be well tolerated, especially in the first 12 hours, and be rapidly eliminated from the vascular compartment. However, patients ingesting T_4 may be well until several days after the ingestion, when peripheral conversion of T_3 is significant and the patient becomes toxic if untreated.

7. Toxicity in children:

a. Enhanced kinetics and metabolism allow children to tolerate overdoses of up to 2.8 gm (45 grains) thyroid extract without symptoms or signs of poisoning.

b. An overdose of 132 grains in a 3-year-old child with only modest symptoms has been reported.

c. A younger child (15 months) taking a similar dose (5 grains/kg) can appear quite toxic.

VIII. Clinical features:

A. Sympathetic overdrive:

1. Tachycardia, palpitations, cutaneous vasodilation, diaphoresis, hypertension, cardiac arrhythmias, myocardial infarction.

2. See also Chapters 47 and 94.

B. Other symptoms: Headache, fever, diarrhea, vomiting, anxiety, agitation, weakness, psychosis, coma, cardiac arrhythmias, dehydration, cardiovascular collapse.

C. Clinical toxicity of T_4 ingestion does not occur for approximately 1 week because of delayed conversion of T_4 to the more clinically potent T_3.

IX. Laboratory findings and evaluation:

A. Thyroid function studies: Although thyroid function tests are of no value in basing treatment or determining prognosis in acute overdose, it is probably wise to order baseline thyroid function studies (serum T_3 and T_4).

B. Other laboratory tests:

1. ECG (see Clinical presentation).

2. Complete blood cell count and blood cultures (rule out infection in presence of hyperthermia).

3. Blood glucose (rule out hypoglycemia in presence of coma, altered mental status).

4. Electrolytes if severe vomiting, diarrhea.

5. May see slight elevation of liver function test values, BUN, and creatinine.

X. General treatment:
   A. Follow APTLS: See Chapter 8.
   B. General management: See Table 90–2 (see Chapter 12 for details).
   C. Supportive care of paramount importance:
      1. Respiratory support (see Chapter 9).
      2. Cardiovascular support:
         a. Cardiac arrest: Follow most recent Advanced Cardiac Life Support guidelines from the American Heart Association (*JAMA* 1986; 255:2841–3044).
         b. Arrhythmias: Follow most recent Advanced Cardiac Life Support guidelines (*JAMA* 1986; 255:2841–3044).
      3. Initiate measures to maintain temperature and fluid and electrolyte balance.
XI. Specific treatment:
   A. Symptoms are readily controlled by beta blockers such as propranolol (40–120 mg PO every 6 hours).
   B. Antithyroid drugs and extracorporeal detoxification are not beneficial and are potentially dangerous.
XII. Prognosis:
   A. Expected response to treatment:
      1. Complete clinical resolution may be expected within 12–48 hours.
      2. Complete chemical resolution in less than a week.
XIII. Special considerations:
   A. Chronic ingestion of large amounts of thyroxine:
      1. May precipitate heart failure, myocardial infarction, arrhythmia, coma, death.
      2. Supportive management.
      3. Most cases occur in paramedical personnel.
XIV. Controversies:
   A. Role of thyrostatic and iodine therapy.

TABLE 90–2.

General Treatment

Treatment	Indicated	Of No Value	Contraindicated
O_2	±		
IV	+		
ECG monitor*	+		
Forced diuresis			X
Acidification			X
Alkalinization		X	
Emesis†/lavage†	+/+		
Charcoal†	+		
Cathartic†	+		

*Usually required for 12–24 hours in pure T_3 ingestions.
†GI decontamination followed by activated charcoal (not necessary if it can be definitely established that <0.5 mg T_4 has been ingested).

    B. Extracorporeal detoxification.

    C. Charcoal and XAD-4 resin hemoperfusion.

XV. Disposition considerations:

    A. Admission considerations:

       1. See General Admission Considerations (Chapters 17 and 18).

       2. All symptomatic patients should be hospitalized.

       3. Suicide risk.

    B. Observation period:

       1. Symptomatic patients should not be observed.

       2. Difficult to make specific recommendations for asymptomatic patients with large ingestions but appropriately treated. Onset of symptoms normally expected within hours. A reasonable observation period would be 6–8 hours for such patients.

    C. Discharge considerations:

       1. General Discharge considerations have been met (see Chapters 17 and 18).

       2. Asymptomatic patients require outpatient observation for 10 days.

       3. If a patient with T_4 ingestion is considered for discharge, particular attention should be paid to close and daily monitoring of symptoms, with appropriate discharge environment where the patient can be continuously observed by responsible adults.

       4. Suicide potential and psychiatric status have been appropriately evaluated.

BIBLIOGRAPHY

Bhasen S, et al: Sudden death associated with thyroid hormone abuse. *Am J Med* 1981; 71:887–890.

Connors J, Thomas J: Thyroid and antithyroid drugs, in Craig C, Sitiel R (eds): *Modern Pharmacology.* Boston, Little Brown & Co, 1982, pp 159–872.

Kulig K, et al: Levothyroxine overdose associated with seizures in a young child. *JAMA* 1985; 254:2109–2110.

Lehrner L, Weir M: Acute ingestion of thyroid hormones. *Pediatrics* 1984; 73:313–317.

Litovitz T, White D: Levothyroxine ingestion in children: An analysis of 78 cases. *Am J Emerg Med* 1985; 3:297–300.

May M, et al: Plasmapheresis in thyroxine overdose: A case report. *J Toxicol Clin Toxicol* 1983; 20:517–520.

Nystrom E, et al: Minor signs and symptoms of toxicity in a young woman in spite of massive thyroxine ingestions. *Acta Med Scand* 1980; 207:135–136.

Roesch C, Becker PG, Sklar S, et al: Management of a child with acute thyroxine ingestion. *Ann Emerg Med* 1985; 14:1114–1115.

White J: Thyroid overdose, in Haddad and Winchester (eds): *Clinical Management of Poisoning and Drug Overdose.* Philadelphia, WB Saunders Co, 1983, pp 950–958.

91

Anticholinergic Agents

Gary M. Oderda, Pharm.D., M.P.H.

I. Route of exposure: Oral, intramuscular, intravenous, transdermal, ocular.
II. Common generic and trade names:
- A. Wide variety of agents produce anticholinergic effects. For some such as antidepressants, anticholinergic effects are not the major mechanism of production of severe toxicity. (See Chapters 63, 65, 92).
    1. Antidepressants: See Chapter 65.
    2. Antihistamines: See Chapter 92. Note wide use in cough and cold products, over-the-counter (OTC) sleep aids, and some OTC analgesics.
    3. Antiparkinsonian medications: benztropine (Cogentin), trihexyphenidyl (Artane).
    4. Antipsychotics: See Chapter 63:
        a. Phenothiazines.
        b. Thioxanthines.
        c. Loxapines.
        d. Butyrophenones.
    5. Antispasmodics: Atropine, dicyclomine (Bentyl), clindinium (Librax).
    6. Scopolamine.
- B. Plants and mushrooms with anticholinergic properties, including:
    1. Jimson weed *(Datura stramonium).* Seeds commonly abused by adolescents to produce hallucinations (Klein-Schwartz W, Oderda G: *Am J Dis Child* 1984; 138:737–739).
    2. Deadly nightshade *(Atropa belladonna).*
    3. Black nightshade *(Solanum nigrum).*
    4. Bittersweet *(Solanum dulcamara).*

5. Jerusalem cherry *(Solanum pseudocapsicum)*.

6. Mushrooms: *Amanita muscaria, Amanita pantherina.*

C. Synthetic atropine substitutes, including:

Adiphenine (Trasentine)   Methantheline (Banthine)
Anisotropine (Valpin)   Methixene (Trest)
Benztropine (Cogentin)   Methscopolamine (Pamine)
Biperiden (Akineton)   Oxybutynin (Ditropan)
Clidnium (Quarzan)   Oxyphencyclimine (Daricon)
Cyclopentolate (Cyclogyl)   Oxyphenonium (Antrenyl)
Dicyclomine (Bentyl)   Pentapiperium (Perium)
Eucatropine   Poldine (Nacton)
Flavoxate (Urispas)   Procyclidine (Kemadrin)
Glycopyrrolate (Robinul)   Propantheline (Pro-Banthine)
Hexocyclium (Tral)   Thiphenamil (Trocinate)
Homatropine   Trihexyphenidyl (Artane)
Isopropamide (Darbid)   Tropicamide (Mydriacyl)
Mepenzolate (Cantil)

III. Pharmacokinetics: See Chapters 63, 65, and 92.

IV. Action: Anticholinergic drugs block action of acetylcholine by competitive inhibition of this neurotransmitter for postsynaptic receptor site. Primarily affects peripheral and CNS muscarinic receptors.

V. Uses: These agents are contained in a vast array of prescription and nonprescription preparations to treat such conditions as depression, allergies (hay fever), irritable bowel syndrome, colds, parkinsonism, and motion sickness.

VI. Toxic mechanism: Results from excessive inhibition of acetylcholine at peripheral and central muscarinic receptors.

VII. Range of toxicity:

A. Toxic dose:

1. Mild anticholinergic effects may be seen at therapeutic or near therapeutic doses for most agents.

2. Children have developed anticholinergic toxicity from ocular instillation of atropine or scopolamine eyedrops. Toxic psychosis was seen in a 6-year-old after use of a transdermal scopolamine patch (Sennhauser, Schwartz: *Lancet* 1986; 2:1033).

3. Toxic doses vary greatly depending on agent involved (see Chapters 63, 65, 92).

B. Fatal dose:

1. Atropine or scopolamine: 10 mg.

2. Other synthetic substitutes: 10–100 mg/kg.

VIII. Clinical features (see also Chapters 63, 65, 92):

A. Peripheral:

1. Skin dry and flushed.

2. Hyperpyrexia common.

3. Hypothermia has been reported after therapeutic use of intravenous atropine.

4. Mydriasis.

5. Urinary retention.

6. Decreased GI motility.

7. Arrhythmias:
   a. Sinus tachycardia common.
   b. Other arrhythmias, particularly those seen with antidepressants and antipsychotics, produced from nonanticholinergic mechanisms.
8. Hypertension.
9. Late hypotension or cardiovascular collapse may also occur.

B. Central:
1. Hallucinations, both auditory and visual, may be seen. May include pricking movements or thrashing about.
2. Psychosis.
3. Seizures.
4. CNS depression including ataxia and coma.
5. Agitation and disorientation.
6. Acute dystonic reactions seen with antipsychotics and antihistamines.

IX. Laboratory findings and evaluation.
A. Serum drug levels: See Chapters 63, 65, 92.
B. Toxicology screen: Many anticholinergics are detected in blood or urine as part of routine toxicology screens. Although these analyses will document presence of an anticholinergic, they are of little value in determining treatment.
C. Other laboratory tests:
1. Arterial blood gases (rule out hypoxia, acidosis in presence of CNS depression, respiratory compromise secondary to impaired ventilation).
2. Complete blood cell count (as part of infection workup in presence of hyperthermia).
3. Serum glucose (with altered mental status).
4. ECG.

X. General treatment:
A. Follow APTLS: See Chapter 8.
B. General management: Table 91–1 (see Chapter 12 for details).

TABLE 91–1.
General Treatment*

Treatment	Indicated	Of No Value	Contraindicated
O$_2$	±		
IV	+		
ECG monitor	+		
Forced diuresis	−		
Acidification	−		
Alkalinization	−		
Emesis/lavage	+/+		
Charcoal	+		
Cathartic	+		

*May differ for specific ingestions; see appropriate chapters.

XI. Specific treatment:
A. Physostigmine (Antilirium): Anticholinesterase:
1. Used in severe anticholinergic poisoning for specific indications:
    a. Severe hallucinations.
    b. Convulsions: Physostigmine should be considered only if standard anticonvulsant therapy (i.e., diazepam) has failed (see Chapter 22).
    c. Hypertension: In most cases anticholinergic hypertension is mild, short-lived, and does not require pharmacologic intervention.
    d. Arrhythmias: Indicated for sinus tachycardia that is hemodynamically compromising.
2. Physostigmine itself may produce significant toxicity:
    a. Severe bradycardia.
    b. Cholinergic crisis.
    c. Asystole has been reported after physostigmine use in tricyclic antidepressant poisoning. The specific role of physostigmine in producing this effect is unclear.
3. Dose:
    a. Adults: Therapeutic trial 2 mg slow IV, no faster than 1 mg/min; 1–2 mg may be repeated in 20 minutes if no response, and then every 15–30 minutes for three to four doses; 1–4 mg can be given as a therapeutic dose.
    b. Children: 0.5 mg slow IV. Can be repeated at 5-minute intervals until cholinergic signs and symptoms are seen (see Cholinergic syndrome, Chapter 47) or maximum of 2 mg. Lowest effective dose should be given as therapeutic dose.
4. **Contraindications** for physostigmine:
    a. QRS interval ≥100 msec.
    b. Evidence of intraventricular conduction defect or heart block.
    c. Although a significant risk exists in the setting of anticholinergic poisoning, atropine may be given cautiously at half the physostigmine dose if severe cholinergic toxicity develops (e.g., profound bradycardia or respiratory depression).
B. Hyperpyrexia: See Chapters 63 and 66.
C. Hypertension: See Chapter 68.
D. Hypotension: See Chapter 10.
E. Seizures: See Chapter 22.
F. Agitation:
1. Protect patient from self.
2. Sedation:
    a. Mild agitation may be treated with diazepam 5–10 mg PO; may be repeated three or four times over next 24 hours. Higher doses are occasionally indicated (e.g., 15–20 mg PO).
    b. Severe agitation: Diazepam 2–5 mg IV initially, titrated upward to· desired sedative response. Generally ≤10 mg is adequate; however, up to 20 mg may be given.
G. Psychosis: If accompanied by severe hallucinations, physostigmine indicated.
H. Dystonic reaction: See Chapter 63.

XII. Prognosis:
   A. Expected response to treatment
      1. Fatality rate in cases of atropine or scopolamine poisoning less than 1%.
      2. Survival for 24 hours associated with full recovery.
      3. Efficacy of physostigmine in reducing mortality in anticholinergic poisoning not established.
XIII. Disposition considerations (see also specific ingestion):
   A. Admission considerations:
      1. See General Admission Considerations (Chapters 17 and 18).
      2. Lethargy, decreased level of consciousness, altered mental status.
      3. Signs of atropinism (tachycardia, postural hypotension, confusion, agitation).
      4. Suicide risk.
      5. ICU: Coma, seizures, arrhythmias, A-V block or other conduction defect, persistent hypotension, uncontrolled hyperpyrexia.
   B. Consultation considerations: See specific chapters.
   C. Observation period: See specific chapters.
   D. Discharge considerations: See specific chapters.

BIBLIOGRAPHY

Klein-Schwartz W, Oderda G: Jimson weed intoxication in adolescents and young adults. *Am J Dis Child* 1984; 138:737–739.

Kulig K, Rumack BH: Physostigmine and asystole. *Ann Emerg Med* 1981; 10:228–229.

Pentel P, Peterson CD: Asystole complicating physostigmine treatment of tricyclic antidepressant overdose. *Ann Emerg Med* 1980; 9:588–590.

Sennhauser FH, Schwartz HP: Toxic psychosis from transdermal scopolamine in a child. *Lancet* 1986; 2:1033.

92

Antihistamines

Gary M. Oderda, Pharm.D., M.P.H.

I. Route of exposure: Oral, intravenous.
II. Common generic names: See Table 92–1.
  A. Medications used in combination with antihistamines:
    1. Acetaminophen: For example:
        Advanced Formula Dristan
        Comtrex
        Periogesic Analgesic Tablets
        Sinulin
        Teldrin Multisystem Allergy Reliever
    2. Aspirin: For example:
        Alka-Seltzer Plus Cold Medicine
        Fiogesic
    3. Ascorbic Acid: Citra Forte Syrup
    4. Atropine: Rutuss tablets.
    5. Codeine:
        Actifed with Codeine
        Ambenyl
        Codimal PH
        Dimetane-DC Cough Syrup
        Phenergan with Codeine
        Phenergen VC with Codeine
    6. Dextromethorphan:
        Albatussin
        Benylin DM
        Benylin DME

TABLE 92–1.

Antihistamines

Class	Generic Name	Usual Single Adult Dose (mg)
H₁ receptor blockers		
Alkylamines	Chlorpheniramine	4
	Brompheniramine	4
Ethanolamines	Diphenhydramine	25–50
	Dimenhydrinate	50
Ethylenediamine	Pyrilamine	25–50
	Tripelenamine	37.5–75
Phenothiazines	Promethazine	25
Piperazines	Hydroxyzine	25
	Cyclizine	50
	Meclizine	25–50
Other	Terfenadine	60
H₂ receptor blockers		
	Cimetidine	300
	Rantidine	150

Codimal DM
Comtrex
Dimetane DX
Phenergan with Dextromethorphan
Quelidrine
Rutuss Expectorant
Scot-tussin Sugar Free Cough and Cold Medicine
Triaminicol Multisystem Cold Syrup
Triaminicol Multisystem Cold Tablets

7. Ephedrine:
   Quelidren
   Rynatuss
8. Guiafenesin:
   Benylin DME
   Rutuss Expectorant
9. Homatropine: Simulin.
10. Hydrocodone:
   Citra Forte Syrup
   Codimal DH
   Rutuss with Hydrocodone
   Triaminic Expectorant DH
11. Methscopolamine:
   Extendryl
   Histaspan-D

12. Phenylephrine:

Advanced Formula Dristan Tablets	Extendryl
	Histaspan-Plus
Advanced Formula Dristan Capsules	Phenergan-VC
	Phenergan-VC with Codeine
Albatussin	Quelidrine
Atrohist Sprinkle	Rynatan
Codimal DH	Rynatuss
Codimal DM	Rutuss with Hydrocodone
Comhist	Rutuss Liquid
Comhist LA	Rutuss Tablets

13. Phenylpropanolamine:
    Alka-Seltzer Plus Cold Medicine
    Sinulin
    Tavist-D
    Triaminic Cold Syrup
    Triaminic Cold Tablets
    Triaminic Expectorant
    Triaminic Expectorant DH
    Triaminicol Multisystem Cold Syrup
    Triaminicol Multisystem Cold Tablets

14. Pseudoephedrine:

Benadryl Decongestant	Fedahist
Benadryl Decongestant Elixir	Isoclor Timesule Capsules
Bromofed	Rondec
Bromofed PD	Rondec TR
Codimal LA	Rutuss Expectorant
Deconamine	Teldrin Multisystem Allergy Reliever
Deconamine SR	
Dimetane DX Cough Syrup	Trinalin

15. Scopolamine: Rutuss Tablets.

III. Pharmacokinetics:
   A. Onset of action: See Table 92–2.
   B. Duration of action:
      1. See Table 92–2.
      2. Variable biological effect lagging several hours behind peak serum levels.
   C. Peak effect: See Table 92–2.
   D. Half-life: See Table 92–2.
   E. Elimination: Classic H_1 antihistamines are distributed to all tissues: they are lipophilic and cross both the blood-brain barrier and placenta. Metabolized in liver by hydroxylation, and inactive metabolites are excreted in urine.
   F. Active metabolites: None.
IV. Action:
   A. Via competitive blocking of histamine receptors.
   B. Local anesthesia.
   C. Cardiac effects (membrane stabilizing).

TABLE 92–2.

Pharmacology of Common Antihistamines

	Half-Life (hr)	Dosing	Peak Levels (hr)	Onset of Effect
Astemizole	20	qd	1–4	2 day
Azatadine	8.7	bid	3	—
Brompheneramine	—	bid-qid	5	15–30 min
Chlorpheneramine	20	bid-tid	—	—
Clemastine	—	bid	2–4	5–7 hr
Cyproheptadine	—	bid-tid	—	—
Dimenhydrinate	—	qid	2	15–30 min
Diphenhydramine	4	tid-qid	2–4	1 hr
Hydroxyzine	3	tid-qid	2	15–30 min
Oxatimide	3.8	bid-tid	—	—
Promethazine	—	qid	—	20 min
Terfenadine	16–22	bid	4–6	1–2 hr

    D. Alpha adrenergic receptor blockade (promethazine [Phenergan]).

    E. Inhibition of scratch-and-flare response.

    F. **H_2 receptor blockers:** Decreased gastric acid secretion.

V. Uses:

    A. Used primarily as cold remedy, premedication for surgical patients, nausea, motion sickness, dystonic reactions from major tranquilizers, sedation.

    B. Over-the-counter sedatives/hypnotics: Rapidly changing market that currently includes only antihistamines: diphenhydramine, pyrilamine, doxylamine.

VI. Toxic mechanism:

    A. Direct H_1 receptor blockade:

        1. Inhibition of vasodilation.

        2. Decrease in capillary permeability.

        3. Cardiac: Inhibition of negative inotropic effects.

        4. Inhibition of nonvascular smooth muscle contractility.

        5. CNS: May observe sedation or stimulation.

        6. Respiratory tract effects (e.g., thickening of bronchial secretions).

        7. Paradoxical histamine release possible with high concentrations.

    B. Indirect effects: Tachycardia (baroreceptor reflex, catecholamine release).

    C. Effects unrelated to receptor blockade: Blockade of cholinergic muscarinic receptors (dose dependent).

    D. Anticholinergic effects not related to H_1 receptor blockade (includes dose-related blockage of cholinergic, muscarinic receptors).

    E. Alpha adrenergic receptor blockade seen with **promethazine**.

    F. **H_2 receptor blockade:** Also causes inhibition of capillary dilation, inhibition of chronotropic effect.

VII. Range of toxicity:

    A. Toxic dose: See Table 92–3.

TABLE 92–3.

Range of Toxicity of Common Antihistamines*

	Minimal Toxicity Expected (mg)	Mild to Moderate Toxicity Possible (mg)
Chlorpheniramine	≥0.5/kg <20 total	≥20
Brompheniramine	≥25 <50 total	≥50
Diphenhydramine	≥5/kg	>100
Doxylamine	≤100 total	
Methapyrilene	≥250	≥500
Pheniramine	<500	

*Immediate-release noncombination products.

  B. Fatal dose: For most antihistamines, 25–250 mg/kg.
VIII. Clinical features:
  A. **H₁ blocking agents:** Clinical effects seen in overdose depend on agent ingested:
    1. Anticholinergic signs and symptoms: See Chapter 91.
    2. Neurologic effects:
      a. Stimulatory: Dyskinesia, acute dystonic reaction, seizures, euphoria, hyperreflexia, hypertension, insomnia, irritability, headache, muscle twitching, nervousness, tachycardia, tremor, vagal stimulation.
      b. Depressive: Ataxia, coma, delirium, dizziness, drowsiness, lethargy, fatigue, lassitude, narcolepsy, somnolence, weakness.
      c. Neuropsychiatric: Confusion, delusions, decreased mental efficiency, impaired judgment, hallucinations, hysteria, mental depression, nightmares.
      d. Peripheral: Areflexia, paralysis, paresthesias, toxic neuritis.
    3. Ears: Labyrinthitis, tinnitus, vertigo.
    4. Eyes: Blurred vision, dilated pupils, diplopia, hypermetropia.
    5. GI: Anorexia, cardiospasm, constipation, diarrhea, nausea, vomiting, heartburn.
    6. Cardiovascular: Cerebral edema, cardiac arrhythmias, hypertension, hypotension, palpitations, shock, syncope, tachycardia, vasovagal phenomenon, cardiorespiratory depression.
    7. Respiratory: Bronchospasm, dry respiratory mucous membranes, nasal congestion.
    8. Genitourinary: Dysuria, increased urinary frequency, urinary retention.
    9. Skin and mucous membranes: Dermatitis, dry mouth, increased perspiration, photoallergic reaction, urticaria.
    10. Other: Hypothermia, renal failure, bone marrow depression.
    11. **Terfenadine** (Seldane) and **astemizole** (Hismanal) are recently

marketed antihistamines that have been reported not to cross the blood-brain barrier and hence do not produce sedation in therapeutic doses. Experience with overdose is limited.

 a. CNS depression, tremors, ataxia, seizures have been seen in animals given large doses.

 b. Hypotension (blood pressure 90/50) not requiring therapy has been reported in a 16-year-old who took 1,500 mg terfenadine.

 c. Torsade de pointes developed in a patient who took 3,360 mg terfenadine, 7,000 mg cephalexin, and 1,200 mg ibuprofen. This patient also developed ventricular fibrillation, which responded to defibrillation and lidocaine.

B. **H$_2$ blocking agents:** Limited overdose experience available.

 1. Major toxic effects expected from acute oral overdoses:

  a. CNS effects: Drowsiness, sedation, depression, confusion, hallucinations, convulsions, coma.

  b. Respiratory depression.

  c. Cardiovascular effects: Hypotension, bradycardia, tachycardia.

  d. Dry mouth, mild epigastric distress.

IX. Laboratory findings and evaluation:

A. Toxicology screen: Some antihistamines are included in toxicology screens. Usually measured qualitatively. Levels not helpful for clinical management.

B. ECG.

C. See Chapter 91.

X. General treatment:

A. Follow APTLS: See Chapter 8.

B. General management: Table 92–4 (see Chapter 12 for details).

XI. Specific management:

A. Physostigmine will reverse anticholinergic effects produced by antihistamines, but should be reserved for specific situations (see Chapter 91).

B. Seizures:

 1. See Chapter 22 for treatment recommendations.

 2. For refractory seizures consider physostigmine (see Chapter 91).

TABLE 92–4.

General Treatment

Treatment	Indicated	Of No Value	Contraindicated
O$_2$	±		
IV	+		
ECG monitor	+		
Forced diuresis		X	
Acidification			X
Alkalinization		X	
Emesis/lavage	+/+		
Charcoal	Repeated doses		
Cathartic	+		

XII. Prognosis:
    A. Expected response to treatment:
        1. **H_1 blocking agents:**
            a. Rare deaths reported.
            b. Patients who live more than 24 hours will probably survive.
        2. **H_2 blocking agents:** Acute ingestion of excessive amounts of cimetidine not associated with significant toxic sequelae.
    B. Expected complications and long-term effects: Rare reactions include leukopenia, agranulocytosis, hemolytic anemia, acute labyrinthitis, dyskinesias.
XIII. Controversies: Physostigmine will reverse anticholinergic effects produced by antihistamines but may itself produce significant complications (see Chapter 91).
XIV. Disposition considerations:
    A. Admission considerations:
        1. See General Admission Considerations (Chapter 18).
        2. Symptomatic.
        3. Suicide risk.
    B. Observation period: Difficult to make recommendations because of great variety of antihistamine preparations with different half-lives, variable individual metabolism of antihistamines, and unpredictable response to treatment.
    C. Discharge considerations:
        1. General discharge considerations have been met (see Chapter 18).
        2. Each patient requires individual consideration. As a general rule, patients should be asymptomatic.
        3. Suicide potential and psychiatric state have been appropriately evaluated.

BIBLIOGRAPHY

Douglas WW: Histamine and 5 hydroxytryptamine (serotonin) and their antagonists, in Gilman AG, Goodman LS, Rall TW, et al (eds): *The Pharmacological Basis of Therapeutics,* ed 7. New York, Macmillan Publishing Co, 1985, pp 605–638.

Krenzelok EP, Litovitz T, Lippold KP, et al: Cimetidine toxicity: An assessment of 881 cases. *Ann Emerg Med* 1987; 16:1217–1221.

Maryland Poison Center Antihistamine Protocol, 1987.

Meredith TJ, Volans GN: Management of cimetidine overdose (letter). *Lancet* 1979; 2:1367.

Smolinske SC: Terfenadine management in Rumack BH (ed): *Poisindex.* Denver, Micromedex, 1987.

Van Rijthoven AW: Cimetidine intoxication (letter). *Lancet* 1979; 2:370.

93

Nonsteroidal Anti-inflammatory Agents

Timothy J. Rittenberry, M.D., F.A.C.E.P.

I. Route of exposure: Oral.
II. Common generic and trade names: See Table 93–1.
III. Pharmacokinetics:
   A. Composition: Derivatives of arylalkanoic acid, indole acetic acid, anthranilic acid, pyrazalone, or oxicam.
   B. Absorption:
      1. Rapid from GI tract.
      2. Ibuprofen 80% absorbed in 0.5–2 hours.
   C. Peak effect: See Table 93–1.
   D. Half-life: See Table 93–1.
   E. Elimination:
      1. Predominantly renal.
      2. Sulindac and indomethacin have significant enterohepatic circulation.
IV. Action: Anti-inflammatory, analgesic, often antipyretic activity.
V. Uses:
   A. Treatment of pain, inflammatory states (e.g., gouty or rheumatoid arthritis).
   B. Generally not recommended for children or infants.
VI. Toxic mechanism:
   A. Exact toxic mechanism unclear but likely related to prostaglandin inhibition:
      1. Decreased renal blood flow related to decreased local prostaglandin E_2 activity may lead to renal injury.

TABLE 93–1.

Nonsteroidal Anti-Inflammatory Drugs

Generic Name	Trade Name	Protein Binding (%)	Half-Life (hr)	Peak Serum Level (hr)	Maximum Adult Dosage (mg/24 hr)	Therapeutic Serum Levels (μg/ml)
Fenoprofen	Nalfon	High	3	2	3,200	40–70
Naproxen	Naproxyn Anaprox	High	10–20	2–4	1,250	30–90
Ibuprofen	Advil Medipren Motrin Rufin Nuprin	95	2	1–1.5	3,200	—
Suprofen	Suprol	High	2–4	2–4	800	—
Mefenamic acid	Ponstel	High	3	2–3	6,000	1–10
Meclofenamate	Meclomen	High	3	1–4	400	10–20
Diflunisal	Dolobid	High	8–12	2–3	1,500	110–120
Indomethacin	Indocin	90	2–11	1	200	—
Sulindac	Clinoril	High	7–18	2	400	3–6
Tolmetin	Tolectin	High	1	1	2,000	—
Piroxicam	Feldene	High	50	3–5	20	—
Phenylbutazone	Butazolidin Azolid	95	60–72	2	600	—
Oxyphenbutazone	Oxalid Tandearil	90	50–75	2–4	600	—

   B. Hypersensitivity reactions may lead to hepatic, renal, or hematopoietic injury.
 VII. Range of toxicity:
   A. See Table 93–2.
   B. Severe toxicity and death uncommon, with few reports. All children to date who have developed serious toxicity have had a history of ingesting >400 mg/kg.
   C. Ibuprofen overdose more common.
VIII. Clinical features:
   A. Common acute symptoms:
     1. GI: Nausea, vomiting, diarrhea, abdominal pain, dyspepsia; bleeding rare.
     2. CNS: Headache, somnolence, dizziness; may progress to seizure or frank coma.
     3. Acute symptoms typically resolve within 24 hours.
   B. Uncommon acute symptoms:
     1. Renal: oliguria, anuria, acute renal failure.
     2. Respiratory: Tachypnea; apnea reported in children and infants.

TABLE 93–2.

Toxicity of Nonsteroidal Anti-inflammatory Agents*

Generic Name	Toxic Dose (gm)
Fenoprofen	60
Naproxen	25
Ibuprofen	0.4/kg†
Mefenamic acid	2.5†
Indomethacin	1.5
	0.175†
Piroxicam	2.5
	0.5‡
Phenylbutazone	2.5
	2.0‡

*From adult cases reviewed in *Poisindex* unless otherwise noted.
†Child.
‡Infant.

3. Hematologic:
   a. Fecal blood loss.
   b. Increased bleeding time.
   c. Bleeding dyscrasias with **indomethacin, phenylbutazone, oxyphenbutazone.**
4. Hepatic: Jaundice with elevation of liver function test values (especially **phenylbutazone, oxyphenbutazone**).
5. Head, eyes, ears, nose, and throat: Decreased hearing acuity, tinnitus, diplopia, visual blurring.
6. Cardiovascular: Hypotension, hypertension, edema secondary to sodium and water retention.
7. Acid-base: Respiratory alkalosis with metabolic acidosis (lactate from hypoperfusion).
C. All have potential for cross reactivity in aspirin-induced syndrome of rhinitis, urticaria, and bronchospasm.
IX. Laboratory findings and evaluation:
A. Blood:
   1. Serum levels not widely available or clinically useful.
      a. A nomogram has been developed to aid in predicting development or worsening of toxicity in both pediatric and adult patients after **ibuprofen** ingestion (Fig 93–1).
         (1) Time coordinates refer to hours after ingestion.
         (2) Plasma levels obtained sooner than 1 hour or later than 12 hours after ingestion cannot be interpreted.
         (3) *Nomogram Prediction of Toxicity Development*

IBUPROFEN NOMOGRAM

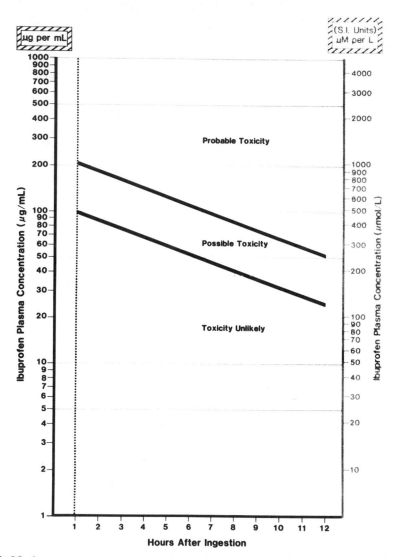

FIG 93–1.
Ibuprofen nomogram (see text for details). (From Hall AH, Smolinske SC, Conrad FL, et al: *Ann Emerg Med* 1986; 15:1308–1313. Used by permission.)

Portion of Nomogram

	Toxicity Probable (%)	Toxicity Possible (%)	Toxicity Unlikely (%)
Severe symptoms	24	17	0
Symptoms	65	33	24
Asymptomatic	35	67	76

(4) Nomogram may aid in predicting which initially asymptomatic or mildly toxic patients have the potential to develop symptoms or more severe symptoms later.

2. Complete blood cell count and spun hematocrit, coagulation profile (prothrombin time, partial thromboplastin time).
3. Blood chemistries.
4. Liver function tests.
5. Cross match and type.
6. Arterial blood gases if indicated (may see significant acidosis in ibuprofen overdose).
7. Baseline urinalysis, BUN, creatinine (potential for renal insufficiency).

X. General treatment:
  A. Follow APTLS: See Chapter 8.
  B. General management: Table 93–3 (see Chapter 12 for details).
  C. Monitor for vital signs, GI bleeding, renal function.

TABLE 93–3.

General Treatment

Treatment	Indicated	Of No Value	Contraindicated
O_2	±		
IV	±		
ECG monitor	±		
Forced diuresis		X	
Acidification			X
Alkalinization		X	
Emesis*	±		
Lavage*	+		
Charcoal†	+		
Cathartic	+		
Dialysis		X	

*Seizures have developed in children who ingested >400 mg/kg; therefore induced emesis should be avoided in children and gastric lavage performed if necessary.

†Inasmuch as there is some evidence for enterohepatic circulation of ibuprofen, multiple doses of activated charcoal might be beneficial in serious poisonings, although this has not been studied.

XI. Specific management:
  A. No specific therapy for ibuprofen overdose.
  B. Treatment is symptomatic and supportive.
  C. No antidotes.
  D. Seizures respond to standard therapy with diazepam (Valium), phenytoin (Dilantin), or phenobarbital (see Chapter 22).
XII. Prognosis:
  A. Expected response to treatment:
    1. Most acute toxicities resolve in 24 hours if symptomatic.
    2. **Phenylbutazone** class **(pyrazolones):** Approximately 10% of severe reactions end in death. If the patient survives for 1 month, recovery is expected.
  B. Expected complications and long-term effects:
    1. GI bleeding.
    2. Renal failure.
    3. Rare reports of esophageal stricture after ibuprofen ingestion.
XIII. Special considerations:
  A. May potentiate effect of other protein-bound drugs **(phenytoin, coumadin, sulfonamides, sulfonylureas).**
  B. **Indomethacin** ingestion associated with significant incidence of psychiatric disturbance (acute psychosis, hallucinosis). May increase lithium levels.
  C. With **ibuprofen,** minimize esophageal exposure with oral fluids.
XIV. Disposition considerations:
  A. Admission considerations:
    1. See General Admission Considerations (Chapters 17 and 18).
    2. Adults: Those who develop symptoms should be admitted and carefully observed until all symptoms have resolved.
    3. Children: (Reported ibuprofen ingestion) >400 mg/kg: gastric lavage and admit for observation.
  B. Observation period:
    1. Adults: 12–24 hours if symptomatic. (This duration of observation is considered inappropriate for most emergency departments.)
    2. Children:
      a. Reliably reported ingestion <200 mg/kg: Ipecac; observe at home.
      b. Reliably reported ingestion between 200–400 mg/kg: Ipecac; observe for at least 4 hours in emergency department.
  C. Discharge considerations:
    1. See General discharge considerations (Chapters 17 and 18).
    2. Children: Ibuprofen <200 mg/kg: Ipecac; observe at home with close and reliable supervision.
    3. Suicide potential and psychiatric status have been appropriately evaluated.

BIBLIOGRAPHY

Court H, Streete P, Volans GN: Acute poisoning with ibuprofen. *Hum Toxicol* 1983; 2:381–384.

Court H, Volans G: Poisoning after overdose with non-steroidal anti-inflammatory drugs. *Adverse Drug React Acute Poisoning Rev* 1984; 3:1–21.

Dreisbach RH, Robertson WO: *Handbook of Poisoning.* Norwalk, Conn, Appleton-Century-Crofts, 1987, p 305.

Haddad LM, Winchester JF: *Clinical Management of Poisoning and Drug Overdose.* Philadelphia, WB Saunders Co, 1983, pp 586–591.

Hall AH, Smolinske SC, Conrad FL, et al: Ibuprofen overdose: 126 cases. *Ann Emerg Med* 1986; 15:1308–1313.

Harchelroad F, Evans TC, Hobbs E: Ibuprofen blood levels vary. *Ann Emerg Med* 1988; 17:186.

Lee CY, Finkler A: Acute intoxication due to ibuprofen overdose. *Arch Pathol Lab Med* 1986; 110:747–749.

Patmas MA, et al: Acute multisystem toxicity associated with the use of nonsteroidal anti-inflammatory drugs. *Arch Intern Med* 1984; 144:519–521.

Perry SJ, Streete PJ, Volans GN: Ibuprofen overdose: The first two years of over-the-counter sales. *Hum Toxicol* 1987; 6:173–178.

Physicians Desk Reference. Raritan, NJ, Medical Economics Co, 1987.

Poisindex. Denver, Micromedex, 1987.

Royer GL, Seckman CE, Welshman IR: Safety profile: Fifteen years of clinical experience with ibuprofen. *Am J Med* 1984; 77(suppl):25–34.

Treatment of patients with ibuprofen overdose (letter). *Ann Emerg Med* 1988; 17:184–185.

94

Sympathomimetic Drugs*

J. Stephen Huff, M.D.

I. Route of exposure: Oral, intranasal, intravenous.
   NOTE: **The following discussion concerns only oral ingestion of sympathomimetic medications in common use.**
II. Common generic and trade names:
   A. Sympathomimetic drugs are found in prescriptions and over-the-counter (OTC) compounds, which frequently contain more than one agent. Illicit use in "look-alike" pills also occurs (see Amphetamines, Chapter 68).
      1. Ephedrine-containing preparations:
         a. Nonprescription drugs:
            HTO Hemorrhoidal Ointment
            Nyquil Nighttime Colds Medicine
            Pazo Hemorrhoidal Ointment and Suppositories
            Vatronol Nose Drops
            Primatene
            Bronkaid Tablets
         b. Prescription drugs:

Amesec	Isuprel Compound Elixir
Azma-Aid Tablets	KIE Syrup
Bronkolixir	Lufylline-EPG
Bronkotabs	Marax
Co-Xan Syrup	Mudraine GG
Derma Medicone-HC	PBZ with Ephedrine
Ointment	Quadrinal

*See also Chapter 68, Amphetamines/Stimulants.

Quelidrine Syrup
Quibron Plus
Rynatuss
T.E.H. Tablets

Tedral
Theophedrizine Tablets
Wyanoids HC Rectal
Suppositories

2. Pseudoephedrine-containing preparations:
   a. Nonprescription drugs:

   Ambenyl-D Decongestant
   Cosanyl Cough Syrup
   CoTylenol Cold Formula
   First Sign
   Multi-Symptom
   Novahistine

   Pseudoephedrine Syrup
   Rhinosyn DM, PD, X
   Ryna C, CX
   Sudafed
   Symptom 2
   Viro-Med+

   b. Prescription drugs:

   Actifed
   Acti-Perm Tablets
   Afrinol
   Anamine
   Brexin
   Chlorafed
   Chlor-Trimeton
   Codimal-L.A.
   Congress Jr.
   Congress Sr.
   Deconamine
   D-Feda
   Dimacol
   Disophrol-Chronotabs
   Drixoral
   Emprazil
   Fedahist
   Fedrazil

   Histalet
   Historal
   Isochior
   Kronofed-A
   Lo-Tussin Syrup
   Nasalspan
   Novafed
   Nucofed
   Polaramine Expectorant
   Poly-Histine-DX
   Rhinafed
   Robitussin DAC, PE
   Rondec
   Sudafed
   Trifed
   Tussend

3. Phenylpropanolamine-containing preparations:
   a. Nonprescription drugs:

   A.R.M.
   Alka-Seltzer Plus
   Allerest
   Anorexin
   Appedrine
   Bayer Children's Cold
      Preparation
   BioSlim T
   C3 Cold Formula
   Children's Hold
   Coffee-Break Cubes
   Comtrex
   Congespirin Cold Medicine
   Contac
   Control Capsules

   Coricidin
   Coryban-D Capsules
   Daycare Cold Medicine
   Dex-A-Diet II
   Dexatrim
   Diadax
   Dorcol
   Fluidex-Plus
   Formula 44D Decongestant
   4-Way Cold Tablets
   Hungrex Plus
   Liqui-Trim
   Novahistine
   Ornacol
   Ornex

P.V.M.
Permathene-12
Pr-Dax 21
Prolamine
St. Joseph Cold Tablets
Sinarest Tablets
Sine-Aid
Sine-off
Sinutab
Slim-One

Sucrets Cold Decongestant
Super Odrinex
Triaminic
Triaminicin
Triaminicol
Tussagesic
Ursinus Inlay-Tabs
Vicks Formula 44D

b. Prescription drugs:

Anatuss
Brocon
Brophentapp T.D. Tablets
Cenadex
Codimal Expectorant
Conex
Decon-Aid TR
Decon-Tuss TR
Dehist
Dephrohist
Dextrotussin Syrup
Dimetrane
Dimetapp
Entex
Flogesic
Histabid
Histalet Forte
Histatapp
Hycomine
Kronohist Kronocaps
Leder-BP
Naldecon
NaprilPlateau Caps

Nilcol
Nolamine
Obestat
Ornade Spansules
Phenatapp
Phenylpropanolamine HCl T.D.
Poly-Histine
Protid
Purebrom Compound
Resaid T.D.
Rhinedecon
Rhinex D-Lay
Rhinolar
Robitussin-CR
Ru-Tuss
S-T Forte Syrup
Sinubid
Sinulin
Tusquelin
Tuss-Ornade
Voxin-PG

4. Phenylephrine-containing preparations:
a. Nonprescription drugs:

Chlor-Trimeton Expectorant
Congespirin
Coricidin
Coryban-D
Demazine
Dristan
4-Way Nasal Spray

Neo-Synephrine
NTZ
Prefrin Liquifilm
Sinex
Sucrets Cold Formula
Trind

b. Prescription drugs:

Albatussin
Anatuss
Brocon

Brophentapp T.D.
Citra Capsules
Codimal

Comhist
Colrex
Dallergy
Dehist
Dimetan
Dimetapp
Donatussin
Duo-Medihaler
Entex
Extendryl
Gustrey Fortis Tabs
Histalet Forte
Histaspan
Histatapp
Histor-D Timecelles
Hycomine Compound
Leder-BP
Naldecon

Napril Plateau Caps
Neotep Granucaps
Pediacof
Phenatapp
Phenergan VC Expectorant
Protid
Purebrom Compound
P-V-tussin Syrup
Quelidrine
Ru-Tuss
Singlet
Sinovan
S-T-Forte
Sulfadrin Nasal Suspension
Tusquelin
Tympagesic
Vicks Sinex

III. Pharmacokinetics:
   A. Onset of action: Within 1 hour.
   B. Plasma half-life: Elimination increased in **acid urine,** with elimination half-life of roughly 2 hours; **alkaline urine** will lengthen elimination half-life up to 10-fold.
   C. Peak effect: For most compounds peak effects are seen between 1 and 3 hours.
   D. Duration of action: Clinical effects generally last less than 8 hours.
   E. Elimination: Major portion of compound excreted unchanged in urine.
   F. Active metabolites: Depends on agent.

IV. Action:
   A. Some compounds are structurally related to amphetamines and literally mimic sympathetic nervous system activity.
   B. These compounds are similar to catecholamines in many ways, but differ in potency and efficacy after oral or nasal administration. Alpha receptor effects predominate. Systolic and diastolic elevations in blood pressure may occur. Ephedrine causes mild bronchial muscle relaxation. Topical administration to the mucosal surfaces causes vasoconstriction. CNS effects vary greatly among compounds.

V. Uses:
   A. **Ephedrine, phenylephrine, pseudoephedrine,** and **phenylpropanolamine** (PPA) utilized as decongestants in both prescription and OTC medications. The drugs are frequently used in combination with each other and in conjunction with other compounds, including antihistamines. PPA is used as an anorectic agent.
   B. Illicit use: Recent reports indicate that illicit use of PPA may be on the rise for its amphetamine-like CNS effects. PPA is also commonly combined with caffeine and ephedrine in "look-alike" capsules (see Chapter 68).

VI. Toxic mechanism: Excessive sympathetic nervous system stimulation.

VII. Range of toxicity:
   A. Toxic dose:
      1. Therapeutic/toxic ratio very low (e.g., for PPA the toxic dose is only three times the dose present in some OTC compounds).
      2. Toxicity is generally dose related, though idiosyncratic reactions occur. Simultaneous use of these compounds may result in greater toxicity than expected from simple summation.
   B. Fatal dose:
      1. Minimum lethal dose unknown.
      2. Mean lethal dose (MLD) for children up to age 2 years:
         Ephedrine: 200 mg
         Phenylephrine: 100 mg
         Phenylpropanolamine (PPA): 200 mg
         Pseudoephedrine: 200 mg
      3. Adult MLD is at least 10 times as high as in children.
VIII. Clinical features:
   A. Signs and symptoms of toxicity:
      1. With high doses, signs and symptoms that may be thought of as sympathetic nervous system overstimulation predominate (see Chapter 68 for clinical description).
      2. PPA may cause bradycardia, thought to result from reflex mechanism.
      3. There are several reports of intracranial hemorrhage, presumably secondary to drug-induced hypertension. Vasculitis is also reported with chronic use.
      4. Clinical effects generally last less than 8 hours.
IX. Laboratory findings and evaluation:
   A. Laboratory testing should be based on clinical situation. Consider complete blood cell count, electrolytes, glucose, BUN, creatinine, calcium, arterial blood gases, urinalysis, ECG.
   B. The enzyme multiplication immunoassay technique (EMIT) for commonly abused amphetamines cross reacts weakly with **ephedrine, pseudoephedrine,** and **PPA**. Thin-layer chromatography will identify the specific compound in question, if necessary.
X. Treatment:
   A. Follow APTLS: See Chapter 8.
   B. General management: Table 94–1 (see Chapter 12 for details).
   C. Anxiety:
      1. A quiet, calm environment is recommended. If needed, can give diazepam 15–20 mg PO.
      2. Avoid haloperidol or chlorpromazine; these lower the seizure threshold. However, for severe agitation major tranquilizers may be necessary.
   D. Seizures: See Chapter 22 for treatment recommendations.
   E. Hypertension:
      1. Short-term treatment of extreme hypertension infrequently required.
      2. Any one of several antihypertensives can be used to treat moderate or severe hypertension:
         a. Nifedipine 10 mg sublingually.

TABLE 94–1.

General Treatment

Treatment	Indicated	Of No Value	Contraindicated
O$_2$	±		
IV	+		
ECG monitor	+		
Forced diuresis		X	
Acidification			X
Alkalinization			X
Emesis/lavage	+/+		
Charcoal	+		
Cathartic	+		

    b. Labetalol 10–80 mg IV.

    c. Propranolol 1 mg IV every minute up to 6 mg. If blood pressure increases even further related to unopposed alpha adrenergic effects, may need to add phentolamine.

    d. If the hypertension worsens, dissolve 50 mg sodium nitroprusside in 2–3 ml 5% dextrose in water. Dilute this in 250–1,000 ml 5% dextrose in water. Do not use any other diluent. Administer the drug initially at 0.5 µg/kg/min by infusion pump or other device that permits precise measurement of the rate of flow. Adjust the rate of infusion upward as necessary, but do not exceed 10 µg/kg/min.

    e. If diastolic pressure rises above 120 mm Hg, give hydralazine HCl (Apresoline) 10–20 mg IM or IV. Monitor blood pressure, and repeat initial dose every hour if necessary.

  F. Ventricular arrhythmias:

    1. Propranolol has been reported effective in slowing supraventricular tachyarrhythmias associated with PPA overdose.

    2. Lidocaine (1.0 mg/kg bolus followed by IV infusion) is recommended by some for frequent or symptomatic ventricular ectopy. Use is controversial because of potential for seizures.

    3. Experience with other antiarrhythmics is limited.

XI. Prognosis:

  A. Expected response to treatment: Toxic symptoms are usually self-limited, generally lasting less than 8 hours.

  B. Expected complications and long-term effects: Prolonged use may result in frank psychosis, with recovery requiring weeks or months.

XII. Special considerations:

  A. Patients taking monoamine oxidase inhibitors are at risk for severe hypertensive reactions when given PPA.

  B. Sympathomimetic agents are often found in fixed-combination preparations, such as with antihistamines, which may be overlooked in the patient with a predominantly sympathomimetic symptom complex.

XIII. Disposition considerations:
  A. Admission considerations:
    1. See General Admission Considerations (Chapters 17 and 18).
    2. Major organ symptoms (e.g., cardiac, CNS).
    3. Agitation, paranoid ideation, threatening behavior unresponsive to anxiolytic therapy.
    4. Suicide risk.
    5. ICU:
      a. Chest pain, regardless of age.
      b. ECG changes suggestive of ischemia or ventricular arrhythmia.
      c. Hypertensive crisis.
      d. Uncontrolled tachyarrhythmia with or without hypotension.
      e. Seizures.
  B. Observation period: Symptoms should clear within 8 hours.
  C. Discharge considerations:
    1. General discharge considerations have been met (see Chapters 17 and 18).
    2. Patients with mild to moderate symptoms can be discharged if all symptoms are resolved within an 8-hour observation period.
    3. Patients with accidental overdose from medication error should be appropriately counseled.
    4. Suicide potential and psychiatric status have been appropriately evaluated.

BIBLIOGRAPHY

Bayer MJ, Maskel L: Abuse and toxicity of over-the-counter stimulants. *Emerg Med Rep* 1983; 4:127–132.

Dreisbach RH, Robertson WO: *Handbook of Poisoning.* Norwalk, Conn, Appleton-Century-Crofts, 1987, p 348.

Haddad LM, Winchester JF: *Clinical Management of Poisoning and Drug Overdose.* Philadelphia, WB Saunders Co, 1983.

Kase CS, et al: Intracerebral hemorrhage and phenylpropanolamine use. *Neurology* 1987; 37:399.

Mariani PJ: Pseudoephedrine-induced hypertensive emergency: Treatment with labetalol. *Am J Emerg Med* 1986; 4:141.

Mueller SM: Neurologic complications of phenylpropanolamine use. *Neurology* 1983; 33:650.

Pentel P: Toxicity of over-the-counter stimulants. *JAMA* 1984; 252:1898.

95

Disulfiram

Carol Jack Scott, M.D.

I. Route of exposure: Oral (250, 500 mg tablets).
II. Common generic and trade names:
  A. Generic name: Tetraethylthiuram disulfide.
  B. Common trade names: Antabuse, Disulfiram tablets.
III. Pharmacokinetics:
  A. Absorption: Rapid but incomplete GI absorption.
  B. Onset of action:
    1. **Disulfiram-ethanol reaction:**
      a. During initiation of therapy, as early as 3 hours; usually within 6 hours.
      b. With standard maintenance doses: symptoms within 5–15 minutes of acquiring a blood alcohol level of 5–10 mg/dl.
    2. **Disulfiram alone:**
      a. May have delay of onset of symptoms up to 12 hours, with maximal symptoms in 24 hours.
  C. Duration of action:
    1. **Disulfiram-ethanol reaction:**
      a. Intensity of reaction begins to decrease after 2 hours but may persist as long as ethanol is present in the blood.
      b. 20% of absorbed disulfiram remains in the body 6 days after single 2 gm dose and can cause disulfiram-ethanol reaction.
  D. Peak effect:
    1. **Disulfiram-ethanol reaction:** Peak intensity of reaction occurs within 20–30 minutes.

    E. Elimination:
        1. 80%–90% metabolized by liver.
        2. 5%–20% excreted unchanged in feces.
        3. Most of the remainder excreted in urine as free and esterified sulfates.
        4. One active metabolite, carbon disulfide, partly excreted by the lungs.
    F. Active metabolite: Carbon disulfide.
 IV. Uses: Indicated for chronic alcoholic who **wants** to remain in a state of enforced sobriety so that supportive therapy and psychotherapy can be applied to best advantage.
  V. Toxic mechanism:
    A. **Disulfiram alone:**
        1. Interference with neurotransmitter activity:
           a. Peripheral: Disulfiram and metabolites inhibit norepinephrine synthesis, which can lead to profound hypotension.
           b. Central: Proposed mechanisms include impaired oxygen consumption, sequestration of copper, accumulation of copper, altered brain catecholamine levels.
        2. Hepatic dysfunction:
           a. Transient decrease in liver enzyme activity.
           b. Cholestatic and fulminate hepatitis have been noted.
    B. **Disulfiram-ethanol reaction:**
        1. Symptoms of disulfiram ethanol reaction have been termed "**acetaldehyde reaction**" because acetaldehyde is causative agent of symptoms. Acetaldehyde accumulates due to competition by disulfiram for acetaldehyde dehydrogenase.
        2. Intensity and duration of reaction are subject to individual variation and are proportional to the dosage of both disulfiram and alcohol.
        3. Intrinsic disulfiram toxic effects also contribute to clinical picture in toxicity.
        4. Disulfiram is not considered to increase toxicity of isopropyl alcohol.
        5. Other disulfiram drug interactions: See Table 95–1.
 VI. Range of toxicity:
    A. Toxic dose:
        1. Disulfiram alone:
           a. Adult:
              (1) Acute: Even though in some patients ingestion of 3 gm has proved toxic, there are reports of patients ingesting as much as 22 gm with favorable outcome.
              (2) Chronic: 125 mg/day for 1–5 years may produce symptoms of toxicity.
              (3) Animal experiments indicate that ingestion by an adult of 30 gm disulfiram as a single dose would produce serious toxicity.
           b. Children:
              (1) As little as 2.5 gm may produce serious toxicity.
              (2) Seven reported cases with doses ranging from 3.25 to 10.0 gm have produced toxic effects.
        2. **Disulfiram-ethanol reaction:**
           a. Toxic effects at therapeutic dosages (purpose is to produce these effects).

TABLE 95–1.

Disulfiram Drug Interactions*

Drug	Mechanism
Antipyrine	Inhibits hepatic mixed-function oxidase catalyzed hydroxylation
Benzodiazepines	Decrease clearance, leading to drug accumulation
Coumarin derivatives	Prolong prothrombin time by decreasing biotransformation of coumarin
Digitalis	Increased toxicity related to hypokalemia in disulfiram-ethanol reaction.
Ethylene dibromide	High incidence of carcinogenicity
Isoniazid	Unknown, leading to neurotoxicity
Metronidazole	Visual and auditory hallucinations
Paraldehyde	Metabolism of this acetaldehyde polymer is blocked at acetaldehyde phase
Phenytoin and congeners	Inhibit metabolism, leading to phenytoin toxicity
Primidone	Enhances primidone conversion to phenobarbital
Tricyclic antidepressants	Potentiate disulfiram-ethanol reaction

*Adapted from Goldfrank L, Flomenbaum NE, Lewin NA, et al: *Toxicologic Emergencies*. Norwalk, Conn, Appleton-Century-Crofts, 1986, p 448.

    b. Can occur in disulfiram-treated patients who consume as little as 7 ml alcohol.

B. Fatal dose:

  1. **Disulfiram alone:** No deaths have been reported from ingestion of disulfiram without ingestion of ethanol.

  2. **Disulfiram-ethanol reaction:**

    a. Death may occur at blood ethanol levels 100 mg/dl after ingestion of as little as 0.5–1.0 gm dilsulfiram.

    b. Deaths have occurred when maintenance doses >500 mg/day were taken and at least 150 mg/kg ethanol ingested.

VII. Clinical features:

A. Side effects of **disulfiram alone** in therapeutic dose range:

  1. Initiation of therapy (up to 2 weeks): Drowsiness, fatigue, dysgeucia,

impotence, acneiform or allergic dermatitis, toxic or hypersensitivity hepatitis.
2. Maintenance therapy: Optic neuritis, peripheral neuropathy, fatal hepatic necrosis, ataxia.
B. Four distinct syndromes are associated with disulfiram toxicity:
1. Child: Acute onset only, approximately 12 hours after ingestion: Lethargy or somnolence, weakness/hypotonia/decreased deep tendon reflexes, vomiting, tachycardia, tachypnea, ketosis disproportionate to degree of dehydration (no associated acidosis).
2. Adult: Acute use:
   a. Encephalopathy characterized by one or all of the following: Depression, hallucinations, agitation, seizures, coma, catatonic-like state, parkinsonism, bizarre ideation; EEG abnormalities.
   b. GI: Nausea, vomiting.
3. Adult: Chronic use:
   a. CNS: Anxiety, slurred speech, depression, Babinski reflex, ataxia, impaired concentration, loss of fine motor coordination; abnormal EEG (consistent with metabolic encephalopathy), parkinsonism
   b. Peripheral neuropathy.
   c. GI: Nausea, vomiting, epigastric pain, diarrhea, hepatitis.
   d. Mouth: metal or garlic taste, sulfur odor on breath.
4. **Disulfiram-ethanol reaction:**
   a. Fully developed symptoms may be seen with blood ethanol levels 50 mg/dl.
   b. Severe symptoms may be noted with ethanol levels 125–250 mg/dl.
   c. Reaction possible up to 2 weeks after discontinuing disulfiram.
   d. Signs and symptoms:
      (1) Mild to moderate reaction: Headache (throbbing), flushing (especially face and trunk), nausea, vomiting, abdominal pain, diaphoresis, thirst, confusion, anxiety, vertigo, blurred vision, dyspnea, hyperventilation, orthostatic hypotension, palpitations, tachycardia, conjunctival injection.
      (2) Severe reaction: Respiratory distress, crushing chest pain, ECG changes of myocardial infarction, hypotension, shock, seizures, ventricular and atrial dysrhythmias, death from cardiovascular collapse.
VIII. Laboratory findings and evaluation:
A. Disulfiram levels:
1. Available but do not correlate with severity of illness; only confirm disulfiram ingestion.
2. Rapid reduction and production of metabolites may yield misleading results if only disulfiram measured.
B. Baseline serum studies:
1. Complete blood cell count (evaluation of fatigue).
2. Potassium (often reduced).
3. Liver function tests (rule out hepatic insufficiency).
4. BUN, creatinine.
5. Serum acetone.

6. Serum and urine ketones.
IX. General treatment:
    A. Follow APTLS: (See Chapter 8).
    B. General management: See Chapter 12 for details.
        1. **Disulfiram alone:** Table 95–2.
        2. Disulfiram-ethanol reaction:
            a. No specific antidote.
            b. 95% oxygen and 5% carbon dioxide (recommended by manufacturer of Antabuse; however, written recommendation not referenced and therapeutic efficacy not documented).
            c. Oral or IV potassium if indicated.
            d. Monitor for signs and symptoms of myocardial ischemia.
X. Specific treatment:
    A. Seizures: Diazepam and phenytoin (see Chapter 22).
    B. Hypotension:
        1. See Chapter 10.
        2. If needed, vasopressor of choice is norepinephrine.
XI. Prognosis:
    A. Expected response to treatment:
        1. **Disulfiram only:**
            a. Outcome in **children** has generally been poor. Of seven reported cases, only three had complete recovery; the others had neurologic sequelae.
            b. **Acute adult** disulfiram use: Complete recovery with resolution of symptoms, usually within weeks, with no adverse sequelae.
            c. **Chronic adult** disulfiram use at therapeutic dosages: 2.2% incidence of reversible toxic encephalopathy.
        2. **Disulfiram-ethanol reaction:** Sudden death may occur up to 24 hours after ingesting ethanol. However, prognosis is good with appropriate supportive care.

TABLE 95–2.

General Treatment

Treatment	Indicated	Of No Value	Contraindicated
O_2	±		
IV	+		
ECG monitor	±		
Forced diuresis		X	
Acidification			X
Alkalinization		X	
Emesis*			X
Lavage	+		
Charcoal†	+		
Cathartic	+		

*No ipecac; all brands contain alcohol.
†Repeat every 4 hours.

    B. Expected complications and long-term effects: Hepatitis, optic neuritis, parkinsonism, peripheral neuropathy, encephalopathy, hypotension, seizures.

XII. Special considerations:

    A. In children, history of disulfiram use may be hard to elicit. Must question adult household members carefully regarding disulfiram use in cases of children with metabolic encephalopathy of unknown origin.

    B. If history of ethanol or alcohol contact absolutely ruled out in patients taking disulfiram, consider cough syrups, sauces, vinegars, elixirs, liniments, and lotions in patients with signs and symptoms suggestive of disulfiram-ethanol reaction.

    C. May potentiate phenytoin toxicity.

    D. Encephalopathy, psychosis: Experimental work has been done with use of 4-methylpyrazone to block alcohol dehydrogenase, thereby decreasing production of acetaldehyde.

    E. Other drugs may act similarly to disulfiram:

        1. Antimicrobial agents:
            Cephalosporins (cefoperazone, moxalactam, cefamandole)
            Chloramphenicol
            Furazolidone
            Griseofulvin
            Metronidazole (Flagyl)
            Quinacrine

        2. Industrial agents:
            Carbon disulfide
            Hydrogen sulfide
            Tetraethyl lead
            Tetramethylthiuram disulfide

        3. Oral hypoglycemic agents:
            Acetohexamide (Dymelor)
            Chlorpropamide (Diabinase)
            Glipizide (Glucotrol)
            Glyburide (DiaBeta, Micronase)
            Phenformin (DBI, no longer available in United States)
            Tolazomide (Tolinase)
            Tolbutamide (Orinase)

        4. Miscellaneous:
            Procarbazine
            Mushrooms *(Corprinus atramentarius, Clitocybe clavipes)*
            Calcium carbimide (Canadian equivalent of Antabuse, Temposil)

        5. Calcium cyanamide:
            Animal charcoal
            Butanal oxime

XIII. Disposition considerations:

    A. Admission considerations:

        1. See General Admission Considerations (Chapters 17 and 18).

        2. **Disulfiram alone:**
          a. All children.
          b. Acute psychosis.

    c. Any complication.

    d. Suicidal risk.

    e. Inability to observe up to 12 hours.

  3. **Disulfiram-ethanol reaction:**

    a. Symptomatic longer than 2 hours with supportive measures

    b. ICU: ECG findings suggestive of myocardial ischemia or cardiac dysrhythmia.

B. Consultation considerations:

  1. Patients who ingest ethanol while taking disulfiram should be seen by alcohol counselor.

  2. Patients with neuropsychiatric symptoms, consider psychiatric or neurology consultation.

C. Observation period:

  1. **Disulfiram only:** Mild to moderate symptoms require minimum of 12 hours of observation.

  2. Adult **disulfiram-ethanol reaction:** May require admission if mild to moderate symptoms last longer than 2 hours.

D. Discharge considerations:

  1. General discharge considerations are met (Chapters 17 and 18).

  2. See also Chapter 25.

  3. Asymptomatic after appropriate observation period.

  4. With disulfiram-ethanol reaction, appropriate alcohol counseling and follow-up should be arranged.

  5. Patients should be told to avoid ethanol up to 2 weeks after discontinuing disulfiram.

BIBLIOGRAPHY

Benitz WE, Tatro DS: Disulfiram intoxication in a child. *J Pediatr* 1984; 105:487–489.

Brown CG: The alcohol withdrawal syndrome. *Ann Emerg Med* 1982; 11:276–280.

Goldfrank LR, Flomenbaum NE, Lewin NA, et al: *Toxicologic Emergencies.* Norwalk, Conn, Appleton-Century-Crofts, 1986, p 447.

Hillbom ME, Shrviharju MS, Lindros KO: Potentiation of ethanol by cyanamide in relation to acetaldehyde accumulation. *Toxicol Appl Pharmacol* 1983; 70:133–139.

Hotson JT: Disulfiram-induced encephalopathy. *Arch Neurol* 1976; 33:141–142.

Kane F: Carbon disulfide intoxication from overdose of disulfiram. *Am J Psychiatry* 1970; 127:690–694.

Kirubabakaran V. Case report of acute disulfiram overdose. *Am J Psychiatry* 1983; 140:1513–1514.

McEvoy GK: Drug Reactions, in *American Hospital Formulary.* Bethesda, Md, American Society of Hospital Pharmacists, 1987, pp 2023–2025.

Rainey JM: Disulfiram toxicity and carbon disulfide poisoning. *Am J Psychiatry* 1977; 134:371–378.

Rumack B: Disulfiram. *Topics in Emergency Medicine.* Rockville, Md, Aspen Systems Corp, 1984; 6:30–37.

Stowell A, Johnsen J, Ripel A, et al: Disulfiram-induced acetonemia. *Lancet* 1983; 1:882–883.

Watson CP, Ashby P: Disulfiram neuropathy. *Can Med Assoc J* 1980; 123:123–126.

Woolley B: Acute disulfiram overdoses. *J Stud Alcohol* 1980; 41:740.

96

Antidiarrheal Agents

J. Andrew Sumner, M.D., F.A.C.E.P.

I. Route of exposure: Oral.
II. Common preparations:
   A. Opioids:
      1. Diphenoxylate with atropine (Lomotil).
      2. Loperamide (Imodium).
      3. Codeine.
      4. Tincture of opium.
      5. Paregoric.
   B. Antisecretory agents: Bismuth subsalicylate (Pepto-Bismol)
   C. Hydrophilic substances: Methylcellulose and adsorbent powders such as kaopectate are nontoxic.
III. Pharmacokinetics:
   A. Opioids:
      1. Slow gastrointestinal motility and prolong transit time, allowing time for absorption of water and electrolytes from the intestinal lumen.
      2. **Codeine** reacts with central opiate receptors that regulate intestinal motility.
      3. **Loperamide** is structurally similar to both haloperidol and diphenoxylate. Effect on GI motility is similar to that of diphenoxylate, and loperamide may decrease intestinal secretion by inactivating the calcium-dependent regulatory protein calmodulin.
      4. **Lomotil** has a chemical structure similar to that of meperidine.
   B. Antisecretory agents: **Bismuth subsalicylate** binds toxins produced by *Vibrio cholera* and *Escherichia coli,* with antimicrobial activity in vitro and

in vivo. Subsalicylate salt is hydrolyzed by coliforms to produce salicylate, which inhibits prostaglandin synthesis responsible for intestinal inflammation and hypermotility. Salicylates may also have antisecretory actions and stimulate reabsorption of fluids by the intestine.

IV. Toxic mechanism: See Chapters 67, 76, 91.

V. Range of toxicity:

A. **Lomotil:**
1. Very narrow range between therapeutic and toxic doses; 10 mg diphenoxylate is equal to 30 mg codeine and represents the maximum daily dose for a child older than 2 years.
2. Toxicity may result from a few tablets, possibly even a single tablet in a child.
3. **Contraindicated** in children younger than 2 years of age.
4. Death has resulted in a 2-year-old child after a 12-tablet ingestion.
5. Toxicity related to narcotic effects, and only rarely is it necessary to specifically treat atropinic effects.

B. **Pepto-Bismol:**
1. Bismuth subsalicylate salt is water insoluble, thus very poorly absorbed, producing almost no bismuth toxicity from a single, large-dose exposure.
2. Doses >0.6–2.0 gm every 6–8 hours could result in GI disturbances, mucous membrane discoloration, renal failure.
3. Recommended daily dose of suspension, 240 ml, contains 2.1 gm **salicylate;** large doses could result in salicylate toxicity.
4. Tablet form contains 350 mg **calcium carbonate,** which occasionally causes hypercalcemia when 2 gm calcium per day are ingested chronically; acute single ingestions of calcium salts may produce mild GI distress, but hypercalcemia has not been reported.

VI. Clinical features:

A. **Lomotil:**
1. Very weak analgesic effect.
2. High doses in the 40–60 mg range produce euphoria and morphine-like physical dependence after chronic administration.
3. Virtually insoluble in aqueous solution, obviating potential for parenteral abuse. Atropine, which is a component, should reduce abuse potential.
4. Lomotil overdose produces mixed narcotic and atropine clinical features:
   a. Early findings (first 3 hours) primarily related to atropine toxicity (see Chapter 91).
      (1) Dilated pupils expected, but often they are miotic as a result of overriding narcotic effects of diphenoxylate.
   b. After 3 hours:
      (1) Respiratory depression with hypotension and hypothermia.
      (2) Urinary retention frequently present, and atropine may be reabsorbed.
      (3) Gastric emptying delayed, and paralytic ileus common.
      (4) Major seizures associated with hypoxia may occur.

B. **Loperamide:**
  1. More serious untoward effects, such as respiratory depression and disturbed level of consciousness, not encountered with usual antidiarrheal doses.
  2. All opioid antidiarrheal agents are likely to produce classic symptoms of respiratory and CNS depression (see Chapter 67).
     a. Toxic megacolon should be considered in patients with inflammatory bowel disease or acute colitis of various origin.
     b. Fluid may be sequestered in dilated loops of bowel when acute infectious diarrhea is present.
     c. Hepatic coma may be precipitated in patients with severe liver disease.
  3. Dystonic reactions are uncommon but have been reported with toxic doses of loperamide, which is chemically structurally similar to haloperidol.
C. **Pepto-Bismol:**
  1. Rarely toxic.
  2. See Range of Toxicity
VII. Laboratory findings and evaluation:
  A. Toxicology screen **may not detect diphenoxylate** because of rapid conversion to diphenoxylic acid. Helpful for other opioids and salicylate level.
  B. Radiographs may show toxic megacolon, free air under diaphragm, dilated bowel loops with air-fluid levels, radiopaque bismuth, pulmonary edema.
  C. See specific chapters for recommendations (Chapters 67 and 76).
VIII. General treatment:
  A. Follow APTLS: (See Chapter 8).
  B. General management: Table 96–1 (see Chapters 12 and 13 for details).

TABLE 96–1.

General Treatment

Treatment	Indicated	Of No Value	Contraindicated
O_2	±		
IV	+		
ECG monitor	±		
Forced diuresis			X
Acidification		X	
Alkalinization		X	
Emesis*	±		
Lavage	±		
Charcoal†	±		
Cathartic‡			X

*Use emesis with precaution; may not be effective with many antidiarrheals containing anticholinergic agents.
†May not be effective with liquid preparations.
‡Most antidiarrhea agents slow gut motility, and toxicity may lead to ileus; best to avoid administering a cathartic.

IX. Specific management:
   A. Specific antiopiate measures with intravenous naloxone (see Chapter 67).
   B. Physostigmine rarely indicated for atropine toxicity, only for life-threatening emergencies such as myoclonic seizures, severe hallucinations, hypertension, arrhythmias (see Chapter 91).
   C. Bladder catheterization indicated because of likelihood of urinary retention and reabsorption of atropine.
   D. Appropriate fluid administration (fluid volume may be sequestered in gut).
   E. Close monitoring for 24 hours because of delayed symptoms and cyclical nature of respiratory depression.
X. Prognosis: Excellent with proper management and early diagnosis.
XI. Disposition considerations:
   A. Admission considerations:
      1. See General Admission Considerations (Chapters 17 and 18).
      2. Most patients should be admitted if symptoms severe, especially if overdose deliberate.
      3. For ingestions with more than one component (narcotic/anticholinergic/salicylates), see chapters on specific ingestions for suggested admission considerations.
      4. Children should be closely observed for 24 hours following Lomotil ingestion.
      5. Suicide risk.
   B. Observation period:
      1. Symptomatic patients with **Lomotil** or **loperamide** overdose should be admitted and not observed in the emergency department.
      2. Asymptomatic patients with **loperamide** or **Lomotil** ingestions should be observed for a minimum of 6 hours.
   C. Discharge considerations:
      1. General discharge considerations have been met (see Chapters 17 and 18).
      2. Asymptomatic.
      3. If overdose a medication error, patient or responsible caregiver understands new instructions for medication use.
      4. Suicide potential and psychiatric status have been appropriately evaluated.

BIBLIOGRAPHY

Rumack B, Temple A: Lomotil poisoning. *Pediatrics* 1974; 53:495–500.

97

Antacids

J. Andrew Sumner, M.D., F.A.C.E.P.

I. Route of exposure: Oral.
II. Common trade names: See Table 97–1.
III. Pharmacokinetics:
   A. Widely variable capacity to neutralize hydrochloric acid in stomach. Used in treatment of peptic ulcer disease and a variety of functional symptoms such as heartburn or indigestion.
   B. Systemic absorbed antacids capable of producing metabolic alkalosis because of appreciable absorption of cationic moiety.
   C. Nonsystemic antacids do not tend to cause systemic alkalosis because cationic moiety in the intestine forms insoluble basic compounds that are not absorbed.
   D. Aluminum hydroxide is used to treat hyperphosphatemia.
IV. Toxic mechanism:
   A. Absorption of HCO_3 (alkalemia).
   B. Magnesium salts (laxative effect) lead to diarrhea and volume loss.
   C. Nephrolithiasis (particularly in renal failure):
      1. Compounds containing $CaCO_3$ (AlternaGEL, Amphojel, Basaljel) in the face of hypercalciuria and alkaluria predipose to nephrolithiasis.
      2. Systemically absorbed antacids with $NaHCO_3$ can have similar effect.
      3. Magnesium trisilicate may lead to kidney stone formation after chronic exposure.
V. Range of toxicity: Low order of toxicity, with rare toxic ingestions. Problems mainly associated with chronic ingestion, particularly in patients with renal failure.

TABLE 97–1.

Composition of Common Antacids

Trade	Active Ingredient		
	$Al(OH)_3$	$CaCO_3$	Other
Single entity			
AlternaGEL	+	−	
Amphogel	+	−	
Basaljel	+	−	
Milk of Magnesia	−	+	
Rolaids			Dihydroxyaluminum, $NaCO_3$
Tums	−	+	
Compound			
Di-Gel	+	+	Simethicone
Gaviscon	+	−	NaAlginate, $MgCO_3$, Alginic acid
Gelusil	+	+	Simethicone
Maalox	+	+	
Maalox Plus	+	+	Simethicone
Mylanta	+	+	Simethicone
Riopan	−	−	Magaldrate*

*Complex of aluminum and magnesium hydroxides.

VI. Clinical features:
   A. Diarrhea (magnesium salts).
   B. Constipation (aluminum salts).
   C. Nephrolithiasis in renal insufficiency.
   D. Dialysis dementia (altered mental status) in renal failure (aluminum salts).
   E. Intestinal obstruction, fecal impaction (aluminum salts).
   F. Milk-alkali syndrome (calcium carbonate plus sodium bicarbonate).
VII. Laboratory findings and evaluation:
   A. Blood:
      1. Arterial blood gases or electrolytes (metabolic alkalosis).
      2. Chemistry: Calcium, magnesium, phosphate (hypercalcemia, hypermagnesemia in renal patients, acute phosphate depletion), BUN, creatinine.
   B. ECG: Arrhythmias secondary to electrolyte disturbances.
   C. Abdominal films: Check for abdominal calcifications, rule out intestinal obstruction.
VIII. General treatment:
   A. Follow APTLS: See Chapter 8.
   B. General management: Table 97–2 (see Chapters 12 and 13 for details).
IX. Specific management: Largely supportive, with correction of alkalosis and electrolyte disturbances.
X. Prognosis:
   A. Expected response to treatment: Generally very good, depending on underlying renal status and associated medical problems.

TABLE 97–2.

General Treatment

Treatment	Indicated	Of No Value	Contraindicated
O_2	±		
IV	+		
ECG monitor	+		
Forced diuresis		X	
Acidification*		X	
Alkalinization			X
Emesis/lavage	± / ±		
Charcoal	±		
Cathartic	–		

*Not indicated for enhanced elimination. Alkalemia is unlikely to be so severe as to require infusion of acid.

XI. Disposition considerations:
   A. Admission considerations: See General admission considerations (Chapters 17 and 18).
   B. Consultation considerations:
      1. Nephrologist or internist for renal failure.
      2. Urology for nephrolithiasis.
      3. General surgeon for intestinal obstruction.
   C. Discharge considerations:
      1. General discharge considerations have been met (see Chapters 17 and 18).
      2. Suicide potential and psychiatric status have been appropriately evaluated.

BIBLIOGRAPHY

Berlyne GM: Aluminum toxicity in renal failure. *Int J Artif Organs* 1980; 3:60–61.

Drake D, Hollander D: Neutralizing capacity and cost effectiveness of antacids. *Ann Intern Med* 1981; 94:215–217.

Dukes MNG: *Meyler's Side Effects of Drugs,* vol 8. Amsterdam, Excerpta Medica, 1975.

Handbook of Nonprescription Drugs, ed 5. Washington, D.C., American Pharmaceutic Association, 1977.

Hewitt GJ, Benham ES: A complication of Gaviscon in a neonate—The gavisconoma. *Aust Paediatr J* 1976; 12:47–48.

Morrissey JF, Barrera RF: Antacid therapy. *N Engl J Med* 1974; 290:550–554.

Peterson WL, Sturdevant RAL, Franke HD: Healing of duodenal ulcer with an antacid regimen. *N Engl J Med* 1977; 297:341.

Townsend CM, Remmers AR, Sarles HE: Intestine: Obstruction from medication bezoar in patients with renal failure. *N Engl J Med* 1973; 288:1058.

98

Antimicrobial Agents

Timothy J. Rittenberry, M.D., F.A.C.E.P.

General Considerations

I. Poisoning from antibiotics rarely causes death.
II. Primary symptom is usually gastrointestinal.
III. Capable of producing hypersensitivity reactions:
    1. Rash (see Chapter 39).
    2. Stevens-Johnson syndrome (e.g., cephalexin, chloroquine, clindamycine, co-trimazole, griseofulvin, isoniazid, penicillins, rifampin, quinine, sulfacetamide sodium, sulfonamides, tetracycline).
    3. Anaphylaxis (see Chapter 24).

Chloramphenicol

I. Route of exposure: Oral, intramuscular, intravenous, otic and ophthalmic ointments and solutions.
II. Common name: Chloromycetin.
III. Pharmacokinetics:
    A. Absorption:
        1. Readily absorbed orally.
        2. Oral bioavailability 75%–90%.
    B. Plasma half-life: 1.5–3.5 hours.
    C. Peak effect: Approximately 2 hours.
    D. Elimination: Inactivated in liver by glucuronidation and hydrolysis; 90% of these products then excreted in urine.

IV. Action:
    A. Interferes with bacterial protein synthesis.
    B. Inhibits mitochondrial protein synthesis and oxidative phosphorylation in mammalian cells.
V. Uses: Broad-spectrum antibiotic.
VI. Toxic mechanism:
    A. Bone marrow depression:
        1. Dose-related, characterized by reticulocytopenia and leukopenia.
        2. Idiopathic aplastic anemia.
VII. Dosage:
    A. Therapeutic dosage:
        1. 50–100 mg/kg/day in patients older than 4 weeks, up to 2 gm.
        2. 50 mg/kg/day in 1–4-week-old infants.
        3. 25 mg/kg/day in preterm and newborn infants.
    B. Toxic dosage: >50–100 mg/kg.
    C. Fatal dose: Report of severe GI symptoms (vomiting, diarrhea) and shock followed by death in neonate given >25 mg/kg/day.
VIII. Clinical features:
    A. Vital signs: Hypotension, hypothermia.
    B. GI: Nausea and vomiting, diarrhea, hepatitis, abdominal distention.
    C. Neurologic: Optic and peripheral neuritis.
    D. Renal impairment.
    E. Hematologic:
        1. Blood dyscrasias (reversible anemia, thrombocytopenia, granulocytopenia): dose dependent, reversible.
        2. Aplastic anemia: 1 in 50,000. Not dose related.
        3. Hemolysis in glucose-6-phosphate dehydrogenase deficiency.
    F. Metabolic acidosis early sign of toxicity.
    G. Other:
        1. Gray (baby) syndrome:
            a. 50–100 mg/kg in preterm and newborn infants.
            b. Abdominal distention, vomiting, pallor, circulatory collapse.
        2. Mucous membrane lesions, toxemia.
IX. Laboratory findings and evaluation:
    A. Serum chloramphenical levels:
        1. 10–20 μg/kg therapeutic.
        2. Serum levels >50 μg/ml associated with increased toxicity.
    B. Complete blood cell count (see Clinical features).
    C. Arterial blood gas and electrolytes (metabolic acidosis early sign of toxicity).
    D. Renal function tests (BUN, creatinine, urinalysis).
    E. Liver function studies (transaminases, bilirubin).
X. Treatment:
    A. Follow APTLS: See Chapter 8.
    B. General management: Table 98–1 (see Chapters 12 and 13 for details).
    C. Specific management:
        1. Symptomatic and supportive.
        2. Maintain urine output 3–6 ml/kg/hr.

TABLE 98–1.

General Treatment

Treatment	Indicated	Of No Value	Contraindicated
O$_2$	±		
IV	+		
ECG monitor	±		
Forced diuresis		X	
Acidification			X
Alkalinization		X	
Emesis/lavage	+/+		
Charcoal	+		
Cathartic	+		
Dialysis*		X	

*No value because of short half-life of drug.

3. Periodic monitoring of complete blood cell count and renal function.
4. Charcoal hemoperfusion may be helpful in deteriorating patient.
5. Consider exchange transfusion in infants.
XI. Prognosis:
   A. One in 50,000 patients develops aplastic anemia.
   B. Other complications: Optic and peripheral neuritis.
XII. Special considerations: Caution should be used in administration of chloramphenicol in patients with liver or kidney injury.
XIII. Disposition considerations:
   A. Admission considerations:
      1. See General Admission Considerations (Chapters 17 and 18).
      2. Serum level >50 µg/ml.
      3. Ingestion >50–100 mg/kg.
      4. Symptomatic.
      5. Metabolic acidosis.
      6. Evidence of myelosuppression.
      7. Suicide risk.
      8. Child abuse or neglect.
   B. Consultation considerations:
      1. Hematologist for consideration of exchange transfusion for massive overdose in infants and children.
      2. Neonatologist for evaluation of gray-baby syndrome.
      3. Nephrologist if hemoperfusion being considered.
      4. Consider neurologist for evaluation of optic and peripheral neuritis.
   C. Observation period: None. All symptomatic patients should be admitted. All asymptomatic patients with significant ingestion should be admitted (see Admission considerations).
   D. Discharge considerations:
      1. General discharge considerations have been met (Chapters 17 and 18).
      2. Insignificant ingestion.

3. Asymptomatic.
4. Appropriate follow-up arranged.
5. Child abuse or neglect has been considered and evaluated.
6. Suicide potential and psychiatric state have been evaluated.

Chloroquine

I. Route of exposure: Oral.
II. Common generic and trade names:
   A. Chloroquine (Aralen).
   B. Related compounds:
     Hydroxychloroquine (Plaquenil)
     Quinacrine (Atabrine)
     Primaquine
III. Pharmacokinetics:
   A. Absorption: Oral bioavailability is 90%
   B. Plasma half-life:
     1. Complex clearance profile:
       a. Triphasic decay with initial half-life of about 5 days.
       b. Half-life of final phase 60 days.
   C. Peak effect: 6 hours.
   D. Elimination: 20% of oral dose excreted in urine.
IV. Action:
   A. Mechanism of action not well defined.
   B. Enzyme inhibition, antihistamine effects, blocks DNA and RNA synthesis.
   C. Concentrated in parasitized erythrocytes.
   D. Primaquine, quinacrine act as oxidants.
V. Uses: Treatment and prophylaxis of malaria, hepatic amebic abscess, and occasionally inflammatory disorders such as rheumatoid arthritis, systemic lupus erythematosus, and other collagen disorders.
VI. Toxic mechanism: Chloroquine has direct toxic effects on myocardium and is the usual mechanism of fatal cardiac arrest.
VII. Range of toxicity:
   A. Therapeutic dose:
     1. Chloroquin:
       a. 500 mg tablet chloraquine (Aralen) contains 300 mg base.
       b. 5 mg base/kg not to exceed 300 mg base per week for chemosuppression, and 1 gm followed by 500 mg/day for 3 days in acute attack.
     2. Primaquine: 26.3 mg/day for 14 days.
   B. Fatal dose:
     1. Chloroquine: 50 mg/kg for adults, 20 mg/kg for children younger than 2 years.
     2. Case reports of death occurring after ingestion of just 1 or 2 tablets.
VIII. Clinical features:
   A. Rapidly progressive. May be fatal in 1–2 hours.
   B. Patients may complain of nausea, vomiting, visual blurring, diplopia.

C. CNS symptoms are prominent and include hyperexcitability, agitation, dizziness, psychosis, seizures.
D. Hematologic abnormalities include methemoglobinemia, hemolysis.
E. Rapid progression may occur, to hypotension, shock, coma, respiratory or cardiac arrest.
F. Irreversible retinal damage has been reported in some patients receiving long-term or high-dose chloroquine therapy. Retinopathy is probably dose dependent. Such patients may be asymptomatic or complain of scotomas, field defects, or misty vision. Patients may also have reversible corneal changes (transient edema or opaque deposits in cornea). These patients may be asymptomatic or complain of visual halos, difficulty focusing, blurred vision.

IX. Laboratory findings and evaluation:
   A. Serum levels: Not useful in acute setting.
   B. Other laboratory tests:
      1. Complete blood cell count (hemolysis)
      2. Methemoglobin level.
      3. Arterial blood gas (if symptomatic).
      4. Electrolytes (vomiting, acidosis, volume depletion).
      5. ECG.

X. General treatment:
   A. Follow APTLS: Chapter 8.
   B. General management: Table 98–2 (see Chapters 12 and 13 for details).
   C. Rapid and aggressive therapy crucial, followed by good supportive care.

XI. Specific management:
   A. Recent work suggests that combining **early mechanical ventilation** with administration of **diazepam and epinephrine** may be effective in treatment of severe chloroquine poisoning. Treatment based on experimental findings that epinephrine counteracts cardiovascular effects of chloroquine and diazepam has been demonstrated experimentally to de-

TABLE 98–2.

General Treatment

Treatment	Indicated	Of No Value	Contraindicated
O$_2$	+		
IV	+		
ECG monitor	+		
Forced diuresis			X
Acidification			X
Alkalinization		X	
Emesis*/lavage	+/+		
Charcoal	+		
Cathartic	+		
Other			

*Caution: Symptoms may progress rapidly; lavage preferred.

crease toxic effects and mortality related to chloroquine (Riou B: *N Engl J Med* 1988; 318:1–6).
B. Seizures and hypotension: See Chapters 10 and 22 for treatment suggestions.
C. Methemoglobinemia: See Chapter 102 for treatment recommendations.
D. Charcoal hemoperfusion of use in deteriorating patient.
E. Hemodialysis, peritoneal dialysis not useful.
XII. Prognosis:
A. Expected response to treatment:
1. Severe chloroquine poisoning usually fatal, with death occurring 1–3 hours after ingestion.
2. Survival for 48 hours is associated with good prognosis.
B. Expected complications and long-term effects:
1. Few permanent complications if good supportive care provided quickly.
2. Possibility of permanent retinal injury.
XIII. Disposition considerations:
A. Admission considerations:
1. See General Admission Considerations (Chapters 17 and 18).
2. All ingestions approaching 50 mg/kg or of unknown amount, regardless of symptoms.
3. All symptomatic patients.
4. Suicide risk.
B. Consultation considerations:
1. Nephrologist for consideration of charcoal hemoperfusion for patients deteriorating despite good supportive measures.
2. Ophthalmology consultation for patients developing or at risk for developing retinopathy.
C. Observation period: None. All patients with chloroquine overdose should be admitted.
D. Discharge considerations: None. All patients with chloroquine overdose should be admitted.

Isoniazid

I. Route of exposure: Oral (tablets and syrup), injectable.
II. Common trade names:
INH
Laniazid
Nydrazid
PIN Forte
Teebaconin
Rimactane
Rifamate.
III. Pharmacokinetics:
A. Absorption: 90% orally absorbed.
B. Plasma half-life: 1–3 hours.

    C. Peak effect: 2 hours (0.7–2 hours in "rapid acetylators").

    D. Elimination:

        1. Predominantly metabolized via acetylation by liver. Both unchanged INH and metabolites are excreted in urine.

        2. Rapid acetylation (autosomal dominant trait) results in serum half-life 0.7–2 hours, compared with 2–4 hours in "slow acetylators" (approximately 60% of all blacks are slow acetylators).

    E. Active metabolites: INH has toxic metabolites.

  IV. Action: Mechanism of action unknown.

   V. Uses: Used independently for chemoprophylaxis of tuberculosis or as part of combination regimen in treating active tuberculosis.

  VI. Toxic mechanism:

    A. Decreases brain gamma aminobutyric acid (GABA) and lowers seizure threshold.

    B. Depletes pyridoxine (vitamin B_6) stores needed for GABA synthesis.

 VII. Range of toxicity:

    A. Toxic dose:

        1. Maximum daily dose: 10 mg/kg or total 300 mg.

        2. 15 mg/kg results in lowered seizure threshold. May induce seizures in patients with previous seizure disorder.

        3. 30–40 mg/kg may result in seizures even without predisposition.

        4. Toxicity at lower doses in patients with preexisting seizure disorder, vitamin B_6 deficiency, chronic alcoholism.

    B. Fatal dose: 30–150 mg/kg if untreated.

VIII. Clinical features:

    A. Typical presentation: Classic triad of "INH overdose syndrome":

        1. Initial lag period of 1–3 hours after ingestion.

        2. Followed by symptoms of nausea, vomiting, dizziness, slurred speech.

        3. After 1–3 hours, generalized seizures, coma, severe metabolic (lactic) acidosis.

    B. Additional findings:

        1. CNS: Altered mentation and depressed sensorium.

        2. Cardiovascular: Tachycardia, hypotension.

        3. Oliguria, acetonuria.

        4. Lactic acidosis, hyperkalemia (mild), hyperglycemia.

        5. Jaundice (chronic exposure).

  IX. Laboratory findings and evaluation:

    A. Serum isoniazid level:

        1. Therapeutic range: 5–8 μg/ml.

        2. Toxicity defined as blood level >30 μg/ml.

        3. Acetylated form not measured.

    B. Other laboratory tests:

        1. Liver function studies (transaminases, bilirubin).

        2. Blood glucose (check for hyperglycemia).

        3. Electrolytes (check for hyperkalemia).

        4. Arterial blood gases, serum lactate level (lactic acidosis).

   X. Treatment:

    A. Follow APTLS: See Chapter 8.

B. General management: Table 98–3 (see Chapters 12 and 13 for details).
C. Respiratory support: See Chapter 9.
XI. Specific management:
  A. Seizures and hypotension:
    1. Pyridoxine: See below.
    2. Diazepam: See Chapter 22 for dosing details.
    3. Hemodialysis.
    4. General anesthesia with halothane or thiopental.
    5. NOTE: **Phenytoin contraindicated:** Interferes with INH metabolism. Has been shown to be ineffective in INH-induced seizures.
  B. Pyridoxine:
    1. Infuse pyridoxine mixed as 5% or 10% solution with D_5W or normal saline over 30–60 minutes.
    2. Goal is to give pyridoxine equivalent by weight to INH ingested (i.e., gram-for-gram bolus of pyridoxine if isoniazid dose known).
    3. Unknown ingestions treated with single dose of 5 gm pyridoxine.
    4. Dose should be repeated in 15 minutes if patient has failed to respond.
  C. Metabolic acidosis: Sodium bicarbonate. Maintain serum pH >7.2.
XII. Special considerations: Both higher incidence and more severe form of toxicity might be expected in slow acetylators.
XIII. Prognosis:
  A. Expected response to treatment:
    1. Acidosis often refractory to treatment.
    2. Survival for 24 hours associated with complete recovery.
    3. Prompt use of pyridoxine can effectively control seizures and may result in rapid regaining of consciousness within 30 minutes–2 hours after administration. Additional anticonvulsants may be unnecessary.
  B. Expected complications and long-term effects: Hepatic injury; may be irreversible.
XIV. Controversies: Some authors have recommended phenobarbital as an alternative to diazepam in treatment of INH-induced seizures; others caution that phenobarbital will increase metabolism of isoniazid to toxic metabolites.

TABLE 98–3.

General Treatment

Treatment	Indicated	Of No Value	Contraindicated
O_2	±		
IV	+		
ECG monitor	+		
Forced diuresis*		X	
Acidification			X
Alkalinization*		X	
Emesis/lavage	+/+		
Charcoal	+		
Cathartic	+		

*Suggested by some authorities but never shown to be clinically effective.

XV. Disposition considerations:
  A. Admission considerations:
    1. See General Admission Considerations (Chapters 17 and 18).
    2. >15 mg/kg ingested.
    3. Symptomatic.
    4. Suicide risk.
  B. Consultation considerations:
    1. Nephrologist if seizures and acidosis not controllable with bicarbonate, pyridoxine, and diazepam, for consideration of dialysis.
    2. Anesthesiologist for seizures unresponsive to emergency department treatment.
  C. Observation period: Cannot make specific recommendations for this drug. Onset of symptoms should occur within 3 hours of ingestion.
  D. Discharge considerations:
    1. General disposition considerations have been met (see Chapters 17 and 18).
    2. Suicide potential and psychiatric status have been appropriately evaluated.

Penicillins and Cephalosporins

  I. Route of exposure: Oral, intravenous.
  II. Pharmacokinetics:
  A. Absorption: Absorbed well orally.
  B. Plasma half-life: 0.5–2 hours.
  C. Peak effect: Approximately 1 hour.
  D. Elimination: Eliminated unchanged by renal tubular excretion.
  E. Active metabolites: After administration of isoxazolyl penicillins (e.g., oxacillin, dicloxacillin).
  III. Action: Inhibition of muramic acid synthesis on bacterial wall.
  IV. Uses: Bacteriostatic or bacteriocidal activity.
  V. Toxic mechanism:
  A. Acute hypersensitivity may occur, with fatal anaphylactic reaction.
  B. In addition, rapid IV infusion of penicillin can lead to hyperkalemia (e.g., potassium benzylpenicillin) and neurotoxicity (may be seen when high doses are administered in presence of diminished renal function).
  VI. Range of toxicity:
  A. Toxicity rare in oral ingestion with normal renal function.
  B. Increased toxicity in parenteral administration with impaired renal function.
    1. 6 gm IV penicillin has caused seizure and coma.
  C. Dermatologic, hematologic, and renal abnormalities with doses of cephaloridine >4 gm/day.
  VII. Clinical features:
  A. Arrhythmias with rapid infusion of potassium salts (e.g., penicillin VK).
  B. Seizures, vertigo, tinnitus, hallucinations, muscle twitching with high doses.

C. Acute renal failure (rare).
D. Hypersensitivity reactions:
   1. Rash (especially with ampicillin).
   2. Respiratory distress (bronchospasm).
   3. Anaphylaxis (particularly in patients given penicillin VK who are also taking beta blockers).
E. GI disturbances.
F. Disulfiram-like reactions possible when ethanol ingested with **moxalactam, cefamandole, cefoperazone.**
G. Toxic psychosis may occur as result of cerebral edema secondary to allergic reaction or as result of inadvertent intravascular administration of **procaine penicillin G.** Reaction after IV administration of procaine penicillin G includes fear of impending death; auditory, visual, and taste disturbances; dizziness; tachycardia, palpitations; confusion, disorientation. Incidence of toxic psychosis secondary to intravascular administration of procaine penicillin G estimated to be between 0.1%–0.3%.
H. Hematologic: Rare events. Includes hemolytic or nonhemolytic anemia, aplastic anemia (extremely rare), eosinophilia, leukocytosis, leukopenia, neutropenia, pancytopenia, nonthrombocytopenic purpura, thrombocytopenia, and thrombotic thrombocytopenic purpura.

VIII. Laboratory findings and evaluation:
A. Serum levels not helpful.
B. Other laboratory tests:
   1. Complete blood cell count (see Clinical features).
   2. Arterial blood gas (with hypersensitivity reactions involving respiratory function). If respiratory compromise present, initiate treatment before obtaining laboratory studies.
   3. Chest radiograph.
   4. Blood glucose (rule out hypoglycemia in presence of mental status changes, seizures).
   5. Electrolytes if severe vomiting, fluid depletion.
   6. Renal function studies (BUN, creatinine).

IX. Treatment:
A. Follow APTLS: See Chapter 8.
B. General management: Table 98–4 (see Chapters 12 and 13 for details).
C. Specific management:
   1. Symptomatic and supportive.
   2. Hemodialysis or hemoperfusion may be useful in deteriorating patient with renal failure.

X. Prognosis: Excellent with good supportive care.

XI. Disposition considerations:
A. Admission considerations:
   1. See General Admission Considerations (Chapters 17 and 18).
   2. Significant symptoms (seizures, altered mental status, protracted vomiting, anaphylaxis).
   3. Suicide risk.
B. Observation period: Difficult to make specific recommendations. Four hours of observations should suffice for most patients who are asympto-

TABLE 98–4.

General Treatment

Treatment	Indicated	Of No Value	Contraindicated
O$_2$	±		
IV	+		
ECG monitor	±		
Forced diuresis		X	
Acidification		X	
Alkalinization		X	
Emesis/lavage	+/+		
Charcoal	+		
Cathartic	+		

matic on presentation. Patients with mild symptoms must be assessed on an individual basis.
C. Discharge considerations:
1. General discharge considerations have been met (see Chapters 17 and 18).
2. Suicide potential and psychiatric status have been appropriately evaluated.

Rifampin

I. Route of exposure: Oral.
II. Common trade names: Rifadin, Rimactane.
III. Pharmacokinetics:
   A. Absorption: 90% absorbed in oral ingestion.
   B. Plasma half-life: 2–5 hours
   C. Peak effect: Peak plasma level in 2–4 hours.
   D. Duration of action: (see Plasma Half-Life for guidelines).
   E. Elimination:
      1. 16% renal excretion; 70% biliary.
      2. Enterohepatic circulation.
IV. Action: Inhibits RNA synthesis.
V. Uses:
   A. Used in combination with other agents for treatment of pulmonary tuberculosis and in asymptomatic carriers of *Neisseria meningitides*.
   B. In overdose and suicide attempt, often taken in combination with other antituberculosis drugs (INH, ethambutol).
VI. Toxic mechanism:
   A. Direct drug-induced hepatotoxicity.
   B. CNS toxicity secondary to drug-induced hepatitis or renal failure.
VII. Range of toxicity:
   A. Therapeutic dose: 10–20 mg/kg/day, not to exceed 600 mg.

B. Toxic dose: Limited experience. Reported toxic ingestions:
   1. 100 mg/kg in a child.
   2. 12 gm in an adult.

VIII. Clinical features:
   A. GI: Nausea, vomiting, diarrhea.
   B. CNS: Drowsiness, headache, dizziness, ataxia, muscular weakness.
   C. Facial edema: Begins 30 minutes–4 hours after ingestion.
   D. Red man syndrome:
      1. Red or orange discoloration of sweat, urine, skin.
      2. Dose dependent.
   E. Hepatotoxicity:
      1. Rare, reversible (1%).
      2. Characterized by jaundice and possible development of hepatorenal syndrome.

IX. Laboratory findings and evaluation:
   A. Plasma rifampin levels: Not useful.
   B. Other laboratory tests:
      1. Liver function studies (transaminases, bilirubin).
      2. Renal function studies (BUN, creatinine, urinalysis).
      3. Blood glucose (rule out hypoglycemia in presence of drowsiness, headache, dizziness, weakness).
      4. Electrolytes (assess fluid, electrolyte status if vomiting, diarrhea severe).

X. Treatment: See Penicillins and Cephalosporins (p. 563).

XI. Prognosis: Excellent with good supportive care.

XII. Disposition considerations:
   A. Admission considerations:
      1. See General Admission Considerations (Chapters 17 and 18).
      2. Very few patients require admission; however, patients with evidence of hepatic or renal toxicity should be admitted for observation.
      3. Suicide risk.
   B. Observation period: See Penicillins and Cephalosporins (p. 563).
   C. Discharge considerations:
      1. General discharge considerations have been met (see Chapters 17 and 18).
      2. Suicide potential and psychiatric status have been appropriately evaluated.

Sulfonamides

I. Route of exposure: Oral, parenteral, topical.

II. Common names:

Mafenide	Sulfamethoxazole
Silver sulfadizine	Sulfasalazine
Sulfacytine	Sulfasuxidine
Sulfacetamide	Sulfathalidine
Sulfadiazine	Sulfisoxazole

III. Pharmacokinetics:
   A. Absorption: Complete oral absorption.
   B. Plasma half-life: 6–8 hours.
   C. Peak effect: 2–4 hours.
   D. Elimination: Free and acetylated sulfonamides excreted in urine.
   E. Active metabolites: Acetylated metabolites seem to be responsible for several side effects, in particular, crystalluria.
IV. Action: Prevents conversion of *para*-aminobenzoic acid (PABA) to folic acid. This is mechanism behind sulfonamide bacteriostatic properties.
   V. Uses: Active against both gram-positive and gram-negative organisms. Particularly useful in urinary tract infections.
VI. Toxic mechanism: Toxicity largely result of hypersensitivity reactions.
VII. Toxicity:
   A. Fatal dose: Deaths have occurred with therapeutic doses of almost all sulfonamides.
VIII. Clinical features:
   A. Drug fever, skin rashes including Stevens-Johnson syndrome, hemolytic anemia, agranulocytosis and thrombocytopenia, renal failure, hematuria.
   B. Toxic aplastic anemia (very rare).
   C. Other rare adverse reactions: Liver necrosis, arthritis, photosensitivity, peripheral neuritis.
   D. Kernicterus in preterm infants.
   E. Methemoglobinemia (overdose).
   F. Hypoglycemia.
IX. Laboratory findings and evaluation:
   A. Complete blood cell count (see Clinical features); type and cross match.
   B. Liver function studies (transaminases, bilirubin).
   C. Renal function studies (BUN, creatinine, urinalysis).
   D. Blood glucose (hypoglycemia).
   E. Methemoglobin level if indicated.
   X. Treatment:
   A. Follow APTLS: Chapter 8.
   B. General management: Table 98–5 (see Chapters 12 and 13 for details).

TABLE 98–5.

General Treatment

Treatment	Indicated	Of No Value	Contraindicated
O$_2$	±		
IV	±		
ECG monitor	±		
Forced diuresis		X	
Acidification		X	
Alkalinization		X	•
Emesis/lavage	+/+		
Charcoal	+		
Cathartic	+		

C. Specific management:
1. Symptomatic and supportive.
2. Treat methemoglobinemia if level greater than 30% or if cyanotic (see Chapter 102).
XI. Prognosis:
A. Expected response to treatment:
1. Renal failure usually resolves completely after approximately 2 weeks.
2. Agranulocytosis successfully treated in 50%–75% of cases.
B. Expected complications and long-term effects: See Clinical features.
XII. Disposition considerations:
A. Admission considerations
1. See General Admission Considerations (Chapters 17 and 18).
2. Very few patients require admission; however, patients with evidence of severe hypersensitivity reaction (e.g., Stevens-Johnson syndrome), hepatic or renal toxicity should be admitted.
3. Suicide risk.
B. Observation period: Asymptomatic patients with sulfonamide ingestions should be observed for several hours in the emergency department.
C. Discharge considerations:
1. General discharge considerations have been met (see Chapters 17 and 18).
2. Remains asymptomatic after observation.
3. Suicide potential and psychiatric status have been appropriately evaluated.

Antimicrobial Agents Without Significant Acute Toxicity

I. Erythromycin:
A. Toxicity following acute overdose rare.
B. Estolate salt associated with reversible hepatic dysfunction:
1. Occurs days after initial dose.
2. Fever, jaundice, abdominal pain, elevated liver function test values, eosinophilia.
II. Metronidazole:
A. Flagyl, Protostat, Metryl.
B. Acute toxicity not reported.
C. Disulfiram-like reaction with ethanol ingestion reported (unsubstantiated by controlled studies).
D. Considered potentially teratogenic in pregnancy.
III. Nitrofurantoin:
A. Acute effects other than GI symptoms rare.
B. Acute cholestatic jaundice; reversible with discontinuation.
IV. Tetracycline:
A. Severe toxicity in overdose rare.
1. Increased intracranial pressure reported with chronic use in infants and adolescents.
2. Maximum oral dosage: 2 gm/day.

B. No specific laboratory studies indicated.
C. Treatment consists of gastric emptying and antacids for gastric irritation.
D. Special considerations:
   1. Complications during pregnancy:
      a. May precipitate hepatic failure.
      b. Causes discoloration of teeth beginning in week 12 of gestation.
      c. Tetracyclines can cause exaggerated sunburn on light-exposed skin. This is a phototoxic reaction and may be accompanied by eczematous or pellagra-like skin changes.

BIBLIOGRAPHY

Ackerman BH, et al: Aminoglycoside therapy. *Postgrad Med* 1984; 75:177.

Beelcy L: Allergy to penicillin. *Br Med J* 1984; 288:511.

Freundlich M, et al: Management of chloramphenicol intoxication in infancy by charcoal hemoperfusion. *J Pediatr* 1983; 103:485.

Mitchell JR, et al: Isoniazid liver injury: Clinical spectrum, pathology and probable pathogenesis. *Ann Intern Med* 1976; 84:181.

Orlowski JP, Paganini EP, Pippenger CE: Treatment of a potentially lethal dose isoniazid ingestion. *Ann Emerg Med* 1988; 17:73–76.

Riou B, Barriot P, Rimailho A, et al: Treatment of severe chloroquine poisoning. *N Engl J Med* 1988; 318:1–6.

Sullivan D, Csuka ME, Blanchard B: Erythromycin ethylsuccinate hepatotoxicity. *JAMA* 1980; 243:1074.

Wong P, et al: Acute rifampin overdose: A pharmacokinetic study and review of the literature. *J Pediatr* 1984; 104:781.

Yarbrough BE, Wood JP: Isoniazid overdose treated with high-dose pyrodoxine. *Ann Emerg Med* 1983; 12:303–305.

99

Cytotoxic and Immunosuppressive Agents

Timothy J. Rittenberry, M.D.

I. Route of exposure: Intravenous, cutaneous, inhalation, intrathecal.
II. Common generic and trade names: See Tables 99–1 and 99–2.
III. Pharmacokinetics: See Table 99–1.
IV. Action:
   A. Wide variety of compounds with spectrum of pharmacologic activity:
      1. Alkylating agents cause cross-linking of DNA. Cellular function disrupted during all stages of cell growth.
      2. Antimetabolite methotrexate inhibits dihydrofolate reductase, preventing 1-carbon transfer reactions and de novo synthesis of DNA and RNA. 5-FU, Ara-C, and 6-MP are activated and falsely incorporated into DNA. They also inhibit enzymes of DNA synthesis, further leading to cell death.
      3. Vinca alkaloids block mitosis by causing metaphase arrest.
      4. Antibiotic agents bind to DNA, blocking DNA transcription or causing DNA fragmentation.
      5. *Cis*-platinum causes DNA cross-linking by complexation.
      6. L-Asparaginase converts extracellular asparagine to aspartic acid, depriving this essential amino acid to certain neoplastic cell lines.
      7. Immunosuppressants inhibit cytotoxic T cell populations.
V. Uses:
   A. Used separately and in various combinations to treat neoplastic disease and graft-versus-host reactions.
   B. Intentional overdose rare. Mostly complications of therapeutic dosage and inadvertent errors in dosage.

570

TABLE 99–1.
Cytotoxic and Immunosuppressive Agents*

Generic Name	Trade Name	Typical Dosage	Metabolism and Excretion	Predominant Toxicity	Comments
Antibiotics					
Doxorubicin	Adriamycin	60 mg/m² IV	50% hepatic with biliary excretion; little renal	Myocardial toxicity (cumulative dose >550 mg/m² in adults, >300 mg/m² in children), myelodepression 10–14 days, tissue necrosis with extravasation	Congestive heart failure may appear during treatment or months after; transient (unrelated) ECG changes; increased toxicity with hepatic disease
Daunorubicin	Cerubidine	60 mg/m² IV	40% biliary, 25% renal	Same as doxorubicin	Same as doxorubicin
Bleomycin	Blenoxane	10–20 U/m² IV	60%–70% renal (unchanged)	Pneumonitis, pulmonary fibrosis (cumulative dose >400 U/m² minimal myelosuppression, hyperpyrexia	Increased toxicity with renal disease
Dactinomycin	Cosmegan	10–15 µg/kg IV	Minimally metabolized; 30% excreted at 7 days	Tissue necrosis with extravasation (1–7 days)	

Continued.

TABLE 99–1 (cont.).

Generic Name	Trade Name	Typical Dosage	Metabolism and Excretion	Predominant Toxicity	Comments
Plicamycin (mithramycin)	Mutamycin	25–30 µg/kg IV	60%–70% recovered at 4 hours (urine)	Myelosuppression, hepatotoxicity	May lead to severe hemorrhagic diatheses, hypocalcemia
Mitomycin-C	Mutamycin	2 mg/m² IV	Hepatic	Myelosuppression (at 1–8 weeks; cumulative effect)	Hemolytic uremic syndrome (at 1–8 weeks; cumulative effect)
Antimetabolites					
Methotrexate	Fotex	2.5–30 mg PO up to 1 gm/m² IV, when used with leucovorin rescue	Up to 90% excreted unchanged by kidney	Myelosuppression (7–14 days), hepatotoxicity, hemorrhagic enteritis, CNS symptoms (intrathecal exposure)	
6-Mercaptopurine	Purinethol	100–200 mg/kg PO	Hepatic	Myelosuppression (at 2–3 days), hepatotoxicity (increased at doses 2.5 mg/kg/day), hyperuricemia	Reversible jaundice in a third; potentiated by allopurinol
Thioguanine	Thioguanine	2 mg/kg PO		Myelosuppression	
Cytarabine	Cytosar-U	100–200 mg/m²	10% excreted in urine unchanged	Myelosuppression	

5-Fluorouracil	Fluorouracil	12 mg/kg IV (not to exceed 800 mg)	60%–80% expired as respiratory CO_2	Myelosuppression, ataxia, mucositis (stomatitis), proctitis, etc	Hemorrhagic diarrhea
Floxuridine	FUDR	0.1–0.6 mg/kg by intraarterial infusion	Same as 5-fluorouracil	Same as 5-fluorouracil	
Alkylating agents					
Cyclophosphamide	Cytoxan	1–5 mg/kg PO up to 1,800 mg/kg IV over 2–5 days	Hepatic	Myelosuppression, cystitis (10%); may impair free water excretion at doses >50 mg/kg	May cause acute myopericarditis
Busulfan	Myeleran	2–8 mg PO	Excreted in urine as methane sulfonic acid	Myelosuppression	Little GI toxicity
Chlorambucil	Leukeran	4–10 mg PO	Hepatic	Myelosuppression (moderate)	Seizures have occurred in children
Carmustine (BCNU)	BiCNU	200 mg/m² IV	60%–70% appears in urine	Myelosuppression (moderate)	CNS toxicity reported
Lomustine (CCNU)	CeeNu	100 mg/m² IV	Same as BCNU	Myelosuppression (delayed)	
DTIC	Dacarbazine	3.5 mg/kg IV	50% appears in urine unchanged	Same as BCNU Severe nausea and vomiting (90%), myelosuppression (moderate)	May induce flulike syndrome
Mechlorethamine	Mustargen	10 mg/m² IV	Completely distributed in minutes	Myelosuppression, marked nausea and vomiting, severe vesication	

Continued.

TABLE 99–1 (cont.).

Generic Name	Trade Name	Typical Dosage	Metabolism and Excretion	Predominant Toxicity	Comments
Melphalan	Alkeran	6 mg PO	15% excreted unchanged in urine	Myelosuppression	Nausea and vomiting infrequent
Vinca Alkaloids					
Vincristine	Oncovin, Vincasar	0.01 mg/kg IV	Hepatic	Neuromuscular toxicity frequent (seizures, weakness, ataxia, hallucinations), severe vesication, myelosuppression (moderate)	Paralytic ileus
Vinblastine	Velban	0.1–0.15 mg/kg IV	Hepatic	Myelosuppression	Less neurological toxicity than vincristine
Miscellaneous					
cis-Platinum	Platinol	100 mg/m^2 IV		Dose-related nephrotoxicity, ototoxicity, marked vomiting, myelosuppression	

L-Asparaginase	Elspar	Up to 1,000 IU/kg IV or IM	Half-life 8–30 hr	Acute hallucinosis, depression, somnolence, disorientation (30%–60%), hepatitis, pancreatitis	May cause delayed encephalopathy; inhibits normal protein synthesis
Procarbazine	Matulane	4–6 mg/kg PO	Hepatic renal	Myelosuppression, marked nausea and vomiting	Disulfiram-type reactions with ethanol; augments effect of CNS depressants
Immunosuppressants					
Azathioprine	Imuran	3–5 mg PO	Significant renal clearance	Myelosuppression, hepatotoxicity	
Cyclosporine	Sandimmune	10–15 mg/kg PO		Renal and hepatic toxicity	

*Essentially all agents capable of causing significant nausea and vomiting.

VI. Toxic mechanism:
   A. Toxic mechanisms are extension of therapeutic actions (see Action).
   B. See Table 99–1.
VII. Range of toxicity:
   A. Small margins of safety.
   B. Efficacy a function of differential toxicity in normal and neoplastic cell lines.
   C. Toxicity at therapeutic dosage the rule.
   D. Many poisonings may not be clinically apparent in single-dose exposure.
   E. See Table 99–1 for selected toxic doses.
VIII. Clinical features (see also Table 99–1):
   A. Acute and severe nausea and vomiting common:
      1. Stimulation of medullary centers.
      2. May lead to weakness, electrolyte imbalance, dehydration.
   B. Myelosuppression:
      1. Leukocytopenia typically begins 5–15 days after exposure, with nadir at 10–14 days.
      2. Granulocytopenia may lead to infection (absolute granulocyte counts $<1,000/mm^3$).
      3. Thrombocytopenia may lead to bleeding.
      4. Recovery in 21–28 days.
      5. Chronic exposure may lead to chronic bone marrow hypoplasia.
   C. Gastrointestinal toxicity:
      1. Stomatitis, glossitis, esophagitis, proctitis, enteritis.
      2. May lead to sanguinous diarrhea with **5-FU.**
   D. Hyperpyrexia with bleomycin from 12–48 hours after exposure.
   E. Hemorrhagic cystitis with **cyclophosphamide:**
      1. May be acute or delayed.
      2. Dysuria, hematuria, frequency.
   F. Renal tubular injury:
      1. **Cyclophosphamide** may inhibit free water excretion, leading to hyponatremia.
      2. **Methotrexate** may precipitate in renal tubule, leading to renal failure.
      3. **Cyclosporine** also causes renal tubular injury.
   G. Hepatotoxicity: **6-Mercaptopurine** and precursor, **azathioprine,** cause hepatocellular necrosis at 1 week–2 years after therapy in 10%–40% of patients.
   H. Pulmonary: "**Busulfan** lung" consists of dyspnea on exertion, cough with interstitial infiltrates 8 months–10 years; aerosolized exposure may cause acute dyspnea or cough.
   I. Skin:
      1. Many are vesicants and may cause necrosis with direct skin exposure.
      2. Alopecia.
      3. Neurotoxicity:
         a. Common with **vincristine, vinblastine.**
         b. Decreased motor strength, cutaneous sensation.
         c. Autonomic dysfunction: constipation, adynamic ileus.

      d. Most severe 2–3 weeks after administration.

      e. Intrathecal exposure of antineoplastic agents may induce seizures.

  J. Cardiac toxicity (**daunorubicin** and **doxorubicin**):

    1. Acutely may cause reversible sinus tachycardia, ST-T wave changes.

    2. Dose-related biventricular failure after 2 weeks–6 months ($>$500 mg/m^2 cumulative dose).

IX. Laboratory findings and evaluation:

  A. Serum levels, except possibly with methotrexate, not useful.

  B. Complete blood cell count, electrolytes, BUN, creatinine, liver function tests, prothrombin time, partial thromboplastin time.

  C. Urinalysis.

  D. Chest radiograph (with pulmonary toxicity).

  E. Arterial blood gas (indicated if pulmonary toxicity, dyspnea).

  F. ECG (indicated if evidence of cardiotoxicity).

X. Treatment:

  A. Follow APTLS: See Chapter 8.

  B. General management of acute and chronic toxicity of oral cytotoxins: See Table 99–2 (see Chapters 12 and 13 for details).

XI. Specific treatment:

  A. No antidotes except for methotrexate (e.g., leucovorin or thymidine rescue).

  B. Management is supportive:

    1. Protracted vomiting treated with phenothiazine preparations (prochlorperazine, thiethylperazine).

    2. Maintain high urine output with methotrexate, *cis*-platinum, cyclophosphamide (3–6 ml/kg/hr).

TABLE 99–2.

General Treatment

Treatment	Indicated	Of No Value	Contraindicated
O$_2$	$\pm$		
IV	$\pm$		
ECG monitor	$\pm$		
Forced diuresis*			X
Acidification		X	
Alkalinization*			X
Emesis†/lavage†	+/+		
Charcoal†	+		
Cathartic†‡	$\pm$		
Dialysis		X	

*May be indicated for methotrexate only. Not generally recommended; even contraindicated for other agents.

†Acute toxicity only. Avoid if vomiting.

‡Many patients with acute ingestion may be taking cyclical therapy with cytotoxins causing diarrhea with potential for severe volume loss. Use cathartics carefully, monitoring volume status.

3. Dialysis not useful. These agents are difficult to remove once systematically distributed:
   a. High lipid solubility.
   b. Active intracellular transport.
   c. High tissue and protein binding.
   d. Short plasma half-lives related to rapid distribution (minutes).
4. Severe thrombocytopenia with bleeding requires platelet transfusions.
5. Broad-spectrum antibiotics indicated in febrile leukopenic patients.
6. Topical exposure must be aggressively rinsed with normal saline solution:
   a. Gloves and protective clothing required for medical personnel.
   b. Breathing apparatus must be used in decontamination if aerosolization of agent a possibility.

C. Methotrexate:
1. Methotrexate deserves special comment because an antidote (leucovorin) exists to treat severe toxicity. Leucovorin neutralizes immediate hematopoietic toxicity.
2. Methotrexate serum level 1×10^{-8} mol/L toxic.
3. Treatment: Administer leucovorin (Citrovorum brand of folinic acid) as soon as possible ("leucovorin rescue"):
   a. Dose should be equal to or higher than methotrexate dose responsible for toxicity.
   b. Maximum 75 mg by IV infusion within 12 hours.
   c. Further dosing with leucovorin can be based on methotrexate serum levels 24 hours after last methotrexate dose:

Methotrexate (10^{-6} mol/L) Serum Level	Leucovorin Dose
0.1–1	10–15 mg/m² q 6 hr × 12 doses
1–5	50 mg/m² q 6 hr until level $<1 \times 10^{-7}$ mol/L
5–10	100 mg/m² q 6 hr until level $<1 \times 10^{-7}$ mol/L

4. Immediate alkaline diuresis enhances excretion:
   a. Add 1–2 ampules $NaHCO_3$ with 20 mEq KCl to 1 L D_5W.
   b. Administer solution at rate sufficient to obtain urine output 3–6 ml/kg/hr and urine pH >7.5.
5. Administration of thymidine (8 gm/m²/day) by continuous infusion may also prevent systemic toxicity.

XII. Prognosis:
A. Expected response to treatment:
1. Prognosis good, with recovery expected in 21–28 days.
2. A 3-year-old child who ingested 2,025 mg methotrexate was treated with leucovorin and had negligible systemic toxicity.
B. Expected complications and long-term effects:
1. Myelosuppression may become apparent days to weeks after exposure.
2. Most antineoplastic agents have carcinogenic potential themselves.

3. Chronic exposure may lead to chronic bone marrow hypoplasia.
XIII. Disposition considerations:
    A. Admission considerations:
        1. Because of potential life-threatening complications, all toxic emergencies resulting from antineoplastic or immunosuppressive agents require hospitalization.
        2. Suicide risk.
    B. Consultation considerations: Oncology or hematology consultation required for evaluation of all patients with signs and symptoms of toxicity.
    C. Observation period: None. All patients with chemotherapeutic or immunosuppressive toxicity should be admitted and not observed expectantly in the emergency department.
    D. Discharge considerations: None. All patients with chemotherapeutic or immunosuppressive toxicity should be admitted.

BIBLIOGRAPHY

Abelson HT, et al: Methotrexate-induced renal impairment: Clinical studies and rescue from systemic toxicity with high-dose leucovorin and thymidine. *J Clin Oncol* 1983; 1:208–216.

Goodman LS, Gilman AB, et al: Chemotherapy of neoplastic diseases, in *Pharmacologic Basis of Therapeutics,* ed 7. New York, Macmillan Publishing Co, 1985, p 1240.

Haddad LM, Winchester JF: *Clinical Management of Poisoning and Drug Overdose.* Philadelphia, WB Saunders Co, 1983, pp 618–635.

Lefrok EA, Pitha J, Rosenheim S: A clinico-pathologic analysis of adriamycin cardiotoxicity. *Cancer* 1973; 3:302.

Physicians' Desk Reference. Raritan, NJ, Medical Economics Co, 1987.

Poisindex. Denver, Micromedex, 1987.

Environmental/Industrial Poisons

100

Carbon Monoxide

Ricardo L. Sanchez, M.D., M.P.H.

I. Route of exposure: Inhalation.
II. Sources:
   A. Incomplete combustion.
      1. All organic fuels are capable of producing carbon monoxide via "incomplete combustion."
      2. Applies to gasoline and diesel engines, charcoal and wood fires, kerosene heaters, home gas and oil appliances, Sterno burners, and housing and industrial fires.
   B. Methylene chloride (see also Table 108–1):
      1. Indirect source: Produced in metabolic degradation.
      2. Methylene chloride is synonymous with dichloromethane, bichloromethane, methane Dichlor, CAS 75-09-2.
      3. Compound found in many paint stripping solutions.
III. Pharmacokinetics:
   A. Absorption: Depends on concentration of CO in inspired air and duration of exposure.
   B. Onset of action: Depends on concentration of CO in inspired air and duration of exposure.
   C. Plasma half-life:
      1. Room air: 4–5 hours.
      2. 100% oxygen: 1.5 hours.
      3. Hyperbaric oxygen at 3 atm: 20 minutes.
   D. Peak effect: Depends on concentration of CO in inspired air and duration of exposure.

E. Duration of action: Depends on concentration of CO in inspired air and duration of exposure and concentration of inspired oxygen. For guidelines, see Plasma Half-Life.

F. Elimination: Resting adults breathing room air will eliminate 50% of CO in 4–5 hours (see Plasma Half-Life above).

G. Active metabolites: Negligible amounts of CO are metabolized to CO_2 in humans.

IV. Sources of exposure:

A. Combustion sources of CO are ubiquitous in the workplace and in the average household.

B. Paint strippers are often used in poorly ventilated areas (methylene chloride).

C. CO is also used in pulmonary function laboratory measurements.

V. Mechanism of toxicity:

A. Cellular hypoxia results from three mechanisms of action:

1. Reduction in oxygen-carrying capacity of blood related to displacement of oxygen by CO from binding sites in hemoglobin. Combines with hemoglobin to form carboxyhemoglobin (COHb).

2. CO has an affinity for hemoglobin 250 times greater than that of oxygen. CO also shifts oxyhemoglobin dissociation curve to the left, making it more difficult for oxygen on the hemoglobin molecule to be given up to the tissues.

3. Inhibition of cellular respiration via poisoning of all heme proteins (myoglobin cytochromes and hyperoxidases).

VI. Range of toxicity: Wide variation in relationship between exposure level and measured percent COHb.

VII. Clinical features (Table 100–1):

A. No pathognomonic feature in the clinical presentation and course of significant CO exposure. Entire spectrum from asymptomatic to unconscious can be expected.

B. Headache, dizziness, nausea, chest pain, fatigue, confusion are often the only abnormalities.

C. Cherry red mucous membranes are rare late finding.

D. Bulla may form in pressure areas.

E. CO-induced rhabdomyolysis and renal failure.

VIII. Laboratory findings and evaluation

A. Blood:

1. Serum levels:

a. COHb measured spectrophotometrically can be used as confirmatory evidence, but **low values do not rule out life-threatening exposure** in the setting of a clear history of exposure.

b. Normal COHb levels:

(1) Nonsmoker: 0.85%.

(2) Smoker: 4%.

(3) Hemolytic anemia: 5%.

2. Arterial blood gas:

a. Normal PO_2, decreased P_{CO_2} (respiratory alkalosis before respiratory depression sets in), severe metabolic (lactic) acidosis (low HCO_3).

TABLE 100–1.

Symptoms of CO Poisoning*

COHb Concentration (%)	Signs and Symptoms†
0–10	None (angina may be noted in patients with coronary artery disease)
10–20	Slight headache, exercise-induced angina, dyspnea on vigorous exertion
20–30	Throbbing headache, dyspnea on moderate exertion
30–40	Severe headache, nausea, vomiting, weakness, visual disturbance, impaired judgment
40–50	Syncope, tachycardia, tachypnea
50–60	Coma, convulsions, Cheyne-Stokes respiration
60–70	Compromised cardiorespiratory function
70–80	Death

*Adapted from Goldfrank LR, Flomenbaum NE, Lewin NA, et al: *Goldfrank's Toxicological Emergencies*. Norwalk, Conn, Appleton-Century-Crofts, 1986, p 665.
†Note that symptoms and prognosis may not correlate well with % CoHb.

    b. Decreased oxygen saturation: Analysis can be misleading unless % O_2 saturation measured rather than calculated. Calculated saturation may look normal.
  3. Electrolytes (increased anion gap metabolic (lactic acidosis).
  4. Other: Complete blood cell count, glucose, BUN, creatinine.
  5. Consider:
    a. Lactate, toxicology screen.
    b. Hyperuricemia, myoglobinuria, and hyperamylasemia have been reported.
 B. Other laboratory tests:
  1. Chest radiograph, ECG, urinalysis.
  2. Serial ECGs and cardiac enzymes may be indicated for several days to rule out myocardial injury.
  3. Methemoglobin level if indicated (e.g., concomitant exposure to nitrogen oxide gases. See Table 102–1).
IX. General treatment:
 A. Follow APTLS: See Chapter 8.
 B. General management: See Table 100–2 (see Chapter 8–10 for details).
 C. Remove patient from area of exposure.
X. Specific treatment:
 A. Respiratory support: Consider intubation in all patients with altered mental status (see Chapter 9).
 B. Hyperbaric oxygen therapy: If available, is the most rapid method for eliminating CO and should be considered for all symptomatic patients,

TABLE 100–2.

General Treatment

Treatment	Indicated	Of No Value	Contraindicated
O_2*	+		
IV	+		
ECG monitor	+		
Forced diuresis		X	
Acidification			X
Alkalinization		X	
Emesis/lavage		X	
Charcoal		X	
Cathartic		X	
Naloxone and glucose†	+		

*100% O_2 single most important intervention. Use tight-fitting face mask with oxygen reservoir at 10 L/min.
†In presence of altered mental status.

and all patients whose estimated peak COHb levels are elevated (see XII. C. below).

    C. Cerebral edema: Fluid restriction. Use of dexamethasone and mannitol are controversial.

    D. Seizures: See Chapter 22 for treatment recommendations.

XI. Prognosis:

    A. Expected response to treatment:

        1. Near universal rapid and effective response to therapy when initiated expeditiously.

        2. Successful reversal of coma has been reported with hyperbaric oxygen therapy initiated as late as 20 hours after exposure.

        3. Several reports of patients requiring repeated hyperbaric treatments over several days before complete resolution of symptoms.

    B. Expected complications and long-term effects:

        1. Most long-term effects related to CNS injury and span the spectrum from personality and affective disorders to memory, sensory, or motor deficits. Many patients present with symptoms weeks or months after apparent complete recovery from CO poisoning episode, particularly if high COHb levels were untreated for several hours.

        2. Comatose patients with initial recovery have a 5%–10% incidence of delayed neuropsychiatric deterioration; approximately two thirds recover. Poor prognosis for complete recovery exists if symptoms of CNS abnormalities continue for 2 or more weeks.

        3. Neurogenic pulmonary edema, brain hypoxic edema, rhabdomyolysis secondary to pressure necrosis, renal failure, hepatic and intestinal injury.

XII. Special considerations:

    A. Coronary artery disease: CO exposure, even at low levels, can act as a precipitating factor in development of angina and myocardial infarction in patients with previously diagnosed or subclinical coronary artery disease.

B. Pregnant patients: Increased fetal vulnerability in the setting of CO exposure normally tolerated by adults.

C. In determining seriousness of exposure and possible peak level, calculations should be based on: time from exposure to time CO level obtained; time and concentration of O_2 therapy; and effects of O_2 concentration on half-life. For example, in an exposed patient, a COHb level of 7 taken after three hours of continuous administration of 100 O_2, probably had a peak level of 28 three hours (2 half-lives) ago.

D. Consider other toxic fumes in exposure (see Chapter 108).

E. Suspect cyanide poisoning from acrylonitrile when a fire victim fails to respond immediately to oxygen treatment or when someone at a fire who is wearing a charcoal mask collapses (charcoal does not filter hydrogen cyanide from the air).

F. If hypoxia persists after administration of oxygen, consider cyanide (see Chapter 101), hydrogen sulfide gas (see Chapter 103), and methemoglobinemia (see Chapter 102).

G. Patients with seemingly normal or only mildly elevated COHb levels, but whose estimated peak COHb level is high, may benefit from hyperbaric treatment to prevent delayed or long-term sequelae. This should be considered even if the patient becomes asymptomatic or only has mild symptoms by the time of the ED evaluation.

XIII. Controversies:

A. Use of corticosteroids and mannitol for cerebral edema. Value in preventing late sequelae unproved.

B. Although hypothermia has been reported as a therapeutic adjunct to oxygen therapy, its use cannot be recommended at this time because of anecdotal nature of reports and potential for further shift of oxyhemoglobin curve to left.

XIV. Disposition considerations:

A. Admission considerations:

1. See General Admission Considerations (Chapters 17 and 18).

2. All symptomatic patients without altered mental status, with COHb levels >25% should be admitted immediately. Estimate COHb level at time of exposure by obtained level and by knowledge of half-life properties and time elapsed by the time the sample was drawn for assay.

3. Patients with COHb levels 10%–25% who remain symptomatic after several hours of ED treatment.

4. COHb level greater than 15% in a patient with a history of cardiac disease.

5. Any patient with altered mental status or sensorium at any time in the period immediately subsequent to CO exposure, even if asymptomatic in the emergency department.

6. Any patients with metabolic acidosis or hypoxia.

7. Any pregnant woman who is symptomatic or has a COHb level greater than 10%.

8. Suicide risk.

9. Considerations for ICU admission:
   a. See Chapter 18.
   b. Patients with altered level of consciousness or levels greater than 25%.
   c. Any patient with acute ECG changes (e.g., ST-T wave abnormalities, atrial or ventricular arrhythmias, premature ventricular contractions, evidence of myocardial ischemia).
   d. Patient requiring respiratory support.
B. Consultation considerations:
   1. Hyperbaric facility for all patients with exposure.
   2. Public health officials (if applicable).
C. Observation period: Patients with initial COHb level 10%–25% who are asymptomatic after treatment and with posttreatment COHb level ≤10% may be discharged after 4–6 hours of observation and after consultation with hyperbaric facility.
D. Discharge considerations:
   1. General discharge considerations have been met (see Chapter 18).
   2. Patients with initial COHb level 10%–25% who are asymptomatic after treatment and with posttreatment COHb level ≤10% may be discharged after 4–6 hours of observation and after consultation with hyperbaric facility.
   3. Patient (and family if possible) has been instructed regarding delayed symptoms and effects, and arrangements for long-term follow-up have been made.
   4. Counseling regarding further home or environmental exposure to CO has been done. Appropriate public health officials notified if necessary. Do not discharge patients who will return to an environment where further exposure may occur.
   5. Caution against excessive physical activity in first few weeks following discharge from the emergency department (increased metabolic activity may result in further tissue injury).
   6. Suicide potential and psychiatric state have been appropriately evaluated.
E. Patient transfer issues:
   1. Care must be taken to ensure that patients with severe CO poisoning are not transferred to a facility with a hyperbaric chamber before they are medically stable.
   2. See Chapter 19.

BIBLIOGRAPHY

Davis SM, Levy RC: High carboxyhemoglobin levels without acute or chronic findings. *J Emerg Med* 1984; 1:539–542.

Ginsberg MD: Carbon monoxide intoxication: Clinical features, neuropathology, and mechanisms of injury. *Clin Toxicol* 1985; 23:281–288.

Goldfrank LR, Flomenbaum NE, Lewin NA, et al: *Goldfrank's Toxicological Emergencies.* Norwalk, Conn, Appleton-Century-Crofts, 1986.

Grace TW, Platt FW: Subacute carbon monoxide poisoning: Another great imitator. *JAMA* 1981; 246:1698–1700.

Hauck, H: Carbon monoxide uptake and the resulting carboxyhemoglobin in man. *Eur J Appl Physiol* 1984; 53:186–190.

Marzella L, Myers RM: Carbon monoxide poisoning. *AFP* 1986; 34:186–194.

Mofenson HC, Caraccio TR, Brody GM: Carbon monoxide poisoning. *Am J Emerg Med* 1984; 2:254.

Myers RAM, Linberg SE, Cowley RA: Carbon monoxide poisoning: The injury and its treatment. *JACEP* 1979; 8:479–483.

Myers RAM, Snyder SK, Emhoff TA: Subacute sequelae of carbon monoxide poisoning. *Ann Emerg Med* 1985; 14:1163–1167.

Myers RAM, Snyder SK, Linberg S, et al: Value of hyperbaric oxygen in suspected carbon monoxide poisoning. *JAMA* 1981; 246:2478–2480.

Naeije R, Peretz A, Cornil A: Acute pulmonary edema following carbon monoxide poisoning. *Intensive Care Med* 1980; 6:189–191.

Olson KR: Carbon monoxide poisoning: Mechanisms, presentation, and controversies in management. *J Emerg Med* 1984; 1:233.

Rumack BH (ed): *Poisindex,* vol 52. Denver, Micromedix, 1988.

101

Cyanide

Paula A. Ryals, M.D., F.A.C.E.P.

I. Route of exposure: Transdermal, oral, inhalation.
II. Common sources:
  A. Plant sources:
    1. Jet beans, chokecherries, cassava beans, Christmas berry, elderberry.
    2. Pits or seeds of apples, peaches, plums, cherries, cherry laurel almonds, apricots, pears.
  B. Other sources:
    1. Fumigation and pesticides (prussic acid).
    2. Industry: Photography, jewelry making, laboratory reagents, ore extracting, electroplating, metal polishing, rubber production, fertilizer.
    3. Home: Silver polish, rat poison.
    4. Fire: Nylon, wool, silk, plastics (polyurethane, acrylonitrile); malfunctioning catalytic converter.
    5. Medicine: Nitroprusside, amygdalin (Laetrile).
  C. Compounds:
    1. Hydrogen cyanide, acrylonitrile, cyanamide, cyanogen chloride, nitroprusside; methyl, ethyl, isopropyl thiocyanates, thanate, lethane; amygdalin, potassium cyanide, calcium cyanide, potassium ferricyanide, cyanates, sodium cyanide.
    2. Laetrile: Trade name for amygdalin, a cyanide-containing compound obtained from crushing and moistening fruit seeds. Laetrile has been championed as vitamin B_{17}, a (not so) harmless treatment for cancer, and has been legalized in some states. Controlled studies have failed to demonstrate its efficacy, and at least one death has been caused by a child taking 1–5 tablets belonging to her father.

D. Injury: *Pseudomonas* infection in burn patients with overwhelming infection produces cyanide.

III. Pharmacokinetics:
   A. Onset of action: Within minutes; more rapid if inhaled.
   B. Half-life: 19 hours.
   C. Elimination: Metabolized in liver by an endogenous enzyme (rhondonase) to thiocyanate.
   D. Active metabolites: Thiocyanate is still toxic, but less so than cyanide.

IV. Uses:
   A. Pest control: Vermicidal fumigant, insecticide, rodenticide, soil sterilization, coyote "glitter."
   B. Industry: Metal polish, electroplating, extracting of silver and gold, removing hair from hides, photography, chemical synthesis, plastics, phencyclidine, synthetic rubber.
   C. Laboratories.
   D. Medicine: Sodium nitroprusside.
   E. Judicial executions.

V. Toxic mechanism: Interferes with intracellular respiration by inhibiting ferric ($Fe(III)$, Fe^{3+}) ion–containing enzymes such as cytochrome oxidase. Also, cyanohemoglobin cannot transport oxygen.

VI. Range of toxicity:
   A. Toxic dose: One report of a man poisoned by eating about 48 apricot kernels that had been roasted at 300° F for 10 minutes.
   B. Fatal dose:
      1. Cyanide is one of the most toxic and rapidly fatal poisons known; 50–100 mg ingested hydrocyanic acid can be fatal.
      2. Inhalation of air with 0.2–0.3 mg/L HCN gas is almost instantly fatal.
      3. Fatal dose of apple, cherry, peach, apricot, plum, jetberry bush, and toyon seeds containing cyanogenetic glycosides such as amygdalin varies from 5–25 seeds for a small child. Only dangerous if seed capsule has been violated.

VII. Clinical features:
   A. Initial symptoms: Giddiness, headache, palpitations, dyspnea, ataxia, coma, seizures, death.
   B. Nausea and vomiting can occur after ingestion of cyanide salts.
   C. Cardiac arrhythmias (atrial fibrillation, premature ventricular contractions, sinus bradycardia) may be noted.
   D. Large exposure may produce one gasping-type breath followed by seizures and death. Aroma of bitter almonds may be detectable on breath or vomitus of victims. Symptoms are sudden and apoplectic.

VIII. Laboratory findings and evaluation:
   A. NOTE: **There is usually insufficient time to obtain laboratory workup before initiating treatment.**
   B. Rapid bedside screening test:
      1. Lee Jones test:
         a. Add $FeSO_4$ crystals to 5–10 ml gastric aspirate, followed by addition of 4–5 ml 20% NaOH. This solution should then be boiled and allowed to cool, at which time 8–10 drops 10% HCl is added. Pres-

ence of cyanide indicated by formation of green-blue precipitate, which intensifies on standing.

    b. False positive result may occur with salicylates, barbiturates, benzodiazepines, phenothiazines, tricyclic antidepressants.

C. Blood:

  1. Arterial blood gas:

    a. (Increased anion gap) Metabolic acidosis (lactate).

    b. Normal PO_2.

    c. Normal calculated oxygen saturation (nomograms used to calculate oxygen saturation assume normal hemoglobin).

    d. Decreased measured oxygen saturation (cyanohemoglobin cannot transport oxygen).

      (1) Difference of 5 between measured and calculated percent oxygen saturation (oxygen saturation gap) suggests poisons such as cyanide, CO, or methemoglobinemia. CO and methemoglobinemia may be excluded by measuring carboxyhemoglobin and methemoglobin levels. Also see Chapters 100 and 102.

    e. Arterial-central venous oxygen difference narrowed (central venous $\%O_2$ saturation may be greater than 70%).

  2. Electrolytes: Elevated anion gap.

  3. Serum lactate: Elevated.

  4. Carboxyhemoglobin and methemoglobin levels if diagnosis in doubt (e.g., fire).

  5. Serum levels:

    a. Cyanide: May take several hours to days to obtain and therefore not useful in acute management. May be important for legal reasons.

    b. Thiocyanate (indicator of amount of cyanide detoxified by naturally occurring enzyme rhodanase).

    c. Methemoglobin (to monitor therapy). Therapeutic methemoglobin levels should not exceed 40%.

IX. General treatment:

A. Follow APTLS: see Chapter 8.

B. General management: See Table 101–1 (Chapter 12 for details).

C. Decontaminate skin if dermal exposure

D. Respiratory support: Intubation may be necessary; consider in all patients with altered mental status (see Chapter 9).

E. Cardiovascular support:

  1. **Cardiac arrest:** Advanced life support should be implemented. Follow most recent Advanced Cardiac Life Support guidelines (*JAMA* 1986; 255:2841–3044).

  2. **Hypotension:** See Chapter 10 for treatment recommendations.

F. Seizures: See Chapter 22 for treatment recommendations.

X. Specific treatment:

A. Adult:

  1. Cyanide Antidote Kit (Eli Lilly & Co., Indianapolis), consists of three parts:

    a. **Amyl nitrite** ampules: Crush and saturate gauze pad, hold 1 inch from victim's nose for 15–30 seconds every minute until you can begin infusion with sodium nitrite.

TABLE 101–1.

General Treatment

Treatment	Indicated	Of No Value	Contraindicated
O₂ (100%)	+		
IV	+		
ECG monitor	+		
Forced diuresis		X	
Acidification			X
Alkalinization		X	
Emesis			X
Lavage*	+		
Charcoal		X	
Cathartic		X	

*Copious; gastric absorption may be delayed.

   b. **Sodium nitrite:** Give 10 ml 3% solution IV over 3–5 minutes. Watch for hypotension. Nitrite therapy converts hemoglobin to methemoglobin, which competes with cytochrome oxidase for cyanide ion and forms a stable cyanomethemoglobin complex. This spares cytochrome oxidase for vital cellular respiratory function.

   c. **Sodium thiosulfate:** Infuse 50 ml 25% solution. This combines with cyanide to form inactive thiocyanate, which is excreted in the urine.

  2. Be prepared to repeat parts b and c if recovery is slow or toxic symptoms recur.

B. Child:

  1. Amyl nitrite inhaler: Crack and inhale 30 sec/min.

  2. See Table 101–2.

  3. May repeat half-dose once.

  4. Monitor methemoglobin to keep level less than 30%.

TABLE 101–2.

Administration of IV sodium nitrite and sodium thiosulfite*

Hemoglobin (gm/dl)	3% NaNO₂ (ml/kg)	25% NaS₂O₃ (ml/kg)
7	0.19	0.95
8	0.22	1.10
9	0.25	1.25
10	0.27	1.35
11	0.30	1.50
12	0.33†	1.65†
13	0.36	1.80
14	0.39	1.95

*From Hall AH, Rumack BH: *Ann Emerg Med* 1986; 15:1071. Used by permission.
†Dose for average child.

XI. Prognosis: In acute poisoning, the patient who survives 4 hours usually recovers.

XII. Special considerations:

    A. Check expiration date of cyanide kit.

    B. Complications of nitrite therapy:

        1. Excess methemoglobinemia causing inadequate oxygen transport. Treat with transfusions of whole blood, **not with methylene blue** (this may release cyanide ion).

        2. Sodium nitroprusside toxicity: May be recognized by increasing acidosis and elevated erythrocyte cyanide and thiocyanate levels.

    C. Very important to distinguish cyanide poisoning from CO intoxication because nitrite therapy will produce up to 40% methemoglobinemia. This is diastrous in hypoxic CO poisoning. CO should be excluded with carboxyhemoglobin level.

    D. New or controversial treatment:

        1. Cobalt salts: Dicobalt-EDTA (Kelocyanor) is available in Europe for treatment of cyanide poisoning. Combines directly with cyanide to form a stable, inactive complex. Kelocyanor has significant cardiac and GI toxicity and can cause electrolyte imbalance.

        2. Hydroxycobalamin (vitamin B_{12a}) used in Europe. Combines with cyanide to form cyanocobalamin (vitamin B_{12}). Toxicity minimal. Used with thiosulfate at dose of 4 gm hydroxycobalamin IV with 8 gm thiosulfate IV over 3–5 minutes. Recommended especially for cyanide poisoning from nitroprusside use and fire.

        3. Rapid methemoglobin inducer, 4-dimethylaminophenol (DMAP) used in Germany for cyanide poisoning. Significant problem with resultant excessive methemoglobinemia.

        4. Hyperbaric oxygen: Evidence for efficacy inconclusive at this time.

XIII. Disposition considerations:

    A. Admission considerations:

        1. See General Admission Considerations (Chapters 17 and 18).

        2. All symptomatic patients should be admitted to ICU for 24–48 hours of observation. Symptoms may recur and can be treated in a manner similar to initial treatment with one-half dose.

        3. Keep antidote kit by bedside.

        4. Suicide risk.

    B. Observation period:

        1. All symptomatic patients should be admitted.

        2. Initially asymptomatic patients with normal examination, vital signs, laboratory tests (particularly arterial blood gas) who continue to show no systemic toxicity from cyanide may be considered for discharge after a minimum of 2 hours of observation in the emergency department.

    C. Discharge considerations:

        1. General discharge considerations have been met (see Chapter 18).

        2. Asymptomatic patients with normal examination who continue to show no systemic toxicity from ingestion after a minimum of 2 hours of observation in the emergency department.

        3. Suicide potential and psychiatric status have been appropriately evaluated.

BIBLIOGRAPHY

Hall AH, Rumack BH: Clinical toxicology of cyanide. *Ann Emerg Med* 1986; 15:1067–1074.
Management of cyanide poisoning (letter). *Ann Emerg Med* 1988; 17:108–109.
Way JL: Cyanide antagonism. *Fundam Appl Toxicol* 1983; 3:383–386.
Way JL, Tamulinas CB, Leund P, et al: Pharmacologic and toxicologic basis for cyanide antagonism. *Proc West Pharmacol Soc* 1984; 27:149–153.
Way JL, Tamulinas CB, Leund P, et al: Recent perspectives on the toxicodynamic basis of cyanide antagonism. *Fundam Appl Toxicol* 1984; 4:S231–S239.

102

Nitrates/Nitrites/Nitroglycerin and Methemoglobinemia

J. Ward Donovan, M.D., F.A.C.E.P.

I. Route of exposure:
   A. Medicinal: Oral, sublingual, transdermal, intravenous.
   B. Industrial: Cutaneous, ocular.
   C. Drug of abuse: Inhalation.
II. Common generic and trade names: See Table 102–1.
III. Pharmacokinetics:
   A. Absorption: Rapid via oral, sublingual, dermal, inhalation routes.
   B. Onset of action: Near immediate.
   C. Half-life:
      1. Parent compound half-lives usually less than 1 hour; metabolite half-lives 1–8 hours.
      2. **Nitroglycerin:** 1–3 minutes (active metabolites 1.8 hours).
      3. Metabolites of **isosorbide dinitrate** and **pentaerythritol tetranitrate:** 10 hours.
      4. Estimated half-life of **methemoglobin:** 55 minutes.
   D. Peak effect: Related to rate and duration of absorption, but usually within 1 hour orally and within minutes by other routes.
   E. Duration of action: Related to rate and duration of absorption.
   F. Elimination: Rapid metabolism in liver by reductive hydrolysis to denitrated metabolites and inorganic nitrites, which are then excreted in urine. First-pass metabolism.
   G. Active metabolites: Some metabolites have pharmacologic activity but effects primarily related to duration of absorption of parent compound. Nitrates metabolized to more toxic nitrites, especially in infants.

TABLE 102–1.

Common Sources and Uses of Nitrates and Nitrites

Sources	Uses
Sodium and potassium nitrites	Fertilizers (contaminated well water)
Sodium and potassium nitrates, nitrates	Vegetables; food preservatives
Sodium nitrite	Cyanide therapy kit; anticorrosive agent
Silver nitrate	Topical burn therapy
Amyl nitrite	Vasodilator; in cyanide kit to induce methemoglobinemia
Bismuth subnitrate	Over-the-counter antidiarrheal agents
Butyl-, isobutyl-, ethyl nitrite (Locker Room, Rush)	Room deodorizers, inhalant intoxicants abused for sexual enhancement
Nitroglycerin (Nitrostat, Nitropaste)	Coronary vasodilator, explosives
Isosorbide dinitrate (Isordil, Sorbitrate)	Vasodilator
Pentaerythritol tetranitrate (Pentrate)	Vasodilator
Erythrityl tetranitrate (Cardilate)	Vasodilator
Ammonium nitrate	Fertilizer

IV. Action:
   A. Vascular smooth muscle relaxants cause vasodilation, marked arteriolar dilation in high doses.
   B. Nitrates are coronary vasodilators.
   C. Smooth muscle relaxation in bronchi, GI tract, biliary system, ureters.
   D. Volatile nitrites enhance penile erection and retard ejaculation.
V. Uses (see also Table 102–1):
   A. Toxicity: Most often seen in inhalant abusers, in infants drinking contaminated well water, and in suicidal ingestions.
VI. Toxic mechanism:
   A. Methemoglobinemia:
      1. Nitrites and to a lesser extent nitrates can cause methemoglobinemia (clinical situation in which >1% of blood has been oxidized to ferric form).
      2. Hemoglobin is continuously oxidized to ferric state in the system; nitrates can accelerate this oxidation.
      3. Methemoglobin is usually generated in subclinical amounts when nitrites or nitrates are inhaled, but significant amounts of methemoglobin can be generated when they are ingested.
      4. Methemoglobin lacks capacity to bind and transport oxygen and in-

creases oxygen affinity in normal reduced hemoglobin (shifts oxygen saturation curve to left).
5. Acute development of methemoglobin levels of 60%–70% can be associated with tissue hypoxia, cardiovascular collapse, death.
B. Other effects related to actions of nitrates or nitrites (see Action), which in toxic amounts are exaggerated.
VII. Range of toxicity:
A. Wide individual variability; infants more sensitive to methemoglobin formation.
B. Toxic dose:
1. Repetitive inhalation for several hours ordinarily necessary to cause significant methemoglobinemia.
2. Medication use (oral, sublingual, transdermal) can result in adverse effects (other than methemoglobinemia) even at therapeutic doses. Light-headedness, syncope, orthostatic hypotension particularly common.
C. Fatal dose:
1. Reported lethal dose by weight of nitrites or nitrates 2–4 gm.
a. Nitroglycerin lethal dose: 2 g.
b. Sodium nitrite lethal dose: 2 g.
2. Ingestion of 10–15 ml isobutyl nitrite product (e.g., in room deodorizer) caused death in a child, but an adult survived ingestion of 12 ml after undergoing methylene blue therapy.
VIII. Clinical features:
A. Methemoglobinemia: Suggested by presence of blue-gray cyanosis **unresponsive to oxygen therapy,** tissue hypoxia with metabolic (lactic) acidosis, chocolate-colored blood. Levels correlate with symptoms (see below).
B. Cardiopulmonary: Vasodilation, skin flushing, orthostatic hypotension, myocardial ischemia, tachycardia, diaphoresis, syncope, coronary vasospasm with acute withdrawal, dyspnea.
C. Headache, nausea and vomiting, abdominal cramps, lethargy, seizures, coma.
D. Severity of poisoning best determined by degree of acidosis and methemoglobinemia.
IX. Laboratory findings and evaluation:
A. Methemoglobin level (methemoglobinemia as percent of total hemoglobin) guides therapy (see below):
1. 15%–30%: Deep cyanosis but usually without symptoms.
2. 30%–45%: Fatigue, weakness, dyspnea, headache, tachycardia.
3. 45%–70%: Stupor and respiratory depression.
4. >70%: Coma, arrhythmias, seizures, death.
5. Anemic patients will have symptoms at lower methemoglobin concentrations because of overall reduction in effective hemoglobin concentration.
B. Arterial blood gas:
1. Characteristic chocolate brown color.
2. Normal PO_2.

3. Decreased P_{CO_2} related to tachypnea.
4. **Decreased measured oxygen saturation** (nomograms used to calculate oxygen saturation assume normal hemoglobin).
5. Decreased HCO_3 related to lactic acidosis.
C. Complete blood cell count, electrolytes.
D. ECG.
E. Spot tests available in emergency department for confirmation of methemoglobinemia:
1. Blood appears chocolate brown on filter paper if methemoglobin level >15%.
2. Addition of 1 crystal potassium cyanate to 1:1000 dilution patient's blood results in color change to pink if methemoglobinemia present.
X. General treatment:
A. Follow APTLS: See Chapter 8.
B. General management: Table 102–2 (see Chapter 12 for details).
C. Respiratory support:
1. See Chapter 9.
2. Cyanosis and tissue hypoxia not corrected until methemoglobinemia adequately treated.
D. Hypotension:
1. Fluids and Trendelenburg position usually correct hypotension.
2. Vasopressors rarely necessary.
3. See Chapter 10.
E. Cutaneous exposure: See Chapter 29.
F. Ocular exposure: See Chapter 28.
XI. Specific treatment:
A. Methylene blue:
1. Methylene blue reduces methemoglobin back to hemoglobin via process involving NADPH-dependent methemoglobin reductase, the enzyme responsible for spontaneous reduction of hemoglobin.
2. Indications: Methemoglobin level 30%–40% and symptomatic.
3. Dose: 2 mg/kg (0.2 ml/kg 1% solution) IV over 5 minutes; may repeat in 1 hour if necessary.

TABLE 102–2.

General Treatment

Treatment	Indicated	Of No Value	Contraindicated
O_2	+		
IV	+		
ECG monitor	+		
Forced diuresis		X	
Acidification			X
Alkalinization		X	
Emesis/lavage	+/+		
Charcoal	+		
Cathartic	+		

    4. Methylene blue is ineffective in NADPH-dependent methemoglobin reductase and G-6-PD deficiency.

  B. Exchange transfusions or hyperbaric oxygen may be helpful in rare severe, unresponsive cases.

  C. Ascorbic acid is used for congenital forms of methemoglobinemia but is not useful for acquired (drug-induced) methemoglobinemia.

XII. Prognosis:

  A. Expected response to treatment: Early, aggressive therapy expected to produce rapid improvement without sequelae.

  B. Expected complications and long-term effects:

    1. Heinz body formation and red blood cell hemolysis may occur, particularly in presence of G-6-PD deficiency.

    2. Methylene blue therapy may cause urine and skin discoloration.

    3. Death.

XIII. Special considerations:

  A. Methylene blue therapy in high doses (cumulative dose >15 mg/kg) may itself cause methemoglobinemia.

  B. Treatment failure with methylene blue raises possibility of enzyme deficiencies (see above) or sulfhemoglobinemia.

  C. Patients seen several hours after exposure have low probability of significant methemoglobin toxicity (unless long-acting nitrates ingested, such as isosorbide dinitrate) and usually do not require methylene blue therapy.

  D. Methylene blue should be avoided in patients with G-6-PD deficiency due to possibility of hemolysis.

XIV. Disposition considerations:

  A. Admission considerations:

    1. See General Admission Considerations (Chapters 17 and 18).

    2. Admit all patients with significant signs or symptoms (hypotension, CNS changes, tachycardia, dyspnea).

    3. Patients with methemoglobin levels greater than 30% should be hospitalized regardless of presence of symptoms.

    4. Unconsciousness at any time in aftermath of nitrite or nitrate overdose; hospitalization until 24 hours after becoming asymptomatic.

    5. Suicide risk.

  B. Consultation considerations:

    1. Hematologist for possible exchange transfusion in extremely symptomatic patients (especially neonates and children) in whom methemoglobinemia is unresponsive to methylene blue.

    2. In ocular exposures, ophthalmologist if ocular symptoms persist despite 15-minute irrigation (see Chapter 28).

    3. Public health authorities if poisoning secondary to environmental or occupational exposure.

  C. Observation period:

    1. Asymptomatic patients with normal examination, with methemoglobin levels less than 30%, may be considered for discharge when a repeat level is less than 15% and they continue to show no systemic toxicity from ingestion after 4–6 hours of emergency department observation.

2. Longer observation period (i.e., at least 6 hours) important in patients who have ingested long-acting nitrates, such as isosorbide dinitrate. Admission is indicated if unable to observe for prolonged period.

D. Discharge considerations:
   1. General Discharge Considerations have been met (see Chapters 17 and 18)
   2. Asymptomatic patients with normal exam, with methemoglobin levels less than 30%, may be considered for discharge when a repeat methemoglobin level is less than 15% and they continue to show no systemic toxicity from the ingestion after 4–6 hours of ED observation.
   3. Drug responsible for methemoglobinemia should be discontinued or dose appropriately reduced in essential medications (e.g., antianginal therapy).
   4. Counseling regarding further home or environmental exposure to nitrites or nitrates should be done. Appropriate public health officials should be notified if necessary. Do not discharge patients who will return to an environment where further exposure may occur.
   5. Suicide potential and psychiatric status have been appropriately evaluated.

BIBLIOGRAPHY

Benowitz NL: Nitrites and nitrates, in Haddad LM, Winchester JF (eds). *Clinical Management of Poisoning and Drug Overdose*. Philadelphia, WB Saunders Co, 1983, pp 882–886.

Curry S: Methemoglobinemia. *Ann Emerg Med* 1982; 11:214–221.

Donovan JW: Methemoglobinemia, in Haddad LM, Winchester JF (eds): *Clinical Management of Poisoning and Drug Overdose*. Philadelphia, WB Saunders Co, 1983, pp 905–909.

Hall AH, Kulig KW, Rumack BH: Drug and chemical-induced methemoglobinemia. *Med Toxicol* 1986; 1:253–260.

Harris JC, Rumack BH, Peterson RG, et al: Methemoglobinemia resulting from absorption of nitrates. *JAMA* 1979;242:2869–2871.

Kaye F: Bedside toxicology. *Pediatr Clin North Am* 1970; 17:522.

103

Sulfides/Sulfites

Robert J. Stine, M.D., F.A.C.E.P.

Sulfides

I. Route of exposure: Inhalation, oral, cutaneous, ocular.
II. Common sources of sulfides:
  A. Hydrogen sulfide (H_2S):
    1. Highly toxic, colorless, flammable gas, has an offensive odor of rotten eggs that may not be perceived in concentrations exceeding 150 ppm because of rapid paralysis of olfactory nerve.
    2. Gas can be released from decaying sulfur-containing organic matter such as fish or manure. Exposure can be from sewage and from chemical reactions involving sulfur-containing acids or sulfur-containing compounds. Gas can be encountered in sewers and septic tanks, in mines, and in industries involved with tanning, metal refining, textile manufacturing, rubber vulcanizing, heavy water production, waste disposal, and oil and gas exploration and processing.
    3. Poisoning can result from exposure to hydrogen sulfide gas liberated by various chemical reactions involving sulfide salts.
  B. Sulfide salts:
    1. Sodium, potassium, ammonium, barium, strontium, calcium sulfide.
    2. Used in a variety of industrial processes (e.g., manufacture of paper and textiles, rubber vulcanizing, photographic developing, metal refining, as a depilatory). Common ingredient in luminous paints.
  C. Carbonyl sulfide (COS):
    1. Toxic gas that is hydrolyzed by water to carbon dioxide and hydrogen sulfide, with the latter being primarily responsible for its toxicity.

2. Gas encountered during destructive distillation of coal or petroleum refining.
D. Carbon disulfide (CS_2): See Table 108–1.
III. Pharmacokinetics:
   A. Absorption:
      1. H_2S gas rapidly absorbed via respiratory tract.
      2. Soluble salts of sulfides absorbed from GI tract. Some sulfide preparations can be absorbed through intact skin.
   B. Onset of action:
      1. H_2S: Exposure to concentrations above 500 ppm can produce life-threatening symptoms and death in 30–60 minutes.
   C. Elimination: Sulfide rapidly detoxified in human body by various oxidative mechanisms with formation of nontoxic products, primarily thiosulfate and sulfate, which are excreted by kidneys.
IV. Toxic mechanism:
   A. Sulfides:
      1. H_2S gas and aqueous solutions of sulfide salts reversibly inhibit respiratory enzyme cytochrome oxidase through complex formation between hydrosulfide (HS^-) anion and ferric iron of cytochrome oxidase.
         a. Systemic toxicity results from anoxia at cellular level. Cellular anoxia leads to depression of CNS, respiratory, cardiac functions.
         b. Anaerobic metabolism results, with secondary metabolic (lactic) acidosis.
      2. Tissue irritants with highly alkaline sulfides (e.g., sodium, potassium, ammonium sulfide) being caustic to tissues.
V. Range of toxicity:
   A. Toxic dose:
      1. H_2S: Systemic toxicity (from cellular anoxia):
         a. >50 ppm: Mild to moderate symptoms.
         b. >200 ppm: Severe symptoms.
      2. Sulfide salts: 10–20 gm elemental sulfur converted in GI tract to sulfides; causes GI irritation and kidney damage.
   B. Fatal dose:
      1. H_2S: >500 ppm can produce rapid loss of consciousness, respiratory paralysis, death. Neurologic sequelae may persist in survivors.
      2. Sulfide salts: 10 gm.
VI. Clinical features:
   A. H_2S:
      1. Local effects:
         a. Result from direct irritant action of gas on tissues, principally membranes of eyes and respiratory tract.
         b. Keratoconjunctivitis, rhinitis, pharyngitis, tracheobronchitis, noncardiogenic pulmonary edema.
         c. GI tract irritation: Nausea and vomiting.
      2. Systemic toxicity:
         a. Primarily result of oxygen deprivation on CNS and heart.
         b. Headache, weakness, dizziness, altered mental status, seizures,

coma, respiratory depression, cardiac arrhythmias, conduction disturbances, hypotension.

    c. Cyanosis common, as is lactic acidosis from anaerobic metabolism.

  B. Sulfide salts:

    1. Tissue irritation or chemical burns can result from contact with aqueous solutions of sulfide salts, depending on alkalinity of solution.

    2. Chemical reactions may release H_2S gas, with findings as above.

VII. Laboratory findings and evaluation:

  A. Arterial blood gases, lactate (assess for hypoxia, lactic acidosis).

  B. Chemistry (electrolytes, renal function, glucose).

  C. Carboxyhemoglobin level if concomitant carbon monxide exposure suspected (e.g., fire).

  D. Methemoglobin level if nitrite therapy instituted, to monitor therapy. Therapeutic methemoglobin levels should not exceed 30%.

  E. Chest radiograph (with respiratory symptoms).

  F. ECG.

VIII. General treatment:

  A. Follow APTLS: See Chapter 8.

  B. General management: Table 103–1 (see Chapter 12 for details).

  C. Inhalation: See Chapters 108 and 111.

  D. Ingestion:

    1. Little available information on management of ingestion of sulfides. It seems appropriate, however, to base therapy on alkalinity of sulfide in question. The following guidelines are suggested:

      a. Low to moderately alkaline sulfides:

        (1) Barium, calcium, strontium sulfide.

        (2) Can be treated with standard procedures to prevent absorption (see Chapter 12).

      b. Highly alkaline sulfides:

        (1) Sodium, potassium, ammonium sulfide.

        (2) These sulfides are caustic substances; thus gastric emptying is not recommended (see Chapter 73).

TABLE 103–1.

General Treatment

Treatment	Indicated	Of No Value	Contraindicated
O_2	+		
IV	+		
ECG monitor	+		
Forced diuresis		X	
Acidification			X
Alkalinization*		X	
Emesis†/lavage†	±/±		
Charcoal	+		
Cathartic†	±		

*Administer HCO_3 if pH <7.2 (metabolic acidosis).
†Depends on alkalinity of substance (see Ingestion below).

(3) In awake patients, dilution with 4–8 oz (120–240 ml) water or milk PO (not to exceed 15 ml/kg in a child), followed by nothing PO, is recommended.

(4) Administration of **activated charcoal** may be of benefit in binding toxic hydrosulfide anion. Patient should otherwise be given nothing PO.

E. Ocular exposure: See Chapter 28.

F. Skin exposure: See Chapter 29.

IX. Specific treatment:

A. Nitrite therapy:

1. Although controversial, nitrite therapy is recommended in potentially serious sulfide poisonings.

2. Nitrites are available in Cyanide Antidote Kit (Eli Lilly & Co., Indianapolis) as amyl nitrite ampules and sodium nitrite solution. **Remember: Sodium thiosulfate, also present in Cyanide Kit, should NOT be given in sulfide poisoning.**

3. Mechanism of effect: Nitrite therapy converts hemoglobin to methemoglobin, which competes with cytochrome oxidase for hydrosulfide ion and forms sulfmethemoglobin complex. This spares cytochrome oxidase for vital cellular respiratory function.

4. Administration:

a. See Chapter 101 (p. 592) for specifics of administering Cyanide Antidote Kit.

b. For persistent or recurrent signs of serious sulfide toxicity, sodium nitrite can be repeated in half dosage.

c. Goal is reversal of sulfide toxicity with methemoglobin level of <30% (requires monitoring).

B. **Hyperbaric oxygen therapy** appears to be of benefit and should be considered in severe cases of sulfide poisoning.

C. Cardiovascular support:

1. **Cardiac arrest:** Advanced life support should be implemented. Follow most recent Advanced Cardiac Life Support guidelines (*JAMA* 1986; 255:2841–3044).

2. Hypotension: See Chapter 10 for treatment recommendations.

D. Seizures: See Chapter 22 for treatment recommendations.

X. Prognosis:

A. Expected response to treatment:

1. H_2S: Prognosis good if the patient is awake within 4 hours.

2. Carbon disulfide: Recovery takes several months and may never be complete.

B. Expected complications and long-term effects: More severe and prolonged the acute neurologic manifestations of toxicity, the greater the chance for permanent neurologic sequelae.

XI. Controversies: **Antidotal therapy:** Although controversial, nitrite therapy is recommended in potentially serious sulfide poisonings.

XII. Disposition considerations:

A. Admission considerations:

1. See General Admission Considerations (Chapters 17 and 18).

   2. Patients with CNS, cardiovascular, pulmonary signs of toxicity or receiving antidotal therapy warrant hospitalization.
   3. Suicide risk.
 B. Consultation considerations: Hyperbaric facility if indicated.
 C. Observation period: Observe patient with minor or no symptoms for minimum of 4–6 hours in emergency department.
 D. Discharge considerations:
   1. General discharge considerations have been met (see Chapter 18).
   2. Asymptomatic patients and patients with minor symptoms and normal examination (except for signs of mild upper airway irritation) may be discharged with medications to alleviate symptoms (e.g., decongestants, sore throat lozenges) after 4–6 hours of observation.
   3. Counseling regarding further home or environmental exposure to toxic sulfides should be done. Appropriate public health officials should be notified if necessary. Do not discharge patients who will return to an environment where further exposure may occur.
   5. Suicide potential and psychiatric state have been appropriately evaluated.
 E. Patient transfer issues:
   1. Care must be taken to ensure that patients with severe hydrogen sulfide poisoning are not transferred to a facility with a hyperbaric chamber before they are medically stable.
   2. See Chapter 19.

Sulfites

  I. Route of exposure: Oral, inhalation, cutaneous, mucous membrane.
 II. Common sources of sulfites:
 A. Sodium and potassium bisulfite.
 B. Sodium and potassium metabisulfite.
 C. Sodium, potassium, calcium, ammonium sulfite.
 D. Sulfur dioxide; also an atmospheric pollutant.
III. Pharmacokinetics:
 A. Absorption: Sulfites well absorbed from GI tract, respiratory tract (sulfur dioxide), and peritoneal cavity (sulfite-containing dialysis solutions).
 B. Elimination: Majority of absorbed sulfites transformed in liver to sulfate, which is excreted in urine.
 IV. Uses:
 A. Sulfites used as antioxidants and preservatives with antimicrobial activity in a variety of foods, beverages, and drugs (including sympathomimetic aerosols).
 B. Used as reducing agents, antiseptics and disinfectants, bleaches in a variety of industrial processes (e.g., bleaching of fabrics, manufacture of paper and dyes, photographic developing).
 C. Sulfur dioxide a by-product of gasoline combustion.

V. Toxic mechanism:
  A. Tissue irritant:
    1. Sulfurous acid formed when sulfur dioxide dissolves in water is responsible for tissue irritation.
  B. Hypersensitivity reactions (particularly in patients with asthma):
    1. Appear to be primarily cholinergic mediated (possibly from activation of respiratory tract receptors by sulfur dioxide) rather than IgE mediated.
VI. Range of toxicity:
  A. Toxic dose:
    1. Acute ingestions of 3.5 mg/kg and 6.0 mg/kg have produced toxic GI and CNS effects, respectively.
    2. Inhalation of sulfur dioxide exceeding 1.6 ppm has caused bronchoconstriction.
    3. Intraperitoneal doses of 5–6 gm/day sodium bisulfite in dialysis fluids has produced CNS stimulation.
    4. Hypersensitivity reactions can occur at much lower doses.
  B. Fatal dose:
    1. Lethal dose: 10–30 gm.
    2. Sulfur dioxide: Acute exposure in high concentration (>1.6 ppm) can cause severe pneumonitis and rapidly lead to death.
VII. Clinical features:
  A. Acute toxic exposure:
    1. Acute ingestion of sulfites:
      a. Associated with nausea, vomiting, diarrhea, abdominal pain, occasionally GI bleeding.
      b. Exposure to large doses of sulfites can result in CNS stimulation, seizures, hypotension, cardiovascular collapse.
    2. Sulfur dioxide:
      a. Very irritating to tissues, particularly mucous membranes.
      b. Depending on concentration of gas and duration of exposure, can produce conjunctivitis, rhinitis, pharyngitis, laryngeal edema, tracheobronchitis, bronchospasm, noncardiogenic pulmonary edema, skin irritation, GI disturbances.
      c. Contact with liquid sulfur dioxide can cause severe ocular injury and frostbite.
  B. Hypersensitivity reactions:
    1. Usually occur in patients with asthma.
    2. Characterized by angioedema, bronchospasm, urticaria, diaphoresis, flushing, tachycardia, hypotension.
VIII. Laboratory findings and evaluation:
  A. Blood:
    1. Arterial blood gases (with respiratory symptoms).
    2. Carboxyhemoglobin level if concomitant carbon monoxide exposure suspected (e.g., fire).
    3. Immediate spun hematocrit (possible GI bleed).
    4. Chemistry (GI, CNS symptoms).

B. Chest radiograph (assess for pneumonitis).

C. Stool hemoccult (assess for GI bleeding).

IX. General treatment:

A. Follow APTLS: See Chapter 8.

B. General management: See Table 103–2 (Chapter 12 for details).

C. Inhalation: See Chapter 108.

D. Ocular exposure: See Chapter 28.

E. Skin exposure:

   1. Treat frostbite with rapid rewarming (by immersing exposed part in water at temperature of 40°–42° C for 15–30 minutes), followed by application of topical antibiotic. Evaluate tetanus immunization. Severe frostbite injuries should be referred to burn specialist.

   2. See Chapter 29.

X. Specific therapy:

A. Bronchospasm:

   1. See Chapter 108 for treatment approach.

   2. If sympathomimetic aerosol therapy used, ensure that preparation does not contain sulfites.

   3. Pulmonary edema:

      a. Careful fluid restriction (avoiding net positive fluid balance).

      b. Positive end-expiratory pressure (PEEP).

B. Hypotension: See Chapter 10 for treatment recommendations.

C. Hypersensitivity reactions (including angioedema): See Chapter 24 for treatment recommendations.

D. Seizures: See Chapter 22 for treatment recommendations.

XI. Prognosis:

A. Expected response to treatment: Prognosis good, given good supportive care.

B. Expected complications and long-term effects:

   1. Rarely, noncardiogenic pulmonary edema.

TABLE 103–2.

General Treatment

Treatment	Indicated	Of No Value	Contraindicated
O₂	±		
IV	+		
ECG monitor	±		
Forced diuresis		X	
Acidification			X
Alkalinization		X	
Emesis*/lavage*	+/+		
Charcoal*	+		
Cathartic*	+		
Dilution†	+		

*For ingestions other than liquid sulfur dioxides or other corrosive-like compounds.
†See Sulfides.

2. Contact with liquid sulfur dioxide can cause severe ocular injury and frostbite.
3. Sulfur dioxide can cause irreversible bronchiolar obstruction or restrictive lung disease.

XII. Special considerations:
   A. Sulfites are potent sensitizers; anaphylaxis can occur from exposure to residues in food or drugs.
   B. Sulfur dioxide may exacerbate chronic obstructive pulmonary disease.

XIII. Disposition considerations:
   A. Admission considerations:
      1. See General Admission Considerations (Chapters 17 and 18).
      2. Patients with upper airway obstruction, persistent bronchospasm, persistent hypotension, seizures, severe GI disturbance, severe ocular injury, frostbite require hospitalization.
      3. Suicide risk.
   B. Consultation considerations:
      1. In ocular exposure, ophthalmologist if symptoms do not resolve after 15 minutes of irrigation.
      2. Burn center for evidence of significant frostbite injury.
   C. Observation period: If asymptomatic or mild upper respiratory or GI symptoms, observe for at least 4–6 hours in the emergency department.
   D. Discharge considerations:
      1. General discharge considerations have been met (see Chapters 17 and 18).
      2. Asymptomatic or mildly symptomatic patients with normal exam (except for signs of mild upper airway irritation) and normal chest radiograph should be observed for 4–6 hours in emergency department; if they remain well, may be discharged without repeat chest radiograph.
      3. Patients with only mild upper respiratory symptoms (e.g., pharyngitis, rhinitis) without objective injury may be discharged with reassurance and medications to alleviate symptoms (e.g., decongestants, sore throat lozenges) after 4–6 hours of observation.
      4. Patients with mild bronchospasm with only minimal wheezing that clears rapidly after sympathomimetic therapy may be discharged with appropriate medications (e.g., metaproterenol inhalant) and follow-up.
      5. Patients suspected of having sulfite hypersensitivity should be discharged with appropriate medications (e.g., bronchodilators if indicated, 2–3 day supply of diphenhydramine) and counseled regarding potential sources of sulfites (e.g., preservatives, foods, beverages). Referral to allergist may be indicated.
      6. Suicide potential and psychiatric state have been appropriately addressed.

BIBLIOGRAPHY

Baker GJ, Collett P, Allen DH: Bronchospasm induced by metabisulphite-containing foods and drugs. *Med J Aust* 1981; 614–617.

Beck JF, Bradbury CM, Connors AJ, et al: Nitrite as an antidote for acute hydrogen sulfide intoxication. *Am Indust Hyg Assoc J* 1981; 42:805–809.

Burnett WW, King EG, Grace M, et al.: Hydrogen sulfide poisoning: Review of five years experience. *Can Med Assoc J* 1977; 117:1277.

Goldfarb G, Simon R: Provocation of sulfite sensitive asthma. *J Allergy Clin Immunol* 1984; 72:135.

Jamieson DM, Guill MF, Wray BB: Metabisulfite sensitivity. Case report and literature review. *Ann Allergy* 1985; 54:121.

Koepke JW, Selner JC, Christopher K, et al: Inhaled metabisulfite sensitivity. *J Allergy Clin Immunol* 1984; 73:135.

Koepke JW, Selner JC, Dunhill AC: Presence of sulfur dioxide in commonly used bronchodilator solutions. *J Allergy Clin Immunol* 1983; 72:504.

Mofenson HC: Hydrogen sulfide, in Rumack, BH (ed): *Poisindex.* Denver, Micromedex, 1987.

Ravizza, AG, Caruga D, Cerchiari EL: The treatment of hydrogen sulfide intoxication: Oxygen vs. nitrites. *Vet Hum Toxicol* 1982; 24:241–242.

Schwartz HJ, Chester EH: Bronchospastic response to aerosolized metabisulfite in asthmatic subjects: Potential mechanisms and clinical implications. *J Allergy Clin Immunol* 1984; 74:511–513.

Smilkstein MJ, Bronstein AC, Pickett HM, et al: Hyperbaric oxygen therapy for severe hydrogen sulfide poisoning. *Ann Emerg Med* 1985; 3:27–30.

Smith RP, Gosselin RE: Hydrogen sulfide poisoning. *J Occup Med* 1979; 21:93.

Smolinske SC: *Sulfites,* in Rumack, BH (ed): *Poisindex.* Denver, Micromedex, 1987.

Stine RJ, Slosberg B, Beacham BE: Hydrogen sulfide intoxication. A case report and discussion of treatment. *Ann Intern Med* 1976; 85:756–758.

Whitecraft DD, Baily TD, Hart GB: Hydrogen sulfide poisoning treated with hyperbaric oxygen. *J Emerg Med* 1985; 3:23–25.

Witek TJ, Schacter EN: Detection of sulfur dioxide in bronchodilator aerosols. *Chest* 1984; 86:594.

104

Hydrocarbons and Petroleum Distillates

Paula A. Ryals, M.D., F.A.C.E.P.

I. Route of exposure: Inhalation, dermal, ingestion (including from food chain), parenteral (although rare, IV injection by drug abusers has been reported).

II. Sources of hydrocarbons:
   A. Hydrocarbon group includes compounds containing carbon and hydrogen.
      1. Aliphatics: Gasoline, kerosene, petroleum naphtha, petroleum ether, mineral seal oil, methane, propane, butane.
      2. Derived from pinewood: Turpentine
      3. Derived from coal tar: Aromatic hydrocarbons: Benzene, toluene, xylene.
      4. Halogenated hydrocarbons: Carbon tetrachloride, trichloroethylene.
      5. Hydrocarbons with other chemical groups added: Insecticides, leaded gasoline, camphor, nitrobenzene.

III. Common names: See Table 104–1.

IV. Pharmacokinetics:
   A. Absorption: Hydrocarbons causing systemic toxicity readily absorbed from lungs, GI tract, occasionally skin.
   B. Onset of action: Nearly immediately after inhalation. After ingestion, varies with product.
   C. Elimination: Excretion of volatile hydrocarbons is pulmonary; soluble metabolites excreted in urine. Other hydrocarbons undergo hepatic metabolism and excretion in feces.

TABLE 104–1.

Chemical and Trade Names

Brand Name	Chemical Type
Magic Pre-Wash	Petroleum distillate
Mobil Oil Cooling System Cleaner	Kerosene
Mobil Oil Fast Flush	Kerosene, orthodichlorobenzene
Napa Balkamp Gasket Remover	Toluene
Old English Furniture Polish	Mineral seal oil
Petit Marine Paint Old Salem	Petroleum distillate
Quaker State Deluxe Motor Oil	Crude oil
Rustoleum Stops Rust	Petroleum naphtha
Scott's Liquid Gold	Petroleum distillate, trichloroethane
Shell Barbecue and Fireplace Lighter Fuel	Petroleum distillate
Shell Carburetor and Combustion Chamber Cleaner	Aromatic petroleum distillate
Shell Furniture Polish	Mineral spirits
Shell Lighter Fluid and Spot Remover	Petroleum naphtha
Shot Laundry Soil and Stain Remover	Petroleum naphtha
Siloo Octane Treatment Gasoline Additive	Methanol, petroleum distillate
Southern Pine Paint Remover	Petroleum distillate
Southern Pine Pure Turpentine	Turpentine
STP Gas Treatment	Mineral spirits, xylene
3-In-1 Household Oil	Petroleum distillate

V. Action: See Toxic mechanism.
VI. Uses:
   A. Commercial: Fuels, paint thinners, shoe polish, degreasers, lighter fluid, laxatives, ointments, dry cleaners.
   B. Commonly abused hydrocarbons: See Table 104–2.
VII. Toxic mechanism:
   A. Tissue damage from hydrocarbon exposure comes from lipid peroxidation and subsequent metabolic acidosis. Hydrocarbons preferentially deposited in fatty tissues (i.e., brain, liver).
   B. Animal studies indicate that ingestion of most aliphatic hydrocarbons without aspiration produces relatively minimal toxicity.
   C. Hydrocarbons causing systemic toxicity after ingestion or inhalation include:
      1. Aromatic hydrocarbons: Benzene, toluene, xylene.

TABLE 104–2.

Commonly Abused Hydrocarbons*

Chemical	Commercial Product
Acetone	Plastic cement
	Model cement
	Fingernail polish remover
Toluene	Plastic cement
	Airplane glue
	Lacquer thinner
	Shoe polish
	Model cement
Xylene	
Gasoline	Motor fuel
Benzene	Rubber cement
	Cleaning fluid
	Tube repair kits
	Liquid solder
Naphtha	Lighter fluid
Hexane	Plastic cement
	Rubber cement
Freons	Aerosol propellant
	Refrigerant
Trichloroethane	Spot remover
	Dry cleaner
Trichloroethylene	Degreaser
	Dry cleaner
	Anesthetic agent
	Rubber cement
	Paint thinner

*From Bryson PD: *Comprehensive Review in Toxicology*. Rockvile, Md, Aspen Systems Corp, 1986, p 294. Used by permission.

2. Halogenated hydrocarbons: Tetrachloroethane, trichloroethane carbon tetrachloride.
3. Other: Freon, pesticides, camphor, heavy metals.
4. Mnemonic for toxic hydrocarbons: "CHAMPS": **C**amphor, **H**alogenated hydrocarbons, **A**romatic, **M**etals (with heavy metal additives), **P**esticides.

D. Intratracheal instillation causes prompt obtundation, respiratory distress, pulmonary hemorrhage.
E. Dermal exposure may lead to CNS effects.
F. IV use can cause pulmonary toxicity.
G. Exact toxic mechanism of chlorinated hydrocarbons such as DDT unknown. Results in widespread focal necrosis in various organs and tissues, especially liver.
H. Risk of aspiration depends primarily on viscosity and surface tension of hydrocarbon (see Table 104–3).

TABLE 104–3.

Viscosity of Aliphatic Hydrocarbons

Aspiration Potential	Description	Examples
Low	High viscosity	Asphalt, mineral oil, baby oil, suntan oil, lubricating oil, petroleum jelly, diesel oil, grease, tar, paraffin
High	Low viscosity	Mineral seal oil, gasoline, kerosene, petroleum, ether, lighter fluid, turpentine, naphtha, mineral spirits

VIII. Range of toxicity:
  A. Toxic dose:
    1. Significant toxicity may be seen after ingestion of at least 1 ml/kg toxic hydrocarbon. Very large amounts (>4–5 ml/kg), however, are necessary for CNS toxicity.
    2. Aspiration of as little as 1 ml may result in severe chemical pneumonitis.
  B. Fatal dose: Benzene is most toxic of the aromatics, and deaths have been reported after an oral dose as little as 15 ml.
IX. Clinical features:
  A. Poisoning most commonly seen in children.
  B. Degree of severity correlates closely with viscosity of ingested product. Danger of aspiration decreases with higher viscosity products (see Table 104–3).
  C. Acute toxicity affects CNS, pulmonary function, cardiac conduction system, and GI tract.
    1. CNS: Obtundation or agitation, euphoria, ataxia, hallucinations, vertigo, nystagmus, tinnitus, diplopia, seizures, chorea, vasomotor instability, fever. Chronic syndromes include cranial and peripheral nerve lesions.
    2. Pulmonary: Coughing, choking, tachypnea, pulmonary edema, hemoptysis, infiltrates, basilar atelectasis, pneumothorax, pneumomediastinum.
    3. Cardiac: Dysrhythmias including asystole, heart block, ventricular fibrillation. Chronically, cardiomyopathy may occur.
    4. GI: Vomiting, occasional bloody diarrhea; elevated liver function tests within hours. Chronic: significant hepatic dysfunction with jaundice.
    5. Renal: Proteinuria, hematuria, renal failure, renal tubular acidosis.
    6. Hematologic: Elevated white blood cell count, hemorrhage, rarely hemolysis. Chronic: aplastic anemia, leukemia.
    7. Dermatologic: Burns, epidermal necrolysis (rare).
X. Laboratory findings and evaluation:
  A. Chest radiograph:
    1. Characteristic findings: Bibasilar infiltrates, atelectasis, hemorrhagic

bronchopneumonia, pulmonary edema, pleural effusion, pneumo-thorax, pneumomediastinum, pneumatoceles.
2. Double gastric fluid level may be noted if glassful of water is consumed first to provide an aqueous layer. As little as 5 ml kerosene in stomach may be detected by this technique (Daffner RH, Jimenex JP: *Radiology* 1973; 106:383–384).

B. Blood:
1. Consider arterial blood gas.
2. Complete blood cell count (leukocytosis), glucose (if altered mental status), electrolytes (may see hypokalemia), BUN, creatinine, liver function studies (PT, PTT, transaminases, bilirubin).

C. Urinalysis (proteinuria, glucose, acetone, hematuria).

D. ECG.

XI. General treatment:
A. Follow APTLS: See Chapter 8.
B. General management: See Table 104–4 (Chapter 12 for details).

XII. Specific treatment:
A. Respiratory support: See Chapters 9 and 108.
B. Arrhythmias:
1. If required, antiarrhythmic therapy should be specific for arrhythmia present.
2. NOTE: **Epinephrine** and other adrenergic drugs **relatively contraindicated** because of hydrocarbon sensitization of conducting system, leading to potential for serious ventricular tachyarrhythmias.

C. Gastric emptying:
1. Highly controversial whether to proceed, and if so which is best technique (gastric lavage versus emesis). (Also see XV. later in this chapter.)

TABLE 104–4.

General Treatment

Treatment	Indicated	Of No Value	Contraindicated
O$_2$	±		
IV	+		
ECG monitor	+		
Forced diuresis*			X
Acidification		X	
Alkalinization		X	
Emesis†/lavage†	±/±		
Charcoal‡		X	X
Cathartic‡			X
Others§			
Dialysis¶	±		

*Best avoided because of potential cardiac toxicity; probably of not much value.
†Controversial (see Gastric emptying).
‡May induce vomiting.
§Wash skin with soap and water if dermal exposure.
¶Effective for certain ingestions.

2. Assure adequate airway, ventilation, stable vital signs prior to any procedure.
3. Gastric emptying considerations:
   a. Syrup of ipecac:
      (1) Indications: Hydrocarbons that can cause systemic toxicity.
         a Toxic petroleum distillates or turpentine, in massive quantity (>4–5 ml/kg).
         b Presence of toxic additive (e.g., heavy metal, pesticide).
         c Aromatic compounds (see Table 104–5).
         d Halogenated compounds (e.g., CCl_4).
         e Camphor.
         f Concomitant ingestion of another toxic substance for which ipecac indicated (e.g., aspirin, acetaminophen).
      (2) Contraindications:
         a Accidental ingestion of petroleum distillate with little potential for systemic absorption or toxicity.
         b Previous unprovoked emesis.
         c Presence of neurologic, respiratory, cardiac abnormalities or absent gag reflex.
         d Standard contraindications for emesis (see Chapter 12).
   b. Gastric lavage:
      (1) Indications:
         a Removal of specific hydrocarbon indicated (see 3.a.1. above), but ipecac-induced emesis contraindicated.
         b Ingestion of another toxic substance for which lavage indicated (e.g., bicarbonate lavage for iron ingestion, starch lavage for iodine).
D. Hemodialysis, hemoperfusion, peritoneal dialysis have been used in carbon tetrachloride, toluene, eucalyptus oil, trichloroethylene poisonings.
XIII. Prognosis:
   A. Expected response to treatment:
      1. General: Mortality less than 1%. Primary cause of death is aspiration resulting in hemorrhagic pneumonitis and pulmonary edema.
      2. Petroleum distillates:
         a. Prognosis determined by extent of pulmonary involvement.
         b. Severe involvement may take weeks to resolve.
      3. Aromatic hydrocarbons:
         a. Survival for 3 days after ingestion associated with good prognosis.
         b. Poor prognosis associated with rapidity of symptom progression and failure to perform gastric decontamination.
         c. Bone marrow suppression associated with poor prognosis in chronic benzene toxicity.
      4. Naphthalene:
         a. Poor prognosis associated with rapidity of symptom progression and presence of coma and seizures.
         b. Renal failure usually resolves by 7–14 days.
      5. Halogenated hydrocarbons:
         a. Carbon tetrachloride: Good prognosis for recovery of renal and he-

patic function. May take several weeks for renal failure to resolve and several months for normal hepatic function to return.

    b. Trichloroethylene: If patient survives for 4 hours, recovery likely.

    c. 1,1,1-Trichloroethane: Survival through acute phase associated with complete recovery.

    d. Tetrachloroethylene: Same as 1,1,1-trichloroethane.

  6. Tetrachloroethane:

    a. Poor prognosis in patients with early hepatic failure and jaundice.

    b. Patients with renal failure usually recover, with full return of kidney function.

  7. Polychlorinated naphthalene and polychlorinated and polybrominated biphenyls: 50% mortality in patients with hepatic failure.

 B. Expected complications and long-term effects:

  1. For petroleum distillates, usually no long-term sequelae.

  2. Hepatic, renal, hematologic derangements may occur hours to days after exposure to hydrocarbons, with potential for systemic toxicity (see above).

  3. Carcinogenic potential exists, with cancer reported to develop months to years later (e.g., some aromatic hydrocarbons, such as benzene).

XIV. Special considerations: Hydrocarbons may have other toxic chemicals added (e.g., insecticides, leaded gasoline, camphor, nitrobenzene). These compounds have toxicity specific to themselves in addition to hydrocarbon base and thus must definitely be removed from stomach.

 A. Halogenated hydrocarbons:

  1. General considerations:

    a. In general, these compounds produce usual constellation of symptoms expected in hydrocarbon poisoning, including GI syndrome, altered mental status, respiratory depression, shock, sensitivity of cardiac conducting system to adrenergic drugs.

    b. Halogenated hydrocarbons more toxic than nonhalogenated hydrocarbons. Chronic syndromes described for workers exposed to fumes usually include renal and hepatic dysfunction.

    c. Specific features of various compounds are listed below. Treatment follows guidelines discussed above with a few additions noted.

  2. Chlorinated hydrocarbons:

    a. These compounds, used as insecticides, are poorly absorbed unless dissolved in organic solvents (kerosene, xylene).

    b. Many are now banned in the United States (e.g., DDT, hetachlor, Kepone, endrin, aldrin). Still in use are lindane, methoxychlor, kethane.

    c. Symptoms of intoxication include nausea, vomiting, apprehension, excitement, muscle tremors, delirium, seizures leading to paralysis and coma.

    d. Treatment includes vigorous GI decontamination with lavage or emesis. Skin decontamination is important. Avoid using oils on skin because they increase absorption. Avoid adrenergic drugs and atropine because they may precipitate arrhythmias.

e. Lindane intoxication requires long-term monitoring of complete blood cell count for myelosuppression.
3. Fluorinated hydrocarbons (Freon): See Table 108–1.
4. Methyl bromide:
   a. Easily penetrates cell membranes and complexes with intracellular proteins.
   b. CNS hyperexcitability prominent, with a syndrome similar to Reye's syndrome described in one child.
   c. Latent period of 12 hours may be noted, followed by acute psychosis, hyporeflexia, tremor, ataxia, seizures, coma.
   d. Careful skin decontamination required because compound can penetrate clothes and rubber gloves.
   e. Pulmonary toxicity: See Table 108–1.
5. Methyl chloride: Causes acute GI symptoms as well as hepatic, renal, hematologic abnormalities. Chronic neurologic syndromes: Ataxia, blurred vision, slurred speech.
6. Ethyl iodide: Depresses CNS and can burn or blister exposed skin.
7. Chloroform:
   a. Initially used as anesthetic until hepatic and cardiac toxicity noted.
   b. Pupils dilated and react sluggishly to light. There is "excitement" phase prior to narcosis.
8. Carbon tetrachloride:
   a. Marked hepatic and renal dysfunction chronically; occasional aplastic anemia from long-term use.
   b. Treatment: Dialysis, hemoperfusion for severe acute intoxication. *N*-acetylcysteine (Mucormyst) may help prevent hepatic damage (see Chapter 77).
   c. See Table 108–1.
9. Methyl chloroform: Prominent CNS depression, shock.
10. Ethylene chlorohydrin:
    a. Exceptionally toxic fumes (exposure limit 1 ppm). Vapor is odorless. Symptoms appear after latent period. Visual symptoms and corneal burns noted occasionally.
    b. Treatment: Decontaminate skin and eyes after exposure.
11. Trichloroethylene:
    a. Prolonged nausea and vomiting, cranial nerve damage (especially trigeminal nerve), cerebellar symptoms, seizures. If exposure combined with ethanol ingestion, may note flushing of face and arms.
    b. See Table 108–1.
12. Tetrachloroethylene: Mucous membrane irritation.
13. Dichloropropane: Pulmonary edema.
14. Methylene chloride:
    a. Produces carbon monoxide following inhalation of methylene chloride vapors.
    b. Treatment: See Chapter 100 and Table 108–1.
B. Aromatic hydrocarbons:
   1. Widely used in industry as solvents and as drugs of abuse (see Table 104–5).

   2. See Table 108–1.
   C. Solvent abuse: See Chapter 108.
XV. Controversies:
   A. Gastric emptying:
      1. Some authors recommend giving ipecac in an awake, alert patient with intact gag reflex if a significant (at least 30 ml or approximately 1 ml/ kg) amount of toxic hydrocarbon has been ingested. Otherwise, if the patient is obtunded, intubate with cuffed endotracheal tube and carefully lavage with 200 ml aliquots fluid.
      2. Other authors cite experimental evidence indicating minimal CNS or pulmonary toxicity for all ingested hydrocarbons and difficulty in estimating volume consumed in a child. In some studies significant aspiration has been noted in patients treated with even cautious gastric lavage. For these reasons they conclude that induction of emesis and even cautious gastric lavage is almost never indicated in pure hydrocarbon ingestions.
      3. Most authors agree that appropriate gastric emptying should be attempted in hydrocarbons combined with additives with the potential for life-threatening complications (e.g., heavy metals, pesticides).
   B. Use of olive or mineral oil to increase viscosity: This may cause lipoid pneumonia if aspirated. Increased incidence of pneumonia has been noted in patients treated with oil. We do not recommend this treatment.
   C. Use of steroids and antibiotics: Not indicated routinely or for prophylaxis.

TABLE 104–5.

Toxicity of Aromatic Hydrocarbons

Compound	Acute Toxicity	Chronic Toxicity
Benzene	Euphoria, dizziness, weakness, headache, tightness, tremor, ataxia, arrhythmia, seizures, coma	Neurasthenia, aplastic anemia, leukemia, blurred vision, cerebral atrophy
Toluene	Same as benzene, plus lacrimation	Abdominal pain, tinnitus, cerebellar degeneration, renal stones, optic neuropathy, rhabdomyolsis, hematemesis, confusion
Xylene	Facial flushing, hepatorenal dysfunction	
Styrene	Mucous membrane irritation, metallic taste, vertigo	Poorly documented but possible teratogenic; CNS effects
Vinyl chloride	Anesthesia; toxic metabolites formed in liver; immunologic syndrome	Acro-osteolysis, angiosarcoma of liver

May be indicated later for positive sputum Gram stain or adult respiratory distress syndrome.

D. Treatment of asymptomatic children with abnormal chest x-ray findings:
   1. Some authorities suggest children can safely be discharged if they remain asymptomatic for 6 hours; others insist on admitting any asymptomatic patient who has or develops abnormal chest x-ray findings.

XVI. Disposition considerations:
   A. Admission considerations:
      1. See General Admission Considerations (Chapters 17 and 18).
      2. Patients should be admitted to the hospital with cardiac monitoring, serial chest films, and at least 24 hours of observation for the following:
         a. Pulmonary symptoms and abnormal chest radiograph on arrival in emergency department.
         b. Symptomatic patients with normal chest radiograph should be observed for 6 hours. If they improve (asymptomatic, normal exam, normal arterial blood gases, normal repeat chest x-ray study), may be safely discharged. However, if symptoms persist or worsen, must be admitted regardless of x-ray findings.
         c. Normal chest radiograph in an asymptomatic patient when reliable home follow-up cannot be assured.
         d. Presence of any clinical signs or symptoms of systemic toxicity including CNS depression, protracted vomiting, fever, hypoxia, dysrhythmias, at any time.
         e. Ingestion has potential for delayed organ system toxicity.
         f. Ingestion of hydrocarbons with potential for systemic toxicity (benzene, nitrobenzene, heavy metals, insecticides, aniline dyes, camphor).
         g. Very large amount ingested (>4–5 ml/kg) of any hydrocarbon.
         h. Suicide risk.
         i. ICU admission considerations:
            (1) Pulmonary symptoms.
            (2) See Chapter 18 for general indications.
   B. Consultation considerations:
      1. Nephrology consultation if hemodialysis or hemoperfusion indicated.
      2. Pulmonary medicine consultation for severe complications secondary to aspiration.
   C. Observation period: 6 hours (in certain well-defined situations; see Discharge considerations).
   D. Discharge considerations:
      1. General discharge considerations have been met (see Chapters 17 and 18).
      2. Asymptomatic patients with normal exam and chest radiograph should be observed for 4–6 hours in the emergency department. If they remain well, may be discharged without repeat chest x-ray study.
      3. Symptomatic patients with normal chest radiograph should be observed for 6 hours. If they improve (asymptomatic, normal exam, normal arterial blood gases, normal repeat chest x-ray study), may be safely discharged. However, if symptoms persist or worsen, must be admitted regardless of x-ray findings.

4. Exceptions to above are for ingestions with potential for significant systemic toxicity or significant delayed effects.
5. Long-term follow-up includes serial complete blood cell counts, renal and hepatic function tests, physical examinations.
6. Suicide potential and psychiatric state have been appropriately addressed.

BIBLIOGRAPHY

Anas N, Namasonthi V, Ginsburg CM, et al: Criteria for hospitalizing children who have ingested products containing hydrocarbons. *JAMA* 1981; 246:840–843.

Banner W, Walson PD: Systemic toxicity following gasoline aspiration. *Am J Emerg Med* 1983; 3:292–294.

Daffner RH, Jimenex JP: The double gastric fluid level in kerosene poisoning. *Radiology* 1973; 106:383–384.

Dice WH, Ward G, Kelley J, et al: Pulmonary toxicity following gastrointestinal ingestion of kerosene. *Ann Emerg Med* 1982; 11:138–142.

Fischman CM, Oster JR: Toxic effects of toluene: A new cause of high anion gap metabolic acidosis. *JAMA* 1979; 241:1713.

Fortenberry JD: Gasoline sniffing. *Am J Med* 1985; 79:740–744.

Hansbrough JF, Zapata-Sirvent R, Dominic W, et al: Hydrocarbon contact injuries. *J Trauma* 1985; 25:250–252.

Kirk LM. Anderson RJ, Martin K: Sudden death from toluene abuse. *Ann Emerg Med* 1984; 13:68.

Kulig K. Rumack BH: Hydrocarbon ingestion. *Curr Topics Emerg Med* 1981; 3:1–5.

Sturmann K, Mofenson H, Caraccio T: Methylene chloride inhalation: An unusual form of drug abuse. *Ann Emerg Med* 1985; 14:903–905.

Wason S, Gibler B, Hassan M: Ventricular tachycardia associated with non-Freon aerosol propellants. *JAMA* 1986; 256:78–80.

Wedin GP, Jones RR: Parenteral administration of hydrocarbons. *Clin Toxicol* 1984; 22:485–492.

105

Camphor

Richard A. Christoph, M.D., F.A.C.E.P.

Camphor is a cyclic ketone of the hydroaromatic turpene group. Originally produced by distilling bark from the camphor tree, it is now synthetically manufactured. It has been available as camphor spirit (10% in alcohol), camphorated oil (20% in cottonseed oil), and camphorated parachlorophenol (35% parachlorophenol and 65% camphor).

I. Route of exposure: Oral, mucous membrane, cutaneous, intramuscular.

II. Common products containing camphor:
>   Camphorated oil
>   Camphor spirits
>   Mentholatum Ointment
>   Ben-Gay Child's Rub
>   Vicks VapoRub
>   Blistix Medicated Lip Ointment
>   Afrin Menthol Nasal Spray
>   Caladryl Cream and Lotion
>   Sinex Decongestant Nasal Spray
>   Vicks Vapo Steam
>   Vicks Inhaler
>   Vicks Throat Lozenges

III. Pharmacokinetics:
   A. Absorption: Rapid absorption from skin and mucous membranes.
   B. Onset of action: 15–20 minutes after ingestion.
   C. Peak effect: Within 90 minutes.
   D. Elimination: Metabolism by hydroxylation and conjugation with glucuronic acid, in liver. Excretion of inactivated camphor metabolites via urine. Some camphor and metabolites excreted by lungs.

E. Active metabolites: None.
IV. Actions: When ingested, camphor is a CNS stimulant with effects ranging from mild excitation to grand mal seizures.
V. Uses:
    A. Rubefacient (topical irritant).
    B. Antipruritic.
    C. Mild topical anesthetic.
    D. Ingredient in paregoric and wide variety of proprietary products intended for external use (liniments), and throat lozenges, nasal sprays, drops.
VI. Toxic mechanism: Stimulates cerebral cortex neurons.
VII. Range of Toxicity:
    A. Toxic dose: Report of 3-year-old with seizures after ingestion of approximately 0.7 gm camphor.
    B. Fatal dose: Highly toxic, with human lethal dose 50–500 mg/kg. One gram has been reported to produce death in 1-year-old; 1 tsp camphorated oil potentially lethal in infants.
VIII. Clinical features:
    A. Eyes:
        1. Mydriasis. Patients may report flickering, darkening, or veiled vision.
        2. Contact with camphor directly on eyes results in irritation but no reports of serious burns.
    B. Respiratory:
        1. Odor of camphor readily apparent.
        2. Postseizure respiratory depression resulting in apnea may cause death.
        3. Tachypnea may be present from central stimulation.
    C. Cardiac: Tachycardia from stimulatory effect.
    D. Gastrointestinal:
        1. Mucosal burning and irritation, nausea and vomiting, abdominal pain shortly after ingestion.
        2. Transient mild elevations of SGOT and lactic dehydrogenase in setting of vomiting and CNS excitation; may mimic clinical pattern of Reye's syndrome.
    E. Renal: Anuria, albuminuria (transient).
    F. CNS:
        1. CNS excitation, tremor, fasciculation, hallucinations, delirium, irritability.
        2. Generalized grand mal **seizures** that **may occur without warning.**
        3. Postconvulsive coma, apnea.
    G. Pregnancy considerations:
        1. Camphor crosses placenta.
        2. One case of fetal death reported.
IX. Laboratory findings and evaluation:
    A. Serum camphor levels: Not generally available, but toxic symptoms appear to correlate with serum levels measured by gas-liquid chromatography.
    B. Initial laboratory assessment: Complete blood cell count (look for moderate leukocytosis), electrolytes, liver function studies (transient elevation of liver transaminases).

    C. Consider chest radiograph (rule out aspiration during seizures), arterial blood gases (with respiratory symptoms), urinalysis.

X. General treatment:
    A. Follow APTLS: See Chapter 8.
    B. General management: Table 105–1 (see Chapter 12 for details).
    C. Do not leave patient unattended.

XI. Specific treatment
    A. General supportive care: See Chapters 8–10.
    B. Seizures: See Chapter 22 for treatment recommendations.
    C. Dialysis:
        1. Several reports of camphor-induced refractory seizures that resolved following lipid dialysis using soybean oil.
        2. Amberlite resin hemoperfusion used successfully in one patient.
        3. Dialysis using one of these methods should be a last resort for life-threatening camphor ingestion with seizures refractory to conventional therapies.

XII. Prognosis:
    A. Expected response to treatment: Most patients recover completely if treatment with good supportive care begins early. Survival for 24 hours associated with complete recovery.
    B. Expected complications and long-term effects: Institution of early appropriate treatment usually effective in preventing long-term CNS sequelae.

XIII. Disposition considerations:
    A. Admission considerations:
        1. See General Admission Considerations (Chapter 18).
        2. History suggestive of ingestion of >0.5 gm camphor in child or >1 gm camphor in adult.
        3. Symptomatic.
        4. Suicide risk.
        5. ICU: Patients exhibiting neurologic symptoms or severe GI symptoms.

TABLE 105–1.

General Treatment

Treatment	Indicated	Of No Value	Contraindicated
O_2	+		
IV	+		
ECG monitor	±		
Forced diuresis		X	
Acidification		X	
Alkalinization		X	
Emesis*			X
Lavage†	+		
Charcoal‡			
Cathartic	+		

*Seizures may occur suddenly without warning.
†Gastric lavage until odor of camphor is undetectable in lavage fluids.
‡Administer activated charcoal 1–2 gm/kg using 240 ml diluent per 30 gm charcoal. Diluent may be water, saline cathartic, or sorbitol.

B. Consultation considerations:
   1. General anesthesia may be necessary for control of seizures unresponsive to standard treatment, as may occur with camphor overdoses.
   2. Consider dialysis for treatment of refractory seizures.
   3. Social worker: In childhood exposure.
C. Observation period: If asymptomatic, 6 hours.
D. Discharge considerations:
   1. General discharge considerations have been met (see Chapters 17 and 18).
   2. Asymptomatic with normal exam after 6 hours of observation.
   3. Suicide potential and psychiatric state have been appropriately addressed
   4. In childhood exposure, home environment has been appropriately assessed and parents counseled.

BIBLIOGRAPHY

Antman E, et al: Camphor overdosage. *NY State J Med* 1978; 78:895–896.

Jimenez JF, et al: Chronic Camphor ingestion mimicking Reye's syndrome. *Gastroenterology* 1983; 84:374–398.

Kopelman R, et al: Camphor intoxication treated by resin hemoperfusion. *JAMA* 1979; 241:727–728.

106

Organophosphates and Carbamates

Richard A. Christoph, M.D., F.A.C.E.P.

Organophosphates

I. Route of Exposure: Oral, cutaneous, inhalation, mucous membrane, injection (rare).
II. Common generic and trade names: See Table 106–1.
III. Pharmacokinetics:
    A. Absorption: Efficiently absorbed from GI tract, through skin, and across pulmonary membranes.
    B. Onset of action:
        1. Immediate after inhalation.
        2. Massive ingestion: 5 minutes.
        3. Onset of toxicity usually within 12 hours, always within 24 hours.
    C. Duration of action: Clinical effects may last for days.
    D. Elimination: Hydrolyzed to alkyl phosphates, with renal excretion of these metabolites.
    E. Parathion has toxic metabolite, paraoxon, produced in liver.
IV. Actions: Organophosphates act by combining with acetylcholinesterase, resulting in inactivation and accumulation of acetylcholine at synapses and myoneural junctions. Initially this linkage is reversible, but ultimately organophosphate-acetylcholinesterase link becomes irreversible.
V. Uses:
    A. Insecticides, pesticides.
    B. Toxic exposure occurs most frequently among children, farmers and unskilled farm workers, suicide victims.

TABLE 106–1.

Organophosphate Insecticides*

Common Name	Produce	Chemical Name
Agricultural insecticides (high toxicity)		
TEPP	Miller Kilmite 40	Tetraethylpyrophosphate
Parathion	Niagara Phoskil Dust	O,O-diethyl O-p-nitrophenyl phosphorothioate
Phosdrin	Mevinphos	Dimethyl-O-(1-methyl-2-carbonmethoxyvinyl phosphate)
Disyston	Disulfoton	Diethyl-S-2-ethyl-2-mercaptoethyl phosphorodithioate
Guthion	Guthion	Dimethyl S-(4-oxo-1,2,3-benzotriazinyl-3-methyl phosphorodithioate)
Animal insecticides (intermediate toxicity)		
Ronnel	Korlan Livestock Spray	O,O-dimethyl O-(2,4,5-trichlorophenyl) phosphorothioate
Coumaphos	Co-Ral Animal Insecticide	Diethyl-O-(3-chloro-4-methyl-7-coumarinyl) phosphorothioate
Chloropyrifos (Dursban)	Rid-A-Bug	O,O-diethyl-O-(3,5,6-trichloro-2-pyridyl) phosphorothioate
Trichlorfon	Trichlorfon Pour On	Dimethyl trichlorohydroxyethyl phosphonate
Household use (low toxicity)		
Malathion	Ortho Malathion 50 Insecticide	Dimethyl-B-(1,2-bis-carboethoxy) ethyl phosphorodithioate
Diazinon	Security Fire Ant Killer	Diethyl-O-(2-isopropyl-6-methyl-4-pyrimidyl) phosphorothioate
Vapona (Dichlorvos, DDVP)	Shell No-Pest Strip	O,O-dimethyl-O-2,2-dichlorovinyl phosphate

*Adapted from Haddad LM, Winchester JF: *Clinical Management of Poisonings and Drug Overdose*, Philadelphia, WB Saunders Co, 1983, p 705.

VI. Toxic mechanism:
  A. Accumulation of acetylcholine transiently stimulates but soon paralyzes conduction through cholinergic synapses in CNS, parasympathetic terminals and some sympathetic terminals (muscarinic effects), somatic nerves and autonomic ganglionic synapses (nicotinic effects).
  B. Cholinergic crisis results, with usual cause of death resulting from respiratory muscular weakness and increased pulmonary secretions.
  C. Organophosphates used as agricultural insecticides are most potent and have highest toxicity. Animal insecticides such as ronnel, coumaphos, chlorpyrifos and trichlorfon are of intermediate toxicity. Malathion and

dichlorvos are of low enough toxicity to be suitable for household use (see Table 106–1).

VII. Range of toxicity (Table 106–2):

    A. Probable minimum lethal dose of parathion: 10–20 mg (mean lethal dose 300 mg, 4 mg/kg).

    B. Report of pediatric death after 2 mg (0.1 mg/kg) dose of parathion.

    C. Exposure to Chlorthion, DEF, malathion, Phostex unlikely to cause fatal poisoning (lethal dose of malathion estimated at 1,375 mg/kg).

VIII. Clinical features:

    A. Onset of clinical symptoms after exposure may vary, depending on route of exposure of specific chemical, but is often within 12 hours and almost always within 24 hours.

    B. Patients may have garlic-like odor on skin and breath.

    C. Initial symptoms predominantly muscarinic. Development of nicotinic

TABLE 106–2.

Common Organophosphates in Order of Decreasing Toxicity

Compound	Fatal Dose (mg/kg)	Compound	Fatal Dose (mg/kg)
TEPP	1.0	Coumophos	15.0
Mipafox	1.0	Fenthion	15.0
Phorate	1.1	Monocrotophos	21.0
Dimefox	1–2	Delnav	23.0
Fensulfathion	2.0	Ethion	27.0
Demeton	2.5	Phosphamidon	27.0
Tetram	3.0	Bomyl	32.0
Parathion*	3.0	Mecarbam	36.0
Paraoxon	3.0	Dichlorvos	56.0
Pirazinon	3.5	Prophos	61.0
Phosdrin	3.7	Methyl demeton	65.0
Gophacide	3.7	Methyl trithion	98.0
Pirazoxone	4.0	Ciodrin	125.0
Sulfatepp	5.0	Aleton	146.0
Folex	5.0	Phosfon	178.0
Isoflurophate	8.0	Dimethoate	215.0
Dyforate	8.0	DEF	325.0
Cyolane	8.9	Naled	430.0
Carbophenothion	10.0	Trichlorphon	450.0
Guthion	10.0	Diazinon	466.0
Schradan	10.0	2-4 DEP	850.0
Zinophos	12.0	Aspon	890.0
Pyrazothion	12.0	Rommell	1,250.0
Disulfeton	12.0	Malathion	1,375.0
Methyl parathion	14.0	Menazon	1,950.0
EPN	14.0	Abate	2,000.0
Dicrotophos	15.0	Phostex	2,500.0

*Report of death in child after 2 mg (0.1 mg/kg).

symptoms and of direct CNS symptoms indicates very severe poisoning. Thus the following clinical effects could be observed:

1. Muscarinic effects (Table 106–3):

   Salivation, sweating   Bradycardia, AV block
   Lacrimation   Hypotension
   Urinary incontinence   Blurred vision
   Defecation, diarrhea   Miosis
   Gastrointestinal symptoms: Bronchospasm
     abdominal cramps,   Bronchorrhea
     tenesmus, nausea, vomiting

2. Nicotinic effects:

   Fasciculations
   Muscle cramps
   Weakness, flaccid paralysis
   Areflexia
   Respiratory failure or arrest
   Tachycardia
   Hypertension

3. CNS effects:

   Headache
   Anxiety
   Ataxia
   Restlessness
   Seizures
   Insomnia, coma
   Areflexia
   Respiratory depression
   Psychosis

   D. May see hypoglycemia.

IX. Laboratory findings and evaluation:

   A. Red cell (erythrocyte) acetylcholinesterase level: ≥25% reduction, diagnostic of organophosphate exposure.

   B. Serum acetylcholinesterase (pseudocholinesterase) level:

      1. Measure if red cell cholinesterase test not available.

TABLE 106–3.

Muscarinic Manifestations:
Useful Acronyms

SLUDGE	or	STUMBLED
Salivation		**S**alivation
Lacrimation		**T**remor
Urination		**U**rination
Defecation		**M**iosis
Gastrointestinal cramps		**B**radycardia
Emesis		**L**acrimation
		Emesis
		Diarrhea

    2. Not as specific as red cell acetylcholinesterase. Will also be reduced in malnutrition, acute infections, anemia, myocardial infarction, dermatomyositis, and 3% of normal patients as a genetic variant.

    3. Send to lab in heparinized tube.

    4. Correlation of serum acetylcholinesterase levels with symptoms (Table 106–4).

  C. Other laboratory tests:

    1. Blood:

      a. Complete blood cell count (leukocytosis with left shift frequently noted).

      b. Electrolytes, arterial blood gases (metabolic acidosis with normal anion gap, compatible with renal tubular acidosis).

      c. Blood glucose (rule out hyperglycemia, hypoglycemia, especially in presence of altered mental status).

      d. Renal and liver function studies (elevation of transaminases).

      e. PT, PTT (prolonged coagulation times).

    2. Chest radiograph: Diverse findings, such as aspiration pneumonitis, atelectasis, pulmonary edema.

    3. ECG: Bradycardia and associated heart block; may develop complex ventricular arrhythmias.

    4. Urinalysis: Hematuria, glycosuria, proteinuria (aminoaciduria), alterations in phosphate resorption, diminished concentrating ability.

X. General treatment:

  A. Follow APTLS: See Chapter 8.

  B. General management: Table 106–5 (see Chapter 12 for details).

  C. NOTE: **Laboratory confirmation of organophosphate exposure should not delay emergency treatment in symptomatic patient. Management should proceed if clinical indications of organophosphate exposure exist.**

  D. External decontamination:

    1. Health care providers should wear gloves to avoid contamination.

    2. Remove all patient's clothing.

    3. Wash patient's skin and hair with soap and water.

TABLE 106–4.

Correlation of Serum Acetylcholinesterase Levels with Symptoms*

% Normal	Symptoms
>50	No symptoms
20–50	Mild poisoning
10–20	Moderate poisoning
<10	Severe poisoning

*From Bryson PD: *Comprehensive Review in Toxicology.* Rockville Md, Aspen Systems Corp, 1986, p 280. Used by permission.

TABLE 106–5.

General Treatment

Treatment	Indicated	Of No Value	Contraindicated
O$_2$	+		
IV	+		
ECG monitor	+		
Forced diuresis		X	
Acidification			X
Alkalinization		X	
Emesis*	+		
Lavage*	+		
Charcoal	+		
Cathartic	+		

*Indicated even if organophosphate is in petroleum distillate base (see Chapter 104).

    4. Wash patient's skin with ethyl alcohol.
    5. See also Chapters 29 and 111.
XI. Specific treatment:
  A. Atropine:
    1. Physiologic antidote (anticholinergic): Affects only muscarinic synapses. Therefore will not counter nicotine effects.
    2. Use with cardiac monitor in place.
    3. Administer atropine **only after respiratory status stabilized** because hypoxia plus atropine may cause ventricular tachycardia.
    4. Administration of atropine is also diagnostic: No clinical signs or symptoms of atropinization after administration of large doses of atropine indicates organophosphate exposure.
    5. Dosage:
      a. Initial dose:
        (1) Adult: 2–5 mg IV.
        (2) Child: 0:05 mg/kg IV
      b. Maintenance dose:
        (1) Adult: 2 mg IV every 15 minutes; can be increased incrementally to 5 mg IV every 15 minutes.
        (2) Child: 0.02 mg/kg IV; can be increased incrementally to 0.05 mg IV every 15 minutes.
    6. Administer atropine until signs of atropinization develop (flushing, dry mouth, dilated pupils).
    7. May require very large quantities (possibly hundreds of milligrams) to achieve adequate atropinization.
    8. After adequate atropinization achieved, begin slow tapering of dose and dosaging intervals after 12–24 hours of treatment.
    9. Signs of excessive atropinization (fever, dilated pupils, delirium, muscle twitching) may occur as organophosphate effects decrease. This is indication to taper atropine dose.

B. Pralidoxime (2-PAM):
1. Indicated for treatment of nicotinic effects such as muscle fasciculation, muscle weakness.
2. Pharmacologic actions:
   a. Cleaves organophosphate-acetylcholinesterase bond, thus reactivating acetylcholinesterase.
   b. Detoxification of organophosphate molecules directly.
   c. Anticholinergic effect.
3. **Must be given before irreversible organophosphate-cholinesterase binding** (and ultimate cholinesterase destruction), which usually occurs within 24–48 hours of exposure. For this reason, pralidoxime may be efficacious only if given within 24 hours after exposure.
4. Dosage:
   a. Adult: 1–2 gm in 250 ml of normal saline IV over 30 minutes.
   b. Child: 25–50 mg/kg IV over 15–30 minutes.
5. May see dramatic reversal of coma, fasciculation, and return to normal strength and well-being. Effects, however, may be temporary, and dose may need to be repeated often.

XII. Prognosis:
A. Expected response to treatment:
1. Pediatric patients: 50% mortality.
2. Adult patients: 10% mortality.
3. Institution of atropine treatment within first 4–6 hours crucial to successful outcome. Death is usually secondary to late recognition or inappropriate or insufficient therapy.
4. Deaths from organophosphate poisoning usually occur within 24 hours of exposure in untreated patients. When death occurs despite treatment, it is likely to occur within 10 days and is usually the result of complications or inadequate atropine therapy (too little or too late).
5. Prognosis significantly influenced by severity of complications (aspiration pneumonia, chemical pneumonitis, adult respiratory distress syndrome (ARDS).
6. If cerebral hypoxia can be avoided, full recovery should occur within 1–2 weeks.
B. Expected complications and long-term effects:
1. Early complications:
   a. Aspiration pneumonia.
   b. Chemical pneumonitis if hydrocarbon distillate vehicle involved.
   c. ARDS.
2. Late complications:
   a. CNS toxicity: Memory impairment, depression, schizophrenia, confusion, peripheral neuropathy, Guillain-Barré syndrome.
   b. Other: Contact dermatitis, ulcerative stomatitis, blood dyscrasias, asthma, pancreatitis with or without pseudocyst formation.

XIII. Special considerations:
A. In setting of acute organophosphate poisoning, **avoid** use of **phenothiazines, reserpine, barbiturates, narcotics, parasympathomimetics,** because of additional depressive effects. **Theophylline, furosemide** also contraindicated.

B. Administration of **epinephrine** may prove dangerous in hypoxic, cyanotic patients with organophosphate poisoning; may precipitate irreversible ventricular fibrillation.

XIV. Controversies:
  A. Hemodialysis and hemoperfusion for organophosphate poisoning.
  B. A new drug, dexetimide, may prove to be superior anticholinergic agent to atropine in organophosphate poisoning.
  C. Scopolamine may also prove beneficial in human organophosphate poisoning.

XV. Disposition considerations:
  A. Admission considerations:
    1. Any symptomatic patient will require hospital admission to a monitored bed for at least 24 hours for monitoring of acute poisoning and effects of atropine and pralidoxime therapy. ICU is the most appropriate setting.
    2. Any asymptomatic patient with potential serious exposure (possible delayed effects).
    3. Suicide risk.
  B. Observation period: Asymptomatic patients should be observed for up to 24 hours (see pharmacokinets, onset of action). This is impractical for most emergency departments and thus admission should be considered in all patients with potential serious exposures.
  C. Discharge considerations:
    1. Delayed toxicity may develop even in asymptomatic patients; therefore, it is probably inappropriate to discharge any patient with potential serious exposure regardless of symptoms or findings.
    2. If only mild exposure, may consider discharge under the following conditions:
      a. General discharge considerations have been met (see Chapter 18).
      b. Counseling regarding further home, occupational, environmental exposure to organophosphates done. Appropriate public health officials notified if indicated. Do not discharge patients who will return to an environment where further exposure may occur.
      c. Suicide potential and psychiatric status have been appropriately evaluated.

Carbamate Insecticides

Carbamate insecticides behave similarly to organophosphates; however, toxicity is usually more benign and of shorter duration. Only important differences are noted here: otherwise see Organophosphates.

  I. Route of exposure: Oral, cutaneous, inhalation, mucous membrane, injection, (rare).
  I.. Common generic and trade names: Most commonly used carbamate insecticides are carbaryl (Sevin), propoxur (Baygon), methomyl (Lannate), aldicarb (Temik). Of these, carbaryl is least toxic and aldicarb most toxic.

III. Pharmacokinetics:
  A. Absorption: Rapid absorption from GI tract, very slow from skin.
  B. Onset of action: Within minutes.
  C. Plasma half-life: 9 hours for carbaryl.
  D. Peak effect: Maximum inhibition of cholinesterase may occur within 1 hour.
  E. Duration of action: 6–8 hours for carbaryl. Note much shorter than for organophosphate insecticides.
  F. Elimination: Metabolites excreted in urine. Enterohepatic recycling of carbaryl metabolites reported to increase half-life in rats.
IV. Actions: This group of insecticides, derivatives of carbamic acid, are reversible cholinesterase inhibitors. As such, they reversibly bind to cholinesterase by carbamylation, which in turn allows accumulation of acetylcholine.
V. Range of toxicity:
  A. Toxic dose:
    1. Case report of moderate symptoms with full recovery in 2 hours after one-time ingestion of 250 mg carbaryl (approximately 2.8 mg/kg).
    2. Case report of Carbofuran in dust causing mild symptoms with full recovery in 2 hours.
  B. Fatal dose: See Table 106–6.
VI. Clinical Features (see also Organophosphates): Clinical toxicity of carbamates differs from organophosphate insecticides in a few, but important ways:
  A. Because of reversibility of cholinesterase inhibition, clinical picture of toxicity is much milder and of shorter duration than that of organophosphates.
  B. Because of poor carbamate penetration into CNS, prominent CNS effects seen with organophosphates is not a problem with carbamates. Thus milder muscarinic effects predominate in carbamate toxicity.
VII. Laboratory findings and evaluation:
  A. Reversibility of cholinesterase bond is such that serum or red cell cholinesterase level may quickly return to normal within a few hours of exposure. Thus reliance on clinical presentation is more important in diagnosis of carbamate poisoning than on lab tests.
  B. Decreased hematocrit if patient has carbamate-induced hemolytic anemia.
VIII. Treatment: Emergency department management of carbamate poisoning identical to that for organophosphates, with some exceptions:
  A. Determination of red cell cholinesterase or pseudocholinesterase levels unnecessary unless dual carbamate-organophosphate exposure suspected.
  B. Usually less atropine necessary and for shorter duration.
  C. Pralidoxime therapy:
    1. Use in carbamate poisonings controversial.
    2. May be ineffective against carbamates because carbamylation bond to cholinesterase enzyme is reversible.
    3. If given in large doses will have additive anticholinesterase effect of its own.
    4. Probably appropriate to use pralidoxime in patients with clinically apparent cholinergic crisis but with unknown exposure (organophosphate vs carbamate) or with suspected organophosphate and carbamate exposure.

TABLE 106–6.

Common Carbamates in Order
of Decreasing Toxicity

Compound	Fatal Dose (mg/kg)
Aldicarb	0.9
Carbofuron	11.0
Isolan	12.0
Methomyl	17.0
Formeturate	20.0
Matocil	21.0
Sok (Bonol)	51.0
Pyrolan	53.0
Dimetilan	64.0
Dimeton	90.0
Baygon	95.0
Mesurol	130.0
Pyramat	200.0
Landrin	208.0
Mobam	234.0
Diallate	395.0
Carbaryl	500.0
Vegadex	850.0
Pebulate	1,120.0
Vernolate	1.625.0
Eptam	1,650.0
Korbutilate	3,000.0
Butylate	4,650.0

IX. Prognosis:
   A. Expected response to treatment:
   a. Excellent prognosis with early institution of atropine therapy and good supportive care.
   b. Recovery far sooner with carbamate toxicity than with organophosphate toxicity with same degree of symptoms.
X. Disposition considerations:
   A. Essentially same as for organophosphates except:
      1. Observation period: for milder cases of carbamate poisoning, even those requiring atropine, observation for 6–8 hours may be sufficient to rule out significant toxicity. If patient remains symptomatic after 6–8 hours of observation, admission is indicated.
      2. Discharge considerations:
         a. General discharge considerations have been met (see Chapter 18).
         b. Asymptomatic with normal exam and vital signs after 6–8 hours of observation.
         c. Suicide potential and psychiatric status have been appropriately evaluated.

BIBLIOGRAPHY

Arena JM: *Poisoning: Toxicology, Symptoms, Treatments,* ed 4. Springfield, Ill, Charles C Thomas, Publisher, 1976.

Becker C, Sullivan JB: Prompt recognition and vigorous therapy for organophosphate poisoning. *Emerg Med Rep* 1986; 7:33–40.

Coye MJ, Barnett PG, Midtling JE, et al: Clinical confirmation of organophosphate poisoning by serial cholinesterase analyses. *Arch Intern Med* 1987; 147:438–442.

Davies JE: Changing profile of pesticide poisoning. *N Engl J Med* 1987; 316:807–808.

Gosselin RE, Smith RP, Hodge HC: *Clinical Toxicology of Commercial Product,* ed 5. Baltimore, Williams & Wilkins Co, 1984.

Haddad LM, Winchester JF (eds): *Clinical Management of Poisoning and Drug Overdose.* Philadelphia, WB Saunders Co, 1983.

Midtling JE, Barnett PG, Coye MJ, et al: Clinical management of field worker organophosphate poisoning. *West J Med* 1985; 142:514–518.

Morgan DP: *Recognition and Management of Pesticide Poisonings,* ed 3. Washington, DC, Environmental Protection Agency, 1982.

Rumack BH: Carbamate insecticides. Poisindex. Denver, Micromedex, 1981.

Senanayake N, Karalliedde L: Neurotoxic effects of organophosphorus insecticides. *N Engl J Med* 1987; 316:761–763.

Tafuri J, Roberts J: Organophosphate poisoning. *Ann Emerg Med* 1987; 16:193–202.

107

Rodenticides and Herbicides

S. Rutherfoord Rose II, Pharm.D.
Gary M. Oderda, Pharm.D., M.P.H.

Strychnine

I. Route of exposure: Oral, intranasal, subcutaneous, intramuscular, intravenous.
II. Common trade names: See Table 107–1.
III. Pharmacokinetics:
   A. Absorption: Rapidly absorbed from nasal passages, GI tract, injection site
   B. Onset of action: Convulsions may occur as early as 15 minutes after oral ingestion or 30 minutes after intranasal administration.
   C. Duration of action: Can be recovered in urine for up to 3 days.
   D. Elimination: Urinary excretion of unmetabolized strychnine; also metabolized in liver by microsomal enzymes.
IV. Action:
   A. Competes with neurotransmitter glycine for specific CNS receptors.
   B. Glycine is involved in inhibition of postsynaptic neurotransmission. Strychnine blockade results in disinhibition and potent CNS stimulation.
V. Uses:
   A. Ingredient in more than 170 commercial products.
   B. Formerly important component of various tonics, analgesics, digestive aids, cold remedies, vitamins, stimulants, sedatives, cathartic pills
   C. Rodenticide (becoming more rare). Intended to be lethal after one exposure.
   D. Adulterant of street drugs.

TABLE 107–1.

Products Containing Strychnine

El Roy Mouse Bait	Kill Mice
Gopher Death	Mole-Nots
Gopher Go	Mouse-Nip
Hot Spring Buttons	Pearson's Gopher Killer
Kilmice	Pearson's Poison Peanut Pellets
Mice Doom Pellets	Sonoma County's Strychnine
Mo-Go	Jackrabbit Poison Bait
Mologen	Sonoma County's Strychnine
Mouse Lure	Linnet Poison
Mouse Seeds	Sonoma County's Strychnine
Dr. Daniel's Colic	Sparrow Poison
Drops	
Dr. Daniel's Equine	
Heave Powder	

VI. Toxic mechanism: With inhibition of neurotransmission blocked in spinal cord, all muscles contract at same time, resulting in severe whole-body spasms.

VII. Range of toxicity:
  A. Fatal dose:
    1. 15–30 mg.
    2. Reports of deaths from as little as 5–10 mg.
    3. Case report of survival after ingestion as large as 15 gm.

VIII. Clinical features:
  A. Restlessness, agitation; increased visual, auditory acuity may occur early.
  B. Principle toxic effect is convulsions as early as 15 minutes after oral ingestion or 30 minutes after intranasal administration.
  C. Patients may remain awake and alert despite whole-body involvement. Hyperreflexia often occurs first, followed by severe muscle spasms, pain, trismus, opisthotonos. Spasms can be triggered by slight stimuli such as sound or sudden motion. Differential diagnosis includes tetanus, hydrophobia (rabies), meningitis, epilepsy, hysteria.
  D. Seizures and severe spasms may result in:
    1. Rhabdomyolysis and potential for renal failure.
    2. Hyperthermia.
    3. Lactic acidosis.
  E. Death results from paralysis of respiratory muscles and resultant hypoxia.

IX. Laboratory findings and evaluation:
  A. Levels of strychnine in gastric contents, urine, blood not helpful clinically.
  B. Blood:
    1. Electrolytes (check for hyperkalemia), Ca^{++} (differential diagnosis of muscle spasms).
    2. Arterial blood gases (hypoxia, acidosis).
    3. Renal function studies (renal failure).
    4. Complete blood count (check for leukocytosis; infection workup).

5. Glucose (rule out hypoglycemia).
6. Serum creatine phosphokinase, myoglobin, phosphate, uric acid (suspect rhabdomyolysis).
C. Other laboratory considerations:
1. Urinalysis and urine dipstick. (If dipstick positive for blood but no red blood cells seen microscopically, suspect myoglobinuria. Also check for pigmented myoglobin casts. See Chapter 48.)
2. Lumbar puncture (if diagnosis in doubt).
3. Chest radiograph.
X. General treatment:
A. Follow APTLS: See Chapter 8.
b. General management: Table 107–2 (see Chapter 12 for details).
C. Treatment based on symptoms rather than amount ingested.
XI. Specific treatment:
A. Respiratory support: See Chapter 9.
B. Gastric decontamination:
1. Once adequate airway management has been achieved and seizures controlled, gastric lavage can be performed with a 1 : 10,000 solution potassium permanganate, which neutralizes strychnine. This can be prepared by dissolving 100 mg tablet in 1 L water. **Emesis absolutely contraindicated** due to possibility of rapid onset of seizures.
2. Lavage can be followed by charcoal and cathartic.
C. Management of complications:
1. **Seizures:**
a. Reduce all sensory stimuli to minimum by placing patient in warm, quiet, darkened room.
b. See Chapter 22 for treatment recommendations.
c. General anesthesia may be necessary to control severe seizures.
2. Rhabdomyolysis: Alkalinization is controversial. See Chapter 70, p. 366.

TABLE 107–2.

General Treatment

Treatment	Indicated	Of No Value	Contraindicated
O$_2$	+		
IV	+		
ECG monitor	+		
Forced diuresis*	±		
Acidification†	±		
Alkalinization†	±		
Emesis‡			X
Lavage§	+		
Charcoal	+		
Cathartic	+		

*May be appropriate if rhabdomyolysis present
†Controversial (see Controversies, below).
‡Rapid change in level of consciousness possible
§See Specific treatment.

3. Hyperthermia: See Chapter 63, p. 309.
4. Lactic acidosis:
   a. Sodium bicarbonate should be administered IV over 5 minutes as needed to reverse severe metabolic acidosis (i.e., pH <7.2).
   b. Keep respiratory component of pH in mind, as major problem may be respiratory acidosis, not metabolic acidosis.

XII. Prognosis:
   A. Expected response to treatment:
      1. Death from respiratory paralysis usually occurs 1–3 hours after ingestion.
      2. Survival past 5 hours associated with excellent prognosis.
      3. Complete recovery usual if patient survives for 24 hours.
   B. Expected complications and long-term effects:
      1. Lactic acidosis, hyperthermia, rhabdomyolysis, renal failure, intractable seizures, death.
      2. No serious long-term complications specifically from strychnine.

XIII. Controversies:
   A. Urinary acidification: Theoretically will enhance elimination, but induces metabolic acidosis in patient already at high risk of severe lactic acidosis. Rhabdomyolysis is further complicated by acidification. Thus risks appear to outweigh benefits.
   B. Urinary alkalinization for rhabdomyolysis is also controversial. See Chapter 70.

XIV. Disposition considerations:
   A. Admission considerations:
      1. Admit all patients with suspected strychnine poisoning.
      2. With complications, ICU is appropriate.
   B. Consultation considerations: Anesthesiologist for seizures unresponsive to emergency department treatment, as may occur with severe strychnine ingestions.
   C. Observation period:
      1. All symptomatic patients should be admitted and not observed expectantly in the emergency department.
      2. Inasmuch as symptoms usually begin 15–30 minutes after ingestion, patients who present hours after alleged ingestion who are asymptomatic, with normal repeat physical examinations and vital signs, may be considered for discharge after 6–8 hours of emergency department observation.
   D. Discharge considerations:
      1. Not appropriate to discharge any patient with suspected strychnine ingestion.
      2. See observation period for disposition of patient presenting hours after alleged ingestion.

Anticoagulants

   I. Route of exposure: Oral, transdermal.
   II. Common trade names: See Table 107–3.

TABLE 107–3.

Anticoagulant Rodenticides*

Hydroxycoumarin types
  Agicide Rat and Mouse Bait
  Banarat Bits
  Banarat Premix
  Black Flag Rat and Mouse Killer
  Black Leaf Mouse Killer Bait
  Black Leaf Ready Mixed Bait
  Black Panther Rat and Mouse Killer
  Brayton's Raticide Cereal Bait
  Cornell WOS Rodenticide
  D-Con Kills Mice
  Fatal Prepared Rat and Mouse Bait
  Geigy Rat and Mouse Bait
  Dr. Hess Warfarat
  Howard Rat Kill Cone
  Howard Ready-to-Use Rat Kill
  Howard Warficide Rat Kill
  Kelly's Red-Mix Rat and Mouse Killer
  Killer Katz
  K-R-O Rat and Mouse Killer
  Lebanon Bait Kills Rats and Mice
  Martin's Mar-Fin Ready Bait
  Mice and Rat Doom
  Myerkill
  Parson's Rat Killer
  Patterson's Mole and Gopher Killer
  Patterson's Rat and Mouse Killer
    (also contains pival)
  Pied Piper for Rats and Mice (also
    contains ANTU)
  Planter's Rat and Mouse Bait
  Rataway
  Rat-B-Gon Rat and Mice Bait
  Rat-Death
  Rat-Kill
  Rat-Nix
  Rat-O-Cide No. 2

Rat-Ola
Ratorex
Rat-Trol Bait
Rax Powder
R-Death Grain Killer
Ro-Do
Rough and Ready Mouse Mix
Safite Rodenticides
Shaple Rat and Mouse Killer
Sla-Rat Prepared
Speckman Deth-Bait
Spray-Trol Brand Rodent-Trol
Stauffer's Brush Killer—Ready to Use
Stauffer's Rodent Bait Cone
Talon G
Twin Light Rat-Away
Voo-Doo 42
Warficide Rat Killer
Wander Rodenticide
WW42
Zord Rodenticide
Indandione types (pival)
  Arwell Rat and Mouse Bait
  Caid
  Chemrat
  Drat
  Eastern States Duocide Mixed Bait
  Green Cross Rat and Mouse Bait
  Dr. Hess Rat and Mouse Killer
  Liphadione
  Microzol
  Patterson's Rat and Mouse Killer
    (also contains warfarin)
  Pivalyn Packets
  Rodent Rid
  Rodent Vev
  Rozol

*From Arena JM: *Poisoning: Toxicology, Symptoms, Treatment* ed 4. Springfield, Ill, Charles C Thomas, Publisher, 1979, pp 173–201.

III. Pharmacokinetics:
  A. Absorption: Rapid after oral administration.
  B. Onset of action: Effects seen within 8–12 hrs after ingestion. Hypoprothrombinemia usually 12–24 hours after ingestion.
  C. Plasma half-life: 40–44 hours (may be days in the case of superwarfarins).
  D. Peak effect: Maximal plasma concentrations reached within 1 hour; peak effects not usually observed until 1–2 days after ingestion.

E. Duration of action: 5 days.
   1. Superwarfarin (e.g., brodifacoum, difenacoum, diphacinone, chlorophacinone) effects can persist for 6 months.
F. Elimination: Metabolites excreted in urine and stool.
G. Active metabolites: Hydroxy metabolites have some anticoagulant activity.

IV. Action: These drugs decrease blood clotting by inhibiting synthesis of vitamin K–dependent clotting factors II, VII, IX, X.

V. Uses:
   A. Anticoagulation:
      1. Therapeutic use in humans in small doses (e.g., deep vein thrombosis, prophylactic anticoagulation of cardiac valve prostheses, transient ischemic attacks).
      2. Rodenticide in larger doses; intended to be chronically toxic so that repeated exposures are necessary to kill rodents. Anticoagulants are by far the most commonly used rodenticides today.

VI. Toxic mechanism:
   A. Induction of anticoagulation leads to bleeding, the most frequent sign of toxicity.
   B. Disruption of capillary membranes may also contribute to hemorrhagic effects.
   C. Single acute ingestions of warfarin rarely cause toxicity. Toxicity, as measured by degree of bleeding, depends on continual ingestion.

VII. Range of toxicity:
   A. Toxic dose:
      1. Warfarin: Acute doses >20–50 mg (0.5 mg/kg) may be expected to prolong prothrombin time (PT).
      2. Superwarfarin: Reports of acute ingestions of 1, 7.5, 25, 75, 90 mg superwarfarin products resulting in bleeding and elevated PT for 6 weeks to more than 6 months despite high-dose vitamin K and plasma infusions.
   B. Fatal dose:
      1. Single doses rarely fatal.
      2. Reports of deaths with the following daily doses:
         a. Warfarin: >5–20 mg/day for >3–5 days.
         b. Dicumarol: 100 mg/day PO.
         c. Ethyl biscoumacetate (Tromexan): 600 mg/day PO.
         d. Phenindione (Danilone, Hedulin): 200 mg/day PO.

VIII. Clinical features:
   A. Internal or external bleeding most common (e.g., melena, epistaxis, bright red blood per rectum, hemetemesis, bruising, ecchymoses, petechiae, purpura, bleeding gums after brushing teeth, hemarthroses, hematuria, hemoptysis, intracerebral bleeding).
   B. Bleeding into airway can result in dysphonia and total airway obstruction.
   C. Patients may complain of flank or back pain.

IX. Laboratory findings and evaluation:
   A. Prothrombin time (PT), partial thromboplastin time (PTT).
   B. Complete blood cell count and immediate spun hematocrit.
   C. Stool Hemoccult test, urinalysis (occult bleeding).
   D. Chest and abdominal radiographs if indicated.

X. General treatment:
  A. Follow APTLS: See Chapter 8.
  B. General management: Table 107–4 (see Chapter 12 for details).
XI. Specific therapy:
  A. Single acute ingestions of few mouthfuls of warfarin product (0.025%–0.05%) or 1 mouthful (approximately 5 gm) superwarfarin (0.005%): No therapy required.
  B. Patients receiving concurrent long-term anticoagulant therapy or repeatedly ingesting rodenticides: Lavage or emesis followed by charcoal and cathartic.
  C. For acute ingestions in patients not receiving long-term anticoagulant therapy, Maryland Poison Control Center protocols (1988) are as follows:
    1. **Observe at home** (calculation example: 15 mg warfarin = 60 gm of 0.025% product):

Warfarin	<15 mg
Hydroxycoumarin	<0.3 mg
Indandione	<5 mg

    It is frequently impossible to determine exact amount of ingestion. Histories should not be relied on even when product containers are available. If there is *any* doubt as to quantity ingested, it is best to take a conservative approach and have the patient brought to the emergency department.
    2. **Induce emesis** with syrup of ipecac at home (see above caution) or in emergency department (no further therapy required):

Warfarin	15–25 mg
Hydroxycoumarin	0.3–0.6 mg
Indandione	5–8 mg

    3. Emergency department evaluation required:

Warfarin	>25 mg
Hydroxycoumarin	>0.6 mg
Indandione	>8 mg

TABLE 107–4.

General Treatment

Treatment	Indicated	Of No Value	Contraindicated
O$_2$	±		
IV	±		
ECG monitor	±		
Forced diuresis		X	
Acidification		X	
Alkalinization		X	
Emesis*/lavage*	+/+		
Charcoal*	+		
Cathartic*	+		

*See Specific therapy.

    D. Therapy to reverse effects of anticoagulant:
       1. Vitamin K (phytonadione, Aquamephyton):
         a. Indications:
           (1) Chronic ingestion.
           (2) Large ingestion.
           (3) Long-acting compound.
         b. Dose: 1–5 mg PO/IM/SC in children; 5–25 mg in adults. May be repeated once.
         c. Goal: Normal PT in case of rodenticide overdose; therapeutic range in patients receiving anticoagulant therapy. Check PT every 8–12 hours until within normal range.
       2. If actively bleeding:
         a. Obtain PT, PTT, complete blood cell count, spun hematocrit immediately. Send type and cross match.
         b. Vitamin K 10–50 mg IV in adults, 0.6 mg/kg in children younger than 12 years, no faster than 1 mg/min.
         c. Fresh-frozen plasma as needed; 250–500 ml in adults.
XII. Prognosis:
    A. Expected response to treatment:
       1. PT should return to normal levels in 24–48 hours with vitamin K therapy.
       2. Reports of deaths up to 2 weeks after serious anticoagulant overdose.
    B. Expected complications and long-term effects: Any complication related to internal hemorrhage, including death.
XIII. Special considerations:
    A. Drugs that potentiate effects of oral anticoagulants:

Acetaminophen	Methylphenidate
Anabolic steroids	Metronidazole
Antibiotics	Miconazole
Aspirin	Nalidixic acid
Cimetidine	Neomycin
Clofibrate	Penicillin
Diazoxide	Phenylbutazone
Disulfiram	Phenytoin
Erythromycin	Propoxyphene
Ethacrynic acid	Sulfinpyrazone
Ethanol	Tetracycline
Glucagon	Thyroxine
Heparin	Tricyclic antidepressants
Indomethacin	Trimethoprim-sulfamethoxazole
Isoniazid	Vitamin E
Monoamine oxidase inibitors	
Mercaptopurine	

XIV. Controversies:
    A. Some authorities do not recommend emesis or lavage for single acute ingestion of regular warfarin compound because of potential for hemorrhage.

B. Use of oral phenobarbital to increase metabolism of superwarfarins in humans has no proved benefit.

C. Administration of oral cholestyramine four times daily may increase warfarin clearance, but further investigation is needed to determine clinical benefit.

XV. Disposition considerations:

    A. Admission considerations:

        1. See General Admission Considerations (Chapters 17 and 18).

        2. Hospitalize all patients with prolonged PT, evidence of active bleeding. PT less than 8–12 hours after ingestion may not reflect severity of poisoning.

        3. History of large ingestion:

            Warfarin: >15–25 mg

            Hydroxycoumarin: >0.3–0.6 mg

            Indandione: >5–8 mg

        4. Suicide risk.

    B. Consultation considerations: Hematologist for any serious bleeding.

    C. Observation period: Most emergency departments are not able to observe patients for sufficient time to obtain repeated coagulation profiles and determine disposition on this basis.

    D. Discharge considerations:

        1. General discharge considerations have been met (Chapters 17 and 18).

        2. Single acute ingestions of a few mouthfuls of warfarin product or 1 mouthful of superwarfarin do not require hospitalization. However, if there is any doubt as to reliability of history, the patient should be admitted.

        3. Asymptomatic patients with normal coagulation profiles on discharge should return within 24 hours for repeat PT, PTT.

        4. Suicide potential and psychiatric status have been appropriately evaluated.

Herbicides: Paraquat and Diquat

I. Route of exposure:

    A. Oral, dermal, ocular, inhalation.

    B. No reported systemic toxicity from inhalation (only epistaxis and throat irritation).

II. Common trade names:

    Chevron Industrial Weed and Grass Killer

    Ortho-Paraquat Cl

    Ortho-Dual-Paraquat

III. Pharmacokinetics:

    A. Absorption:

        1. GI absorption slow and prolonged (10% in first 24 hours).

        2. Dermal absorption may result in systemic effects and is enhanced through abraded skin.

B. Onset of action: Symptoms may be present within a few minutes to hours of ingestion.

C. Peak effect: Peak serum levels in first few hours.

D. Duration of action: Although little paraquat is found remaining in serum after first day, appearance of lung damage may be delayed for up to a week.

E. Elimination: Distributed to all body tissues but actively concentrated by alveolar cells of lungs; excreted by kidneys. These agents are inactivated by contact with soil.

IV. Action: Acts as oxidation-reduction couple reducing molecular oxygen to toxic free radical "superoxides," which in turn may generate H_2O_2, hydroxyl radical, and single oxygen. These can react directly with cellular components and with membranes by lipid peroxidation and thiol oxidation.

V. Uses:

A. Herbicides.

B. Greater than 60% of toxic exposures are suicide attempts.

VI. Toxic mechanism:

A. See Action.

B. Concentration of toxic free radicals in lung, liver, heart, kidneys produces necrosis.

C. Most important toxic effects of free radicals are in lungs, where resulting progressive fibrosis is the leading cause of death. This process is oxygen dependent.

D. Concentrated solutions (20%–40%) are corrosive, as opposed to solutions which are less than 1% used for home and garden.

VII. Range of toxicity:

A. Toxic dose: Toxic symptoms may occur from ingestions as small as 3/4 tsp.

B. Fatal dose:

1. Paraquat: 10–15 ml 20%–40% solution.

2. Diquat: Deaths have been reported from ingestions as small as 30 mg/ kg.

VIII. Clinical features:

A. Paraquat:

1. Three phases of disease. Time of onset, rate of progression, severity of each stage roughly dose related.

a. Early:

(1) Acute respiratory distress related to pulmonary hyperemia and congestion occurs immediately after severe poisoning.

(2) Acute ingestion causes burning of mouth and throat.

(3) Strong irritant action at areas of contact; maximum at 12–24 hours.

(4) Skin: Inflammation, formation of vesicles, loss of nails.

(5) Cornea, conjunctiva: Severe inflammation and potential scarring and ulceration.

b. Mid-course:

(1) Renal and hepatic failure.

(2) May last a few days, then gradually resolve. In mild poisoning

        may be transient or not appear at all. Usually appears 3–5 days after ingestion in moderate poisoning.

      (3) Myocarditis, epicardial hemorrhages, adrenal necrosis possible.

    c. Late:

      (1) Respiratory failure despite no apparent pulmonary abnormalities may be observed during first several days after ingestion.

      (2) Pulmonary edema and hemorrhage become evident and are replaced by progressive fibrosis until patient dies of hypoxia.

      (3) Pulmonary symptoms secondary to fibrosis may not occur until 6 weeks after ingestion, when all other systems have returned to normal.

    2. Dermatitis follows topical exposures.

    3. Death usually results from progressive respiratory failure.

  B. Diquat: Diquat produces fewer pulmonary effects but is more likely to cause lethargy, coma, cerebral hemorrhage, severe acute renal failure, with proteinuria noted 2–6 days after exposure. Treatment is the same as for paraquat.

IX. Laboratory findings and evaluation:

  A. Rapid screening test for paraquat:

    1. Add 2 ml 1% sodium dithionite in 1N sodium hydroxide to 10 ml urine. Blue color indicates presence of paraquat.

    2. Not sensitive to concentration <1 μg/ml.

  B. Serum paraquat levels:

    1. Plasma concentration less than 2.0, 0.3, 0.1 μg/ml at 4, 10, 24 hours, respectively, associated with good outcome.

    2. Serum level greater than 0.2 μg/ml at 24 hours and 0.1 μg/ml at 48 hours usually associated with poor or fatal outcome.

    3. However, recent work suggests that blood and urine concentrations measured prior to initiation of treatment may not correlate with degree of toxicity.

  C. Other useful laboratory tests:

    1. Electrolytes (must observe closely because treatment may involve 2–3 days of cathartic therapy).

    2. Renal function tests (BUN, creatinine).

    3. Arterial blood gases (with respiratory symptoms).

    4. Hepatic function tests (transaminases, bilirubin).

    5. Chest radiograph (pulmonary edema).

    6. ECG (sinus tachycardia may suggest myocarditis).

    7. Urinalysis (proteinuria, oliguria).

X. General treatment:

  A. Follow APTLS: See Chapter 8.

  B. General management: Table 107–5 (see Chapter 12 for details).

  C. Remove and discard all contaminated clothing. Irrigate eyes, wash skin, hair, nails repeatedly with soap and water (see Chapters 28, 29, and 111).

  D. Hospital personnel should have gowns, gloves, and masks.

  E. Monitor respiratory and hydration status closely.

XI. Specific management:

  A. No antidote exists. Early elimination from the body is essential to survival.

TABLE 107–5.

General Treatment

Treatment	Indicated	Of No Value	Contraindicated
O₂*			X
IV	+		
ECG monitor	+		
Forced diuresis†	+		
Acidification		X	
Alkalinization		X	
Emesis‡/lavage‡	+/+		
Charcoal‡§	+		
Cathartic§	+		

*WARNING: **Supplemental oxygen may potentiate pulmonary toxicity. Early intubation and ventilation with positive-pressure breathing has been suggested as a method of administering lower concentrations of oxygen while maintaining adequate arterial oxygen pressure. It is suggested that supplemental oxygen therapy with concentrations above 21% be used only when arterial oxygen pressure falls below 40 mm Hg.**
†Initiate early.
‡Avoid if evidence of corrosive GI injury.
§Activated charcoal and cathartic have been shown to be equally as effective as Fuller's earth or bentonite, which are often not available in many hospitals. Continue per nasogastric tube for 2–3 days. This may cause massive diarrhea and requires close fluid and electrolyte monitoring and support.

  B. Hemodialysis:
    1. In patients with evidence of renal failure.
    2. Most effective if started within 12 hours of ingestion.
  C. **Hemoperfusion** with charcoal or fuller's earth **(not resin)** has been successful in enhancing elimination and improving survival if initiated early and repeated until toxin is no longer detected in the blood.
  D. Total gut irrigation:
    1. Relatively new therapy.
    2. Solution (see below) administered by pump through nasogastric tube for 3–4 hours at 75 ml/min.
    3. Solution consists of 1 L warmed distilled water with NaCl 6.14 gm, KCl 0.75 gm, Na Bicarbonate 2.94 gm.
    4. Massive diarrhea is sequelae. Therefore close monitoring of hemodynamic and electrolyte status is best done in ICU.
  E. Evidence of corrosive GI injury (see Chapter 73 for management suggestions).
XII. Prognosis:
  A. Expected response to treatment:
    1. One series reported 85%–95% mortality.
    2. Following massive ingestion, death may occur within a few hours or days, secondary to multiple organ failure.
    3. Delayed pulmonary symptoms imply very poor prognosis.
  B. Expected complications and long-term effects:
    1. Renal, hepatic, pulmonary failure.

2. **Pulmonary symptoms may not occur until 6 weeks after ingestion,** by which time the patient usually has seemingly fully recovered.

XIII. Special considerations:

A. High concentrations of oxygen accelerate lung damage and supplemental oxygen should not be administered until need becomes critical ($Po_2 <$ 40 mm Hg). Management of hypoxia with paraquat poisoning is extremely difficult.

B. Marijuana may be contaminated with toxic quantities of paraquat, particularly if grown in Mexico.

1. However, no reports of paraquat toxicity associated with smoking marijuana.

2. Potentially dangerous if ingested in cookies, brownies.

XIV. Controversies:

A. Steroids, immunosuppressives, fibrinolytic agents, superoxide dismutase, vitamin E, considered ineffective.

B. More research needed before plasmapheresis can be recommended.

XV. Disposition considerations:

A. Admission considerations:

1. All known or suspected ingestions.

2. ICU admission considerations:

a. If total bowel irrigation to be undertaken, should admit to ICU to closely monitor volume status.

b. Respiratory compromise.

c. Consider if dialysis required.

3. Suicide risk.

B. Consultation considerations:

1. Nephrology consultation if hemodialysis or hemoperfusion indicated.

2. Ophthalmology for ocular exposures if symptoms do not resolve after 15 minutes of ocular irrigation.

3. Dermatology if dermatitis from skin exposure.

4. GI consultation for endoscopy, if indicated.

5. Surgeon for evidence of GI perforation.

6. Hypoxic patient with evidence of paraquat-induced pulmonary injury may require consultation with pulmonary medicine specialist.

7. Information on paraquat can be obtained from Poison Information Service, Chevron Chemical Co. (415) 233-3737.

C. Observation period: Not appropriate to observe. All patients should be admitted.

D. Discharge considerations: Not appropriate to discharge. All patients should be admitted.

BIBLIOGRAPHY

Bismuth C, Gardiner R, Dally S, et al: Prognosis and treatment of paraquat poisoning: A review of 28 cases. *J Toxicol Clin Toxicol* 1982; 19:461–474.

Blain P, Nightingale S, Stoddart J: Strychnine poisoning: Abnormal eye movements. *J Toxicol Clin Toxicol* 1982; 19:215–217.

Boyd RE, Brennan P, Deng J, et al: Strychnine poisoning. *Am J Med* 1983; 74:507–512.

Decker WJ, et al: Two deaths resulting from apparent parenteral injection of strychnine. *Vet Hum Toxicol* 1982; 24:161.

Fisher H, Clements J, Wright R: Enhancement of oxygen toxicity by the herbicide paraquat. *Am Rev Respir Dis* 1973; 107:246–252.

Fristedt B, Sterner N: Warfarin intoxication from percutaneous absorption. *Arch Environ Health* 1965; 11:205–208.

Gaudreault P, et al: Efficacy of activated charcoal in the treatment of oral paraquat intoxication. *Ann Emerg Med* 1985; 14:123–125.

Harsanyi L, Nemeth A, Lang A: Paraquat (gramoxone) poisoning in southwest Hungary, 1977–1984: Toxicological and histopathological aspects of group intoxication cases. *Am J Forensic Med Pathol* 1987; 8:131–134.

Hoffman S, Jederkin R, Korzets Z, et al: Successful management of severe paraquat poisoning. *Chest* 1983; 84:107–109.

Jones EC, Growe GH, Naiman SC: Prolonged anticoagulation in rat poisoning. *JAMA* 1984; 252:3005–3007.

Lipton RA, Klass EM: Human ingestion of a "superwarfarin" rodenticide resulting in prolonged anticoagulant effect. *JAMA* 1984; 252:3004–3005.

McCarthy L, Speth C: Diquat intoxication. *Ann Emerg Med* 1983; 12:394–396.

Maini R, Winchester JF: Removal of paraquat from blood by haemoperfusion over sorbent materials. *Br Med J* 1975; 3:281–282.

Maron BJ, Krupp JR, Tune B: Strychnine poisoning successfully treated with diazepam. *J Pediatr* 1971; 78:697–699.

Murdoch DA: Prolonged anticoagulation in chlorphacinone poisoning. *Lancet* 1983; 1:355–356.

Okonek S, et al: Successful treatment of paraquat poisoning: Activated charcoal per os and "continuous hemoperfusion." *J Toxicol Clin Toxicol* 1982; 19:807.

Onyeama HP, et al: A literature review of paraquat toxicity. *Vet Hum Toxicol* 1984; 26:494.

Renowden S, Westmoreland D, White JP, et al: Oral cholestyramine increases elimination of warfarin after overdose. *Br Med J* 1985; 291:513–514.

Swissman N, Jacoby J: Strychnine poisoning and its treatment. *Clin Pharmacol Ther* 1964; 5:136–140.

108

Toxic Inhalants

Robert J. Stine, M.D., F.A.C.E.P.

I. Route of exposure: Inhalation, mucous membrane, ocular.
II. Common sources:
   A. Toxic inhalants comprise a variety of noxious gases and particulate matter in gaseous suspension that are capable of producing bodily injury.
   B. Exposure can be intentional (e.g., solvent abuse, suicide attempt) or accidental (e.g., industrial accident) and can occur in a variety of settings (e.g., workplace, home, during transport of toxic materials).
   C. See Table 108–1 for a more complete listing of sources of toxic inhalants.
III. Pharmacokinetics: See Table 108–1.
IV. Uses: See Table 108–1.
V. Toxic mechanisms (see also Table 108–1):
   A. Simple asphyxiation:
      1. Physiologically inert gases that produce hypoxia by displacing oxygen from inspired air (e.g., acetylene, argon, butane, carbon dioxide, ethane, ethylene, helium, hydrogen, methane [natural gas], neon, nitrogen, propane, propylene).
      2. Morbidity and mortality related to degree and duration of hypoxia, with death imminent at oxygen concentration of 5% or less.
   B. Local irritation:
      1. Direct tissue injury, principally involving eyes and mucosa of the respiratory tract (e.g., acrolein, ammonia, chlorine, chloroacetophenone, dibenzoxazepine, formaldehyde, hydrogen chloride, hydrogen fluoride, O-chlorobenzylidene malononitrile, ozone, phosgene, sulfur dioxide).
      2. Extent of injury determined by intrinsic properties of the gas, its concentration, and duration of exposure.

TABLE 108–1.
Toxic Inhalants

Agent	Major Sources	Toxicologic Mechanism*	Toxic Effects†	Specific Therapy‡	Prognosis
Acetone	Industrial and household cleaners; dyes; nail polish remover	Local irritation, systemic toxicity	Eye irritation; tracheobronchitis; skin irritant; CNS disturbances; respiratory depression; hyperglycemia, ketosis	Decontamination; respiratory support	Survival for 48 hours usually followed by recovery
Acrolein	Manufacture of plastics, rubber, textiles, resins	Local irritation	Conjunctivitis; rhinitis, pharyngitis; tracheobronchitis	Decontamination; respiratory support	Survival for 4 hours usually followed by recovery
Acrylonitrile	Manufacture of acrylics, rubber, adhesives; fumigant; chemical intermediate in synthesis of antioxidants, pharmaceuticals, dyes	Systemic toxicity (cellular asphyxiation related to inhibition of cytochrome oxidase by cyanide)	Dyspnea; CNS disturbances; cardiovascular disturbances; lactic acidosis; pulmonary edema; GI disturbances; conjunctivitis; carcinogen	Respiratory support; cardiovascular support; administration of sodium nitrite and sodium thiosulfate; hyperbaric chamber	
Ammonia	Refrigerants; fertilizers; manufacture of plastics, pesticides, detergents, fertilizers, explosives; petroleum refining	Irritation	Conjunctivitis; corneal injury; rhinitis; pharyngitis; laryngeal edema; laryngospasm; bronchospasm; tracheobronchitis; pulmonary edema; chemical burns	Decontamination; respiratory support	Survival for 48 hours usually followed by recovery Permanent blindness frequent after eye contact

Arsine	Metal refining, smelting; semiconductor industry	Systemic toxicity	Hemolytic anemia; acute renal failure; arrhythmias; hypotension; GI disturbances; conjunctivitis	Decontamination; cardiovascular support; exchange transfusion, hemodialysis	
Benzene	Paints; varnish removers; petrols; adhesives; industrial solvent; manufacture of chemicals, dyes, nylon, lacquers, styrene, varnishes	Systemic toxicity (sensitization of myocardium to catecholamines); local irritation	Arrhythmias; CNS disturbances; seizures; respiratory depression; hematologic disorders; mucous membrane, skin irritation; pulmonary edema	Decontamination; respiratory support; cardiovascular support	Acute: Survival for >3 days usually followed by recovery; prognosis poor with rapidly progressive symptoms and lack of response to hydrocarbon removal. Chronic: Decrease in bone marrow cellularity or peripheral cell count correlated with poor prognosis
Cadmium	Ore smelting; metal alloying, welding; electroplating	Local irritation systemic toxicity	Conjunctivitis; tracheobronchitis; pulmonary edema; metal fume fever; renal dysfunction; anemia; emphysema	Decontamination; respiratory support; (?)chelation therapy	
Carbon	Combustion products; foundry work; mining	Simple asphyxiation	Dyspnea; cyanosis; CNS disturbances; cardiovascular disturbances	Respiratory support	Survival for >4 days associated with recovery

Continued.

TABLE 108–1 (cont.).

Agent	Major Sources	Toxicologic Mechanism*	Toxic Effects†	Specific Therapy‡	Prognosis
Carbon disulfide	Insecticide; fumigant; solvent in rubber and rayon industries; degreasing agent	Local irritation; systemic toxicity	Conjunctivitis; tracheobronchitis; CNS disturbances; seizures; respiratory failure; GI disturbances; skin irritation; chemical burns	Respiratory support; decontamination; (?)urea, pyridoxine infusion	Gradual improvement over several months; complete recovery may never occur
Carbon monoxide	Foundry work; petroleum refining; mining; product of incomplete combustion	Systemic toxicity (chemical asphyxiation related to formation of carboxyhemoglobin	Dyspnea; CNS disturbances; cardiovascular disturbances	Respiratory support; hyperbaric oxygen	Complete recovery unlikely if symptoms of mental deterioration persist for 2 weeks
Carbon tetrachloride	Adhesives; spot removers; fumigant; synthesis of refrigerants, solvents, aerosol propellants	Systemic toxicity (sensitization of myocardium to catecholamines, cellular toxin); local irritation	CNS disturbances; seizures; cardiovascular disturbances; respiratory depression; hepatic, renal injury; GI disturbances; conjunctivitis; skin irritation	Decontamination; respiratory support; cardiovascular support; hemodialysis, N-acetylcysteine	Complete return of liver and kidney function in 2–12 months; renal function may return spontaneously after 2–3 weeks in anuric patients
Chlorine	Bleaching of cloth and paper; manufacture of plastics, chlorinated chemicals; water purification; disinfection of sewage, swimming pools	Local irritation	Conjunctivitis; keratitis; rhinitis; pharyngitis; tracheobronchitis; pulmonary edema; chemical burns; GI disturbances	Decontamination; respiratory support	Death may occur up to 24 hours after exposure, from circulatory failure

Chloroacetophenone	Mace, tear gas	Local irritation	Ocular pain, blepharospasm, lacrimation; ocular ulceration; skin irritation; chemical burns; laryngospasm; pulmonary edema; GI disturbances	Decontamination; respiratory support	Severe eye injury may result in morbidity up to 15 years after exposure
Chromium fumes	Electroplating; metal welding	Local irritation; systemic toxicity	Keratoconjunctivitis; nasal ulceration; tracheobronchitis; chemical pneumonitis; pulmonary edema; chemical burns; asthma; pneumoconiosis; metal fume fever; hepatic, renal injury; hematologic disorders	Decontamination; respiratory support; forced diuresis; urinary alkalinization	Progression to anuria associated with poor prognosis
Copper fumes, dust	Metal welding	Local irritation; systemic toxicity	Eye irritation; chemical pneumonitis; skin irritation; chemical burns; metal fume fever; CNS disturbances	Decontamination; respiratory support; chelation therapy (if systemic toxicity)	
Dibenzoxazepine	Riot-control agent	Local irritation	Ocular pain, blepharospasm, lacrimation; rhinitis; skin irritation; chemical burns; laryngospasm; pulmonary edema; GI disturbances	Decontamination; respiratory support	

Continued.

TABLE 108–1 (cont.).

Agent	Major Sources	Toxicologic Mechanism*	Toxic Effects†	Specific Therapy‡	Prognosis
Fluorinated hydrocarbons (Freon)	Refrigerants; aerosol propellants; industrial solvents; fire extinguishers; local anesthetics	Systemic toxicity (sensitization of myocardium to catecholamines); asphyxia during inhalation; local irritation	Arrhythmias; conjunctivitis; pharyngitis; bronchospasm; tracheobronchitis; pulmonary edema (from thermal degradation products); frostbite (from escaping compressed gas)	Decontamination; respiratory support; cardiovascular support; provide calm, quiet environment; rapid rewarming of frostbite	Intentional inhalation from aerosol cans results in death so sudden that no treatment possible
Formaldehyde	Disinfectants; fumigants; adhesives; deodorants; emission from urea-formaldehyde foam insulation; wood products; embalming fluid	Local irritation	Conjunctivitis; rhinitis; pharyngitis; laryngeal edema; tracheobronchitis; pulmonary edema (uncommon); GI disturbances; chemical burns; hypersensitivity dermatitis; asthma	Decontamination; respiratory support	Survival for >48 hours usually associated with recovery
Gasoline (mixture of hydrocarbons and additives)	Gasoline production, use	Systemic toxicity (sensitization of myocardium to catecholamines); local irritation	Arrhythmias; CNS disturbances; seizures; respiratory depression; pulmonary edema; GI disturbances; lead poisoning	Decontamination; respiratory support; cardiovascular support	Extent of pulmonary involvement after 24 hours indicates severity; >30% pulmonary infiltration resolves in 2–4 weeks
Hydrogen chloride	Organic chemical synthesis; dye making	Local irritation	Keratoconjunctivitis; rhinitis; pharyngitis; laryngospasm; laryngeal edema; tracheobronchitis; pulmonary edema	Decontamination; respiratory support	Persistent esophageal strictures in 95% of survivors In one series 30% of persons who ingested acid died

Agent	Sources/Uses	Mechanism/Toxicity	Signs and Symptoms	Treatment	Prognosis
Hydrogen cyanide	Fumigant; ore extracting processes; electroplating	Systemic toxicity (cellular asphyxiation related to inhibition of cytochrome oxidase)	Dyspnea; CNS disturbances; cardiovascular disturbances; lactic acidosis; pulmonary edema; GI disturbances	Decontamination; respiratory support; administration of sodium nitrite, sodium thiosulfate; hyperbaric oxygen	Survival for 4 hours usually followed by recovery
Hydrogen fluoride	Glass and metal etching; petroleum industry; manufacture of integrated circuits	Local irritation; direct cellular poison	Ocular injury; laryngeal edema; chemical pneumonitis; pulmonary edema; chemical burns	Decontamination; respiratory support; calcium gluconate injections SC (except eye)	Survival for 3–4 days usually followed by recovery
Hydrogen sulfide	Oil and gas exploration and processing; metal refining; textile manufacturing; rubber vulcanizing; heavy water production; tanning industry; waste disposal: sewers, septic tanks; mines	Systemic toxicity (cellular asphyxiation related to inhibition of cytochrome oxidase); local irritation	CNS disturbances; cardiovascular disturbances; seizures; respiratory depression; lactic acidosis; keratoconjunctivitis; rhinitis; pharyngitis; tracheobronchitis; pulmonary edema; GI disturbances	Decontamination; respiratory support; cardiovascular support; administration of nitrites; hyperbaric oxygen	Survival for 4 hours usually followed by recovery
Magnesium fumes, dust	Metal welding, alloying; mining	Systemic toxicity; local irritation	Metal fume fever; upper respiratory tract irritation (dust); skin ulcerations (particles)	Decontamination	

Continued.

TABLE 108–1 (cont.).

Agent	Major Sources	Toxicologic Mechanism*	Toxic Effects†	Specific Therapy‡	Prognosis
Manganese fumes, dust	Foundry work; battery making; metal welding; mining	Systemic toxicity	Metal fume fever; CNS disturbances; psychosis; pneumonitis	Antiparkinsonian drugs	Recovery possible if immediate removal from exposure occurs before CNS symptoms; EDTA will not prevent CNS deterioration
Mercury fumes	Ore smelting; electrolysis; heating of mercury compounds	Local irritation; systemic toxicity	Conjunctivitis; necrotizing bronchiolitis; pneumonitis; pulmonary edema; metal fume fever; neuropsychiatric disturbances; gingivostomatitis; GI disturbances; renal failure	Respiratory support; chelation therapy; hemodialysis	Acute: Recovery likely with appropriate treatment Chronic: CNS recovery may never be complete in cases of chronic exposure, especially to alkyl mercury compounds
Methane	Natural gas; mining	Simple asphyxiation	Dyspnea; cyanosis; CNS disturbances; cardiovascular disturbances	Respiratory support	
Methyl bromide	Fumigant	Local irritation; systemic toxicity	Tracheobronchitis; pulmonary edema; chemical burns; CNS disturbances; seizures; psychosis; arrhythmias; GI disturbances; renal failure; hepatic injury	Decontamination; respiratory support; cardiovascular support; (?)chelation therapy	Survival for 48–72 hours usually followed by complete recovery, but neurotoxic effects may persist for months

Substance	Sources/Uses	Mechanism	Clinical Findings	Treatment	Comments
Methylene chloride	Paint removers; solvent in aerosol products; fumigants; dyes; varnishes, lacquers	Systemic toxicity (cellular asphyxiation related to its metabolite, carbon monoxide); anesthesia	CNS disturbances; respiratory depression; eye irritation; chemical pneumonitis; irritation; chemical burns	Decontamination; respiratory support; 100% oxygen, hyperbaric oxygen	Intestinal luminal narrowing may occur secondary to erosions
Natural gas	Petroleum refining; mining; heating; cooking	Simple asphyxiation	Dyspnea; cyanosis; CNS disturbances; cardiovascular disturbances	Respiratory support	
Nitrogen	Underwater work; mining	Simple asphyxiation	Dyspnea; cyanosis; CNS disturbances; cardiovascular disturbances	Respiratory support	Survival for 24 hours usually followed by complete recovery
Nitrogen oxides (NO, NO_2, N_2O, N_2O_3, N_2O_4, N_2O_5)	Electric arc welding electroplating; metal etching; dynamite blasting; silage (silo-filler's disease); reaction of nitric acid and organic matter; nitrous fumes	Local irritation, systemic toxicity (chemical asphyxiation related to formation of methemoglobin)	Tracheobronchitis; laryngeal edema; pulmonary edema; bronchiolitis obliterans; CNS disturbances; symptoms of methemoglobinemia (usually minor)	Respiratory support; methylene blue (see p. 54 for dosage); corticosteroids for bronchiolitis obliterans	
Organophosphates	See Chapter 106	See Chapter 106	See Chapter 106	See Chapter 106	See Chapter 106
O-chlorobenzylidene malononitrile	Tear gas	Local irritation	Ocular pain, blepharospasm, lacrimation; skin irritation; laryngospasm; GI disturbances	Decontamination; respiratory support	Permanent eye injury unlikely; pulmonary edema may be noted 12–24 hours after exposure
Osmium tetroxide fumes	Alloy making; platinum hardening	Local irritation	Conjunctivitis; rhinitis; tracheobronchitis; chemical pneumonitis	Decontamination; respiratory support	

Continued.

TABLE 108–1 (cont.).

Agent	Major Sources	Toxicologic Mechanism*	Toxic Effects†	Specific Therapy‡	Prognosis
Ozone	Arc welding; air, exhaust, sewage, water treatment	Local irritation	Conjunctivitis; rhinitis; pharyngitis; tracheobronchitis; pulmonary edema (uncommon); GI disturbances	Decontamination; respiratory support	Maximum respiratory effects may be seen 12–24 hours after exposure
Phosgene	Synthesis of polyurethane, isocyanates, polycarbonate resins, dyes, pharmaceuticals; thermal decomposition of chlorinated hydrocarbons	Local irritation	Conjunctivitis; pharyngitis; tracheobronchitis; pulmonary edema; chemical burns	Decontamination respiratory support	Survival for 24 hours associated with complete recovery
Propane	Cooking, heating	Simple asphyxiation	Dyspnea; cyanosis; CNS disturbances; cardiovascular disturbances	Respiratory support	Extent of pulmonary involvement indicates severity after first 24 hours; Infiltration of >30% of lung volume resolves in 2–4 weeks; no long-term pulmonary effects

Substance	Uses	Mechanism/Toxicity	Clinical features	Treatment	Remarks
Sulfur dioxide	Bleaching agent; ore smelting; manufacture of paper, chemicals; preservative; refrigerant; fumigant; disinfectant; burning of fossil fuels, sulfur-containing materials	Local irritation	Conjunctivitis; rhinitis; pharyngitis; laryngeal edema; bronchospasm; tracheobronchitis; pulmonary edema; GI disturbances; skin irritation; chronic lung disease	Decontamination; respiratory support	
Toluene	Paints, adhesives; varnishes, lacquers; paint thinners; solvent in chemical, rubber, paint, pharmaceutical industries	Systemic toxicity; (?)sensitization of myocardium to catecholamines; asphyxia during inhalation; ocal irritation	Neuropsychiatric abnormalities; muscle weakness; GI disturbances; renal dysfunction; electrolyte disturbances; metabolic acidosis; arrhythmias; seizures; rhabdomyolysis; conjunctivitis; tracheobronchitis	Decontamination; respiratory support; cardiovascular support; fluid, electrolyte repletion	Death may occur up to 3 days after acute poisoning
Toluene diisocyanate	Manufacture of polyurethane, adhesives, insulation material, plastics	Local irritation; sensitization; systemic toxicity	Conjunctivitis; keratitis; tracheobronchitis; bronchospasm; GI disturbances; skin irritation; CNS disturbances; chronic lung disease	Decontamination; respiratory support	Survival for 24 hours usually followed by complete recovery
Trichloroethane	Adhesives; spot removers; cleaning agents; paint removers; typewriter corrective fluid; degreasing agent	Systemic toxicity (sensitization of myocardium to catecholamines, CNS narcosis); local irritation	Arrhythmias; respiratory depression; CNS disturbances; seizures; transient hepatic, renal dysfunction; GI disturbances; conjunctivitis; skin irritation	Decontamination; respiratory support; cardiovascular support	Survival after initial anesthetic effects usually followed by complete recovery

Continued.

TABLE 108-1 (cont.).

Agent	Major Sources	Toxicologic Mechanism*	Toxic Effects†	Specific Therapy‡	Prognosis
Trichloroethylene	Adhesives; varnishes, lacquers; spot removers; typewriter correction fluid; degreasing agent; industrial solvent	Systemic toxicity (sensitization of myocardium to catecholamines, CNS narcosis); local irritation	Arrhythmias; respiratory depression; CNS disturbances; seizures; cranial nerve disorders; hepatic injury; renal failure; GI disturbances; conjunctivitis; pulmonary edema; skin irritation	Decontamination; respiratory support; cardiovascular support	Survival for 4 hours usually followed by complete recovery
Vanadium fumes, dust	Glass, ceramic, alloy making; welding electrodes; catalyst in chemical industry	Local irritation; systemic toxicity	Conjunctivitis; rhinitis; tracheobronchitis; pulmonary edema; asthma; GI disturbances; dermatitis (with green fume fever; psychiatric disturbances	Decontamination; respiratory support; (?)chelation therapy	
Vinyl chloride	Manufacture of plastics (e.g., polyvinyl chloride)	Systemic toxicity	CNS disturbances (large doses); acro-osteolysis; hepatic fibrosis; hepatic angiosarcoma	Decontamination; respiratory support	Symptoms related to osteo-acrolysis do not improve after removal from exposure, although there is some radiographic improvement

Zinc chloride fumes	Metal soldering; dry cell making; textile finishing	Local irritation	Ocular injury; tracheobronchitis; pulmonary edema; chemical burns	Decontamination; respiratory support	Mortality from pulmonary edema 10%–40%
Zinc oxide fumes	Metal welding; melting or heating of metallic zinc	Systemic toxicity	Metal fume fever	Respiratory support	Recovery likely if symptoms mild after first 6 hours; death may occur up to 1 week after ingestion in severe poisonings

*Specific mechanisms of toxicity given in parentheses where applicable.

†Toxic effects vary depending on concentration of inhalant and duration of exposure.

‡Specific therapy depends on clinical situation. Supportive care (including advanced life support) and symptomatic therapy (e.g., administration of analgesic, antipyretic, antiemetic) should be provided as needed.

Decontamination: (1) removal of victim's clothing (with care to avoid contamination of personnel), (2) copious irrigation of eyes with saline solution or water, (3) thorough washing of affected skin with soap and water.

Respiratory support: (1) airway management, (2) aggressive pulmonary toilet, (3) administration of supplemental oxygen (100% initially); (4) administration of bronchodilators (i.e., beta sympathomimetic agents, theophylline) unless contraindicated, (5) assisted ventilation, (6) use of positive end-expiratory pressure (PEEP) as appropriate. Beta adrenergic agonists are contraindicated in intoxications involving hydrocarbons that sensitize myocardium to catecholamines. Corticosteroids are useful in treating severe bronchospasm, hypersensitivity reactions, and bronchiolitis obliterans; however, they are of questionable benefit in chemical pneumonitis and should be avoided in smoke inhalation.

Cardiovascular support: (1) specific antiarrhythmic therapy if needed, (2) treatment of hypotension (i.e., volume infusion, application of military antishock trousers [MAST] or administration of a vasopressor [e.g., dopamine] as appropriate), (3) treatment of myocardial ischemia. Volume infusion and use of MAST contraindicated in presence of pulmonary edema; vasopressors should be avoided if possible in intoxication involving agents that sensitize myocardium to catecholamines.

3. Primary determinant of site of respiratory tract injury is the aqueous solubility of the gas.
   a. Highly soluble agents are well absorbed in the upper respiratory tract, producing rhinitis, pharyngitis, laryngeal edema, tracheobronchitis (e.g., ammonia, chlorine, formaldehyde, hydrogen chloride, ozone, sulfur dioxide).
   b. Low-solubility agents tend to be distributed to the lower airways and alveoli, producing chemical pneumonitis, noncardiogenic pulmonary edema, bronchiolitis obliterans (e.g., nitrogen dioxide, phosgene).
C. Systemic toxicity:
   1. Adverse effects on various organ systems via varied mechanisms (see Table 108–1), including:
      a. Impairment of oxygen delivery to cells (e.g., carbon monoxide).
      b. Impairment of oxygen utilization by cells (e.g., hydrogen cyanide, hydrogen sulfide).
      c. Sensitization of myocardium to endogenous catecholamines (e.g., certain hydrocarbons).
      d. Direct organotoxicity (e.g., vinyl chloride).
   2. Systemic effects depend on toxic mechanism(s) and organ system(s) involved (see Table 108–1).
D. Combination of above mechanisms.
E. Hypersensitivity reaction from inhalation of an antigen that causes an immune response.
VI. Clinical features (see also Table 108–1):
A. Simple asphyxiants:
   1. Signs and symptoms are those of hypoxia (e.g., tachypnea, tachycardia, altered mental status, cyanosis, cardiac arrhythmias, seizures, coma).
   2. Features generally appear when inert gas comprises about 20% of inspired air or when oxygen concentration declines to about 15%.
B. Irritant gases:
   1. Injury may range from irritation to chemical burns, with eyes and mucosa of the respiratory tract the most sensitive to injury.
   2. Site of pulmonary injury depends on water solubility of the gas (see Toxic mechanisms).
C. Systemic toxins:
   1. Chemical asphyxiants:
      a. Produce signs and symptoms of tissue hypoxia, predominantly CNS and cardiovascular (e.g., carbon monoxide, hydrogen cyanide, hydrogen sulfide; see Chapters 100, 101, 103, respectively).
   2. Hydrocarbons that sensitize myocardium to endogenous catecholamines (e.g., halogenated hydrocarbons) can precipitate cardiac arrhythmias and sudden death.
   3. Other agents can produce various effects, depending on their organotoxicity (see Table 108–1).
D. Hypersensitivity reactions:
   1. Immediate (asthma, anaphylaxis, chemosis, urticaria).

    2. Delayed, usually by 4–6 hours:

      a. Hypersensitivity pneumonitis, generally associated with exposure to organic dusts (e.g., fungal spores, animal proteins).

      b. Characterized by presence of dyspnea and cough, constitutional symptoms (e.g., fever, chills, malaise, anorexia), pulmonary infiltrates.

VII. Laboratory findings and evaluation:

  A. Arterial blood gases.

  B. Chest radiograph.

  C. Pulmonary function tests useful in quantitating extent of pulmonary dysfunction.

  D. Other useful studies, depending on clinical situation, include: serum electrolytes, glucose, creatinine; hepatic function tests; ECG; urinalysis.

  E. Specific toxicologic studies should be obtained as needed:

    1. Carboxyhemoglobin level indicated in patients exposed to fire or smoke or having CNS signs or symptoms of unknown cause.

  F. In select situations (e.g., smoke inhalation), bronchoscopy can be useful in diagnosing and determining extent of pulmonary tract injury and in removing debris.

  G. Xenon lung scanning is a sensitive means of diagnosing pulmonary injury in victims of smoke inhalation.

  H. Fluorescein staining or slit lamp examination useful in assessing for ocular injury.

VIII. General treatment:

  A. Follow APTLS: See Chapter 8.

  B. General management: Table 108–2 (see Chapters 8–10 for details).

  C. Decontamination:

    1. Eye exposure: Irrigate exposed eyes with copious amounts of water or saline solution (see Chapter 28 for treatment recommendations).

    2. Skin exposure: Remove victim's clothing (with care to avoid exposure to personnel) and wash exposed areas with soap and water (see Chapter 29 for management approach).

TABLE 108–2.

General Treatment

Treatment	Indicated	Of No Value	Contraindicated
O$_2$	+		
IV	+		
ECG monitor	+		
Forced diuresis*		X	
Acidification		X	
Alkalinization		X	
Emesis/lavage		X	
Charcoal		X	
Cathartic		X	

*Except in severe chromium intoxication (see Table 108–1).

IX. Specific treatment (see also Table 108–1):
  A. Pre-hospital: See Chapter 111.
  B. Hospital:
    1. Mainly supportive and symptomatic, with specific measures as appropriate.
    2. Respiratory support of primary importance:
      a. **Airway:** Endotracheal intubation indicated in the presence of upper airway edema or burns, inadequate ventilation, copious pulmonary secretions, status epilepticus, or depressed level of consciousness.
      b. See Chapter 9.
      c. Provide vigorous pulmonary toilet as needed. May require endotracheal intubation. Bronchoscopy can be helpful in removing pulmonary debris.
    3. Bronchospasm:
      a. Beta adrenergic agonists:
        (1) Epinephrine 0.3–0.5 ml (0.01 ml/kg in child) of 1:1,000 solution SC every 20–30 minutes for up to three doses.
        (2) Aerosol therapy:
          a Isoetharine (Bronkosol): 0.5 ml 1% isoetharine diluted with normal saline solution or diluent to 3.0 ml and administered by nebulized inhalation treatment or low-pressure intermittent positive pressure breathing (IPPB) over 15–20 minutes.
          b Metaproterenol (Alupent): 0.3 ml 5% metaproterenol diluted with normal saline solution or diluent to 3.0 ml and administered by nebulized inhalation treatment or low-pressure IPPB over 15–20 minutes.
        (3) NOTE: These agents are **contraindicated** in inhalations involving substances that sensitize myocardium to catecholamines (e.g., halogenated hydrocarbons).
      b. Aminophylline:
        (1) 5–7 mg/kg IV over 20–30 minutes.
        (2) Initial maintenance infusion 0.5 mg/kg/hr (up to 1.25 mg/kg/hr in children).
      c. Corticosteroids:
        (1) Methylprednisolone 0.5–1.0 mg/kg IV every 6 hours) in severe, persistent bronchospasm. (Children: 1–2 mg/kg IV every 6 hours.)
        (2) Hydrocortisone 0.5–1.0 gm IV every 6 hours. (Children: 4–5 mg/kg IV every 6 hours.)
        (3) NOTE: Steroids should be avoided in smoke inhalation (see Corticosteroids, below).
    4. Pulmonary edema:
      a. Careful fluid management (avoid net positive fluid balance).
      b. Positive end-expiratory pressure (PEEP).
      c. Morphine sulfate **contraindicated.**
    5. Corticosteroids:
      a. Useful in treating hypersensitivity reactions (e.g., asthma, hypersensitivity pneumonitis) and bronchiolitis obliterans.

       b. These agents are of questionable benefit in treating chemical pneumonitis.

       c. **Contraindicated in smoke inhalation** because of associated increase in morbidity and mortality.

   6. Antibiotics indicated only when there is evidence of infection; not recommended for prophylaxis.

   7. Cardiovascular support:

       a. **Cardiac arrest:** Advanced life support should be implemented. Follow most recent Advanced Cardiac Life Support guidelines. (*JAMA* 1986; 255:2841–3044).

       b. Hypotension:

          (1) See Chapter 10 for treatment recommendations.

          (2) Avoid sympathomimetics if possible in intoxications involving toxins that sensitize myocardium to catecholamines (e.g., halogenated hydrocarbons).

X. Prognosis: See Table 108–1.

  A. Expected Response to Treatment

   1. Toxic inhalations: Usual outcome for patients with toxic inhalation injuries who do not die of asphyxia and who are supported successfully throughout acute phase is recovery without residual functional impairment.

   2. Hypersensitivity reactions: Symptoms of hypersensitivity pneumonitis generally resolve within 12–24 hours following removal of the patient from the antigenic source.

  B. Expected complications and long-term effects:

   1. Toxic inhalations:

       a. Airway obstruction and less often restrictive impairment; particularly true for exposures to nitrogen oxides, ammonia, sulfur dioxide.

       b. Residual bronchiolitis obliterans may accompany nitrogen dioxide toxicity.

       c. Disorders such as bronchiolitis obliterans, bronchostenosis, bronchiectasis may be seen in victims of smoke inhalation.

   2. Hypersensitivity reactions: Prolonged or repeated antigenic exposure can result in a chronic form of the disease, with irreversible pulmonary damage (fibrosis).

XI. Special considerations:

  A. Hydrogen cyanide: See also Chapter 101.

   1. Should be suspected when fire victim fails to respond immediately to oxygen treatment or when someone at a fire who is wearing a charcoal mask collapses (charcoal does not filter hydrogen cyanide from air).

   2. If the patient survives the first four hours after exposure, recovery is likely. However, neurologic sequelae may persist.

  B. Always consider concomitant carbon monoxide intoxication in any toxic inhalation and especially in smoke inhalation and exposure to fires. If signs of tissue hypoxia persist after administration of oxygen, consider exposure to cyanide, hydrogen sulfide gas, or methemoglobinemia.

  C. Lacrimators:

   1. Potent irritants used for riot control and self-defense. Most common

agents are chloroacetophenone (Mace, tear gas), *O*-chlorobenzylidene, malononitrile, dibenzoxazepine.

2. These agents produce immediate ocular burning (with blepharospasm and lacrimation) and skin irritation. In high concentrations, chemical burns (including corneal ulcerations), laryngospasm, pulmonary edema can occur.

3. Treatment consists of decontamination (i.e., irrigation of eyes and washing of involved skin) and supportive and symptomatic care as needed.

D. Metal fumes:

1. Consist of a gaseous suspension of oxidized metallic particles. Inhalation of these fumes can occur during welding, smelting, galvanizing of a variety of metals (e.g., aluminum, antimony, beryllium, brass, cadmium, chromium, cobalt, copper, iron, magnesium, manganese, mercury, nickel, selenium, silver, tin, vanadium, zinc). Toxicity results from local irritant or systemic effects of fumes.

2. Clinical manifestations are varied, depending on the metal involved (see Table 108–1), and include signs and symptoms of pulmonary tract injury (e.g., rhinitis, tracheobronchitis, chemical pneumonitis, pulmonary edema) and a syndrome known as metal fume fever.

   a. Metal fume fever is characterized by sudden onset (usually within 4–8 hours of exposure) of thirst, metallic taste in the mouth, fever, chills, malaise, myalgias, headache; pulmonary signs and symptoms may be present if the metallic oxide also has irritant properties. The course of metal fume fever is generally benign, with resolution in 24–48 hours.

3. Treatment of these entities includes supportive and symptomatic care (e.g., administration of supplemental oxygen, bronchodilators, analgesic, antipyretic as needed). Steroids are of questionable benefit in treating pulmonary tract injury.

E. Smoke inhalation:

1. Smoke is a complex mixture of heated gases and coated carbon particles representing products of combustion and pyrolysis. Smoke can contain a variety of hazardous materials, depending on the substances undergoing thermal degradation (Table 108–3).

2. Inhalation of smoke can lead to injury by (1) simple asphyxiation, (2) thermal damage to tissues, (3) local irritation, (4) systemic toxic effects.

3. Clinically, there may be skin and airway burns (usually confined to upper airway), signs and symptoms of chemical injury to the respiratory tract (e.g., laryngeal edema, tracheobronchitis, chemical pneumonitis, noncardiogenic pulmonary edema), and various systemic signs related to hypoxia and toxic effects of the specific products of combustion present in the smoke.

4. Bronchoscopy and xenon lung scanning are useful in diagnosing and determining extent of pulmonary tract injury.

5. Treatment is intensive supportive care (e.g., airway management, administration of supplemental oxygen and bronchodilators, assisted ven-

TABLE 108–3.

Toxic Components of Smoke

Agent	Source
Acrolein	Acrylics, cellulose, polyolefins
Aldehydes	Cotton, paper, wood
Ammonia	Nylon, silk, wool
Carbon dioxide	Carbon-containing matter
Carbon monoxide	Carbon-containing matter, incomplete combustion
Chlorine	Plastics
Hydrogen chloride	Chlorinated acrylics, polyvinyl chloride, retardant-treated materials
Hydrogen cyanide	Nylon, paper, polyacrylonitrile, polyurethane, silk, wool
Hydrogen fluoride	Fluorinated hydrocarbons
Hydrogen sulfide	Hair, hides, wool
Isocyanates	Polyurethane
Nitrogen oxides	Celluloid, fabrics, wallpaper, wood
Phosgene	Chlorinated hydrocarbons, plastics, polyvinyl chloride
Styrene	Polystyrene
Sulfur dioxide	Sulfur-containing material

tilation, use of PEEP). Concomitant carbon monoxide toxicity should always be suspected, and if present treated appropriately. With evidence of upper airway injury, intubate early; it may become too difficult once significant edema develops. Specific treatment is based on identified material (see Table 108–1). Steroids have been shown to be detrimental and should be avoided.

F. Solvent abuse:
   1. Refers to recreational use of organic solvents. Methods include inhaling solvent from a plastic bag ("bagging") or from a saturated cloth ("huffing"). Commonly abused substances are presented in Table 108–4.
   2. Solvent abuse is most common in adolescent youths.
   3. Toxicity and clinical manifestations are varied, depending on toxic agent(s) involved (see Table 108–1):
      a. Neuropsychiatric disturbances predominate.
      b. Sudden death can occur.
      c. Sensitization of myocardium to endogenous catecholamines can occur.
      d. Inhalation of leaded gasoline can cause irreversible neurologic symptoms (see Chapter 109).
   4. Diagnosis of solvent abuse can be confirmed by detection of solvents in blood or by detection of metabolites in urine (e.g., hippuric acid [toluene], methylhippuric acid [xylene], phenol [benzene], trichloro-

acetic acid and trichloroethanol [trichloroethane, trichloroethylene], mandelic and phenylglyoxylic acids [styrene]).

5. Treatment involves providing a protective, calm environment for patients who are hallucinating and appropriate supportive care as needed. Psychiatric or drug abuse counseling is important.

XII. Disposition considerations:

    A. Admission considerations:

        1. See General Admission Considerations (Chapters 17 and 18).

        2. Generally, symptomatic patients (other than those with mild upper airway irritation; e.g., pharyngitis, rhinitis) should be admitted for 24–48 hours of observation. These include patients with:

            a. Dyspnea on room air, hypoxemia.

            b. Evidence of lower airway involvement (e.g., wheezing, rales, infiltrates on chest film).

            c. Upper airway edema, inflammation (e.g., stridor, dysphagia, dysphonia).

            d. Upper airway burns, thermal injury.

            e. Tracheobronchitis.

            f. Potentially serious systemic signs.

        3. If there is serious doubt that the patient is reliable or does not have easy access to a health care facility, hospitalization for observation is advised.

        4. Suicide risk.

    B. Intensive Care Admission Considerations: See Chapter 18.

TABLE 108–4.

Solvent Composition of Products Abused*

Product Inhaled	Chemical Constituents
Glues, adhesives	Toluene, benzene, xylene, acetone *N*-hexane, trichloroethylene, tetrachloroethylene, 1,1,1-trichloroethane, carbon tetrachloride, toluene
Gasoline (petrol)	Hydrocarbons, tetraethyl lead
Aerosols	Fluorocarbons
Lighter refills	Butane
Acrylic paint	Toluene
Paints, varnishes, lacquers	Trichloroethylene, methylene chloride, toluene
Dyes	Acetone, methylene chloride
Nail polish remover	Acetone, amyl acetate

*From Haddad LM, Winchester JF (eds): *Clinical Management of Poisoning and Drug Overdose.* Philadelphia, WB Saunders Co, 1983, p 802. Used by permission.

C. Consultation considerations:
   1. Potential need for eye, nose, throat or pulmonary consultation for laryngoscopy or bronchofibroscopic examination.
   2. Hyperbaric facility if indicated (e.g., carbon monoxide toxicity (see Chapter 100).
D. Observation period: If patient is asymptomatic or has mild upper respiratory symptoms, observe for at least 4–6 hours in emergency department.
E. Discharge considerations:
   1. General disposition considerations have been met (see Chapters 17 and 18).
   2. Asymptomatic patients with normal exam and chest x-ray should be observed for 4–6 hours in emergency department; if they remain well, may be discharged without repeat chest x-ray study.
   3. Patients with only mild upper respiratory symptoms without objective injury (e.g., pharyngitis, rhinitis) may be discharged with reassurance and symptomatic medications (e.g., decongestants, sore throat lozenges) after 4–6 hours of observation.
   4. Public health officials have been notified.
   5. Disposition environment is safe from re-exposure.
   6. Patient is discharged in the company of a responsible adult if it is easy to return or if there is easy access to other appropriate medical care should an untoward event occur.
   7. Suicide potential and psychiatric state have been appropriately addressed.

BIBLIOGRAPHY

Dula DJ: Metal fume fever. *JACEP* 1978; 7:448–450.

Fischman CM, Oster JR: Toxic effects of toluene: A new cause of high anion gap metabolic acidosis. *JAMA* 1979; 241:1713.

Fortenberry JD: Gasoline sniffing. *Am J Med* 1985; 79:740–744.

Goldfrank LR, Flomenbaum NE, Lewin NA, et al (eds): *Goldfrank's Toxicologic Emergencies,* ed 3. Norwalk, Conn, Appleton-Century-Crofts, 1986.

Haddad LM, Winchester JF (eds): *Clinical Management of Poisoning and Drug Overdose.* Philadelphia, WB Saunders Co, 1983.

Haggerty M, Soto-Greene M, Reichman LB: Caring for victims of toxic gas inhalation: Emergency treatment and in-hospital management. *J Crit Illness* July 1987; 77–87.

Kirk LM, Anderson RJ, Martin K: Sudden death from toluene abuse. *Ann Emerg Med* 1984; 13:68.

Montague TJ, Macneil AR: Mass ammonia inhalation. *Chest* 1980; 77:496–498.

Rumack BH (ed): *Poisindex.* Denver, Micromedex, 1987.

Streicher HZ, Gabow PA, Moss AH, et al: Syndromes of toluene sniffing in adults. *Ann Intern Med* 1981; 94:758–762.

Summer W, Haponik: Inhalation of irritant gases. *Clin Chest Med* 1981; 2:273–286.

Wason S, Gibler B, Hassan M: Ventricular tachycardia associated with non-Freon aerosol propellants. *JAMA* 1986; 256:78–80.

109

Heavy Metals

Paula A. Ryals, M.D., F.A.C.E.P.

Arsenic

   I. Route of exposure: Oral, inhalation.
  II. Common forms of arsenic:
      Elemental arsenic
      Arsenic trioxide
      Arsine gas
      Arsenic acid
      Arsenates (pentavalent)
      Arsenites (trivalent)
      Arsphenamine
      Acetarsone
      Methane arsonic acid
      Cacodylic acid (dimethyl arsenic acid)
      Roxarsone (28% elemental arsenic; used in animal feeds)
      Ant and rat poisons
      Other organic forms
 III. Pharmacokinetics:
     A. Absorption: Rapid.
     B. Onset of action: Minutes to hours after oral ingestion.
     C. Elimination: Natural elimination via urine, feces, sweat.
  IV. Action: See Toxic mechanism.
   V. Uses:
     A. Used in industry, agriculture, ceramic trades.
     B. Herbicide, rodenticide, insecticide, fungicide, tanning agent, glass.

C. Most common cause of acute heavy metal poisoning.

D. Vehicle for homicidal and suicidal use.

VI. Toxic mechanism:

    A. Disruption of cellular metabolism through combination with sulfhydryl enzymes.

    B. Arsenate uncouples oxidative phosphorylation.

VII. Fatal dose: Approximately 120 mg.

VIII. Clinical features:

    A. Acute exposure:

        1. Initially GI: Dysphagia, burning in throat, garlic odor on breath, symptoms of severe gastroenteritis such as abdominal pain, nausea, vomiting, diarrhea, fluid depletion.

        2. GI symptoms followed by: cyanosis, dyspnea, hypotension, ventricular arrhythmias, delirium, coma, seizures.

        3. Later effects in survivors include acute tubular necrosis and hemolysis with eosinophilia.

        4. Acute inhalation exposure may result in pulmonary edema.

    B. Chronic exposure (2–8 weeks after ingestion, or ongoing exposure):

        1. Exfoliative dermatitis, hyperpigmentation, Aldrich-Mees lines in nails, painful polyneuritis, neurasthenia, memory impairment, cancer of skin or lung, excessive salivation, cirrhosis, weight loss, anemia.

IX. Laboratory findings and evaluation:

    A. Blood:

        1. Serum level: Normal <7 μg/dl.

        2. Complete blood cell count; chemistry values, including amylase, liver function studies, arterial blood gases.

    C. Abdominal radiograph; heavy metals such as arsenic are radiopaque.

    D. Chest radiograph (in presence of pulmonary findings).

    E. ECG (arrhythmias).

    F. Hair analysis difficult and unreliable.

X. General treatment:

    A. Follow APTLS: See Chapter 8.

    B. General management: Table 109–1 (see Chapters 8–10 for details).

TABLE 109–1.

General Treatment

Treatment	Indicated	Of No Value	Contraindicated
O$_2$	+		
IV	+		
ECG monitor	+		
Forced diuresis		X	
Acidification		X	
Alkalinization		X	
Emesis/lavage	+/+		
Charcoal*	±		
Cathartic		X	

*Controversial.

XI. Specific management:
  A. Mild symptoms (acute exposure):
    1. Chelation therapy with **dimercaprol** (BAL) IM: 2–3 mg/kg/dose every 8–12 hours for 24 hours, then every 12–24 hours for 10 days.
  B. Severe symptoms (acute exposure):
    1. **Dimercaprol** 3–5 mg/kg/dose every 8–12 hours for 24 hours, then every 12 hours for 10 days.
    2. Discontinue chelation when urine arsenic <50 μg/dl (24-hour urine specimen collection).
  C. Chronic exposure
    1. D-Penicillamine 20–40 mg/kg/dose, given 4 times daily up to maximum of 1 gm/day for 1 week followed by no treatment for 1 week.
    2. Repeat chelation if urine arsenic >50 μg/dl after the second week.
  D. Hemodialysis if renal failure present.
XII. Prognosis:
  A. Expected response to treatment:
    1. Prognosis related to:
      a. Early initiation of chelation therapy.
      b. Initial severity.
    2. In acute arsenic poisoning, survival for more than 1 week associated with complete recovery.
    3. Complete recovery from chronic arsenic poisoning may require 6 months–1 year.
  B. Expected complications and long-term effects: See Clinical features.
XIII. Special considerations:
  A. Arsine gas:
    1. Colorless, nonirritating, garlic odor; frequently produced in industrial settings.
    2. Well absorbed by lungs; produces hemolysis, jaundice, abdominal pain, hemoglobinuria.
    3. Chelation therapy ineffective in arsine gas poisoning, and treatment is by exchange transfusion or hemodialysis.
    4. See also Table 108–1.
XIV. Disposition considerations:
  A. Admission considerations: All patients with suspected or documented exposure.
  B. Consultation considerations:
    1. Dialysis service if renal impairment present.
    2. Public health officials, industrial physicians should be consulted if indicated.
  C. Observation period: None; observation inappropriate.
  D. Discharge considerations: None; all patients should be admitted.

Iron

See Chapter 88.

Lead

I. Route of exposure:
    A. Inorganic lead poisoning:
        1. Oral:
            a. Children: Ingestion of pica, leaded paint, or newsprint.
            b. Family members: Drinking from lead-glazed pitchers, often obtained as souvenirs from less developed countries; lead pipes.
        2. Inhalation: Adult welders or battery makers.
    B. Organic lead poisoning:
        1. Inhalation: Lead gasoline.
        2. Dermal.
II. Common forms: See Uses.
III. Pharmacokinetics:
    A. Absorption:
        1. Inhalation: Absorption is rapid, although symptoms may not occur unless exposure is prolonged.
        2. GI: Children absorb 50% of ingested dose, adults only 10%.
        3. Dermal: Poor except in case of organic lead.
    B. Onset of action: Effects may arise acutely, but poisoning is generally chronic.
    C. Half-life: Kidneys: 7 years; Bone: 32 years.
    D. Duration of action: Poisoning is usually chronic, months to years.
    E. Elimination: Extremely slow excretion. Eliminated through nails, sweat, hair, bile, urine. Also deposited in teeth, bones, kidneys.
IV. Action: Lead combines with sulfhydryl groups on proteins and partially inhibits enzymatic action in heme synthetic pathway.
V. Uses:
    A. Industrial: Smelters, battery recycling plants, auto body paintshops, painters.
    B. Other sources: Paint, dirt, newsprint, lead pipes, pottery, batteries, gasoline, fumes from burning of old painted wood, moonshine whiskey.
VI. Toxic mechanism:
    A. Lead combines with sulfhydryl groups on proteins and partially inhibits enzymes in heme synthetic pathway.
    B. Anemia results from decreased heme synthesis and interference with sodium-potassium ATPase pump in red blood cell membranes, resulting in increased fragility and decreased survival.
    C. Chronic nephritis, myocarditis, direct CNS cytotoxic effect.
    D. Crosses placenta; associated with premature rupture of membranes and premature delivery.
VII. Range of toxicity:
    A. Toxic dose: Accumulation and toxicity occur if >0.5 mg/day absorbed.
    B. Fatal dose: Estimated to be 0.5 gm absorbed lead.
VIII. Clinical features:
    A. Acute presentation:
        1. Symptoms: Table 109–2.

TABLE 109–2.

Symptoms of Acute Lead Toxicity

Age	Mild Symptoms	Severe Symptoms
Toddler	Anorexia, occasional vomiting, irritability, lethargy, refusal to play	Slurred speech, anemia, persistent vomiting, peripheral neuropathy, stupor, ataxia, convulsions, coma
Child	Learning regression; others similar to toddler's symptoms, above	
Adolescent, Adult	Colicky abdominal pain, constipation, limb pain, hypertension	Renal failure, headache, memory loss

    2. Laboratory findings:
      a. Anemia (Hgb <10 gm/dl), basophilic stippling.
      b. Increased urinary aminolevulinic acid (ALA), coproporphyrins
      c. Opacities on abdominal radiographs.
      d. Blood lead level >60 μg/dl, erythrocyte protoporphyrin (EP) 7–10 times normal (>35 μg/dl).
  B. Chronic lead ingestion:
    1. Symptoms: Nonspecific aches and pains, wrist and ankle drop, chronic nephritis.
    2. Laboratory findings:
      a. Anemia (Hgb <10 gm/dl), basophilic stippling.
      b. Increased urinary ALA.
      c. Lead lines in long bones.
      d. Blood lead level 30–60 μg/dl, erythrocyte porphyrin (EP) <7 times normal.
  C. Organic lead poisoning:
    1. Caused by inhaling leaded gasoline.
    2. Symptoms can develop after 1 week of heavy use, and include irritability, restlessness, bradycardia, hypotension, tremor, confusion, chorea, mania. May be irreversible.
IX. Laboratory findings and evaluation:
  A. Indications for screening blood lead and erythrocyte porphyrin (EP) levels:
    1. Children with pica; anemia; hyperkinetic behavior; neurologic disease, including seizures.
    2. Children living in houses built before 1940; test early in the second year of life.
    3. Symptomatic as described above.

B. Levels:
   1. Serum lead level >25 μg/dl abnormal.
   2. Symptoms usually seen with levels >80–100 μg/dl.
   3. Free EP level >35 μg/dl abnormal.
C. Blood or bone marrow smear for basophilic stippling; also, complete blood cell, reticulocyte counts.
D. Radiographs:
   1. Long bones for lead lines in children. Lead lines consist of areas of increased density at ends of growing bones, present in chronic poisoning in children (most common ages 2–5 years). Multiple bands represent repeated episodes of poisoning.
   2. Abdominal radiographs may reveal opaque particles, especially in rectosigmoid areas, if paint or other lead products have been ingested recently.
X. General treatment:
   A. Follow APTLS: See Chapter 8.
   B. General management: Table 109–3 (see Chapters 8–10 for details).
XI. Specific management:
   A. Chelation therapy for acute poisoning:
      1. Acute encephalopathy: Start with BAL 75 mg/m^2 IM every 4 hours. After 4 hours start continuous infusion of CaNa$_2$-EDTA 1,500 mg/m^2/day. Therapy with BAL and CaNa$_2$-EDTA should be continued for 5 days; interrupt therapy for 2 days, then continue with both for 5 additional days. If blood lead level remains high, other cycles may be needed, depending on blood lead rebound.
      2. Symptomatic, without encephalopathy: Start with BAL 50 mg/m^2 IM every 4 hours. After 4 hours start CaNa$_2$-EDTA 1,000 mg/m^2/day, preferably by continuous infusion or in divided doses IV. Therapy with CaNa$_2$-EDTA should be continued for 5 days. BAL may be discontinued after 3 days if blood lead <50 mg/dl. Interrupt therapy for 2

TABLE 109–3.

General Treatment

Treatment	Indicated	Of No Value	Contraindicated
O$_2$	±		
IV	±		
ECG monitor	±		
Forced diuresis		X	
Acidification		X	
Alkalinization		X	
Emesis	±		
Lavage*	+		
Charcoal	+		
Cathartic	+		

*Preferred in possible severe toxicity.

days, then treat for 5 additional days (including BAL) if blood Pb remains high. Other cycles may be needed, depending on blood lead rebound.

B. Chronic poisoning: D-Penicillamine 20–40 mg/kg/day (maximum 1 gm) may be given for 3–6 months. EDTA also effective.

C. In presence of impaired renal function, dialysis is mandatory.

XII. Prognosis:

A. Expected response to treatment:

1. Mortality in patients with lead encephalopathy has been as high as 25%.

2. Effect of EDTA on prognosis in lead encephalopathy has not been determined.

3. Complete recovery from lead poisoning may take up to 1 year.

B. Expected complications and long-term effects: Approximately 50% of patients surviving episodes of lead encephalopathy have permanent neurological deficits.

XIII. Special considerations:

A. Lead poisoning in childhood may be subacute and chronic, leading to developmental delay and subtle neurologic deficit.

B. Toxicity from tetraethyl and tetramethyl lead does not respond to chelation treatment.

XIV. Disposition considerations:

A. Admission considerations:

1. See General Admission Considerations (Chapters 17 and 18).

2. Symptomatic.

3. Blood lead levels >60 µg/dl or free EP >5 µg/gm Hgb, regardless of symptoms.

4. Radiopaque material on flat plate or lead lines in knees, wrists.

B. Consultation considerations:

1. Nephrology consultation if dialysis indicated (e.g., if impaired renal function develops).

2. In adults with chronic toxicity, refer to neurologist for performance of nerve conduction velocities.

3. Social worker, for children with toxicity.

C. Observation period: None.

D. Discharge considerations: None; all patients with suspected or proved toxicity should be admitted.

Mercury

I. Route of exposure: Ingestion, inhalation, intravenous, intramuscular, transdermal, mucous membrane, aspiration.

II. Common forms:

Mercury vapor

Elemental mercury

Inorganic mercury salts (e.g., mercuric chloride)
Organic mercury salts (e.g., methyl mercury)
III. Pharmacokinetics:
    A. Absorption:
        1. Inhalation of mercury vapor: 100%.
        2. Inorganic salts: 15% absorbed from GI tract.
        3. Organic salts (e.g., methyl mercury): Completely absorbed from GI tract.
        4. Elemental mercury (e.g., quicksilver, thermometer mercury): Not absorbed in GI tract; eliminated in feces.
    B. Onset of action:
        1. Inhalation: Within few hours of exposure to mercury vapor.
        2. Inorganic mercury (e.g., mercuric chloride): Toxicity develops within few minutes, from corrosive qualities.
        3. Organic mercury: Onset of symptoms from methyl mercury may occur weeks to months after exposure.
    C. Half-life: See Table 109–4.
    D. Duration of action: May be chronic (weeks, months, years).
    E. Elimination: See Table 109–4.
IV. Action: See Toxic mechanism.
V. Uses:
    A. Elemental: Manufacture of thermometers, batteries, electrical appliances, lamps, jewelry.
    B. Inorganic salts: Manufacture of explosives, fireworks, dyes.
    C. Organic salts: Fungicides, pesticides, insecticides.
VI. Toxic mechanism:
    A. Binds to sulfhydryl radicals on proteins, leading to inhibition of several enzymes. CNS, in particular, affected.
    B. Soluble mercuric salts toxic to all cells by depressing cellular enzymatic mechanisms by combining with sulfhydryl (–SH) groups. Renal glomeruli and tubules are specifically injured in course of mercury excretion, leading to acute tubular necrosis and uremia.
    C. Mercuric chloride also has direct irritant effect on tissues.
    D. Inhaled mercury vapor causes acute pneumonitis.
VII. Range of toxicity:
    A. Toxic dose:
        1. Elemental mercury has no toxic effect when ingested.
        2. Mercurous chloride and organic antiseptic mercurials, such as merthiolate, are relatively nontoxic because of poor absorption.
    B. Fatal dose:
        1. Mercuric salts, such as mercuric chloride, between 1–4 gm, with 0.5 gm reported to have produced death.
        2. Single fatal dose of mercurous chloride and organic antiseptic mercurials such as merthiolate, 2–4 times fatal dose of soluble inorganic mercury salts such as mercuric chloride.
VIII. Clinical features: See Table 109–4.
 IX. Laboratory findings and evaluation:

TABLE 109–4.

Features of Mercury Poisoning

Poisoning	Elemental	Inorganic	Organic
Route of exposure	Vapor, via lungs	GI, dermal	GI, dermal
Tissue of distribution	Lungs, CNS	Kidneys, liver, marrow, spleen RBCs, lungs, GI, skin	Hemoglobin binding, CNS, renal, hepatic
Clearance half-life (excretion) (days)	60 (reticuloendothelial system)	40 (urine, stool)	70 (hepatorenal, bile)
Clinical effects	Interstitial pneumonitis, acute respiratory failure, chronic tremors, erethism	Dermatitis, salivation, gingivitis, colitis, renal failure, dementia, nausea, vomiting, gastroenteritis, proteinuria, uremia, hematuria	Diverse neurologic deficits (dysarthria, ataxia, paresthesias, sensory loss, tunnel vision, mental status changes (erethism: emotional instability, lethargy, memory loss)

A. Blood and urine mercury levels:
   1. Toxic levels:

	Abnormal	Symptomatic
Blood (μg/dl)	>4	>500
Urine (μg/L)	>20	>300

   2. Blood levels not always reliable in either acute or chronic exposure.
B. Hair analysis:
   1. Good for assessing chronic exposure (poor for acute exposures).
   2. >400–500 μg/gm associated with neurotoxicity.
C. Chest radiograph, arterial blood gases, if history of inhalation exposure
D. Renal function studies, urinalysis, electrolytes, if severe fluid depletion from vomiting.
X. General treatment:
  A. Follow APTLS: See Chapter 8.
  B. General management: Table 109–5 (see Chapters 8–10 for details).
  C. Chelation therapy:
    1. Acute poisoning:
      a. Dimercaprol (BAL) 3–5 mg/kg every 4 hours for 2 days, then 2.5–3 mg/kg every 6 hours for 2 days, then every 12 hours for 7 more days.
      b. Alternatively, D-penicillamine:
        (1) Children: 100 mg/kg/day in four divided doses (maximum 1 gm/day).

TABLE 109–5.

General Treatment

Treatment	Indicated	Of No Value	Contraindicated
O$_2$	±		
IV	±		
ECG monitor	±		
Forced diuresis		X	
Acidification		X	
Alkalinization		X	
Emesis	+		
Lavage*	+		
Charcoal	+		
Cathartic	+		
Demulcent†			

*For mercuric chloride and other mercury salts, lavage may be performed with sodium formaldehyde sulfoxylate (20 gm ampule), which reduces them to metallic mercury, which is less soluble.
†Milk or egg white immediately after ingestion.

    (2) Adults: 250 mg PO 4 times a day.
    (3) Contraindications: Penicillin allergy, renal failure (unless hemodialysis).
  c. *N*-Acetyl-D,L-penicillamine has been reported to be more effective than D-penicillamine. Available on investigational basis from Aldrich Chemical Co., Milwaukee. Contraindications the same as for D-penicillamine.
  d. Continue chelating agent until urine mercury level <50 µg/L.
  2. Chronic poisoning: D-Penicillamine 20–40 mg/kg/day (maximum 1 gm/day).
  3. In presence of impaired renal function, hemodialysis is mandatory to speed removal of mercury-dimercaprol complex.
XI. Prognosis:
  A. Expected response to treatment:
    1. Prognosis for recovery excellent if dimercaprol given for at least 1 week.
    2. CNS deficits may never return to normal despite optimal therapy, particularly with organic mercury compounds.
  B. Expected complications and long-term effects:
    1. Long-term neurological disability common after poisoning from ethyl or methyl mercury.
    2. Esophageal, gastric, intestinal stenosis may occur after mercuric chloride ingestion.
XII. Special considerations:
  A. Disk battery ingestion:
    1. Release of mercuric oxide, resulting in severe GI tract corrosion, hematemesis, bloody diarrhea, shock secondary to volume loss.
    2. Treatment is by removal with water-soluble contrast enema under

fluoroscopy, followed by D-penicillamine. May require endoscopy, gastrotomy or laparotomy.

3. Neurologic symptoms from organic mercury poisoning (e.g., methyl mercury) may not be reversible with chelation therapy.

B. Mercury fumes: See Table 108–1.

XIII. Controversies:

A. EDTA has been recommended by some for treatment of mercury poisoning; however, it binds poorly to mercury and has potential for nephrotoxicity and therefore probably should not be used.

B. Other experimental and investigational agents:

1. 2,3-Dimercaptopropane-1-sulfonate, an investigational drug, has been effective in two cases of inorganic mercury poisoning.

2. DMSA (meso-dimercaptosuccinic acid) and DMPS (2,3-dimercapto-1-propane sulfonic acid sodium salt).

3. Polythiol resin to trap organic mercury in gut in order to interrupt enterohepatic circulation.

4. DTT (dithiothreitol).

5. Hemoperfusion column of agarose polymercaptol microsphere beads.

XIV. Disposition considerations:

A. Admission considerations:

1. See General Admission Considerations (Chapters 17 and 18).

2. Any significant exposure to mercury vapor or inorganic mercury salts requires admission.

3. Ingestion of elemental mercury (usually from swallowing part of a broken thermometer) does not require admission unless GI transit is abnormally delayed.

4. Exposure to even small amounts of organic mercury compounds usually requires admission and always requires long-term treatment with careful follow-up.

B. Consultation considerations:

1. GI and surgical consultation required for stenotic lesions of esophagus secondary to mercuric chloride and for button battery ingestions.

2. Dialysis service should be consulted if impaired renal function develops.

C. Observation period: None; observation not appropriate.

D. Discharge considerations:

1. None; all patients with mercury toxicity should be admitted.

2. Patients with documented oral ingestion of metallic mercury may be discharged because no systemic absorption occurs.

Other Heavy Metal Poisoning Syndromes and Diseases

I. Clinical effects:

A. Metal fume fever:

1. Copper, magnesium, manganese, silver, vanadium, zinc, aluminum, antimony, beryllium, brass, cadmium, chromium, cobalt, iron, mercury, nickel, selenium, tin.

2. See Chapter 108.

B. Occupational asthma: Aluminum, chromium, cobalt, nickel, selenium, vanadium.

C. Chronic obstructive pulmonary disease, interstitial pneumonitis: Aluminum, beryllium, cadmium, chromium, cobalt, selenium, titanium, tungsten, vanadium

D. Dermatitis: Antimony, beryllium, chromium, cobalt, gold, magnesium, nickel.

E. Renal dysfunction: Cadmium, gold, manganese, selenium, vanadium.

F. Hepatic dysfunction: Antimony, chromium, gold, selenium.

G. GI syndrome: Antimony, thallium, cadmium, vanadium.

H. CNS, psychiatric: Cobalt, gold, manganese, thallium, vanadium.

I. Hematologic dysfunction: Antimony, cobalt, gold.

II. Special remarks on selected heavy metals:

A. Antimony: Similar to arsenic poisoning.

B. Beryllium: Sarcoidlike syndrome.

C. Cadmium:
1. Cancer of prostate gland, anosmia, yellow teeth.
2. See also Table 108–1.

D. Chromium (trivalent):
1. Low toxicity, hexavalent-irritant, corrosive.
2. See also Table 108–1.

E. Manganese:
1. Parkinson's disease, acute psychosis.
2. See also Table 108–1.

F. Thallium: Ophthalmologic changes, hair loss.

BIBLIOGRAPHY

Done AK, Peart AJ: Acute toxicities of arsenical herbicides. *Clin Toxicol* 1971; 4:343–355.

Elhassani S: The many faces of methylmercury poisoning. *J Toxicol Clin Toxicol* 1982; 19:875–906.

Gerhardt R, Crecelius E, Hudson J: Moonshine-related arsenic poisoning. *Arch Intern Med* 1980; 140:211–213.

Green VA, Wise GW, Callenbach J: Lead poisoning. *Clin Toxicol* 1976; 9:33–51.

Kulig K, Rumack CM, Rumack BH, et al: Disk battery ingestion: Elevated urine mercury levels and enema removal of battery fragments. *JAMA* 1983; 249:2502–2504.

Oehme F: British anti-lewisite (BAL), the classic heavy metal antidote. *Clin Toxicol* 1972; 5:215–222.

Peterson RG, Rumack BH: D-Penicillamine therapy of acute arsenic poisoning. *J Pediatr* 1977; 91:661–666.

Piomelli S, Rosen JF, Chisolm JJ, et al: Management of childhood lead poisoning. *J Pediatr* 1984; 105:527.

Zepp EA, Thomas JA, Knotts GR: The toxic effects of mercury. *Clin Pediatr* 1974; 13:783–787.

110

Halogens

James J. Walter, M.D., F.A.C.E.P.

Iodine

I. Route of exposure: Oral, inhalation, cutaneous, transdermal, mucous membrane, ocular, intravenous.

II. Common generic and brand names:
   A. Tinctures (alcoholic extract of a drug):
      1. USP tincture (2% I_2 and 2.4% NaI in 50% alcohol).
      2. Strong iodine tincture (7% I_2 and 5% KI in 83% alcohol).
   B. Lugol's solution (5% I_2 and 10% KI in aqueous solution).
   C. Iodophors (complexed with organic carrier): Povidone-iodine (10% solution contains 1% available iodine).
   D. Iodide salts or iodinated glycerol (Organidin) for use as expectorant.
   E. I_2-containing organic compounds used as radiographic contrast agents.

III. Pharmacokinetics:
   A. Absorption: Little free iodine absorbed from GI. Most of element that reaches blood is in iodide form. When used as a topical agent, iodine solution and iodophor are not well absorbed when applied to intact skin, except in neonates and when denuded (e.g., burns).
   B. Onset of action: Immediate onset of local corrosive action.
   C. Elimination: After absorption, free iodine is trapped in thyroid gland to be used in biosynthesis of iodinated thyroid hormone. Iodide not concentrated in thyroid gland is eliminated by renal excretion. When ingested, free iodine is rapidly converted to iodide by food present in stomach and intestine.
   D. Metabolites: Iodide ion is noncorrosive and relatively harmless and plays no role in the toxicity of acute iodine poisoning.

IV. Action:
  A. Used in biosynthesis of iodinated thyroid hormone.
  B. Adult requirement for iodine is 150 μg/day.
V. Uses:
  A. Therapeutic:
    1. Topical antiseptic with low tissue toxicity. Antiseptic effect derives from free iodine present in iodine tinctures, Lugol's solution, iodophors (complex of iodine with carrier), ointment.
    2. Iodide salts and iodinated glycerol used as expectorants.
    3. Iodide salts in combination with antithyroid drugs have a role in preoperative treatment of acute hyperthyroidism, because doses >6 mg/day inhibit thyroid hormone synthesis (Wolff-Chaikoff effect).
    4. Iodide is used to protect thyroid gland after accidental exposure to radioactive isotopes of iodine.
  B. Other: Added to commercial table salt.
VI. Toxic mechanism:
  A. Ingested iodine:
    1. Toxicity related almost entirely to its highly corrosive effect on mucosa of GI tract. Similar to acid corrosives, it acts directly on cells, precipitating protein. Necrosis and ulceration of GI tract result, with intense symptoms of pain and vomiting.
    2. Other organ system toxicity:
      a. Usually secondary to corrosive gastroenteritis and its consequences: massive fluid loss into gut, circulatory collapse, acidosis, aspiration.
      b. Iodine also seems to exert direct systemic effects on organ systems, and absorption of free iodine may play a role in organ system damage seen with acute iodine poisoning:
        (1) Acidosis, CNS deterioration, and death have been reported from povidone-iodine used in mediastinal irrigation.
        (2) Renal failure has been seen with this iodophor used topically for significant burns.
        (3) Intravascular hemolysis.
    3. Iodide salts ingested acutely are noncorrosive and relatively harmless. Iodinated glycerol (Organidin) likewise has not been reported to cause any serious problems.
    4. In general, iodophors are lower in toxicity and less caustic than iodine tinctures and Lugol's solution.
  B. Topical:
    1. Iodine solution and iodophor are not well absorbed when applied to intact skin. However, serious toxicity (acidosis, nephrotoxicity, thyroid suppression) has occurred with application of these agents to neonates, patients with burns greater than 20% of body surface, or when used for prolonged irrigation.
    2. Hypersensitivity: Reaction to topical application can occur, with skin eruption and constitutional symptoms.
  C. Inhalational exposure to iodine vapors can cause irritation to mucous membranes and respiratory symptoms.
  D. Parenteral: Anaphylactoid reactions to intravenous iodine compounds.

E. Chronic intoxication: Prolonged ingestion leads to:
1. Symptom complex known as iodism (see Chronic intoxication below).
2. GI symptoms.
3. Hypothyroidism.

VII. Range of toxicity: Although there is wide variability, mean lethal dose of free iodine for adults is 2–4 gm (1–2 oz of strong tincture).

VIII. Clinical features:
A. Acute intoxication:
1. Gastrointestinal:
   a. Burning abdominal pain and vomiting seen in virtually all cases of significant iodine ingestion.
   b. Diarrhea is common and may be bloody.
   c. Perforation may occur.
   d. Patients may note mouth and esophageal pain, as well as thirst and metallic taste. Brown staining of buccal membranes may be seen.
   e. Blue-colored emesis will be present if there is starch in the stomach, converting iodine to iodide.
2. Neurologic: Headache, dizziness, delirium, stupor, coma.
3. Cardiovascular: Hypotension, tachycardia, shock.
4. Respiratory: Laryngeal edema, aspiration, respiratory distress.
5. Renal: Nephritis with oliguria or anuria is a sequel to shock, intravascular hemolysis, or perhaps the toxic effect of free iodine and may become apparent in 1–3 days.
6. Endocrine: Transient thyroid dysfunction.

B. Hypersensitivity: See Toxic mechanism.

C. Topical:
1. Superficial burns if exposure to strong tincture or solution.
2. If absorbed transdermally, can cause same clinical picture as ingestion.

D. Inhalant: Respiratory irritation and adult respiratory distress syndrome.

E. Chronic intoxication:
1. Toxic syndrome called iodism results from chronic iodide exposure. Severity is dose related (see below).
2. Symptoms: Salivation, metallic taste, coryza, conjunctivitis, headache, laryngitis, bronchitis, stomatitis, parotitis, enlargement of submaxillary glands, lymphadenopathy, anorexia, weight loss, skin rash.

IX. Laboratory findings and evaluation:
A. Serum iodine levels: Not helpful; they give information on levels of iodide and small amounts of protein-bound iodine, which have no role in organ system injury. Pathophysiology of iodine toxicity centers round corrosive gastroenteritis and its attendant complications.

B. Other laboratory tests:
1. Complete blood cell count with immediate spun hematocrit (intravascular hemolysis, GI bleed).
2. Chemistry: electrolytes, renal function (volume depletion) glucose.
3. Arterial blood gases (respiratory symptoms, metabolic acidosis, shock).
4. Lactate level if acidotic.
5. ECG (with cardiovascular findings).
6. Stool Hemoccult test.

7. Upright chest radiograph (look for evidence of perforation, respiratory symptoms).
8. Urinalysis: Protein, casts, red cells, leukocytes.

X. General treatment:
  A. Follow APTLS: See Chapter 8.
  B. General management: Table 110–1 (See Chapters 8–10 for details).
  C. Close monitoring and support of cardiorespiratory status.

XI. Specific treatment:
  A. Gastric decontamination:
    1. Immediate therapy includes administration of milk, flour solution (2 tbsp in 500 ml water) or eggwhite solution to absorb iodine. May give milk every 15 minutes to relieve gastric irritation.
    2. Gastric lavage or emesis not indicated initially if esophageal injury suspected. Lavage should be withheld until esophagus and stomach are examined by endoscopy.
    3. If no esophageal injury, perform gastric lavage with the following:
      a. Solution of starch in water (15 gm corn starch in 500 ml water) to absorb remaining iodine. Lavage should be continued until gastric aspirate is no longer blue.
      b. If available, may give Na thiosulfate 100–200 ml of 1%–5% solution to convert remaining iodine to harmless iodide. Repeat until clear.
      c. If starch or Na thiosulfate not readily available, iodine is readily absorbed by charcoal. Avoid if endoscopy planned.
    4. Administer cathartic if no esophageal or gastric injury.
  B. Volume depletion, hypotension (see also Chapter 10):
    1. Include GI bleed as potential source of volume loss.
  C. Saline diuresis will promote excretion of iodide as chloride competes with iodide for reabsorption by renal tubules.

TABLE 110–1.

General Treatment

Treatment	Indicated	Of No Value	Contraindicated
O₂	±		
IV	+		
ECG monitor	+		
Forced diuresis		X	
Acidification		X	
Alkalinization		X	
Emesis*/lavage*	±/±		
Charcoal*	±		
Cathartic*	±		
Blood typing and screen†	+		

*See Specific treatment below.
†Send to blood bank

 D. Supportive treatment in anticipation of renal failure:
   1. Monitor urinary output, perform frequent urinalysis.
   2. Dialysis if renal failure develops.
 E. Acute corrosive effects: See Chapter 73.
 F. Ocular exposure: See Chapter 28.
 G. Dermal exposure: See Chapter 29.
 H. Toxic inhalant: See Chapter 108.
 I. Hypersensitivity reactions (including anaphylaxis) to iodinated contrast agents: See Chapter 24.
 J. Chronic intoxication:
   1. Discontinue medication.
   2. Treat symptoms.
XII. Prognosis:
 A. Expected response to treatment:
   1. In lethal intoxication, death usually occurs within first 48 hours, from hypovolemic shock, acidosis, pulmonary complications secondary to corrosive gastroenteritis.
   2. Although accidental or intentional ingestion of iodine is not uncommon, fatalities are rare.
   3. No reported fatalities from iodochlorhydroxyquin or iodide poisoning.
 B. Expected complications and long-term effects: Late esophageal and pyloric strictures may occur.
XIII. Disposition considerations:
 A. Admission considerations:
   1. See General Admission Considerations (Chapters 17 and 18).
   2. Evidence of GI injury.
   3. Signs and symptoms suggestive of systemic toxicity (see Clinical features)
   4. Suicide risk.
 B. Consultation considerations:
   1. GI consultation for early endoscopy if GI symptoms present. (Endoscopy may determine safety of gastric decontamination procedures).
   2. Surgical consultation for severe GI bleeding, bowel perforation.
   3. Consider burn unit for serious topical burns.
   4. Ophthalmology for ocular exposure.
   5. Nephrology consultation may be helpful if renal failure develops.
 C. Observation period: Asymptomatic patients with normal exam, no evidence of GI hemorrhage, and who continue to show no systemic toxicity from ingestion after 4–6 hours of observation in the emergency department may be discharged.
 D. Discharge considerations:
   1. General discharge considerations have been met (see Chapters 17 and 18).
   2. Asymptomatic with normal exam after sufficient observation.
   3. Suicide potential and psychiatric status have been appropriately evaluated.

Bromide

I. Route of exposure: Oral, inhalation, cutaneous (with ethylene dibromide, methyl bromide).

II. Common generic and trade names: See Table 110–2.

III. Pharmacokinetics:

    A. Plasma half-life: Approximately 12 days.

    B. Peak effect: In absence of vomiting, peak serum levels of Br^- are seen within 2 hours after ingestion of bromide salts, but may be delayed up to 10 hours after ingestion of organic Br^- compound (e.g., carbromal).

    C. Duration of action: Very long; see Half-life.

IV. Action:

    A. Bromide has a similar distribution pattern to Cl^-. The body attempts to maintain a constant total halide concentration in extracellular fluids by adjustment of renal absorption. Since Br^- is absorbed more quickly in the renal tubule than is Cl^-, it gradually displaces Cl from body fluids and accumulates when ingested chronically. Because of rapid tubular reabsorption, elimination half-life of Br^- is extremely long.

    B. Neurologic effects of Br^- are thought to be related to nerve cells being particularly sensitive to membrane-stabilizing effects of extracellular Br^-.

V. Uses:

    A. In the United States, bromides have been removed from all over-the-counter sedatives-hypnotics since the mid- to late 1970s. Classic bromide-containing products such as Nervine (80% bromide) are no longer avail-

TABLE 110–2.

Bromide-Containing Compounds

Compound	Trade Name	Bromide (%)	Therapeutic Use
Brompheniramine melate	Dimetane Drixoral Others	25	Antihistamine
Bromocriptine	Parlodel		Hormonal disorders, Parkinson's disease
Dexbrompheniramine	Drixoral SA Disophrol Chronotab SA	25	Antihistamine
Dextromethorphan hydrobromide	Cheracol Nyquil Robitussin DM	23	Nonnarcotic antitussive
Acetylcarbromal*	Sedamyl	29	Sedative
Carbromal*	Obral Carbrital	34	Sedative
Quinine hydrobromide*	Bromoquinine	17	Muscle relaxant in cold preparations

*Not available in U.S.

able. Bromo-seltzer (previously 67% bromide) has not contained bromide since the early 1970s.

B. Bromides are still found in numerous nonprescription and prescription cough syrups and cold preparations (see Table 110–2), but in such small quantities as to present no risk for intoxication.

C. The liquid ethylene dibromide and the gaseous methyl bromide used as fumigants and in industry are considerably more toxic than the bromide ion alone.

VI. Toxic mechanism:

A. Toxicity of the Br⁻ ion is dependent on total halide intake. A patient on a high salt diet can tolerate an amount that might produce severe poisoning in a salt-restricted patient.

B. Neural tissue is particularly sensitive to Br⁻, accounting for prominent CNS depression.

C. Direct irritation to GI mucosa.

D. Dangerously narrow margin between therapeutic and toxic blood levels leading to their discontinuation on the market.

E. Chronic ingestion frequently leads to a neurotoxic syndrome called bromism, which at one time accounted for over 2% of admissions to mental hospitals. Bromides have since been replaced by more effective, less toxic agents, as noted above.

F. Ethylene dibromide and methyl bromide are caustic to skin. Severe exposures to these compounds can also produce widespread systemic toxicity and death by mechanisms unrelated to bromide ion.

VII. Range of toxicity:

A. Toxic dose:

1. 1–3 gm sodium bromide causes sedation. Acute ingestions of more than 5 gm can produce GI and CNS toxicity.

2. Toxic bromide levels can readily be reached with therapeutic doses taken daily over a period of weeks.

B. Fatal dose:

1. 20–30 gm bromide as an acute oral dose may be lethal in adults, secondary to CNS depression, GI toxicity, aspiration.

VIII. Clinical features:

A. Acute intoxication:

1. Acute Br⁻ intoxication is rare because large amounts of ingested Br⁻ are irritating to the GI tract and emesis occurs almost immediately, preventing significant absorption.

2. Main features are severe GI symptoms and CNS depression.

3. Ethylene dibromide: CNS, pulmonary, hepatic, and renal dysfunction with intractable acidosis. Systemic toxicity from inhalation, oral ingestion, or skin exposure.

4. Methyl bromide: Primarily CNS, pulmonary toxicity (see Table 108–1).

5. Both ethylene dibromide and methyl bromide can cause serious cutaneous injury.

B. Chronic intoxication: Major toxicity is **bromism,** a chronic, insidious syndrome with neurologic and occasionally dermatologic manifestations.

1. Diagnosis should be considered in patients with:

a. Obscure neuropsychiatric illnesses.

b. Especially if associated with acneiform skin lesions.

c. A decreased or narrow anion gap (Cl^- levels variably elevated).

2. Signs and symptoms:

a. Neuropsychiatric: Confusion, impaired memory, drowsiness, headache, irritability, psychosis, weakness, tremors, incoordination, dysarthria, papilledema, changes in deep tendon reflexes, extensor plantar response. If intake continued, stupor and coma may develop.

b. Gastrointestinal: Anorexia, weight loss, constipation.

c. Dermatologic: Dermatitis in 25% of patients with chronic bromism. Usually an acneiform eruption ("bromide rash").

IX. Laboratory findings and evaluation:

A. Serum bromide level:

1. Elevated level confirms diagnosis.

2. Acute intoxication: levels usually not markedly elevated secondary to vomiting and resultant poor absorption.

3. Chronic intoxication: Usually correlated with Br^- level of at least 150 mg/dl, although toxicity may occur at levels as low as 100 mg/dl. Levels >300 mg/dl may be lethal. Fairly good correlation between Br^- levels and symptoms, although debilitated and elderly patients may show severe signs of toxicity with relatively low serum levels.

4. With chronic inhalation exposure to methyl bromide a bromide level greater than 5 mg/dl signifies toxicity.

B. Other laboratory tests:

1. Electrolytes: Cl^- levels may be falsely elevated (bromide is measured as Cl by technique), especially in relatively acute ingestions. Elevated Cl^- level and **decreased anion gap** are classic findings in Br^- intoxication (see Chapter 48).

2. Arterial blood gases (rule out acid-base disorder, hypoxia).

3. Liver function tests, particularly in ethylene dibromide poisoning (transaminases, bilirubin).

4. Renal function tests (BUN, creatinine), urinalysis.

5. Blood glucose, calcium.

6. Complete blood cell count.

7. Other laboratory studies dictated by clinical findings (e.g., skull films if suspected head trauma, head CT, lumbar puncture).

X. Treatment:

A. Follow APTLS: See Chapter 8.

B. General management: Table 110–3 (see Chapters 8–10 for details).

XI. Specific treatment:

A. Acute intoxication:

1. Sodium chloride administration:

a. If patient awake and alert, may administer 2–3 gm NaCl tablets PO 3–4 times a day with copious amounts of water (at least 4 L/day).

b. Saline diuresis:

(1) Administer normal saline solution or D_5 1/2 NS IV.

(2) Furosemide 1 mg/kg (maximum 40 mg) IV push. Furosemide assures adequate urine output and hastens Br^- excretion.

(3) Goal: Urine output 3–6 ml/kg/hr.

TABLE 110–3.

General Treatment

Treatment	Indicated	Of No Value	Contraindicated
O$_2$	±		
IV	±		
ECG monitor	±		
Forced diuresis‡	+		
Acidification			X
Alkalinization		X	
Emesis/lavage	+/+		
Charcoal*	+		
Cathartic†	±		
Hemodialysis‡	Effective		

*Charcoal not likely to be of use with anions such as inorganic Br⁻ but should be used if there is any question of multiple-drug ingestion, often the case.
†May be used if there are active bowel sounds.
‡See Specific Treatment, below, for indications.

  c. Clinical half-life of Br⁻ decreased to 30–60 hours with oral NaCl and to 24 hours with normal saline plus furosemide.
  d. Continue NaCl administration until Br⁻ level decreased to <100 mg/dl and symptoms begin to clear.
 2. Hemodialysis may be used in severe, life-threatening intoxication when saline diuresis cannot be used. It has reduced the half-life of Br⁻ to 1–2 hours.
 B. Chronic intoxication:
  1. In chronic bromism, administer NaCl or ammonium chloride tablets 2–3 gm PO three or four times a day with copious amounts of water.
  2. Oral NaCl may be required for 1–4 weeks in chronic bromism, since neurologic symptoms are often slow to resolve.
  3. Continue Cl⁻ administration until Br⁻ level decreased to 100 mg/dl and symptoms begin to clear.
 C. Ethylene dibromide and methyl bromide: The most critical intervention is strict decontamination to reduce cutaneous absorption. Otherwise, treatment is supportive. (See Chapter 29 for treatment of skin exposure.)
XII. Prognosis:
 A. Expected response to treatment:
  1. Prognosis excellent if chloride therapy instituted and good supportive care provided.
  2. Time to full recovery may be prolonged, up to six months.
 B. Expected complications and long-term effects:
  1. Hepatic failure in ethylene dibromide poisoning.
  2. Neuropsychiatric dysfunction in chronic bromism.
XIII. Disposition considerations:
 A. Admission considerations:
  1. See General Admission Considerations (Chapters 17 and 18).
  2. Acute ingestions >10 gm suggest potential for serious toxicity or death.
  3. Serum levels >100 mg/dl in chronic ingestion (lower levels in those with underlying health problem or restricted salt intake).

4. Symptomatic.
5. Evidence of impaired renal function.
6. Suicide risk.
B. Consultation considerations:
1. Nephrologist if hemodialysis indicated.
2. Dermatologist for evaluation of severe topical dermal injury or severe dermatitis of chronic bromism.
C. Observation period:
1. Symptomatic patients should be admitted and not observed expectantly in the emergency department.
2. Asymptomatic healthy patients with serum levels <100 mg/dl may be considered for discharge if they continue to show no systemic toxicity after 6–8 hours of emergency department observation. (True for both acute and chronic ingestions.)
D. Discharge considerations:
1. General discharge considerations have been met (see Chapters 17 and 18).
2. Asymptomatic with normal exam.
3. Suicide potential and psychiatric status have been appropriately evaluated.

Fluoride

I. Route of exposure: Oral, ocular, inhalation, transdermal (e.g., hydrofluoric acid burns).
II. Common generic and trade names: See Table 110–4.
III. Pharmacokinetics:
A. Absorption: Fluoride ion readily absorbed from GI tract, lung, skin. When highly soluble compounds such as NaF are ingested, absorption of fluoride in GI tract is rapid and complete. Bioavailability approaches 100%.
B. Peak serum levels: One-half hour.
C. Plasma half-life: 2–9 hours (variable because of differences in extent of skeletal incorporation.
D. Duration of action: Serum fluoride levels after significant ingestion usually return to normal within 24 hours.
E. Elimination: Major route of fluoride excretion is via renal clearance, dependent primarily on urinary flow.
IV. Action:
A. Fluoride forms insoluble salts with calcium, magnesium, and other cations.
B. Fluoride is an avid seeker of calcified tissue (bone, teeth) and immediately begins to incorporate into bone in part as fluorapatite. Percentage of dose deposited in bone is dependent on turnover rate of skeletal components and on previous fluoride exposure. Children with active bone growth or persons unexposed to fluorinated water incorporate up to 75%. An especially marked effect occurs in patients with end-stage renal disease, with fluoride uptake into bone approximately 100%.

TABLE 110–4.

Fluoride-Containing Compounds

Compound	Form	Product Type	Trade Name	Fluoride Concentration (mg/ml)
NaF	Drop	Dietary supplement	Pediaflorluride	0.5
				2.25
	Tablet	Dietary supplement	Poly-Vi-Florluride	0.25–1
			Florvite	
	Rinse	Mouthwash	Phos-Flur	0.2 (0.04% NaF)
			Point-Two Dental Rinse	1(0.2% NaF)
	Paste	Toothpaste	Crest	1.1 (0.24% NaF)
SnF$_2$	Rinse	Mouthwash		0.25 (0.09%) SnF$_2$
(stannous fluoride)				
	Paste	Toothpaste	Aim	1 (0.4% SnF$_2$)
NaFPO$_4$ (MFP)	Rinse	Mouthwash		0.2 (0.15% MFP)
	Paste	Toothpaste	Colgate Aqua Fre	1 (0.76% MFP)

    C. Very slow backdiffusion of fluoride from bone does not cause or add to toxicity.

V. Uses:

    A. Fluoride in drinking water represents largest single amount of daily intake (average 0.5–1.5 mg/day).

    B. Fluoride solution applied directly to newly erupted teeth appears effective in reducing caries.

    C. Combined with calcium, vitamin D, or estrogen, fluoride may have a role in treatment of osteoporosis. When given in pharmacologic doses, fluoride not only becomes incorporated into crystal lattice of hydroxyapatite in bone, but also increases new bone formation.

    D. Inorganic fluoride salts most commonly found in:

        1. Insecticides, rodenticides (NaF).

        2. Dental hygiene products (NaF, SnF$_2$, NaFPO$_4$).

        3. Fluorinated water.

    E. Fluoride also sold as liquid or tablet (NaF) for dietary supplementation (see Table 110–4).

    F. Other common form is hydrogen fluoride, a highly corrosive acid (gaseous or in solution) used in industry (see Chapter 108).

VI. Toxic mechanism:

    A. Toxicity of inorganic fluoride salt depends on its solubility. NaF which readily dissociates is responsible for most acute poisoning. Roach powder and rodenticides may contain 30%–80% NaF.

    B. Although judicious fluoride intake has beneficial effects on developing dental enamel, fluoride is a direct and powerful cellular toxin when taken in acute overdose and causes profound musculoskeletal disease when excessive quantities are ingested chronically. Pathophysiology and clinical presentation of acute and chronic intoxication are distinct.

C. Acute intoxication:
   1. Ingested fluoride ion reacts with gastric acid to produce corrosive hydrogen fluoride.
   2. In acute ingestion, fluoride acts as a cellular poison. It inhibits glycolytic and other enzyme systems and depresses tissue respiration.
   3. Cellular effects lead to a decrease in vasomotor tone, impairment of nerve conduction, direct interference with cardiac contractility. The respiratory center, initially stimulated, may ultimately be depressed or paralyzed in severe intoxication.
   4. Hypocalcemia:
      a. Acute fluoride ingestion can rapidly lower ionized calcium levels by binding available calcium resulting in profound hypocalcemia.
      b. Sharp decline in serum concentration of calcium can be seen within 10 minutes of ingestion.
      c. Normal calcium levels usually reestablished within several hours, but hypocalcemia occasionally persists up to 24 hours.
      d. By binding to calcium and other cations, fluoride interferes with many homeostatic enzyme systems.
   5. It has been assumed that profound hypocalcemia is responsible for arrhythmias and delayed cardiovascular collapse leading to death. More likely, combination of hypocalcemia and hyperkalemia promotes myocardial irritability and is the basis of cardiotoxicity in acute fluoride intoxication.

D. Chronic intoxication ("fluorosis"):
   1. Musculoskeletal and systemic disease can be produced after chronic ingestion of excessive fluoride.
   2. May occur in those consuming water with very high fluoride concentration or in industrial workers with chronic inhalation exposure. Severe symptoms from chronic industrial exposure, termed "crippling fluorosis," probably no longer occur.
   3. Hemodialysis patients have been found to have bone concentrations of fluoride significantly higher than normal. The consequences of this excessive fluoride are unknown, but fluoride perhaps exacerbates osteomalacia and osteosclerosis in some dialysis patients.

VII. Range of toxicity:
   A. Toxic dose (acute toxicity):
      1. Minimum toxic or lethal dose not well established. Wide variation in individual response.
      2. Acute ingestion of 3–5 mg/kg fluoride will usually produce only gastrointestinal symptoms; ingestion of >5 mg/kg risks systemic toxicity (hypotension, weakness, paresthesias, muscular irritability).
      3. Significant toxicity unlikely from household dental hygiene products.
         a. Household dentifrice products not allowed to contain more than 264 mg NaF (120 mg fluoride) per tube or bottle.
         b. Mouthwashes or toothpaste containing NaF or SnF_2 hazardous only

if large volumes are ingested (e.g., 25 kg child would have to ingest 200 ml of a 0.2% NaF rinse or 200 gm toothpaste to risk serious toxicity).

    c. Amount (mg/kg) of fluoride ingested should be calculated in all dentrifice ingestions.

B. Fatal dose (acute toxicity):

    1. Acute ingestion of 30–60 mg/kg fluoride likely to be fatal if untreated.

    2. Single dose of 5–10 gm NaF in adult is lethal without treatment (2.2 mg NaF = 1 mg fluoride).

    3. In small children, as little as 200 mg NaF may be fatal.

C. Chronic toxicity:

    1. Musculoskeletal and systemic symptoms can be produced after many years with intake exceeding 6-10 mg/day fluoride.

    2. Continuous use of water containing >2.5 ppm will result in mottling of dental enamel in 80%.

VIII. Clinical features:

A. Diagnostic complex: History of possible insecticide, rodenticide, dentifrice, dietary supplement ingestion, with predominant GI symptoms, depressed mental state, hyperreflexia, muscular irritability, suggests acute fluoride intoxication.

B. Acute clinical presentation:

    1. Gastrointestinal: Hydrogen fluoride causes hemorrhagic gastroenteritis with vomiting, diarrhea, abdominal pain, dysphagia, salivation, hematemesis.

    2. Cardiovascular: See Toxic mechanism.

    3. Respiratory: Initially shallow rapid respirations, followed by respiratory depression.

    4. Neurologic:

        a. Symptoms secondary to acute hypocalcemia: Headache, weakness, paresthesia, hyperreflexia, muscular irritability, spasms, tetany, rarely seizures.

        b. Depressed level of consciousness suggests absorption of at least 50% lethal dose.

    5. Acute inhalation of HF or F_2 gas:

        a. Intense inflammation of tracheobronchial tree, with coughing and respiratory distress for several hours.

        b. Respiratory symptoms classically return after 1–2 day latent period and persist for 1–4 weeks.

        c. Noncardiogenic pulmonary edema may develop.

        d. See Table 108–1.

    6. Hydrofluoric acid burns:

        a. Special consideration should be given to patient with skin exposure to hydrofluoric acid.

        b. This inorganic acid is used widely in industry and research in solution concentrations as high as 70%.

        c. Skin exposure results in rapid, intensely painful, deep burns.

        d. Inhalation of hydrofluoric acid vapors results in oropharyngeal and lower respiratory tract mucosal ulcerations, with respiratory distress and pulmonary edema occurring within minutes.

      e. Fatal systemic fluorosis from transdermal fluoride absorption has been reported. Fluoride ion can induce systemic hypocalcemia of profound proportions resistant to replacement therapy, myocardial necrosis, chemical pneumonitis and hemorrhagic pulmonary edema.

  C. Chronic clinical presentation:

     1. Fluorosis: Characterized by weight loss, weakness, myalgia, anemia, brittle bones, stiff joints, dental mottling (if ingested during enamel formation).

     2. Bony changes consist of thickening of bony cortex, formation of numerous exostoses, calcification of ligaments and tendons.

     3. Dental fluorosis ranges from discrete hypopigmented areas to dark discoloration and pitting of enamel.

IX. Laboratory findings and evaluation:

  A. Serum and urinary fluoride levels

     1. Little data available correlating fluoride levels with toxic effects in acute ingestion. Level declines rapidly as fluoride deposited in bone.

     2. Lethal levels reportedly >3 mg/L.

     3. In chronic industrial exposure, useful to follow urinary fluoride levels every 6 months. Maintaining urinary fluoride levels <5 mg/dl will avoid development of fluorosis.

  B. Other laboratory tests:

     1. Blood chemistry: Need to carefully follow Ca^{++} (hypocalcemia) and potassium (hyperkalemia) levels for first 24 hours; also check for hypomagnesemia.

     2. Complete blood cell count with immediate spun hematocrit (may see decreased total RBC and WBC, falling Hct with GI bleed).

     3. Arterial blood gases (metabolic [lactic] acidosis, inhalants, respiratory symptoms).

     4. ECG (arrhythmias, hyperkalemia).

     5. Chest radiograph (with toxic inhalants: pneumonitis, noncardiogenic pulmonary edema).

     6. Stool Hemoccult test.

X. General treatment:

  A. Follow APTLS: See Chapter 8.

  B. Prompt recognition is vital because of rapid development of symptoms and need for immediate specific therapy. Because cardiovascular collapse may be caused by irreversible hyperkalemia, and because extent of potassium efflux from cells is directly related to duration of fluoride contact, early removal of fluoride may be life-saving.

  C. General management: Table 110–5 (see Chapters 8–10 for details).

  D. Monitor respiratory status and ECG closely.

  E. Hypotension: See Chapter 10.

XI. Specific treatment:

  A. Ingestions:

     1. Goal is to reduce corrosive action of HF in GI tract, prevent absorption, restore intravascular volume, treat hypocalcemia.

     2. For ingestions <5 mg/kg, only need to give milk to relieve GI symptoms.

TABLE 110–5.

General Treatment: Acute Toxicity

Treatment	Indicated	Of No Value	Contraindicated
O_2*	±		
IV	+		
ECG monitor	+		
Forced diuresis†	+		
Acidification			X
Alkalinization†	+		
Emesis			X
Lavage†	+		
Charcoal		X	
Cathartic			X
Diluent†	+		
Other‡	+		

*Indicated in toxic inhalants.
†See Specific treatment.
‡Blood typing and screen.

3. For ingestions >5 mg/kg:
    a. Administer a solution of 5 ml $CaCl_2$ mixed in 1 L water or milk, orally or via gastric tube to precipitate CaF_2:
        (1) Adults: 200 ml.
        (2) Children: 50–100 ml.
    b. **Antacids** (with aluminum) also effective in binding fluoride.
    c. Remove stomach contents with **gastric lavage.** Although lavage is controversial in acid ingestions, it is recommended here because of potential toxicity of fluoride ion.
    d. After initial lavage has been completed, several ounces lime water or antacid should be given orally at frequent intervals.
    e. Activated charcoal may be tried but is not likely to be of benefit because of small size of dissociated fluoride ion. Use is primarily recommended because of high incidence of multiple-drug ingestions along with fluoride.
    f. In significant ingestion or if symptoms of hypocalcemia develop (e.g., tetany), administer 0.1–0.2 ml/kg (5 ml in children) 10% calcium gluconate IV up to 10 ml over 10–15 minutes with cardiac monitoring. May repeat in 20–30 minutes if symptoms reappear.
    g. IV D_5 0.45 NS with 1 ampule $NaHCO_3$ to induce **alkaline diuresis** (>2 ml/kg/hr) is most effective way of removing absorbed fluoride.
4. Arrhythmias:
    a. If required, antiarrhythmic therapy should be specific for arrhythmia present.
    b. Quinidine may be an effective therapy for combination of hyperkalemia and ventricular arrhythmias, but has only been tested in animal models.

c. If hyperkalemia induced, treat hyperkalemia (see Electrolyte Disturbances).
5. Electrolyte disturbances:
   a. Hyperkalemia: Treat with standard approach (glucose, insulin, HCO_3^-, Ca^{++}).
   b. Hypocalcemia: Administer 10–20 ml (0.5 ml/kg in children) 10% calcium gluconate IV over 10–15 minutes with cardiac monitoring.
   c. Hypomagnesemia:
      (1) 10% magnesium sulfate 1–2 gm IV or 15 minutes. May also be given IM. Children 25–50 mg/kg/dose every 4–6 hours for 3–4 total doses. Infants: 20 mg/kg. Should be given slowly IV followed by 100 mg IM every 12 hours until magnesium level is normal.
      (2) Intravenous route should be reserved for patients requiring immediate control of seizures or tetany.
   d. Treatments may be ineffective until fluoride levels are reduced. In such instances, **cation exchange resins or dialysis** may be only effective means of reversing fluoride-induced hyperkalemia.
6. Renal insufficiency: Hemodialysis with fluoride-free dialysate should be considered in presence of associated renal insufficiency.
B. Inhalation injury: See Chapter 108.
C. Topical exposure to hydrogen fluoride:
   1. See Chapters 29 and 73.
   2. Remove clothing; wash burned areas with copious amounts of water.
   3. Treat in prehospital setting with iced soaks or wet dressing of alcohol or an alcohol solution of quarternary ammonium compound (benzethonium, benzalkonium chloride).
   4. For mild burns, continue step 3. Observe closely for 1–4 hours.
   5. For burns involving a skin surface area >25 sq in, ECG and serum electrolytes including serum calcium should be obtained.
   6. If hypocalcemia exists or is suspected because of prolonged Q-T interval, 10–20 ml 10% calcium gluconate (100–200 mg calcium) may be administered IV over 10–15 minutes and electrolytes closely monitored.
   7. For severe burns inject 10% calcium gluconate solution directly into affected skin areas, with or without local or regional anesthesia. Injections should be performed with a 30-gauge needle, and no more than 0.5 ml calcium gluconate should be injected per square centimeter. Injections should extend 0.5 cm beyond margin of the burn.
   8. After calcium gluconate injections, and with suitable local or regional anesthesia, careful debridement of affected areas should be carried out. Involved nails should be removed.
   9. Severely burned areas should be elevated, magnesium oxide ointment applied (alternatively, A & D ointment may be used), and covered with bulky dressing.
   10. If pain recurs, additional calcium gluconate injections can be given as above. Reconstructive procedures should be planned when appropriate.

XII. Prognosis:
   A. Expected response to treatment:
      1. In lethal ingestion, death usually occurs in 2–4 hours secondary to respiratory paralysis and cardiovascular collapse.
      2. Prognosis good if patient survives more than 24 hours after ingestions and 4 days after inhalation injuries. Time to recovery, however, may be prolonged.
      3. Prognosis for stomach and esophageal burns same as for acids (see Chapter 73).
   B. Expected complications and long-term effects:
      1. See Chronic Clinical Presentation.
      2. Recovery may take more than a year after removal in chronic exposure.
XIII. Special considerations:
   A. Delayed cardiovascular collapse often refractory to conventional therapy. Vasopressors, for example, are often not effective in animal models.
   B. Treatment of fluoride-induced hyperkalemia with glucose, insulin, bicarbonate may be ineffective until fluoride levels are reduced. In such instances cation exchange resins or dialysis may be the only effective means of reversing fluoride-induced hyperkalemia.
XIV. Controversies:
   A. Reports in animal experiments of boron used effectively to bind fluoride at cellular level.
   B. Reports of inducing metabolic alkalosis to enhance renal excretion of fluoride.
   C. Reports of effective removal of fluoride by cation exchange resins, apheresis.
XV. Disposition considerations:
   A. Admission considerations:
      1. See General Admission Considerations (Chapters 17 and 18).
      2. Ingestions >5 mg/kg associated with potential for serious toxicity or death.
      3. All symptomatic patients.
      4. Findings on endoscopy even if asymptomatic.
      5. Even if initial symptoms are relieved by treatment, should probably admit for observation, as with any caustic.
      6. Patients with hydrofluoric acid skin burns should be admitted if they have:
         a. Burns involving skin surface area >25 sq in.
         b. Hypocalcemia (existent or suspected because of prolonged Q-T interval).
      7. Suicide risk.
   B. Consultation considerations:
      1. Endoscopist if signs and symptoms of severe esophageal or stomach injury.
      2. General surgeon for GI bleed, severe GI symptoms, or physical findings.
      3. Nephrologist if hemodialysis indicated.
      4. Burn specialist for severe hydrofluoric acid burns.

C. Observation period: Difficult to make recommendations. Probably not appropriate for any significant fluoride ingestion.
D. Discharge considerations:
   1. General Discharge Considerations have been met (see Chapters 17 and 18).
   2. Asymptomatic throughout course, with normal examination and vital signs.
   3. Suicide potential and psychiatric status have been appropriately evaluated.

BIBLIOGRAPHY

Baer R, Harris H: Types of cutaneous reactions to drugs. *JAMA* 1967; 202:150.

Bayless J, Tinanoff N: Diagnosis and treatment of acute fluoride toxicity. *J Am Dent Assoc* 1985; 110:209.

Berman L, Taves D, Mitra S, et al: Inorganic fluoride poisoning: Treatment by hemodialysis. *N Engl J Med* 1973; 289:922.

Carney M: Five cases of bromism. *Lancet* 1971; 2:523–524.

Chabrolle J, Rossier A: Danger of iodine skin absorption in the neonate. *J Pediatr* 1978; 93:158.

Dela Cruz F, Brown DH, Leiken JB, et al: Iodine absorption after topical absorption. *West J Med* 1987; 146:43–45.

Dominguez RA: Bromide intoxication: A persistent problem. *J Kentucky Med Assoc* Sept 1978; 438.

Elin R, Robertson E, Johnson E: Bromide interferes with determination of chloride by each of four methods. *Clin Chem* 1981; 27:778.

Elsair J, Mead R, Denine R: Boron as a preventive antidote in rabbits: Its action on fluoride and calcium-phosphorus metabolism. *Fluoride* 1980; 13:129–138.

Fried FE, Malek-Ahmedi P: Bromism: Recent perspectives. *South Med J* 1975; 68:220–222.

Glick PL, Gugleilmo J, Tranbaugh RF, et al: Iodine toxicity in a patient treated by continuous povidone-iodine mediastinal irrigation. *Ann Thor Surg* 1985; 39:478–480.

Hine CH: Methyl bromide poisoning: A review of 10 cases. *J Occup Med* 1969; 11:1–10.

Iberti T, Patterson B, Fisher C: Prolonged bromide intoxication resulting from a gastric bezoar. *Arch Intern Med* 1984; 144:402–403.

Letz GA, Pond SM, Osterloh JD, et al: Two fatalities after acute occupational exposure to ethylene dibromide. *JAMA* 1984; 252:2428–2431.

McIvor ME: Delayed fatal hyperkalemia in a patient with acute fluoride intoxication. *Ann Emerg Med* 1987; 16:1165–1167.

McIvor ME, Baltazar RF, Beltran J, et al: Hyperkalemia and cardiac arrest from fluoride exposure during hemodialysis. *Am J Cardiol* 1983; 51:901–902.

McIvor ME, Cummings CC, Mower MM, et al: The manipulation of potassium efflux during fluoride intoxication: Implications for therapy. *Toxicology* 1985; 37:233–239.

McIvor ME, Cummings CE, Mower MM, et al: Sudden cardiac death from acute fluoride intoxication: The role of potassium. *Ann Emerg Med* 1987; 16:777–781.

Maes V, Huygens L, DeKeyser J, et al: Acute and chronic intoxication with carbromal preparations. *J Tox Clin Toxicol* 1985; 23:341.

Mayer TG, Gross PL: Fatal systemic fluorosis due to hydrofluoric acid burns. *Ann Emerg Med* 1985; 2:149–153.

Peitsch J, Meakins JL: Complications of povidone-iodine absorption in topically treated burn patients. *Lancet* 1976; 1:280.

Shewmake SW, Anderson BG: Hydrofluoric acid burns. *Arch Dermatol* 1979; 115:593–596.

Smith G: Toxicity of fluoride containing dental preparations: A review. *Sci Total Environ* 1985; 43:41.

Strubelt O, Iven H, Younes M: The pathophysiological profile of acute cardiovascular toxicity of sodium fluoride. *Toxicology* 1982; 24:313–323.

Tepperman PB: Fatality due to acute systemic fluoride poisoning following a hydrofluoric acid skin burn. *J Occupat Med* 1980; 22:691–692.

Thornton E: Sleep aids and sedatives. *JACEP* 1977; 6:408.

Trump DL, Hochberg MC: Bromide intoxication. *Johns Hopkins Med J* 1976; 138:119–123.

White JW: Hydrofluoric acid burns. *Cutis* 1984; 34:241–244.

Yolken R, Konecny P, McCarthy P: Acute fluoride poisoning. *Pediatrics* 1976; 58:90–93.

111

Hazardous Chemicals in Industry and Environment

Paula A. Ryals, M.D., F.A.C.E.P.

Hazardous materials (those constituting a threat to people, animals, plants, or the environment) are nearly ubiquitous in the industrial setting. Often the diagnosis of occupational poisoning requires a careful history and a high index of suspicion. Hazardous material emergencies usually involve unknown substances or unknown concentrations of chemicals that have been identified as highly dangerous.

Many hazardous materials may not be toxic per se but may present the danger of fire or explosion if not carefully handled. Some compounds, such as polyurethane, are nontoxic unless burned, when cyanide gas may be released. If the composition of building materials is not known, victims overcome by smoke should be treated for carbon monoxide poisoning and possible toxic gas inhalation.

I. Risk groups:
   A. Workers: Especially in industrial and transportation sectors.
   B. Law enforcement personnel: On scene first, especially road accidents involving hazardous material spills.
   C. Firefighters: Hazardous materials involved in about 20% of their calls.
   D. Public: Widespread ignorance of risks; may require evacuation.
   E. The media: Anxious to cover rapidly breaking news stories, may unconsciously or purposefully disregard safety lines.
   F. Emergency medical technicians: Tend to focus on search, rescue, and medical needs of individual patients without regard to potentially dangerous environmental conditions around accident site.
   G. Hospital personnel: Few have significant experience with hazardous material management.

II. Route of exposure:
   A. Oral, dermal, transdermal, mucous membrane.
   B. Burns (fire or caustics).
   C. Radiation.
III. Common types of hazardous chemicals:
   Solvents (hydrocarbons)
   Heavy metals
   Carbon monoxide
   Cyanide
   Caustics, corrosives
   Formaldehyde
IV. Types of injuries caused by hazardous materials:
   A. Thermal, including electrical and other burns.
   B. Radiation-related injuries; important factors are type of radiation, distance of patient to source, time of exposure, degree of shielding.
   C. Asphyxiation: Toxic gases can displace oxygen in the environment causing asphyxiation as well as airway or pulmonary irritation.
   D. Chemical, especially pesticides and organophosphates.
   E. Biological agents: Acquired immune deficiency syndrome (AIDS) virus, hepatitis, other infectious diseases.
V. Clinical features:
   A. Emergency medical personnel should note and record any smell reported by patients or rescuers. Color of liquids, powders, gases may be important information. In unknown exposure, examiner should search for diagnostic or suggestive signs during physical examination. The two most common routes of injury from hazardous chemicals are skin contact and inhalation. If the injury is from smoke inhalation, knowledge of what was burning may aid in the diagnosis. Burning plastics may release hydrogen halides. Incomplete combustion produces carbon monoxide. Phosgene is released from the burning of carbon tetrachloride, trichloroethylene, and other halogenated hydrocarbons.
   B. Very few specific physical findings are unique to toxic exposure. Common signs and symptoms encountered in industrial poisonings include:
      1. Respiratory symptoms: Choking or burning in chest, bronchospasm, rhinorrhea, rales, dyspnea, wheezing.
      2. GI syndromes: Nausea, vomiting, diarrhea, hepatic dysfunction.
      3. Renal dysfunction.
      4. Central and peripheral nervous system syndromes: Headache, lassitude, tremor, peripheral neuropathy. Chronic exposure to toxins can increase incidence of malignancy.
   C. Gaseous exposure: See Chapter 108.
   D. Dermal exposure: See Chapter 29.
   E. Ocular exposure: See Chapter 28.
   F. Radiation: See Chapter 112.
   G. Explosion:
      1. Any of the above.
      2. Burns.
      3. Major or minor trauma.

VI. Laboratory findings and evaluation:
    A. Arterial blood gases, including carboxyhemoglobin
    B. Complete blood cell count.
    C. Electrolytes, including calcium.
    D. BUN, creatinine.
    E. Blood glucose.
    F. Urinalysis.
    G. Blood and urine toxicology screen.
    H. Further studies such as methemoglobin, RBC pseudocholinesterase, chest radiograph, ECG may be indicated.
    I. Gaseous exposure: See Chapter 108.
    J. Dermal exposure: See Chapter 29.
    K. Radiation: See Chapter 112.
VII. General management:
    A. On-site treatment:
       1. Identification of material:
          a. Assess fire, explosion, radiation potential as early as possible. Such hazard assessment is imperative before attempting to rescue and triage casualties.
          b. May be difficult in some circumstances (e.g., fire at a chemical plant with multiple substances).
          c. In the event of a hazardous material accident, information resources to be consulted should be identified beforehand. (e.g., hospitals, toxicologists, poison information center; see Table 111–1).
          d. Safe perimeters for containment, decontamination, triage, and treatment must be established at outset, with all approaches and movement occurring upwind from chemical spill. Except for basic resuscitative measures (opening airways, CPR and dressings for hemorrhage), all medical care should take place outside contaminated area.
       2. Personal safety precautions:
          a. Self-contained breathing devices or filter masks should be available when toxic gases or particulates are encountered.
          b. Impermeable protective clothing (e.g., suits, gloves, boots, helmets) should be used in handling certain very toxic materials.
          c. Showers, eye irrigation.
       3. Field stabilization:
          a. Must take place outside of the contaminated zone.
          b. See APTLS (Chapter 8).
          c. Protect cervical spine if trauma has occurred.
          d. May be dangerous to use open Ambu-Bag system to assist ventilations because more toxic fumes may be bagged into the victim's lungs. Do not withhold if patient is apneic or has agonal respirations and no other assisted ventilation is available.
          e. Remove all clothing and copiously wash all exposed areas with water or other decontamination solutions if available. Rare exceptions to this rule are exposure to agents that react violently with water (e.g., chemical may ignite, explode, or produce toxic fumes with

TABLE 111–1.

Agencies Potentially Involved in Hazardous
Materials Emergencies*

Environmental Protection Agency
Military National Guard
Natural Resources
Fire Department
Police Department
Fish and Game Commission
Highways/Transportation Department
Flood Control
Harbor Commission/Port Authority
Public Health Department
Rescue Squad
Civil Defense
Conservation
Forestry
Water Resources
Public Safety
Public Works
Federal Emergency Management Agency
Referral Hospital Regional (EMS) Poison Center
Centers for Disease Control

*From Haddad LM, Winchester JF: *Clinical Management of Poisoning and Drug Overdose.* Philadelphia, WB Saunders Co, 1983. p 251. Used by permission.

water), such as chlorosulfonic acid, titanium tetrachloride, calcium oxide, or agents insoluble in water, such as phosphorus.

   f. It is important that adequate communication between incident site and medical control site (usually a hospital) be maintained and that receiving health care facility be adequately forewarned that they will be receiving chemically contaminated patients. Important information to convey includes: number of victims, chemical agent(s) involved, circumstances underlying exposure, extent of exposure, therapeutic measures rendered at the scene and en route to hospital.

B. Hospital treatment:

   1. Ideally, patients should be brought initially to a special, predesignated decontamination suite containing:

     a. Shower with container to hold drainage water.

     b. Separate outside entrance and exit into emergency department.

   2. Rescuers and victims should remove all clothing, which should be bagged and discarded safely.

   3. Hospital personnel should have gowns, gloves, masks, and occasionally self-contained breathing devices.

4. After rescuers and victims are thoroughly rinsed, they may leave decontamination suite and enter emergency department for definitive care. Hospital personnel leave gowns, gloves, etc., in contaminated area. Remember to irrigate eyes and skin if contaminated and give 100% O_2 for inhalation exposure.

C. **Do not forget assessment of suicide potential, either as cause of accident or guilt secondary to causing it.**

D. Consider other drug ingestions concurrent with industrial or environmental exposure. Accidents may occur because other drugs have been ingested.

VIII. Specific management: See specific chapters.

TABLE 111–2.

Sources of Information Concerning Emergency Response*

Bombing investigations (FBI) and terrorist bombing	(202) 324-4664
Bureau of Explosives	(202) 835-9500
Centers for Disease Control	(404) 452-4100
Chemical Transportation Emergency (CHEMTREC)	(800) 424-9300 (continental USA) (202) 483-7616 (outside continental USA)
Department of Energy (DOE) Information Hotline (Nuclear)	(301) 353-5555†
Destruction of explosives and destructive devices	(800) 424-9555†
National Response Center (U.S. Coast Guard) (Environmental Protection Agency)	(800) 424-8802†
Pesticide Lab (Environmental Protection Agency)	(800) 531-7790
Pesticide Incident Monitoring System	(800) 292-7664 (Texas)
Pesticide Safety Team Network (PSTN): Call CHEMTREC	(800) 424-9300†
ACFX Rail Car	(314) 724-7850
GATX Rail Car	(312) 621-6200
NATX Rail Car	(312) 648-4000
UTLX Rail Car	(312) 431-3111
US Coast Guard, Pollution Response Branch	(800) 424-8802*

*From Haddad LM, Winchester JF: *Clinical management of poisoning and drug overdose.* Philadelphia, WB Saunders Co, 1983, p 252. Used by permission.

†**EMERGENCY NUMBERS, FOR EMERGENCY USE ONLY!**

IX. Prognosis: See specific chapters.
X. Special considerations:
   A. Many hazardous materials may not be toxic per se but may present danger of fire or explosion if not carefully handled.
   B. Polyurethane is a compound that is nontoxic unless burned, in which case cyanide gas may be released.
   C. If composition of building materials is not known and victims are overcome by smoke, treat for carbon monoxide poisoning and possible toxic gas inhalation.
   D. **Transportation accidents** involving vehicles carrying hazardous materials require special care and expertise:
      1. If scene involves derailed train cars, wrecked and burning trucks, fire, explosions in factories, it is easy to concentrate so intently on the hazardous materials that other hazards presented by these situations are overlooked.
      2. Rescuers, fire or police personnel may be overcome by toxic fumes as they rush to the site without adequate protective clothing.
      3. Important to identify the content before approaching:
         a. Read diamond-shaped placard on side of truck or railroad car. Use binoculars to read sign prior to approach.
         b. Note characteristics of chemical spill: color, odor, consistency.
         c. If it is safe to do so, obtain shipping papers from cab of truck or from train personnel (Table 111–2).
XI. Sources of information concerning emergency response:
   A. Poison Control Center.
   B. Health hazard information usually readily available from company supervisors or medical departments. National Institute of Occupational Safety

TABLE 111–3.

Teams Capable of Emergency Response to Chemical Spills*

Centers for Disease Control (CDC).	(404) 452-4100
CHLOREP (Chlorine Emergency Plan), with access through CHEMTREC	
Coast Guard National Strike Force, with access through National Response Center	(800) 424-8801
Dow Chemical Company	(517) 636-4400
DuPont Company	(302) 774-7500
Environmental Response Team, available through Environmental Protection Agency	(215) 597-9898
National Agricultural Chemical Association Pesticide Safety Team Network, with access through CHEMTREC	
National Response Center (U.S. Coast Guard)	(800) 424-8802
U.S. Army Technical Escort Center Chemical Emergency Response Team, Department of the Army Operations Center	(703) 521-2185

*From Haddad LM, Winchester JF: *Clinical management of poisoning and drug overdose.* Philadelphia, WB Saunders, 1983, p. 253. Used by permission.

and Health (NIOSH) sets exposure limits for all hazardous materials and mandates appropriate protective gear and monitoring systems.

C. Excellent reference is *Guidebook for Hazardous Materials Incidents: Emergency Response Guidebook,* Department of Transportation Publication 5800.3, Washington, DC, 1984. Available from US DOT Materials Transportation Bureau. Attn: DMT-11, Washington, DC 20036.

D. Obtain specific information concerning handling spills of hazardous materials from emergency numbers noted in Table 111–2.

E. Resources available in planning for hazardous materials emergencies:
   1. Planning Guide and Checklist for Hazardous Materials, Federal Emergency Management Agency, Washington, DC.
   2. U.S. Coast Guard Chemical Hazard Response Information System. Available through National Response Center, (800) 422-8802.
   3. NIOSH/OSHA Pocket Guide to Chemical Hazards, U.S. Government Printing Office, Washington, DC 20402.

F. Often, special expertise is needed to control hazardous material leak and to arrange long-term monitoring of environment (see Table 111–3).

G. See Tables 111 1 and 111–2.

BIBLIOGRAPHY

Burton BT, Bayer MJ: Hazardous materials. *Top Emerg Med* 1985; 7:1–70.

Leonard RB: Community planning for hazardous materials. *Top Emerg Med* 1986; 7:55–64.

MMWR 1983; 32(suppl 1).

National Response Team: *Hazardous Materials Emergency Planning Guide.* Washington, DC, March 1987.

Stutz DR, Ricks RC, Olsen MF: *Hazardous Materials Injuries: A Handbook for Pre-hospital Care.* Greenbelt, Md, Bradford Communications Corp, 1982.

US Congress, Office of Technology Assessment: *Transportation of Hazardous Materials,* OTA-SET-304. Washington, DC, US Government Printing Office, July 1986.

112

Radiation

Harlan A. Stueven, M.D., F.A.C.E.P.
David Roberts, M.D., F.A.C.E.P., A.B.M.T.

I. Route of exposure:
   A. Contamination:
      1. Radioactive material becomes physically attached to skin or clothes.
      2. Contaminated patient is potential health threat to medical personnel and other patients, yet risk of actual morbidity and mortality is minimal.
   B. Incorporation: Radioactive material is inhaled, ingested, or contaminates open wound.
   C. Irradiation:
      1. Patient has been exposed to flux of radioactive particles.
      2. **Such patients do not become "radioactive" and pose no danger** to staff unless also physically contaminated by radioactive materials.
II. Radiation physics:
   A. Radioactive refers to loss of either particles (alpha or beta) or energy (gamma rays) from spontaneously decaying unstable atoms.
   B. Alpha particles are heavy particles with range of a few centimeters in air and cannot penetrate skin. Thus alpha-emitting contamination is not a hazard to open wounds or when inhaled or ingested.
   C. Beta particles are similar to electrons, with a range of several meters in air and a few millimeters in tissue, and pose a biological threat both internally and externally.
   D. Gamma rays and X rays are electromagnetic energy with a range of many meters in air and many centimeters in tissue, and like beta particles constitute a biological threat both internally and externally.
III. Action: Radiation produces intracellular ionization.

IV. Uses: Nuclear power, isotope production, chemistry laboratories, medical (e.g., radiation therapy for cancer).
V. Toxic mechanism: Toxic effects of radiation are a result of intracellular ionization and formation of free radicals. These free radicals cause breaks in DNA and RNA strands, leading to cellular and chromosomal changes. Such changes may be passed on to progeny or result in cell death or inability to replicate. Tissues most affected are brain, GI tract, bone marrow.
VI. Radiation dose effects: See Table 112–1.
VII. Laboratory findings and evaluation:
   A. Baseline complete blood cell count:
      1. Absolute lymphocyte count obtained 48 hours after exposure is important predictor of prognosis:
         a. >1,500: Prognosis good.
         b. 500–1,500: Prognosis fair.
         c. <500: Prognosis poor.
   B. Baseline electrolytes: May be significant vomiting, leading to fluid/electrolyte imbalance.
   C. Beta human chorionic gonadotropin. May be helpful to identify pregnant women for counseling.
   D. Assays of blood and urine for measurement of radioactivity in cases of internal contamination.
VIII. Treatment:
   A. Determine if patient contaminated, using Geiger-Mueller instrument with special window.
   B. Monitor patient for radioactivity, preferably in ambulance. If radioactive, notify receiving emergency facility to allow them to prepare for patient.
   C. Emergency department treatment:
      1. Cordon off route of patient into department.
      2. Prepare examination room: Remove extraneous equipment and supplies; close ventilation and plumbing system unless self-contained.
      3. All health care personnel should don surgical dress and use sterile technique.
      4. Remove patient's clothes in ambulance and place in sealed plastic bag.
      5. Thorough patient decontamination:
         a. Wash patient with soap and water.
         b. Catch effluent in containers; do not use abrasives for cleansing; continue until nares, ear canals, mouth, all body parts are no longer radioactive.
   D. Treatment for ingested radioactive material:
      1. Gastric lavage should be performed, with gastric contents measured for radioactivity and sent for toxicologic screening.
      2. Chelation therapy may be considered for ingested isotopes:
         a. Radioactive iodine in GI tract may be blocked by 2–3 drops potassium iodide in water.
         b. Radioactive strontium may be precipitated in gut by aluminum phosphate gel.
         c. Radium may be precipitated by barium sulfate.
   E. Inhalation of radioactive material: Treat as though irradiated.

TABLE 112–1.
Acute Radiation Syndrome*

Dose Range (rem)	Syndrome Type	Symptoms	Lymphocytes (Day 2)	Platelets (Day 30)	Treatment	Prognosis
0–25	None	None	Normal	Normal	None	
25–100	None	Mild prodromal	Normal or slightly depressed relative to baseline	Normal or slightly depressed relative to baseline	None necessary	
100–200	Hematopoetic (mild)	Prodromal nausea, vomiting	50% reduction	25%–50% reduction	Symptomatic	Recovery expected
200–400	Hematopoetic (moderate)	Prodromal latent period; definite hematologic derangement; some nausea, vomiting	75% reduction	50%–75% reduction	Supportive; antibiotics; blood products	Some mortality; most recover
400–600	Hematopoetic (severe); some GI	Marked prodromal; latent period; marked hematologic derangement; nausea, vomiting, diarrhea; prostration; bleeding; infection	90% reduction	90% reduction	Supportive; fluids; antibiotics; blood products; marrow transplants; stem cell transfusion	50% or more mortality

| 600–1,000 | GI | Marked prodromal; shortened latent period; marked nausea, vomiting, diarrhea; prostration; coma; death; hematologic derangement depends on survival time | Essentially absent | Essentially absent | All of above or expectant | Mortality increases to 100% above 900 rems; mean survival 1 mo |
| 5,000 | CNS | N/A | N/A | N/A | N/A | Death within 2 days, usually hours |

*From Milroy WC: Management of irradiated and contaminated casualty victims. *Emerg Med Clin North Am.* 1984; 2:667–686.

F. Treatment for radioactive material incorporated into open wounds:
   1. Thorough irrigation and cleansing.
   2. Consider surgical debridement, saving all tissue in appropriate containers.
G. Transfusions, bone marrow transplants, aggressive management of infections indicated.

IX. Prognosis:
   A. Expected response to treatment: See Table 112–1.
   B. Expected complications and long-term effects: Potential long-term effects from whole body irradiation include leukemia; thyroid, breast, lung cancer.

X. Disposition considerations:
   A. Admission considerations:
      1. See General Admission Considerations (Chapters 17 and 18).
      2. Patients with intermediate exposure should be admitted and placed in protective isolation; have fluid and electrolyte imbalances corrected; and have peripheral blood counts and bone marrow aspirations performed regularly.
      3. If absolute lymphocyte count <1,200 or less than 50% of baseline at 48 hours, patient should be admitted with reverse isolation precautions.
      4. Suicide risk.
   B. Consultation considerations:
      1. Hematologist for all admitted patients; patients discharged should be referred to an internist for follow-up complete blood cell count in 48 hours.
      2. Radiation safety officer or health physicist must be a member of decontamination team.
      3. Appropriate governmental authorities should be notified, including state agencies, Department of Energy Regional Coordinating Office for Radiological Assistance.
      4. Major source of information and advice on management of radiation accidents available 24 hours per day from Radiation Emergency Assistance Center/Training Site (REAC/TS), Oak Ridge Associated Universities, Oak Ridge, TN; (615) 576-3131.
   C. Discharge considerations:
      1. General disposition considerations have been met (see Chapters 17 and 18).
      2. Asymptomatic patients may be discharged only if the following criteria have been satisfied.
         a. WBC and platelet counts are normal.
         b. Proper decontamination protocols have been followed.
         c. Arrangements for follow-up CBC in 48 hours have been made.
      3. Suicide potential and psychiatric status have been appropriately evaluated.
   D. Transfer issues:
      1. Indications for transfer to a specialized radation treatment center:
         a. High-dose total body or local radiation >100 rem.

b. Residual radioactive contamination of wounds.
c. Significant internal contamination.
d. Presence of illness that complicates care of irradiated patient.

BIBLIOGRAPHY

Leonard RB, Rick RC: Emergency department radiation accident protocol. *Ann Emerg Med* 9:462–470.

Milroy WC: Management of irradiated and contaminated casualty victims. *Emerg Med Clin North Am* 1984; 2:667–686.

Richter LL, Berk HW, Teates CD, et al: A systems approach to the management of radiation accidents. *Ann Emerg Med* 1980; 9:303–309.

Saenger EL: Radiation accidents. *Ann Emerg Med* 1986; 15:1061–1066.

113

Venoms

Edward J. Otten, M.D.

I. Sources of exposure: See Table 113–1.

Snake Venoms

Most venomous snake bites are from snakes of the family Crotalidae, the pit vipers. Coral snakes (family Elapidae) are responsible for the majority of the remainder of snake bites. These distinctions are important because different antisera are available for treatment. Over 95% of snake bites are attributable to pit vipers, and discussion focus is primarily on these.

   I. Snake identification: See Figure 113–1.

  II. Range of toxicity:

     A. Toxic and fatal doses depend on:

        1. Potency of venom.

        2. Amount of venom injected.

        3. Size and health of person bitten.

        4. NOTE: **Dead snakes may still pose a hazard because exposure to fangs may result in envenomation.**

     B. Onset of symptoms is variable, depending on species of snake. Most signs or symptoms appear within 4 hours.

 III. Clinical features:

     A. Minimal: Local edema, ecchymosis, pain. Few if any systemic symptoms or signs. Minimal if any laboratory abnormalities.

     B. Moderate: Severe pain, swelling beyond area of bite, some systemic symptoms and signs (nausea, vomiting, diaphoresis, orthostatic hypotension), abnormal laboratory values.

TABLE 113–1.

Sources of Venom Exposure

Common Name	Scientific Name	Location	Mechanism of Envenomation	Toxin	Symptoms and Signs	Management
Rattlesnakes	Crotalus sp (32 species)	US (except Maine, Alaska, Hawaii) Mexico, South America	Bite	Enzymes, polypeptides, crotoxin, other	Pain, edema, erythema, numbness, tingling around mouth, shock, renal failure, coagulation abnormal	Crotalid polyvalent antivenin,* supportive care, local wound care
Water moccasin	Agkistrodon sp	Southeast US	Bite	Enzymes, polypeptides	Same as rattlesnake	Same as rattlesnake
Copperhead	Agkistrodon sp	South Central and Eastern US	Bite	Enzymes, polypeptides		
Massasauga	Sistrurus sp	Midwest US	Bite	Enzymes, polypeptides	Pain, edema, nausea	Same as rattlesnake
Pigmy rattlesnake	Sistrurus sp	Southeast US	Bite	Enzymes, polypeptides		
Coral snake	Micrurus sp	Southeast US, Texas	Bite	Neurotoxin	Lethargy, paralysis, weakness, diplopia	Coral snake antivenin,* respiratory support
Sonoran coral snake	Micruroides sp	Arizona	Bite	Neurotoxin	Headache, weakness	Supportive as indicated; no antivenin available
Gila monster, beaded lizard	Helodema sp	Arizona, Mexico	Bite	Multiple enzymes	Pain, edema, weakness	Supportive; no antivenin
Sea snake	Hydrophid sp, Enhydrina sp	Coastal Southern California, Mexico, Pacific and Indian Oceans	Bite	Neurotoxin, myotoxin	Weakness, ptosis, trismus, muscle spasms, myoglobinuria	Sea snake antivenin*

(Continued.)

TABLE 113–1 (cont.).

Common Name	Scientific Name	Location	Mechanism of Envenomation	Toxin	Symptoms and Signs	Management
Exotic snakes (imported into US)	Elapids, viperids, crotalids, others	South America, Asia, Africa, Australia	Bite	Enzymes, neurotoxins, other	Variable	Supportive as indicated; call Antivenin Index (1-602-626-6016) for location of nearest antivenin*
Black widow spider	Latrodectus sp	US except Alaska	Bite	Neurotoxin	Muscle spasms, pain, headache, hypertension, paresthesias, shortness of breath	Calcium gluconate 10% IV, diazepam for muscle relaxation, antivenin* available but should be given rarely, ice packs
Brown recluse spider	Loxosceles sp	Southern US, South America	Bite	Enzymes, sphingomyelinase, other	Necrotic skin lesion, rash, disseminating intravascular coagulation, renal failure	Dapsone 50 mg bid for skin lesion, antivenin under development, supportive measures
Imported spiders	Phoneutria sp Atrax sp, others	South America, Australia	Bite	Enzymes, neurotoxins	Variable	Antivenin available for Australian funnel web spider; otherwise, supportive care
Arizona bark scorpion	Centruroides sculpturatus	Arizona	Sting	Neurotoxin	Pain, salivation, nausea, vomiting, sweating, respiratory arrest	Antivenin* available, call Antivenin Index (1-602-626-6016); supportive measures

Common name	Genus/species	Location	Mechanism	Toxin	Symptoms	Treatment
Bees, wasps, hornets	Apidae, vespidae, bombidae, sphecidae	US	Sting	Melitin, lipids, polypeptides, enzymes, kinins, histamines, other	Pain, erythema, edema, anaphylaxis, respiratory arrest, urticaria	Remove stinger, local ice, epinephrine, antihistamines, steroids, dopamine for severe reactions, supportive measures
Fire ants, army ants	Solenopsis sp, others	Southern US, Central and South America, Mexico	Sting	Alkaloids	Burning pain, itching, erythema, edema, allergic reaction, anaphylaxis	Local cold packs, epinephrine, antihistamines, supportive care
Ticks	Dermacentor sp	US, Canada	Bite	Neurotoxir	Ascending paralysis	Remove tick, supportive care
Caterpillars	Lepidoptera sp	Worldwide	Urticating hairs	Enzymes, polypeptides	Pain, erythema, allergic reactions	Local care, steroid cream, analgesics, supportive care
Blister beetles, conenose bugs, wheel bugs, assassin bugs, centipedes	Coleoptera sp, Hemiptera sp, Scolopendra sp	Worldwide	Spray, sting, bite	Cantharide, serotonin, many others	Pain, burning, erythema, pruritus, vesicles, allergic reactions	Local wound care, analgesics
Platypus	Ornithorhyncus sp	Australia	Sting	Proteins	Pain, edema	Supportive care
Shrew marine animals	Blarina sp Fishes (see Chapter 114)	Eastern US	Bite	Proteins	Pain, edema	Supportive care

*Antivenin is horse serum derivative, and **all patients must be tested for horse serum sensitivity before administering.** All antivenin should be given intravenously. Amounts based on severity of bite and response of patient. Expert assistance should be obtained if unfamiliar with use of antivenin.

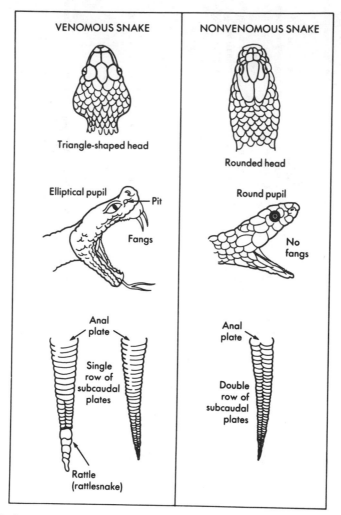

FIG 113–1.
Identification of venomous and nonvenomous snakes. (From Rosen P, et al: *Emergency Medicine: Concepts and Clinical Practice.* St Louis, CV Mosby Co, 1988, p 983. Used by permission.)

    C. Severe:
       1. Marked local and systemic symptoms and signs: weakness, bradycardia or tachycardia, shock, severe coagulopathy, renal glomerulitis, pulmonary vascular congestion, massive edema.
       2. Neurotoxic symptoms: Dizziness, numbness, tingling, visual disturbances, seizures, fasciculation. More common with *Elapid* [coral snake] bites.

3. Significant abnormalities in laboratory values (see Laboratory findings and evaluation).

IV. Laboratory findings and evaluation:
   A. Blood tests:
      1. Complete blood cell count, electrolytes, BUN, creatinine.
      2. Coagulation studies: PT, PTT, platelets, fibrinogen, fibrin degradation products.
      3. Creatine phosphokinase (rhabdomyolysis).
      4. Arterial blood gases.
      5. Type and cross match.
   B. ECG.
   C. Urinalysis (e.g., myoglobinuria).
V. General treatment:
   A. Follow APTLS: See Chapter 8.
   B. General management: See Table 113–2.
   C. Tetanus prophylaxis.
VI. Specific treatment: See Table 113–1.
   A. Patient bitten by a pit viper who is more than 1 hour from a medical facility may have a constricting band, **not a tourniquet,** applied to an extremity proximal to the bite, with splinting. Band should be at least 1 inch wide and loose enough to admit a finger underneath; should not compromise blood flow.
   B. Wound should be cleaned, irrigated with sterile saline solution, appropriate tetanus immunization given. Antibiotic should be started, preferably one effective against *Staphylococcus* (e.g., Augmentin).
   C. Ice or cryotherapy contraindicated.
   D. Steroids are of no value for acute snake bite.
   E. Fasciotomy should not be done unless compartment pressures are elevated, as for any traumatic injury.
   F. Indications for antivenom:
      1. For pit viper bite, number of vials of antivenin (Wyeth) required depends on grade of envenomation:

No envenomation (dry bite)	No antivenin
Mild envenomation (local edema and pain only)	None to 5 vials
Moderate envenomation (pain, edema beyond site, other systemic manifestations such as nausea, vomiting, orthostatic hypotension)	Up to 20 vials
Severe envenomation (shock, severe coagulopathy, massive edema)	20 or more vials

      2. All patients should be tested for equine serum sensitivity prior to initiation of antivenin therapy. Patients with history of previous exposure or allergy to horse serum should receive antivenom only if in danger of losing life or limb. If this dangerous procedure is undertaken, diluted aliquots of antivenin can be administered by slow IV drip. This should be undertaken only in the intensive care setting. Although po-

TABLE 113–2.

General Treatment

Treatment	Indicated	Of No Value	Contraindicated
O$_2$	±		
IV	+		
ECG monitor	+		
Forced diuresis		X	
Acidification			X
Alkalinization			X
Emesis/lavage		X/X	
Charcoal		X	
Cathartic		X	
Dialysis*	+		

*If renal failure present.

tentially dangerous, some authors recommend epinephrine infusion in such cases.

    G. Shock: See Chapter 10 for treatment recommendations.

VII. Prognosis:

    A. Usually excellent for patients with envenomation despite significant soft tissue injury (edema, pain, hemorrhagic blebs).

    B. Patients with systemic effects (hypotension, renal failure, decreased level of consciousness, pulmonary edema) should recover with appropriate supportive care.

    C. Adequate, early, specific antiserum treatment (if indicated) will reduce mortality from all snake bites below 10%.

VIII. Special considerations:

    A. Injudicious use of incision, suction, ice, tourniquets in the field has resulted in severe complications (e.g., lacerated tendons, nerves, arteries, wound contaminated by saliva, ischemic injury). Tissue necrosis may result from overaggressive use of ice.

    B. Treatment of snake bites remains controversial. Use of and indications for antivenin, steroids, surgical procedures are source of great disagreement.

    C. Immunologic tests for detection of snake venom and venom antibodies such as enzyme-linked immunoassay (ELISA) and radioimmunoassay (RIA) should be obtained if possible. Wound aspirate, serum, urine can be used for venom detection. Unfortunately, more work is necessary to improve specificity of these tests and to shorten running times. Nonspecificity and cross-reactivity of snake venoms is also a problem with these tests.

IX. Disposition considerations:

    A. Admission considerations:

        1. See General Admission Considerations (Chapters 17 and 18).

        2. Any person bitten by a pit viper (with moderate to severe envenomation) or any other venomous snake should be admitted for at least 24 hours.

3. Any person receiving antivenin should be admitted and monitored. Antivenin is best administered in ICU.
B. Consultation considerations:
   1. Local zoologist or herpetologist for aid in snake identification.
   2. Local zoo, university department of biology.
   3. National index is maintained by the Arizona Poison Control Center, (602) 626-6016, for locating type-specific antivenins to use in exotic venomous snake bites.
   4. International *Antivenin Index* lists medical consultants and internationally available antivenins.
   5. Surgical consultation if bite wound excision is indicated or if patient develops compartment syndrome from severe edema.
C. Observation period:
   1. Any person with snake bite should be observed in the emergency department for a minimum of 4 hours.
      a. Pit viper envenomation suspected: If any sign of envenomation occurs during observation, bite should be graded and treated appropriately.
      b. Non–pit viper symptoms (particularly neurologic): Supportive care indicated until snake can be physically identified or perhaps ELISA performed, if available.
   2. Patients with minimal envenomation can often be discharged after 24 hours. (This duration of observation may be inappropriate for many emergency departments.)
D. Discharge considerations:
   1. Patients with no symptoms or laboratory abnormalities after a period of 4 hours may be safely discharged with instructions to return immediately if any problem arises.
   2. Manifestation of bite confined to immediate area around bite.
   3. Patient should be seen again within 24 hours for follow-up.

Gila Monster

I. Range of toxicity: toxic and fatal doses unknown, but presumably comparable with some snake venoms.
II. Treatment:
   A. Supportive.
   B. No antivenom.
III. Prognosis: Mortality about 1% in adults, about 5% in children.

Black Widow Spider

I. Range of toxicity: Toxicity of venom probably greater than that of most snake venoms, but spider injects only a minute amount of poison.
II. Clinical features:
   A. Bite may not be immediately noticed, but extreme pain and muscle rigidity soon follow.

    B. Other signs and symptoms include fever, chills, urinary retention, priapism, hyperactive reflexes, sweating, nausea, vomiting, hypertension.

III. Treatment:
    A. Cold packs applied to bite.
    B. Salicylates, opioids for pain control.
    C. Calcium gluconate, 0.1–0.2 ml/kg 10% solution IV, up to a total of 10 ml, can be used to decrease cramping. Hydrocortisone, 100 mg IV, intravenous muscle relaxants (e.g., methocarbamol) or diazepam may be necessary.
    D. An antivenin is available (Merck, Sharpe & Dohme) and after testing for horse serum sensitivity can be administered in severe reactions according to package insert.

IV. Prognosis: Death from spider bite in previously well individuals is unlikely. Recovery usually complete within a week.

 V. Disposition: Hospitalization required, but is usually brief.

Brown Recluse Spider

   I. Brown recluse spider belongs to the family Loxoscelidae. Adult body is usually 7–12 mm long and 3–5 mm wide. A violin-shaped dark marking located on dorsal surface is characteristic.

  II. Range of toxicity: Very rarely, death has been reported as a result of disseminated intravascular coagulation (DIC) and its attendant renal failure (Vorse M, et al: *J Pediatr* 1972; 80:1035).

III. Clinical features:
    A. Initial bite may be painless.
    B. Symptoms: Pain, pruritus, malaise, chills, sweats, GI upset, myalgias, dizziness, dyspnea, headache. Systemic symptoms more common in children.
    C. Signs: Erythema, cellulitis, rash, hemorrhagic blister, angioedema, urticaria, lymphangitis. Severe cases may be characterized by cutaneous necrosis, shock, coma.
    D. Other: Hemolysis, thrombocytopenia, DIC, renal failure.

IV. Laboratory findings and evaluation:
    A. Currently there are no diagnostic tests to confirm brown recluse envenomation. Diagnosis based on history, symptoms, characteristic appearance of bite wound.
    B. CBC if patient has fever, chills, evidence of hemolysis, thrombocytopenia; and should be obtained prior to initiation of dapsone therapy (dapsone reported to rarely cause hemolytic anemia or methemoglobinemia).

 V. Treatment:
    A. Elevation and ice packs applied intermittently for symptomatic relief; antihistamine for relief of pruritis.
    B. Dapsone 100 mg PO twice a day for 2 weeks.
    C. Erythromycin if evidence of infection (e.g., cellulitis).
    D. Surgical excision if evidence of cutaneous necrosis.
    E. Steroid therapy if systemic symptoms (e.g., venom-induced hemolysis).

VI. Prognosis: Healing of necrotic areas may require 6–8 weeks. Death extremely uncommon, usually occurs in first 48 hours.

VII. Special considerations:
- A. Dapsone may produce hemolytic anemia in persons with G-6-PD deficiency, and very rarely methemoglobinemia.
- B. Avoid heat, because increased temperature increases activity of toxin and may significantly worsen initially minor bites.

VIII. Controversies:
- A. Although steroids, heparin, antibiotics, surgical excision, antihistamines, dapsone, expectant observations have been reported to be effective, insufficient number of cases have been reported to conclude that any of these are helpful.
- B. Although produced experimentally, brown recluse antivenin is not available commercially.

IX. Disposition: Hospitalization rarely indicated for brown recluse spider bites unless accompanied by systemic effects or complications.

Scorpion

I. Treatment:
- A. Symptomatic and supportive.
- B. Cold packs applied to bite.
- C. Salicylates, opioids for pain control.
- D. Antivenin available for *Centruroides* species from Arizona Poison Center.

II. Prognosis:
- A. Fatalities rare except in children younger than 6 years of age.
- B. Rapid progression of symptoms in first 2–4 hours after sting indicates poor outcome.
- C. Survival for 48 hours ordinarily followed by recovery, although deaths have occurred 4 days after sting.

BIBLIOGRAPHY

Amitai Y, Mines Y, Aker M, et al: Scorpion stings in children: A review of 51 cases. *Clin Pediatr* 1985; 24:136.

Arnold RE: Controversies and hazards in the treatment of pit viper bites. *South Med J* 1979; 72:902.

Bernstein B, Ehrlich F: Brown recluse spider bites. *J Emerg Med* 1986; 4:457–462.

Emergency department management of poisonous snakebites. *Bull Am Coll Surg* May 1981; 19–22.

King LE: Spider bites. *Arch Dermatol* 1987; 123:41–43.

King LE, Rees RS: Dapsone treatment of a brown recluse spider bite. *JAMA* 1983; 250:648.

Kitchen CS, Van Mierop: Envenomation by the eastern coral snake *(Micrurus fulvius fulvius)*: A study of 39 victims. *JAMA* 1987; 258:1615–1618.

Minton SA: Present tests for detection of snake venom: Clinical applications. *Ann Emerg Med* 1987; 16:937.

Moss HS, Binder LS: A retrospective review of black widow spider envenomation. *Ann Emerg Med* 1987; 16:188–192.

Otten EJ: Antivenin therapy in the emergency department. *Am J Emerg Med* 1983; 1:83–93.

Otten EJ: Venomous animal injuries, in Rosen P, et al: *Emergency Medicine: Concepts and Clinical Practice.* St Louis, CV Mosby Co, 1987.

Otten EJ, McKimm D: Venomous snakebite in a patient allergic to horse serum. *Ann Emerg Med* 1983; 12:624–627.

Rauber A: Black widow spider bites. *J Toxicol Clin Toxicol* 1983; 21:473.

Rees R, Campbell D, Rieger E, et al: The diagnosis and treatment of brown recluse spider bites. *Ann Emerg Med* 1987; 16:945–949.

Rimsza ME, Zimmerman DR, Bergeson PS: Scorpion envenomation. *Pediatrics* 1980; 66:298.

Russell F: Snake venom poisoning. Philadelphia, JB Lippincott Co, 1985.

Sullivan JB: Past, present and future immunotherapy of snake venom poisoning. *Ann Emerg Med* 1987; 16:938–944.

Timms PK, Gibbons RB: Latrodectism: Effects of the black widow spider bite. *West J Med* 1986; 144:315–317.

Vorse M, Seccareccio P, Woodruff K, et al: DIC following fatal brown spider bite. *J Pediatr* 1972; 80:1035.

Watt CH: Poisonous snakebite treatment in the United States. *JAMA* 1978; 240:654–656.

Wong RC, Hughes SE, Voorhees JJ: Spider bites. *Arch Dermatol* 1987; 123:98–104.

114

Marine Life

Daniel L. Savitt, M.D.

Foodborne Marine Toxins

Ciguatera Poisoning (Table 114–1)

  I. Route of exposure:
  A. Clinical syndrome produced by eating large carnivorous fish containing ciguatoxin.
  B. Most common fishborne poisoning.
  II. Common sources:
  A. Toxin *(Gambierdiscus toxicus),* produced by a dinoflagellate, ultimately concentrated in fish, which are then eaten by humans.
  B. Most commonly found in large barracuda, grouper, snapper, surgeon fish, pompano, mackerel, butterfly fish, sea bass, perch, although over 400 species have caused ciguatera poisoning.
  III. Pharmacokinetics:
  A. Onset of action: Symptoms begin 30 minutes–4 hours after ingestion; may be as long as 30 hours later.
  IV. Actions: Ciguatoxin alters membrane permeability to sodium.
  V. Toxic mechanism: Altered membrane permeability to sodium results in blockade of nerve conduction.
  VI. Range of toxicity:
  A. Toxic dose: Not clearly documented. Cannot be estimated by amount of fish or species ingested.
  B. Fatal dose: LD_{99} in mice 0.5 μg/kg.

TABLE 114–1.
Foodborne Marine Toxins

Type of Poisoning	Agent/Species	Toxin	Laboratory Features	Signs and Symptoms	Management
Ciguatera	Large tropical carnivorous fish, most commonly barracuda, grouper, snapper	Ciguatoxin, maitotoxin, others Five component; heat and acid stable; produced by *gambierdiscus toxicus*, a pinoflagellate, and concentrated in food chain Onset of symptoms within 1 hour; may become more severe over next 6 hours	Toxin may be identified in fish by RIA CIE, ELISA	Gastrointestinal distress shortly after meal Neurologic symptoms of perioral paresthesias, dysesthesias, malaise, hypotension, bradycardia, rarely respiratory failure and death Reversal of hot/cold sensation and late pruritis with alcohol consumption characteristic	Gastric emptying and charcoal administration; avoid magnesium-based cathartics Symptomatic IV fluids, antiemetics, antidiarrheal agents, atropine IV for bradycardia, calcium gluconate 1–3 gm IV/24 hr for severe cases; avoid opiates Persistent neurologic symptoms may respond to amitriptyline 25 mg PO twice a day Hypotension not responsive to fluids; use dopamine Discharge if symptomatically improved Admit if dehydrated, persistent GI distress, unusual or severe neurologic symptoms
Paralytic shellfish	Shellfish in temperate and tropical seas	Saxitoxin, gonyautoxin Neurotoxin produced by *Gonyaulaux* sp, a dinoflagellate that blooms, discoloring water and producing a "red tide"		GI distress shortly after meal Neurologic features: Perioral paresthesias, sensation of floating, weakness, visual signs,	Gastric lavage with 2% $NaHCO_3$, activated charcoal; supportive therapy based on presentation Intubation and mechanical ventilation for respiratory

Type	Species/Source	Mechanism/Onset	Symptoms	Treatment
		Onset of paresthesias within minutes; rapid progression to paralysis may occur	flaccid paralysis with respiratory failure	failure Patients with any significant neurologic signs or symptoms should be admitted Those with delayed presentation or very mild symptoms may be discharged
Scomboid	Decomposition of members of tuna family en route to market	Histamines produced by various bacteria Onset of symptoms shortly after ingestion	Edema, pruritus, flushing, bronchospasm, hypotension Fish often have metallic or peppery taste	Gastric emptying, IV diphenhydramine and cimetidine in standard doses, IV hydration if indicated Most patients will respond to therapy and may be discharged when symptomatically improved
Pufferfish	Pufferfish, *fugu* sp, *arothron* sp, others	Neurotoxin (tetrodotoxin) concentrated in gonads but present in many organs; interferes with sodium conductance Onset of symptoms shortly after ingestion occasionally may be delayed several hours	Perioral paresthesias, GI distress, dysphagia, hypotension, respiratory failure, coma, death Up to 60% mortality	Gastric lavage and charcoal administration Intensive supportive care based on presentation Admission advised for any confirmed ingestion
Hallucinogenic fish	Surgeon fish, *Acanthurus* sp, others	Poorly characterized Onset of symptoms within 2 hours of ingestion	Visual and auditory hallucinations following meal	Gastric emptying and charcoal administration Parenteral benzodiazepines to control agitation Symptomatically improved patients may be discharged

VII. Clinical features:
   A. Syndrome of GI symptoms (nausea, vomiting, diarrhea, abdominal cramps) occurring shortly after ingestion, sudden onset of diaphoresis, neurologic symptoms of peripheral paresthesias and dysesthesias.
   B. Other frequent symptoms and signs include malaise, arthralgias, myalgias, hypotension, bradycardia.
   C. **Pathognomonic:** Reversal of hot and cold sensation and severe pruritis following alcohol ingestion.
   D. In severe poisoning: Paralysis, seizures, respiratory arrest.
   E. Symptoms may last from days to weeks.
VIII. Laboratory findings and evaluation:
   A. Electrolytes, BUN, creatinine (volume loss).
   B. Amylase, liver function studies, urinalysis (assessment of abdominal pain).
   C. ECG (see Clinical presentation).
   D. CBC (general assessment of infection).
   E. Blood glucose (rule out hypoglycemia in presence of malaise).
   F. Arterial blood gases, chest film if respiratory distress.
IX. Treatment:
   A. Follow APTLS: See Chapter 8.
   B. General management: Table 114–2 (see Chapter 12 for details).
   C. Most cases can be managed symptomatically; rare cases proceed to respiratory failure and death.
   D. Intravenous hydration, antiemetic, and antidiarrheal therapy will ameliorate most symptoms.
   E. Symptomatic bradycardia should be treated with atropine. Severe cases may benefit from intravenous calcium gluconate 1–3 gm over 24 hours.
X. Prognosis:
   A. Expected response to treatment: Full recovery without sequelae.
   B. Expected complications and long-term effects: Rarely, neurologic symptoms may persist for months.
XI. Special considerations: Long-term complications of persistent neurologic sequelae have been successfully managed with amitriptyline 25 mg twice a day.

TABLE 114–2.

General Treatment

Treatment	Indicated	Of No Value	Contraindicated
O_2	±		
IV	+		
ECG monitor	+		
Forced diuresis			X
Acidification			X
Alkalinization		X	
Emesis/lavage	+/+		
Charcoal	+		
Cathartic			X

XII. Disposition considerations:
- A. Admission considerations:
  1. See General Admission Considerations (Chapters 17 and 18).
  2. Diagnosis uncertain.
  3. Significant volume loss, hypotension, evidence of shock.
  4. Neurologic symptoms including bradycardia.
- B. Consultation criteria: Persistent neurologic symptoms may require neurologic consultation.
- C. Observation period: Difficult to make specific recommendations. Degree of toxicity cannot be estimated from amount of fish ingested. Each case should be assessed separately.
- D. Discharge criteria:
  1. General discharge considerations have been met (see Chapters 17 and 18).
  2. No evidence of significant toxicity (e.g., hypotension, bradycardia, neurologic symptoms) after sufficient observation.
  3. Patient able to take fluids orally.

Paralytic Shellfish Poisoning (see Table 114–1)

- I. Route of exposure: Oral.
- II. Common sources of toxin:
  - A. Several dinoflagellate or plankton species, most notably *Gonyaulaux* sp, produce responsible toxin.
  - B. Enormous population growth of these dinoflagellates at certain times of year produces discoloration of ocean (known as "red tide").
  - C. Toxin concentrated in shellfish (clams, oysters, mussels, scallops), which are then eaten by humans.
- III. Pharmacokinetics:
  - A. Absorption: Toxin rapidly absorbed from GI tract.
  - B. Onset of action: Toxicity normally appears within 30 minutes of ingestion; can be delayed for up to 10 hours.
- IV. Toxic mechanism: Toxin produced by dinoflagellates is saxitoxin, which inhibits neuromuscular transmission by blocking sodium channels in nerve tissue and skeletal muscle, resulting in muscle paralysis.
- V. Range of toxicity:
  - A. Fatal dose:
    1. Death can result from only 0.5–1.0 mg.
    2. Fatalities have been reported resulting from ingestion of only one mussel, clam, or oyster.
- VI. Clinical features:
  - A. Shortly after eating toxin-containing shellfish patients complain of perioral paresthesias, tremor, dysarthria, dysphagia, ataxia, sensation of "floating," weakness, visual changes, seizures, occasionally flaccid paralysis.
  - B. Cardiac conduction defects may develop.
  - C. Respiratory failure secondary to paralysis may develop.
  - D. Mental status remains normal.

VII. Laboratory findings and evaluation:
   A. Arterial blood gases (rule out hypoxia, acidosis, if patient has respiratory difficulty).
   B. Chest radiograph (respiratory symptoms or findings).
   C. ECG.
VIII. Treatment:
   A. Follow APTLS: See Chapter 8.
   B. General management: See Table 114–3 (see Chapter 12 for details).
   C. Following general measures, treatment is supportive.
   D. Intubation and mechanical ventilation may be required.
   E. In setting of cardiac depression or hypotension, **activated charcoal hemoperfusion** may be helpful.
IX. Prognosis:
   A. Mortality 1–10%.
   B. Survival for 12–24 hours after ingestion associated with complete recovery.
X. Disposition considerations:
   A. Admission considerations: Admission threshold must be low. All patients with known or suspected paralytic shellfish poisoning should be admitted.
   B. Consultation considerations: Nephrologist should be consulted if activated charcoal hemoperfusion being considered.
   C. Observation period: Not appropriate to observe.
   D. Discharge considerations: Not appropriate to discharge. All patients with known or suspected poisoning should be admitted.

Scromboid Poisoning (see Table 114–1)

   I. Route of exposure: Oral.
  II. Common sources of exposure: Scromboid can develop after ingestion of affected mackerel, tuna, bonito, albacore, skipjack, mahi-mahi (dolphin fish).

TABLE 114–3.

General Treatment

Treatment	Indicated	Of No Value	Contraindicated
O_2	±		
IV	+		
ECG monitor	+		
Forced diuresis			X
Acidification			X
Alkalinization		X	
Emesis	−		
Lavage*	+		
Charcoal	+		
Cathartic	+		

*Gastric lavage with 2% $NaHCO_3$ solution.

III. Pharmacokinetics:
    A. Onset of action: Symptoms occur within minutes to hours.

IV. Toxic mechanism:
    A. Free histadine in fish muscle is converted to histamine and saurine by marine microflora (e.g., *Morganella morganii*) containing enzyme histadine decarboxylase.
    B. Conversion to histamine is enhanced in setting of improper refrigeration of fish.
    C. Histamine released into circulation causes widespread peripheral dilation and increased permeability of capillaries, marked loss of plasma from the circulation.
    D. This may result in urticaria, respiratory difficulty, anaphylactic shock.

V. Range of toxicity: Fish containing at least 20 mg histamine/100 gm tissue are reported to produce toxic symptoms.

VI. Clinical features:
    A. Affected fish frequently have a metallic or peppery taste.
    B. After consumption of such fish, patients may develop symptoms of immediate-type hypersensitivity or anaphylaxis: edema, pruritis, flushing, bronchospasm, hypotension.

VII. Laboratory findings and evaluation:
    A. Diagnosis confirmed by elevated urine, serum, histamine levels.
    B. ECG.
    C. Chest radiograph (If respiratory symptoms).

VIII. Treatment:
    A. Follow APTLS: See Chapter 8.
    B. General management: See Table 114–4 (Chapter 12 for details).
    C. Antihistamines:
        1. Diphenhydramine 50 mg IV.
        2. Cimetidine 300 mg IV.
        3. Follow with oral diphenhydramine to prevent relapse.

TABLE 114–4.

General Treatment

Treatment	Indicated	Of No Value	Contraindicated
O$_2$	+		
IV	+		
ECG monitor	+		
Forced diuresis		X	
Acidification			X
Alkalinization*		X	
Emesis/lavage†	±/+		
Charcoal	+		
Cathartic	+		

*Of no value for purpose of elimination. Administration of HCO$_3$ may be required for severe metabolic acidosis.
†Preferred.

    D. Bronchospasm:

       1. **Bronchodilators:**

         a. **Epinephrine:** 0.3–0.5 mg (0.01 mg/kg in child) of 1:1,000 solution SC every 20–30 minutes for up to three doses.

         b. **Nonsulfite-containing sympathomimetic aerosol therapy** (e.g., albuterol, metaproterenol).

         c. **Aminophylline:** 6 mg/kg IV over 20–30 minutes, followed by maintenance infusion of 0.5–1.0 mg/kg/hr.

       2. **Corticosteroids** (e.g., methylprednisolone, 0.5–1.0 mg/kg IV every 6 hours), if severe, persistent bronchospasm.

    E. Hypotension: See Chapter 10 for treatment recommendations.

  IX. Prognosis: Prognosis excellent with good supportive care; most patients show improvement after a few hours of treatment with antihistamines.

   X. Disposition considerations:

    A. Admission considerations: Patients with persistent symptoms, shock, or requiring intensive respiratory treatment should be admitted. Patients with neurologic signs or symptoms or unclear diagnosis should be admitted.

    B. Observation period: Symptoms generally last 4–6 hours.

    C. Discharge criteria:

       1. General discharge criteria have been met (Chapter 18).

       2. No evidence of significant toxicity (e.g., urticaria, bronchospasm, hypotension) after sufficient observation.

       3. Patient able to take fluids orally.

Pufferfish Poisoning (see Table 114–1)

    I. Route of exposure: Oral.

   II. Common sources of toxin:

    A. Occurs mainly in Japan, where it is called "fugu."

    B. Other names: Balloon fish toxin, blow fish toxin, globefish toxin, puffer fish toxin, swellfish toxin, toadfish toxin, tetrodotoxin (TTX), maculotoxin (MTX), tarichatoxin, triturus embryonic toxin.

  III. Pharmacokinetics:

    A. Absorption: Toxin rapidly absorbed from GI tract, within 5–15 minutes.

    B. Onset of action: Symptoms appear within 5–45 minutes after ingestion; may be delayed for 3 hours.

    C. Plasma half-life: Half-life of toxin between 30 minutes–4 hours.

  IV. Toxic mechanism:

    A. Toxicity related to tetrodotoxin, a neurotoxin found throughout the body of the fish but concentrated in the gonads.

    B. Toxin interferes with sodium-potassium pump in neurons, resulting in blockade of neuromuscular transmission.

    C. This results in respiratory depression and vasodilation.

   V. Range of toxicity:

    A. Toxic dose: Not established.

    B. Fatal dose: 8–10 µg/kg may be fatal.

  VI. Clinical features:

    A. After consuming toxic fish, patient may develop perioral paresthesias, GI distress (nausea, vomiting, diarrhea, abdominal pain), dysphagia, dysphonia, headache, diaphoresis.

    B. More severe symptoms may then develop, including cardiac arrhythmias, fasciculations, ascending paralysis, seizures, hypotension, respiratory failure, coma.

VII. Laboratory findings and evaluation:

    A. Arterial blood gases.

    B. Complete blood cell count.

    C. Chest radiograph (with respiratory distress)

    D. Electrolytes if vomiting, diarrhea severe.

    E. ECG.

VIII. Treatment:

    A. Follow APTLS: See Chapter 8.

    B. General management: Table 114–5 (see Chapter 12 for details).

IX. Prognosis: Mortality 60% in some series.

X. Disposition considerations:

    A. Admission considerations: All patients with pufferfish poisoning should be admitted.

    B. Consultation considerations: Gastroenterology consultation if endoscopy indicated to remove ingested fish parts.

    C. Observation period: Not appropriate to observe.

    D. Discharge considerations: Not appropriate to discharge: All patients with pufferfish poisoning should be admitted.

Hallucinogenic Fish Poisoning (see Table 114–1)

I. Most commonly caused by surgeon fish and a few other tropical species. Toxicity characterized by auditory and visual hallucinations and neurologic symptoms. Supportive treatment may be aided with benzodiazepines if required.

TABLE 114–5.

General Treatment

Treatment	Indicated	Of No Value	Contraindicated
O$_2$	+		
IV	+		
ECG monitor	+		
Forced diuresis		X	
Acidification			X
Alkalinization*		X	
Emesis/lavage†	+/+		
Charcoal	+		
Cathartic‡	+		

*Not indicated to hasten elimination. HCO$_3$ may be required in severe acidemia.

†May require endoscopy to remove ingested fish.

‡Avoid if diarrhea present.

TABLE 114–6.

Hazardous Marine Chordates

Common Name	Species	Location	Mechanism of Envenomation	Toxin	Symptoms and Signs	Management
Shark	Many	Temperate and tropical seas	Direct trauma from bite	None	Hemorrhagic shock, other signs based on location of trauma	Control of bleeding, resuscitation from shock, surgical debridement, tetanus toxoid as indicated, prophylactic penicillin or cephalosporin, treatment of documented infection based on culture. Admission based on surgical requirements
Stingray	*Dasyatis* sp, others	Temperate and tropical seas worldwide, Amazon basin	Sting from spine at base of tail, usually when stepped on	Multicomponent: serotonin, enzymes. Rapid onset of pain	Local pain and edema, weakness, GI irritability, tachycardia, muscle spasm, hypotension	Wound debridement and irrigation; soak extremity in hot water (100°–110° F) for up to 90 min for pain control. Local anesthetics, systemic analgesics. Tetanus toxoid as indicated. Deep wounds should be treated with prophylactic cephalosporin. Do not close puncture wounds. Admission rarely indicated

Organism	Species	Distribution	Mechanism	Venom	Symptoms	Treatment
Moray eel	*Gymnothorax* sp., others	Temperate and tropical seas	Direct trauma from bite	None	Local pain and bleeding	Local wound care as indicated
Catfish	Many	Fresh and saltwater worldwide	Envenomation from dorsal and pectoral spines	Multicomponent Rapid onset of pain	Local pain and bleeding	Local wound care as indicated
Scorpion fish	Many	Temperate and tropical seas	Envenomation from dorsal spine when handled or stepped on	Multicomponent, protein based	Rapid onset of pain; immediate progression to other symptoms such as severe and debilitating local pain, edema, nausea, weakness, chest and abdominal pain, hypotension, syncope	Hot water immersion of extremity (100°–110° F) for up to 90 min for pain relief Appropriate supportive care based on signs and symptoms Admission indicated if antivenin administered or severe symptoms
Lion fish	*Pterois* sp	Tropical seas except Caribbean	Same as Scorpion fish	Same as Scorpion fish	Same as Scorpion fish	Same as Scorpion fish
Stone fish	*Synanceja* sp	Tropical seas except Caribbean	Same as Scorpion fish	Same as Scorpion fish	Same as Scorpion fish (death reported with stone fish)	Same as Scorpion fish Antivenin available for stone fish (in US from Seaworld of Ohio, San Diego, and some local aquaria.
Sea snakes	See Chapter 113					

TABLE 114–7.

Hazardous Marine Invertebrates

Common Name	Species	Location	Mechanism of Envenomation	Toxin	Symptoms and Signs	Management
Coral	Many	Tropical, worldwide	Contact	Protein, multicomponent	Pain, slow healing wounds, onset over first 24–48 hr	Wash and irrigate Wet to dry dressings Topical antibiotic or tetracycline paste Outpatient management usually sufficient
Molluscs						
Cone shell	Conus sp	Tropical, worldwide	Bite	Neurotoxin	Pain at site, paresthesias, dysphagia, respiratory failure, death Rapid progression of symptoms following bite	Incise wound until bleeding Local anesthetics or systemic analgesics for pain Supportive care as appropriate Admission for patients with neurologic signs or systemic symptoms
Blue-ring octopus	Octopus lunaltus	Australia	Bite	Neurotoxin	Pain and edema at site, perioral anesthesia, myoclonus, paralysis, respiratory failure, death Onset of symptoms within 5–30 min	Supportive care as appropriate Mechanical ventilation if appropriate Admission for other than local symptoms

	Species	Distribution		Mechanism	Clinical features	Treatment
Echinoderms Sea urchin, Starfish	Many	All seas	Contact	Mechanical	Pain and inflammation at site	Remove spines manually or with adhesive tape; Hot water (100°–110° F) immersion of extremity for pain; Surgery may be required for granuloma formation; Outpatient management usually sufficient
Bristleworm	*Eurythoe* sp, *Hermodice* sp	Tropical, worldwide	Contact	Mechanical	Pain and inflammation at site	Remove spines with adhesive tape; Oral analgesics
Coelenterates Fire coral	*Millepora* sp	Tropical, worldwide	Contact	Multicomponent	Pain and edema at site, muscle spasm, hypotension, bronchospasm, arrhythmias, laryngeal edema, death	Wash involved areas with **sea water**
Sea anemones	Many	All seas	Contact	Same as fire coral	Same as fire coral	Wash involved areas with alcohol or 5% acetic acid; slurry of baking soda applied topically effective for some species; Papain topically, hot water immersion for pain; Shave off tentacles with razor; Diphenhydramine and topical steroids for local reactions

(Continued.)

TABLE 114–7 (cont.).

Common Name	Species	Location	Mechanism of Envenomation	Toxin	Symptoms and Signs	Management
						Calcium gluconate 1.0 gm IV for muscle spasm Supportive care as appropriate Admission if severely symptomatic
Jellyfish	Many	All seas	Contact	Enzymes, proteins	Systemic signs proportional to magnitude of envenomation Onset of symptoms immediately following contact	Same as Sea anemone
Portugese man-o-war	*Physalia* sp	Tropical, Atlantic and Pacific oceans	Contact	Same as jellyfish	Same as jellyfish	Same as sea anemone
Box jelly	*Chironex* sp	Australia	Contact	Same as jellyfish	Same as jellyfish	Specific antivenom available in Australia Admission frequently required, especially for pediatric patients

Hazardous Chordates

I. See Table 114–6.
II. Laboratory findings and evaluation:
  A. Soft tissue radiograph or xerogram may reveal retained foreign body.

Hazardous Invertebrates

I. See Table 114–7.
II. Laboratory findings and evaluation:
  A. Soft tissue radiograph or xerogram may reveal retained foreign body.

BIBLIOGRAPHY

Auerbach PS, Yajko DM, Nassos PS: Bacteriology of the freshwater environment: Implications for clinical therapy. *Ann Emerg Med* 1987; 16:1016–1022.

Burnett JW, Calton GJ: Jellyfish envenomation syndromes updated. *Ann Emerg Med* 1987; 16:1000–1005.

Burnett JW, Calton GJ, Burnett HW, et al: Loreal and systemic reactions to jellyfish stings. *Clin Dermatol* 1987; 5:14–28.

Davis RT, Villar LA: Symptomatic improvement with amitripytline in Ciguatera fish poisoning. *N Engl J Med* 1986; 315:65.

Emerson DL, Balbraith RM, McMillan JP, et al: Preliminary immunologic studies of Ciguatera poisoning. *Arch Intern Med* 1983; 143:1931–1933.

Etkind P, Wilson ME, Gallagher K, et al: Bluefish-associated scromboid poisoning. *JAMA* 1987; 258:3409–3410.

Halstead BW, Vinei JM: Venomous fish stings. *Clin Dermatol* 1987; 5:29–35.

Kasdan ML, Kasdan AS, Hamilton DL: Lionfish envenomation. *Plast Reconstr Surg* 1987; 80:613–614.

Kizer KW, McKinney HE, Auerbach PS: *Scorpaenidae* envenomation. *JAMA* 1985; 253:807–810.

Morris JG, Lewin P, Hargett NT, et al: Clinical features of ciguatera poisoning. *Arch Intern Med* 1982; 142:1090–1092.

Sims JK: A theoretical discourse on the pharmacology of toxic marine ingestions. *Ann Emerg Med* 1987; 16:1006–1015.

Sims JK, Ostman DC: Pufferfish poisoning: Emergency diagnosis and management of mild human tetrodotoxication. *Ann Emerg Med* 1986; 15:1094–1098.

Williamson JA: The blue-ringed octopus bite and envenomation syndrome. *Clin Dermatol* 1987; 5:127–133.

115

Mushrooms

Michael S. Jastremski, M.D.

More than 5,000 varieties of mushrooms exist in the United States of which 100 can be toxic. Although mushrooms are an unusual cause of acute poisoning, the emergency physician needs to maintain a high index of suspicion because of the potential for a fatal outcome. Mushroom poisoning should be considered in the differential diagnosis of acute gastroenteritis or central nervous system dysfunction, especially in small children, wild-food connoisseurs, and recreational mushroom abusers. Wild mushrooms grow best in the spring and fall, so mushroom poisoning is more likely during these seasons. Table 115–1 summarizes the salient characteristics of the eight groups of toxic mushrooms. Figure 115–1 outlines a reasonable course when there is a high index of suspicion of acute mushroom poisoning.

I. Route of exposure: Oral.
II. Common and scientific names: See Table 115–1.
III. Range of toxicity: Deaths have been reported from ingestion of part of a single mushroom from highly toxic species.
IV. Clinical features: See Table 115–1.
V. Laboratory findings and evaluation:
   A. Electrolytes, blood glucose, liver function studies (transaminases, bilirubin), BUN, creatinine, CBC, prothrombin time (PT), partial thromboplastin time (PTT).
   B. Arterial blood gases, if indicated.
   C. If possible, offending mushroom should be obtained and identified. Identical mushrooms from the area where the mushroom was picked should be collected, wrapped in waxed paper, brought to the emergency department, and saved in a refrigerator (not where food is ordinarily kept!) for subsequent identification should symptoms develop.

TABLE 115–1.

Poisonous Mushrooms

| Group | Species | Toxin | Clinical Presentation | | Treatment |
			Signs and Symptoms	Onset	
1	*Amanita* spp *Conocybefilaris*	Cyclopeptides, amanitotoxins	Latent period	6–24 hr	Intensive supportive care
	Galerina spp *Lepiotaheluncola*		Gastroenteritis phase: nausea, vomiting, diarrhea, cramps, dehydration	6–24 hr Lasts 12–24 hr	Gastric emptying (activated charcoal) Thioctic acid 50– 150 mg every 6 hr IV with glucose
			Remission period	Lasts up to 24 hr	(children: 5–50 mg); efficacy has not been proven
			Hepatic and renal failure	Often death in 4–7 days Recovery takes weeks	Penicillin G 250 mg/kg/day continuous IV infusion Steroids Consider plasma exchange or hemoperfusion Hemodialysis for renal failure

(Continued.)

TABLE 115–1 (cont.).

Group	Species	Toxin	Clinical Presentation		Treatment
			Signs and Symptoms	Onset	
IA	*Cortinarious* spp	Orellanine and Orelline Cyclopeptides	Gastroenteritis, usually mild Latent period Renal failure	First day Days to weeks Usually reverses	Same as group I if recognized early Hemodialysis if not recognized until renal failure
II	*Amanita* spp	Muscimol, ibotenic acid	Hallucinations, intoxicated state Anticholinergic Dry mouth Warm flushed skin Dilated pupils Tachycardia Hypertension	30–120 min Resolves in 8–24 hr	Observation: Almost always self-limited without specific intervention Avoid sedatives Physostigmine 1–2 mg IV bolus (children: 0.5 mg) only if hemodynamic compromise or seizures refractory to standard anticonvulsant therapy

	Species	Toxin	Symptoms	Onset/Duration	Treatment
III	*Gyromitra* spp *Paxina* spp *Sarcospmaera coronaria*	Gyromitrin, monomethylhydrazine	Gastroenteritis Methemoglobinemia Hemolysis CNS stimulation: delerium, seizures, coma	6–24 hr Duration ranges from resolution in 24 hours to death in 5–7 days, depending on severity	Intensive support Methylene blue 1–2 mg/kg IV Transfusion Pyrodoxine 25 mg/kg IV, repeated as needed based on CNS status (up to 5 gm)
IV	*Beletus* spp *Inocybe* spp	Muscarine	Cholinergic activation Sweating Salivation Blurred vision Cramps Emesis Urinary incontinence Bradycardia Hypotension	30–120 min Duration 6–24 hr	IV hydration Atropine 1–2 mg (children: 0.01 mg/kg) IV repeated as needed until symptoms resolve
V	*Corprinus ayramentarius* *Clitocybe clavipes*	Coprine	Antabuse effect if alcohol ingested Flushing and sweating Parasthesias Nausea and vomiting Hypotension Metallic taste	May occur up to 1 week after eating mushrooms Syndrome starts 30–60 min after alcohol consumed Recovery in 2–4 hr	Avoid ethanol Most cases resolve quickly without specific treatment General supportive care for severe cases

(Continued.)

TABLE 115–1 (cont.).

Group	Species	Toxin	Clinical Presentation		Treatment
			Signs and Symptoms	Onset	
			Chest tightness Dyspnea Coma in severe cases ECG changes		Rule out myocardial infarction if ECG changes
VI	*Psilocybe* spp *Gymdopila* spp *Conocybe cyanopus* *Strophans coronilla*	Psilocybin, psilocin	Hallucinations Hyperkinesis Weakness Drowsiness Rarely, "bad trip"	30–60 min Duration 4–6 hr	Reassurance Benzodiazepines

   D. Spot test for amatoxins in mushrooms:
1. Drop of liquid is expressed from fresh mushroom onto lignin-containing paper and then allowed to dry.
2. Drop of concentrated hydrochloric acid (10–12 N) is added to dried liquid from mushroom.
3. If amatoxins are present, blue color develops within 1–2 minutes (longer if amatoxins present in low concentration).
4. If mushroom too dry to express fluid, may be crushed in absolute methanol, then placed on lignin-containing paper.

   E. Potential sources of information regarding poisonous mushrooms: State health department, university botany department.

VI. General treatment:

   A. Follow APTLS: (See Chapter 8).

   B. General management: Table 115–2 (see Chapter 12 for details).

VII. Specific treatment:

   A. See Figure 115–1.

   B. When no specimen is available for identification, treatment based on clinical presentation.

   C. Thioctic acid, a Krebs' cycle coenzyme, has not been tested in a controlled clinical trial but has been reported to reduce mortality from amantadine poisoning in a number of case reports. Thiocetic acid is not generally available, but regional poison control center or state health department may be able to supply it.

   D. See Table 115–1.

VIII. Prognosis:

   A. Expected response to treatment:
1. Most patients do well with symptomatic treatment only.
2. Potentially fatal mushrooms often produce first symptoms more than 6 hours after ingestion. However, do not conclude that nontoxic species was ingested by early onset of symptoms; patient may have ingested several different species of mushrooms.
3. *Amanita phalloides* and other hepatotoxic mushrooms have case fatality rate approaching 50% if untreated. If appropriate treatment is

TABLE 115–2.

General Treatment

Treatment	Indicated	Of No Value	Contraindicated
O$_2$	+		
IV	+		
ECG monitor	+		
Forced diuresis		X	
Acidification			X
Alkalinization		X	
Emesis/lavage	+/+		
Charcoal	+		
Cathartic	±		

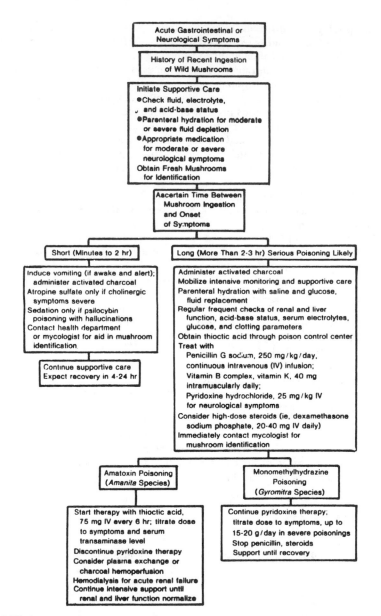

FIG 115–1.
Treatment algorithm for mushroom poisoning. (From Hanrahan JP, Gordon MA: *JAMA* 1984; 251:1057–1061. Used by permission.)

TABLE 115–3.
Disposition Considerations in Mushroom Poisoning

Group	Toxin	Disposition
I	Cyclopeptides Amanitotoxins	Always admit to ICU.
IA	Orellanine and orelline cyclopeptides	Admit for hemodialysis or charcoal hemoperfusion
II	Muscimol Ibotenic acid	Observe in emergency department. Most patients will be able to go home in 6–8 hours after symptoms resolve. If seizures or hemodynamic compromise, admit to hospital.
III	Gyromitrin Monomethylhydrazine	Admit to hospital (ICU for severe cases).
IV	Muscarine	Observe in emergency department until symptoms resolve, then discharge to home. Admit if still symptomatic after 6–8 hours.
V	Coprine	Observe in emergency department until symptoms resolve, then discharge to home. Admit for cardiac monitoring if ECG changes.
VI	Psilocybin Psilocin	Observe in quiet area until symptoms resolve, then send home.
VII	Unknown	Each case must be considered on an individual basis.

instituted early, good supportive care provided, and no major complications ensue, recovery is usual.

IX. Disposition considerations:
  A. Admission considerations:
    1. See General Admission Considerations (Chapters 17 and 18).
    2. See Table 115–3.
  B. Consultation criteria: May require help of a mycologist for aid in mushroom identification (contact local Health Department).

BIBLIOGRAPHY

Hanraham JP, Gordon MA: Mushroom poisoning. *JAMA* 1984; 251:1057–1061.
Lampe KF, McCann M: Differential diagnosis of poisoning by North American mushrooms, with particular emphasis on *Amanita phalloides*–like intoxication. *Ann Emerg Med* 1987; 16:956–962.

Lincoff G, Mitchel DH: *Toxic and Hallucinogenic Mushroom Poisoning.* New York, Van Nostrand Reinhold, 1977.

Olson KR, Woo OF, Pond SM: Treatment of mushroom poisoning. *JAMA* 1984; 252:3130–3132.

Parish RC, Doering PL: Treatment of *Amanita* mushroom poisoning: A review. *Vet Hum Toxicol* 1986; 28:318–322.

Rumack BH, Peterson RG: Diagnosis and treatment of mushroom poisoning. *Top Emerg Med* 1979; 1:85.

Vesconi S, Langer M, Iapichino G, et al: Therapy of cytotoxic mushroom intoxication. *Crit Care Med* 1985; 13:402.

116

Botanical Toxicity

Harlan A. Stueven, M.D., F.A.C.E.P.
David Roberts, M.D., F.A.C.E.P., A.B.M.T.

I. Route of exposure: Oral, cutaneous.
II. Common and botanical plant names: See Tables 116–1 through 116–3.
III. Toxic mechanism (See also Table 116–4): Several mechanisms; not all are known:
   A. Calcium oxalate crystals: Prototype **Dumbcane;** causes primarily oropharyngeal pain, burning, inflammation.
   B. GI symptoms:
      1. Toxalbumin: Prototype castor bean.
      2. Glycoalkaloids: Prototype Jerusalem cherry.
      3. Colchicine: Prototype autumn crocus.
   C. Cardiac glycosides, prototype lily-of-the-valley; causes cardiac and GI toxicity.
   D. Belladonna alkaloid: Prototype jimson weed; causes anticholinergic symptoms.
   E. Miscellaneous other toxins may cause:
      1. Direct GI irritation.
      2. Nicotine-like actions.
      3. Cause chemical irritation to skin.
      4. Centrally mediated emesis, stimulation, depression, hallucination.
      5. Direct hepatotoxic, cyanogenic, hematologic toxicity.
IV. Clinical features (See also Table 116–4):
   A. Patient with botanical poisoning often does not know the plant that caused the symptoms, will give vague description or improper common name. Consequently, symptoms and physical exam may be only clue to cause.

751

TABLE 116–1.

Nontoxic Houseplants*

Common Name	Botanical Name
African violet	*Saintpaulia ionantha*
Aluminum plant	*Pilea cadierei*
Aralia false	*Dizygotheca elegantissima*
Baby's tears	*Helxine soleirolii*
Begonia	*Begonia semperflorens*
Bird's nest fern	*Asplenium nidus*
Boston fern	*Tradescantia*
Bridal veil	*Tradescantia*
Christmas cactus	*Zygocactus truncatus*
Coleus	*Coleus blumei*
Corn plant	*Dracena fragrans*
Creeping Charlie	*Pilea nummularifolia* or *Plectranthus australis*
Creeping Jenny	*Lysimachia nummularia*
Donkey tail	*Sedum morganianun*
Emerald ripple	*Peperomia caperata*
Fiddleleaf fig	*Ficus lyrata*
Gardenia	*Gardenia radicans*
Grape ivy	*Cissus rhombifloria*
Hawaiian ti	*Cordyline terminalis*
Hen and chicks	*Echeveria* or *Sempervivium tectorus*
Jade plant	*Crassula argentea*
Lipstick plant	*Aeschynanthus lobbianus*
Mother-in-law tongue	*Sansevieria trifasciata*
Monkey plant	*Ruella makoyana*
Parlorpalm	*Chamaedorea elegans*
Peacock plant	*Calathea*
Piggy-back plant	*Tolmiea menziestii*
Pink polka dot plant	*Hypoestes sanguinolenta*
Prayer plant	*Maranta leuconeura*
Rosary bead plant	*Ceropegia woodii*
Rubber plant	*Ficus elastica*
Sensitive plant	*Mimosa pudica*
Snake plant	*Sansevieria trifasciata*
Spider plant	*Chlorophytum comosum*
String of hearts	*Creopegia woodii*
Swedish ivy	*Pextranthus australis*
Umbrella plant (Schefflera)	*Brassaia actinophylla*
Wandering Jew	*Tradescantia albiflora* or *Zebrina pendula*

Wax plant	*Hoya carnosa* or *H. exotica*
Weeping fig	*Ficus benjamina*
Zebra plant	*Alphelandra squarrosa*

*From Goldfrank LR, et al: *Goldfrank's Toxicologic Emergencies.* Norwalk, Conn, Appleton-Century-Crofts, 1986, pp 581–582. Used by permission.

B. History:
  1. Time from ingestion to symptoms:
     a. Immediate mouth symptoms suggest dumbcane *(Dieffenbachia* or *Philodendron).*
     b. Significantly delayed GI symptoms suggest *Abrus* or *Ricinus.*
  2. Skin:
     a. Itching, burning, redness, vesicle after hours to days suggest poison ivy, oak, sumac, elder, dogwood *(Toxicodendron).*
     b. Hemorrhagic rash suggests exposure to sap of *Agave.*
  3. Mouth, pharynx:
     a. Pain, oral edema, mucous membrane blistering suggest *Dieffenbachia, Philodendron, Caladium,* Jack-in-the-pulpit *(Arisaema),* elephant ear *(Colocasia).*
     b. Caustic burns suggest rosary pea *(Abrus).*
  4. Gastrointestinal:
     a. Nausea, vomiting, diarrhea, crampy abdominal pain suggest tulips,

TABLE 116–2.

Poisonous House Plants*

Common Name	Botanical Name
Asparagus fern	*Asparagus officinalis*
Bird of paradise	*Strelitzia regirae*
Boston ivy	*Parthenocissus quinquelfolia*
Creeping Charlie	*Glecoma hederacea*
Emerald duke, majesty, red princess	*Philodendron hastatum*
Glacier ivy	*Hedera glacier*
Heartleaf, parlor ivy	*Philodendron cordatum*
English ivy	*Hedera helix*
Nephythytis arrowhead vine	*Syngonium podophyllum albolineatum*
Pothos	*Scindapsus aureus*
Saddleleaf	*Philodendron selloum*
Umbrella plant	*Cyperus alternifolius*

*From Goldfrank LR, et al: *Goldfrank's Toxicologic Emergencies.* Norwalk, Conn, Appleton-Century-Crofts, 1986, pp 581–582. Used by permission.

TABLE 116–3.

Poisonous Plants Outside the Home*

Poisonous plants and flowers	Poisonous trees and shrubs
Amaryllis	Apple
Autumn crocus	Black locust
Bleeding heart	Buckeye, horse chestnut
Daffodil	Chinaberry tree
Foxglove	Cherry (choke)
Glory lily	Elderberry
Hyacinth	Gingko
Hydrangea	Sandbox tree
Iris	Yew
Larkspur	Poisonous wildflowers of woods
Lily-of-the-valley	
Monkshood	Bloodroot
Narcissus	Hellebore (false)
Nicotiana (cultivated)	Jack-in-the-pulpit
Primrose	Mayapple
Spider lily	Skunk cabbage
Poisonous ornamental plants and flowers	Water hemlock
	Poisonous wildflowers of fields
American ivy	
Atropa belladonna	Buttercup
Azalea	Death camas
Common privet	Jimsonweed
Daphne	Nettles
English ivy	Nightshade
Golden chain	Poison hemlock
Honeysuckle(?)	Tobacco (wild)
Jessamine (yellow, Carolina)	
Lantana	
Oleander	
Rhododendron	
Wisteria	
Yew	

*From Goldfrank LR, et al: *Goldfrank's Toxicologic Emergencies.* Norwalk, Conn, Appleton-Century-Crofts, 1986, pp 581–582. Used by permission.

poke root, holly berries, Mexican bird of paradise, desert potato, poinsettia *(Euphorbia)*, spurges, *Solanum.*

5. CNS:
   a. Stimulation suggests tobacco or nicotine, coffee, tea, cocaine.
   b. Depression suggests marijuana, peyote.
   c. Immediate seizures suggest water hemlock *(Cicuta).*
   d. Paralysis suggests poison hemlock *(Conium),* nicotine in later stages, yellow jessamine.

TABLE 116–4.

Plants Commonly Involved in Poisoning*

Name	Poisons Part of Plant, Active Principle if Known	Clinical Findings	Treatment
Arum family: Calla lilly, elephant ear, Jack-in-the-pulpit (Dieffenbachia, Caladium, Alocasia, Colocasia, Philodendron, Arisaema triphyllum)	All parts (oxalates and other toxins)	Severe irritation of mucous membranes, nausea and vomiting, diarrhea, salivation Rare systemic effects	Give demulcents: milk, oil, cooling drinks
Oleander (Nerium oleander)	All parts (oleandrin)	As for digitalis (see Chapter 81)	As for digitalis (see Chapter 81)
Pokeweed (Phytolacca americana)	All parts, especially root (saponins, glycoproteins)	Burning in mouth, stomach; persistent vomiting, diarrhea; slowed respiration, weakness	Remove ingested poison
Rhubarb (Rheum spp)	Leafy part (oxalic acid)	Nausea, vomiting, diarrhea, abdominal pain; reduced urine formation, hemorrhages	As for oxalic acid
Solanaceae Blue nightshade (Solanum dulcamara)	Leaves and fruit (solanine)	Abdominal pain, vomiting, diarrhea, mental and respiratory depression, hypothermia or fever, delirium, slow or fast pulse, shock	Maintain respiration and circulation; remove ingested poison
Black nightshade (Solanum nigrum)	Leaves and unripe berries (solanine)		
Jerusalem cherry (Solanum pseudo-capsicum)	Leaves and unripe berries (solanine)		
Potato (Solanum tuberosum)	Green tubers, new sprouts (solanine)		
Yew (Taxus)	Wood, bark, leaves, seeds (taxine)	Nausea, vomiting, diarrhea, abdominal pain	Remove ingested poison
Baneberry (Actaea spp)	All parts	Nausea, vomiting, diarrhea, shock	Remove ingested poison by activated charcoal, gastric lavage, or emesis; treat symptoms

(Continued.)

TABLE 116–4 (cont.).

Name	Poisons Part of Plant, Active Principle if Known	Clinical Findings	Treatment
Betelnut (*Areca catechu*)	Seed (arecoline)	Vomiting, diarrhea, difficult breathing, impaired vision, convulsions	Give atropine, 2 mg SC; repeat as necessary; remove poison (as for baneberry)
Bird of paradise (*Caesalpinia gilliesii, Poinciana spp*)	Seed pod	Nausea, vomiting, diarrhea	Give milk, beaten eggs, liquid petrolatum; replace fluids; remove poison (as for baneberry)
Bleeding heart (*Dicentra spp*)	All parts (alkaloids)	Ataxia, respiratory depression, convulsions	Remove poison (as for baneberry)
Bloodroot (*Sanguinaria spp*)	All parts (sanguinarine)	Vomiting, diarrhea, shock, coma	Remove poison (as for baneberry)
Boxwood (*Buxus sempervirens*)	Leaves, twigs	Nausea, vomiting, convulsions	Remove poison (as for baneberry)
Buckeye, horse chestnut (*Aesculus spp*)	Seed (glycoside)	Nausea, vomiting, weakness, paralysis	Remove poison (as for baneberry)
Burning bush (*Euonymus atropurpureus*), spindle tree (*Euonymus eropaea*)	Fruit, leaves	Nausea, vomiting, diarrhea, weakness, chills, coma, convulsions	Remove poison (as for baneberry)
Calabar bean (*Physostigma venenosum*)	Bean (physostigmine)	Dizziness, faintness, vomiting, diarrhea, pinpoint pupils	Remove poison (as for baneberry)
Celandine (*Chelidonium majus*)	All parts (chelidonine)	Nausea, vomiting, coma	Remove poison (as for baneberry)
Cherry (*Prunus spp*)	Seed, leaves (amygdalin)	Stupor, vocal cord paralysis, twitching, convulsions, coma from chewing seeds (see cyanide poisoning, Chapter 101)	Remove poison (as for baneberry); treat cyanide poisoning (see Chapter 101)
Chinaberry (*Melia azedarach*)	Fruit, leaves	Nausea, vomiting, diarrhea, paralysis	Remove poison (as for baneberry)

Plant	Toxic parts	Symptoms	Treatment
Chrysanthemum	All parts (resin)	Exudative dermatitis from sensitivity	Wash skin
Corn cockle (*Agrostemma githago*)	Seeds (githagin)	Nausea, vomiting, respiratory depression	Remove poison (as for baneberry)
Crowfoot family Christmas rose (*Helleborus niger*)	All parts (helleborin, related alkaloids)	Severe GI irritation with vomiting, diarrhea	Remove poison (as for baneberry)
Crowfoot, buttercup (*Ranunculaceae*)	All parts		
Marsh marigold (*Calthapalustris*)	All parts		
Daffodil (*Narcissus pseudonarcissus*)	Bulb	Nausea, vomiting, diarrhea	Remove poison (as for baneberry)
Daphne	All parts	Stomatitis, abdominal pain, vomiting, bloody diarrhea, weakness, convulsions, kidney damage	Remove poison, treat shock and seizures
Elderberry (*Sambucus* spp)	Leaves, shoots, bark, roots (cyanogenic glycoside)	Dizziness, headache, nausea, vomiting, respiratory stimulation, tachycardia, convulsions	Remove poison (as for baneberry); treat cyanide poisoning (see Chapter 101)
Finger cherry (*Rhodomyrtus macrocarpa*)	Fruit	Complete and permanent blindness within 24 hr	Remove poison (as for baneberry)
Glory lily (*Gloriosa superba*)	All parts (gloriosine, colchicine)	Vomiting, diarrhea, fall of blood pressure, alopecia	Remove poison (as for baneberry); maintain blood pressure
Holly (*Ilex* spp)	Berries	Vomiting, diarrhea, narcosis	Remove poison (as for baneberry)
Hyacinth	Bulb	Nausea, vomiting	Remove poison (as for baneberry)
Hydrangea	All parts (possibly cyanogenic)	Gastroenteritis; observe for symptoms of cyanide poisoning	Remove poison (as for baneberry); treat cyanide poisoning (see Chapter 101)
Indian tobacco (*Lobelia inflata*)	All parts (lobeline)	Progressive vomiting, weakness, stupor, tremors, pinpoint pupils, unconsciousness (see nicotine, Chapter 68)	Remove poison (as for baneberry); give artificial respiration; give atropine, 2 mg sc

(Continued.)

TABLE 116–4 (cont.).

Name	Poisons Part of Plant, Active Principle if Known	Clinical Findings	Treatment
Iris (*Iridaceae*)	Root	Nausea, violent diarrhea, abdominal burning	Remove poison (as for baneberry)
Jessamine (*Gelsemium sempervirens*)	All parts (gelsemine, related alkaloids)	Muscular weakness, convulsions, sweating, respiratory failure	Remove poison (as for baneberry); give atropine, 2 mg SC every 4 hr; artificial respiration
Jetberry (*Rhodotypos scandens*)	Berries (cyanogenic glycoside)	Like cherry (see Cyanide, Chapter 101)	Remove poison (as for baneberry). Treat cyanide poisoning (Chapter 101)
Jute (*Corchorus olitorius, Corchorus capsularis*)	Fibrous stem	Asthmatic attacks, rhinitis from sensitivity	Avoid further exposure
Laburnum, golden chain (*Laburnum anagyroides*), Kentucky coffee berry (*Gymnocladus dioica*)	Leaves, pod, seeds (cytisine)	Burning in mouth and abdomen, nausea, severe vomiting, diarrhea, prostration, irregular pulse and respiration, delirium, twitching, unconsciousness; renal damage may occur	Remove poison (as for baneberry)
Lantana (*Lantana camara*)	All parts (lantanin)	Photosensitization with great increase in injury from sunlight	Avoid sunlight
	Green fruit	Vomiting, lethargy, cyanosis, coma, dilated pupils, slowed respiration	Remove poison (as for baneberry); administer O$_2$
Laurel (*Kalmia* spp)	All parts (andromedotoxin)	Salivation, increased tear formation, nasal discharge, vomiting, convulsions, slow pulse, low blood pressure, paralysis	Remove poison (as for baneberry)
Lily-of-the-valley (*Convallaria* spp)	All parts (digitalis-like)	See Digitalis (Chapter 81)	See Digitalis (Chapter 81)
Locust (*Robinia pseudoacacia*)	Seed (robin)	Same as for castor bean	Same as for castor bean
Lupin, lupine (*Lupinus* spp)	All parts, especially berries (lupinine and related alkaloids)	Paralysis, weak pulse, depressed breathing, convulsions	Remove poison (as for baneberry); give artificial respiration; treat convulsions

Manchineel (*Hippomane mancinella*)	Sap	Severe irritation, blistering, peeling of skin from contact with sap	Wash with soap and water or alcohol
Mango (*Mangifera indica*)	Skin of fruit, sap of tree	Dermatitis, nausea, vomiting, diarrhea	Do not eat peel; avoid contact with sap
Mexican poppy (*Argemone mexicana*)	Leaves, seeds (alkaloids)	Vomiting, diarrhea, cardiac and visual effects	Remove poison (as for baneberry)
Mistletoe (*Phoradendron flavescens*)	All parts, especially berries	Vomiting, diarrhea, slowed pulse similar to digitalis	Treat as for digitalis (see Chapter 81)
Moonseed (*Menispermum canadense*)	Fruit (alkaloid)	Nausea, vomiting, mechanical injury	Remove poison (as for baneberry)
Nutmeg (*Myristica fragrans*)	Seeds (myristicin)	Hallucinations, delirium, convulsions	Remove poison (as for baneberry)
Physic nut (*Jatropha spp*)	Seed	Nausea, vomiting, bloody diarrhea, unconsciousness	Remove poison (as for baneberry)
Poinsettia (*Euphorbia pulcherrima*)	Leaves, stems, sap	Irritation, vesication, gastroenteritis	Remove poison (as for baneberry); wash sap from skin with soap and water
Primrose (*Primula spp*)	Stems, leaves (primin)	Skin reddening and irritation, itching, swelling, blistering on contact with plant	Wash skin with rubbing alcohol after handling plant
Privet (*Ligustrum vulgare*)	Berries, leaves	GI irritation, renal damage, fall in blood pressure	Remove poison (as for baneberry)
Rayless goldenrod (*Aplopappus heterophyllus*), snakeroot	All parts (tremetol)	Drinking milk from animals that have been fed white snakeroot or rayless goldenrod causes nausea, loss of appetite, weakness, severe vomiting, jaundice from liver damage, constipation, convulsions; there may be oliguria or anuria from kidney damage	Treat liver damage, anuria
Rhododendron	All parts (andromedotoxin)	Salivation, increased tear formation, nasal discharge, vomiting, convulsions, slowing of pulse, lowering of blood pressure, paralysis	Remove poison (as for baneberry)

(Continued.)

TABLE 116–4 (cont.).

Name	Poisons Part of Plant, Active Principle if Known	Clinical Findings	Treatment
Sweet pea (*Lathyrus* spp)	All parts, especially seeds	Paralysis, weak pulse, depressed breathing, convulsions	Remove poison (as for baneberry); give artificial respiration; treat convulsions
Tung nut (*Aleurites fordii*)	Seed (sapotoxin)	Nausea, vomiting, abdominal pain, weakness, fall in blood pressure, shallow respiration	Remove poison (as for baneberry)
Wisteria	All parts	Gastric upset, vomiting	Remove poison (as for baneberry)
Yellow oleander (*Thevetia* spp)	All parts (Digitalis-like)	See Digitalis (Chapter 81)	See Digitalis (Chapter 81)

*From Dreisbach RH, Robertson WO: *Handbook of Poisoning.* Norwalk, Conn, Appleton-Century-Crofts, 1987, pp 498, 500–503. Used by permission.

6. Cardiovascular:
    a. Atrioventricular conduction defects of heart block suggests lily-of-the-valley *(Convallaria)*, foxglove *(Digitalis)*, oleander *(Nerium)*, yellow oleander *(Theretia)*, mistletoe.
    b. Hypotension may result from *Pieris, Phoradendron, Veratrum*. Hypertension may result from *Brugmansia* or *Datura*. Arrhythmias may result from *Aconitum*.
7. Anticholinergic symptoms may suggest jimsonweed *(Datura)*, deadly nightshade *(Atropa)* and henbane *(Hyoscyamus)*, muscimol/ibotenic acid class of mushrooms.
8. Cellular asphyxia: Dyspnea, tachycardia, altered level of consciousness may suggest cyanide intoxication secondary to amygdalin consumption from fruit pits, especially apricot and peach.
C. Classification of common toxic plants: Patients may describe the plant. Color of leaf, flower, or fruit may suggest cause.
    1. Colored leaves:
        a. Red: Poinsettia *(Euphorbia)*.
        b. Variegated: Dumbcane *(Dieffenbachia, Philodendron)*, Snow on Mountain *(Euphorbia)*.
    2. Flowers:
        a. Red: Glory, lily *(Gloriosa, Rhododendron)*, red angel's trumpet *(Brugmansia)*, belladonna lily *(Amaryllis)*.
        b. Yellow: Yellow oleander *(Thevetia)*, buttercup, butter daisy, cursed crowfeet *(Ranunculus)*, golden chain *(Laburnum)*, yellow jessamine *(Gelsamium)*.
        c. Purple: Crocus *(Colchium)*, pasque flower *(Anemone)*, foxglove *(Digitalis)*, monkshood *(Aconitum)*, mescal bean *(Sophora)*, jimson weed *(Datura)*, *Wisteria*.
        d. White: Crocus *(Colchium)*, baneberry *(Actaea)*, windflower (anemone); lily-of-the-valley *(Convallaria)*, horse nettle *(Solanum)*, *Pieris, Rhododendron*, poison hemlock *(Conium)*, water hemlock *(Cicuta)*, red angel's trumpet *(Brugmansia)*, jimson weed *(Datura)*, daffodil *(Narcissus)*, chokecherry *(Prunus)*, pokeweek *(Phytolacca)*.
    3. Berries or fruit:
        a. Red: English yew, Japanese yew *(Taxus)*, baneberry *(Actaea)*, lily-of-the-valley *(Convallaria)*, bittersweet, Jerusalem cherry *(Solanum)*, holly *(Ilex)*, rosary pea *(Abrus)*, chokecherry *(Prunus)*.
        b. Green: *Euphorbia, Hippomane*.
        c. White: Baneberry *(Actaea)*.
        d. Black: Nightshade *(Solanum)*, black cherry *(Prunus)*, pokeweed *(Phytolacca)*.
        e. Yellow: Horse nettle *(Dolanum)*, May apple *(Podophyllum)*.
        f. Variegated: Castor bean *(Ricinus)*.
V. Laboratory findings and evaluation:
A. Laboratory aids are of limited value in diagnosing plant poisoning, but the following should be obtained or monitored in selected poisonings:
    1. CBC and smear: **Intravascular hemolysis** suggests castor bean *(Ricinus)* and rosary pea or jequirity bean *(Abrus)*.

2. PT, PTT, platelets: **Bleeding diathesis** suggests coumarins or pennyroyal oil *(Mentha)*.
3. BUN, creatinine: Renal failure suggests rhubarb leaves or crocus *(Colchicum)*.
4. Liver function studies, PT: **Liver failure** suggests pyrrolizidine poisoning *(Boragineceae)*, found in some herbal teas; cyclopeptide class of mushrooms *(Amanita phalloides)*.
5. **Elevated serum cyanide** suggests amygdalin from fruit pits.
6. Electrolytes if vomiting, diarrhea severe.

VI. General treatment:
  A. Follow APTLS: See Chapter 8.
  B. General management: Table 116–5 (see Chapter 12 for details).

VII. Specific treatment:
  A. Skin: Wash skin and clothes with soapy water, followed by antihistamines and topical corticosteroids for severe dermatitis.
  B. Mouth, pharynx: Milk, popcicles, etc., may be used as soothing agents; antihistamines and corticosteroids may help reduce swelling.
  C. GI: Symptomatic; replace fluid and electrolyte losses.
  D. Cardiac: Symptomatic bradycardia or tachycardia, hypertension or hypotension and arrhythmias should be treated by standard means. Cardiac glycoside poisoning may require Fab fragment antibodies (see Chapter 81).
  E. CNS: Hallucinations may be controlled by reassurance; severe CNS excitation or seizures may require intravenous diazepam 5–10 mg.
  F. Anticholinergic symptoms: See Chapter 91 for treatment recommendation.

VIII. Disposition considerations:
  A. Admission considerations:
    1. See General Admission Considerations (Chapters 17 and 18).
    2. Admission should be considered in those with severe oropharyngeal

TABLE 116–5.

General Treatment

Treatment	Indicated	Of No Value	Contraindicated
O$_2$	±		
IV	±		
ECG monitor	±		
Forced diuresis		X	
Acidification		X	
Alkalinization		X	
Emesis	+		
Lavage*	±		
Charcoal	+		
Cathartic	+		

*Gastric lavage probably has lesser value, particularly if leaf fragments are ingested.

symptoms, severe GI symptoms associated with dehydration, suspected cardiac glycoside ingestion, or sympathomimetic plant intoxication.
3. Suicide risk.
B. Consultation considerations: If plant identification difficult, may want to consult local poison center or botanist at local college or university.
C. Observation period: Cannot make general recommendation because of great variety of plants with different effects.
E. Discharge considerations:
1. General discharge considerations have been met (see Chapters 17 and 18).
2. Each patient requires individual consideration.
3. Suicide risk and psychiatric state have been appropriately evaluated.

BIBLIOGRAPHY

Arena J: Plants that poison. *Emerg Med* 1981; 13:25–57.
Epstein WL: Plant-induced dermatitis. *Ann Emerg Med* 1987; 16:950–955.
Kingsbury JM: Phytotoxicology, in Doull J, Kloassen CD, Amdur MO (eds): *Casarett and Doull's Toxicology*. New York, Macmillan Publishing Co, 1980.
Kunkel DB, Spoerke DG: Medical Toxicology. *Emerg Med Clin North Am* 1984; 2:133–144.
Lampe KF, McCann MA: *AMA Handbook of Poisonous and Injurious Plants*. Chicago, American Medical Association, 1985.
Yarbrough B: Plant poisoning: A comprehensive management guide. *ER Rep* 1983; 3:13–18, 19–24.

117

Food Poisoning

Harlan A. Stueven, M.D., F.A.C.E.P.
David Roberts, M.D., F.A.C.E.P., A.B.M.T.

I. Symptoms of foodborne disease often have insidious onset and are constitutional. Unless suspicion is high, the cause may be missed.
II. There are some geographic predilections for certain foodborne diseases, but persons living in almost any section of the United States could be subject to any foodborne illness.
III. Differential diagnosis:
   A. Herbicides and insecticides that may have been sprayed on plants, such as paraquat and organophosphates.
   B. Insecticides containing toxins such as arsenic and thallium.

Botulism

I. Route of exposure: Oral.
II. Sources of exposure:
   A. Reported from ingestion of home canned foods and vegetables, particularly smoked or pickled.
   B. Honey and intestinal flora can be causes in infants.
III. Onset of action: 8–22 hours.
IV. Toxic mechanism:
   A. Ingestion of food contaminated by feces or soil.
   B. Causative organism: *Clostridium botulinum,* a spore-forming, anaerobic, gram-positive bacillus that produces toxin.
   C. Toxin binds rapidly and irreversibly to peripheral neuromuscular junction, preventing release of acetylcholine and achieving presynaptic block, resulting in muscle paralysis.

V. Range of toxicity:
   A. Most poisonous substance known. Lethal dose is 1 picogram (10^{-9} mg)/ kg, or 0.1–1.0 μg total dose of toxin.
   B. As little as 0.1 ml contaminated food may be fatal.
VI. Clinical features:
   A. GI symptoms after 24 hours.
   b. Descending bilateral symmetric motor paralysis:
      1. Diplopia, dysphoria, dysphagia (bulbar palsy).
      2. Respiratory insufficiency.
   C. Infants (average age 16 weeks) may have weakness, constipation, hypotonia, diminished sucking reflex.
VII. Laboratory findings and evaluation:
   A. No laboratory test available to diagnose botulism in emergency department; diagnosis is clinical. Confirmation comes from botulism in mouse injected with patient's serum or suspect food.
   B. Stool, serum, vomitus, gastric contents, suspect food may be positive for spores or toxin. Specimens should be refrigerated.
   C. Wounds may be cultured anaerobically.
   D. Arterial blood gases, chest radiograph if ventilatory impairment.
VIII. General treatment:
   A. Follow APTLS: See Chapter 8.
   B. General management: Table 117–1 (see Chapter 12 for details).
IX. Specific management:
   A. Aggressive airway management and ventilatory support may be required.
   B. Trivalent antitoxin (A, B, E) should be administered to all patients. If unavailable in hospital pharmacy, trivalent antitoxin is available from Centers for Disease Control (see Consultation considerations for phone number of CDC).
      1. Dose: 1–2 vials IV; repeat in 4 hours.
      2. Desensitization may be required if patient hypersensitive to horse

TABLE 117–1.

General Treatment

Treatment	Indicated	Of No Value	Contraindicated
O$_2$	+		
IV	+		
ECG monitor	+		
Forced diuresis		X	
Acidification			X
Alkalinization		X	
Emesis		X	
Lavage*	±		
Charcoal		X	
Cathartic*†	±		

*Lavage and catharsis may remove spores or toxin from GI tract.
†Caution in face of diarrhea and volume depletion.

serum. Epinephrine should be administered if patient develops signs of anaphylaxis.

X. Prognosis:
   A. Expected response to treatment:
      1. Case fatality rates in literature range from 50%–70% in untreated patients. Use of antitoxin and good supportive therapy can reduce mortality to 10%–25%.
      2. Serum sickness from antitoxin reported 5%–10%.
      3. Total recovery with adequate supportive care usually occurs even in severe cases, although this may take several months to a year.
      4. Mortality in infants less than 5%.
   B. Expected complications and long-term effects:
      1. Acute: CNS hypoxia, aspiration pneumonia, death.
      2. Chronic: Residual neurologic disability and weakness, dysgeusia, dry mouth, constipation, dyspepsia, arthralgia, exertional dyspnea, abnormal pulmonary function testing.
XI. Special considerations: Penicillin probably does not prevent germination of spores in gut, nor is it effective against toxin-produced food poisoning. It is indicated in treatment of infant and wound botulism, because these are caused by active infection with *C. botulinum.*
XII. Controversies:
   A. Guanedine HCl has been used with little success. Not routinely recommended.
   B. Empiric therapy with penicillin probably ineffective in treatment of *C. botulinum* food poisoning.
XIII. Disposition considerations:
   A. Admission considerations:
      1. Any patient with symptoms of botulism or suspected exposure should be hospitalized.
      2. ICU:
         a. Respiratory compromise.
         b. Evidence of neurologic impairment.
   B. Consultation considerations: State health department and Centers for Disease Control in Atlanta should be notified of any case of suspected botulism.
   A. CDC: (404) 329-3311 (information) (404) 329-3644 (evenings, nights)

Other Foodborne Agents of Disease

I. Route of exposure: Oral.
II. Sources of exposure:
   A. Suspect food may give a clue to organism causing foodborne disease.
   B. Foods commonly involved in foodborne diseases:
      1. Beef, chicken, turkey (common organisms: *Salmonella, Clostridium perfringens, Staphylococcus, Campylobacter fetus*).
      2. Ham (common organism: *Staphylococcus*).

3. Pork (common organisms: *Trichinella, Staphylococcus, Salmonella*).
4. Seafood (common organisms: *Salmonella, Vibrio parahaemolyticus*).
5. Bakery, dairy products (common organisms: *Staphylococcus, Salmonella*).
6. Honey products (common organism: *Clostridium botulinum* in infants).
7. Chinese food (causative agent: monosodium glutamate).

III. Onset of action:
  A. Time from ingestion to onset of symptoms is often a clue to causative agent:
    1. Less than 2 hours:
      Monosodium glutamate
      Some mushroom toxins (see Chapter 115).
      Foodborne marine toxins (see Chapter 114):
        Puffer fish toxin
        Scromboid toxin
        Shellfish toxin
    2. 2–8 hours:
      Bacillus cereus
      Ciguatoxin
      Staphylococcus aureus
    3. 8–14 hours:
      B. cereus
      Clostridium perfingens
      Some mushroom toxins (see Chapter 115).
    4. More than 14 hours:
      Escherichia coli
      Clostridium botulinum
      Salmonella
      Shigella
      Streptococcus (group A)
      Trichinella
      Vibrio sp

IV. Toxic mechanism: foodborne agents of disease cause symptoms by two mechanisms:
  A. Invasion: Colonization leads to invasion of lamina propria of bowel wall and subsequent fluid production or bloody diarrhea.
    1. Prototype infections caused by *Salmonella* or *Shigella.*
    2. Other common agents effecting disease via invasion: *Campylobacter fetus, Streptococcus faecalis, Yersinia enterocolitica,* invasive *E. coli.*
  B. Toxin production: Absorption leads to activation of adenyl cyclase, production of cyclic adenosine monophosphate (cAMP) and fluid.
    1. Prototype seen in food poisoning secondary to staphylococcal enterotoxin.
    2. Other common agents effecting disease via toxin: Enterotoxigenic *E. coli, C. botulinum, Vibrio cholera, C. perfringens, B. cereus.*
    3. *S. aureus* toxin also has direct effect on CNS.

V. Clinical features:
  A. Symptoms:
    1. General: Nausea, vomiting, diarrhea, abdominal cramps.
    2. Specific:
       a. Flushing, headache, paresthesias suggest fish toxins.
       b. Pharyngitis suggests *Streptococcus*.
       c. Diplopia with or without descending bulbar palsy suggests *C. botulinum*.
       d. Wheezing may implicate food allergy or sulfites.
    3. Rapid progression to death may occur with certain agents (e.g., *V. cholera*).
  B. Other family or group members eating same foods may develop symptoms at similar time after ingestion.
  C. Physical examination:
    1. Vital signs:
       a. Severe poisonings may cause varying degrees of dehydration, prostration, shock.
       b. In toxin-mediated diseases, temperature may be normal.
       c. In invasive disease, temperature often elevated.
    2. Skin:
       a. Urticaria suggests scromboid toxin.
       b. Orbital edema suggests *Trichinella*.
    3. Neurologic:
       a. Loss of proprioception suggests puffer fish toxin, paralytic shellfish (see Chapter 114).
       b. Symmetric descending motor paralysis suggests *C. botulinum*.
       c. Hot and cold reversal suggests ciguatera poisoning.
    4. Lymphadenopathy suggests *Brucella, Toxoplasma*.
VI. Laboratory findings and evaluation:
  A. Complete blood count:
    1. Leukocytes:
       a. Often not elevated in toxin-mediated diseases.
       b. May be increased with invasive organisms.
    2. Eosinophilia suggests *Trichinella*.
  B. Electrolytes: Abnormalities nonspecific but may be consistent with dehydration.
  C. Stool:
    1. Evidence of occult or severe bleeding and stool leukocytes may be found in invasive diseases and may be helpful in differentiating from toxin-mediated disease.
    2. Cultures should be obtained in patients with severe signs or symptoms lasting more than 1 week.
  D. Examination and culture of incriminated foods for heavy metals, toxins, and larvae may reveal source.
VII. General treatment:
  A. Follow APTLS: See Chapter 8.
  B. General management: Table 117–2 (see Chapter 12 for details).

C. Control severe vomiting by administration of antiemetic such as prochlorperazine 10 mg IM every 4 hours as needed.

D. Diarrhea: Usually generally self-limited; should not be suppressed unless severe and unremitting.

VIII. Specific management:

A. If vomiting and diarrhea are severe, maintain fluid and electrolyte balance by intravenous administration of fluid.

1. To 1 L 5% dextrose in 0.5N saline solution (adult) (1 L 5% dextrose in 0.25N saline solution [child]) add 50 mEq NaHCO and 10–20 mEq KCl. This provides per liter:

	Adult	Child
Na (mEq)	117	80
Cl (mEq)	85–95	47–57
HCO (mEq)	44	44
K (mEq)	10–20	10–20
Dextrose (gm)	50	50

2. **NOTE: If significant vomiting is present, NaHCO should not be added and more KCl may be required.**

B. Antibiotic therapy recommended against the following organisms:

1. ***Shigella:*** Trimethoprim-sulfamethoxazole is drug of choice.

2. ***Entamoeba histolytica*** (amebiasis), ***Giardia:*** metronidazole.

3. ***Salmonella:*** Usually not treated unless underlying illness or severe systemic toxicity. If serious conditions exist, treat with chloramphenicol.

4. ***Campylobacter:*** Usually not treated unless underlying illness or severe systemic toxicity. If serious conditions exist, treat with erythromycin.

5. ***Yersinia:*** Usually not treated unless underlying illness or severe systemic toxicity. If serious conditions exist, treat with gentamicin.

C. Outpatient rehydration therapy:

1. Oral fluids as tolerated for 12–24 hours before beginning regular diet.

TABLE 117–2.

General Treatment

Treatment	Indicated	Of No Value	Contraindicated
O₂	±		
IV	+		
ECG monitor	±		
Forced diuresis			X
Acidification			X
Alkalinization		X	
Emesis/lavage		X/X	
Charcoal		X	
Cathartic			X

   2. Oral rehydration formula for diarrhea:
      a. Prepare two separate glasses of liquids:
         (1) Glass 1:
               8 oz fruit juice (orange, apple, other) rich in potassium
               ½ tsp honey or corn syrup (contains glucose, necessary for
                  absorption of essential salts)
               1 pinch table salt (contains sodium and chloride)
         (2) Glass 2:
               8 oz water (carbonated or boiled)
               ¼ tsp baking soda (contains sodium bicarbonate)
   3. Drink alternately from each glass until thirst is quenched. Supplement
      as desired with carbonated beverages, water, tea made with boiled or
      carbonated water.
   4. When diarrhea has stopped for 24 hours, begin cereal and rice prod-
      ucts, applesauce, ripe bananas (avoid other fruits until this diet toler-
      ated). Next can add legumes and fruit, and later meat. Milk and other
      dairy products should be reintroduced last.
   5. Breast-fed infants should continue feeding and receive plain water as
      desired while receiving these rehydration solutions.
IX. Prognosis:
   A. General: Excellent prognosis, with only 1% fatality rate noted in litera-
      ture. Survival for 48 hours associated with complete recovery.
   B. Specific organisms:
      1. *Shigella:*
         a. Generally self-limited disease, but excretion in stool may continue
            for weeks.
         b. Relapse rate of 10% if untreated.
      2. *Salmonella:* Antidiarrheals and antibiotics may prolong excretion and
         carrier state for months.
      3. *Staphylococcus:* Generally responsive to symptomatic therapy, but
         fatality rate may be as high as 4% in debilitated patients.
X. Special considerations:
   A. Notify local health department of any suspected food poisoning.
   B. See also Chapters 114–116.
XI. Disposition considerations:
   A. Admission considerations:
      1. See General Admissions Considerations (Chapters 17 and 18).
      2. Admission should be considered in cases of severe volume depletion,
         significant electrolyte abnormalities, evidence of sepsis, shock, paraly-
         sis.
      3. Inability to tolerate oral intake.
      4. Underlying debility.
   B. Observation period: Patients with significant volume depletion will re-
      quire intravenous hydration, antinausea medication, observation for 2–3
      hours or until can take sufficient fluids orally to keep up with needs.
   C. Discharge considerations:
      1. General discharge considerations have been met (see Chapters 17 and
         18).

2. Most patients can be discharged after ruling out severe dehydration, significant electrolyte abnormalities, significant GI bleeding, evidence of sepsis, shock, paralysis.
3. Particular care should be taken that appropriate follow-up is arranged.

BIBLIOGRAPHY

Arnon SS, Midura TF, Damus K, et al: Honey and other environmental risk factors for infant botulism. *J Pediatr* 1979; 94:331–336.

Cherington M: Botulism: Ten-year experience. *Arch Neurol* 1974; 30:432–437.

Donta ST: Food Poisoning, in Braude AI (ed): *Medical Microbiology and Infectious Disease.* Philadelphia, WB Saunders Co. 1981, p 1034.

Foster EM: Foodborne hazards of microbial origin. *Fed Proc* 1978; 37:2577–2581.

MacDonald KL, Spengler RF, Hathaway CL, et al: Type A botulism from sauteed onions: Clinical and epidemiological observations. *JAMA* 1985; 1275–1278.

Puggiari M, Cherington M: Botulism and guanidine. *JAMA* 1978; 240:2276–2277.

Schmidt-Nowara WW, Samet JM, Rasario PA: Early and late complications of botulism. *Arch Intern Med* 1983; 143:451–456.

Tacket CO, Shandera WX, Mann JM, et al: Equine antitoxin use and other factors that predict outcome in type A foodborne botulism. *Am J Med* 1984; 76:794–798.

Commercial Products

118

Bleaches, Soaps, Detergents

Robin M. Cuddy, M.D.

Cleaning products have in common the presence of a surfactant, which is the principal determinant of toxicity. A surfactant is anionic when the net charge is negative, and cationic when the net charge is positive. An electrically neutral surfactant is nonionic. In most household products the surfactants are either anionic or nonionic. Cationic surfactants are used in disinfectants, industrial or institutional products, and fabric softeners.

Toxicity is also determined by other ingredients in the product, such as inorganic salts (phosphates, carbonates, silicates, sodium citrate), proteolytic enzymes, fabric softeners, sudscontrolling agents, bleaches, perfumes, soil-redeposition inhibitors, and colorants.

Anionic and Nonionic Detergents and Soaps

  I. Route of exposure: Oral, cutaneous, mucocutaneous, ocular, inhalation.
 II. Common trade names:
     Tide Laundry Detergent
     Bold Laundry Detergent
     Cheer Laundry Detergent
     Ajax Laundry Detergent
III. Absorption: Not absorbed to any great extent.
 IV. Action: See Toxic mechanism.
  V. Uses: Commercial use, laundry detergent, hand soap bars.

VI. Toxic mechanism:
  A. Local corrosive effects likely only with certain types of products:
    1. Anionic detergents, which include soaps, irritate skin by removing oils, which leads to papular dermatitis.
    2. Nonionic detergents are only slightly irritating.
  B. Neither type has significant systemic toxicity.
  C. Water softeners (polyphosphates, tripolyphosphates, pyrophosphates): When added to laundry detergents can bind calcium and cause hypocalcemia; can also increase irritant effect.
  D. Local tissue irritation of GI tract mucous membranes.
VII. Range of toxicity:
  A. Toxic dose: Maximum safe amount for children may be estimated at 0.1–1.0 gm/kg.
  B. Fatal dose: LD_{50} 1–5 gm/kg.
VIII. Clinical features:
  A. Can irritate skin and mucosal membranes.
  B. Ingestion can cause nausea, vomiting, diarrhea, oropharyngeal irritation. Spontaneous emesis will normally occur within an hour if toxic dose ingested.
  C. Eye exposure generally causes momentary eye irritation.
IX. Laboratory findings and evaluation:
  A. Electrolytes (when ingestion associated with protracted vomiting).
  B. Consider hypocalcemia if product contains water softeners.
X. Treatment:
  A. Follow APTLS: See Chapter 8.
  B. Dilute with milk or water.
  C. Emesis or lavage generally not indicated and may be harmful.
  D. Examine mucosal surfaces. Esophagoscopy generally not indicated unless product is indeed caustic (federal regulations require labeling) or there is clinical evidence of caustic ingestion (stridor, drooling, dysphagia, oral burns).
  E. Skin exposures can be treated by flushing skin with water. Eyes should be irrigated with water for 15 minutes. If pain or irritation persists, consider ophthalmology consultation.
XI. Prognosis: No deaths from ingestion reported.
XII. Disposition considerations:
  A. Admission considerations:
    1. See General Admission Considerations (Chapters 17 and 18).
    2. Patients with protracted vomiting or diarrhea should be admitted.
    3. Suicide risk.
  B. Consultation criteria;
    1. If eye pain or irritation persists despite 15 minutes of irrigation, obtain ophthalmology consultation.
    2. GI consultation for endoscopy if indicated.
    3. Psychiatric consultation for any patient who attempted suicide.
  C. Observation period: If spontaneous emesis has not occurred within 2 hours, it is unlikely a toxic dose has been ingested and no further treatment is required.

D. Discharge considerations:
1. Discharge considerations have been met (see Chapters 17 and 18).
2. Suicide potential and psychiatric status have been appropriately evaluated.

Cationic Detergents

I. Route of exposure: Oral, cutaneous, mucocutaneous, ocular, inhalation.
II. Common generic and trade name: Benzalkonium (Zephiran).
III. Uses: Commercial detergents, antiseptic.
IV. Toxic mechanism: Toxicity of cationic detergents consists of interference with many cellular functions, which results in vomiting, confusion, restlessness, possible cardiovascular collapse, convulsions, coma, respiratory and other muscle weakness, and even death.
V. Doses:
A. Toxic dose:
1. Systemic toxicity and death have been reported with ingestions estimated at 30 mg/kg.
2. Corrosive effects have been seen with greater than 7.5% concentration.
B. Fatal dose: 1–3 gm.
VI. Clinical features:
A. Cationic detergents can cause nausea, vomiting, abdominal pain, hemorrhagic necrosis of GI tract, CNS depression, seizures, cardiovascular collapse.
B. Eye exposure can cause irritation or serious corneal damage, depending on concentration of product.
VII. Laboratory findings and evaluation:
A. CBC and spun hematocrit (if evidence of GI bleeding).
B. Ca^{++}, electrolytes, renal function tests.
C. Blood glucose (rule out hypoglycemia in presence of CNS depression).
D. Stool Hemoccult test.
E. Type and cross match blood if indicated.
VIII. Treatment:
A. Follow APTLS: See Chapter 8.
B. General management: See Table 118–1 (see Chapter 12 for details).
C. Dermal exposure: Flush with water.
D. Ocular exposure: Irrigate with water for 15 minutes. If irrigation or pain persists, consult ophthalmologist.
E. Diarrhea is treated symptomatically.
IX. Specific management:
A. Administration of milk or activated charcoal followed by cathartic.
B. Esophagoscopy should be done within 24 hours when history indicates definite ingestion of caustic concentration or when stridor, dysphagia, drooling, oral burns are present.
C. Seizures: See Chapter 22 for treatment recommendations.
D. In rare instances, complex phosphate builders, not commonly used now,

TABLE 118–1.

General Treatment

Treatment	Indicated	Of No Value	Contraindicated
O$_2$	±		
IV	+		
ECG monitor	±		
Forced diuresis		X	
Acidification			X
Alkalinazation		X	
Emesis*/lavage*	± / ±		
Charcoal*	±		
Cathartic*	±		
Hemodialysis		X	

*Contraindicated in presence of esophageal injury.

produce dangerous hypocalcemic tetany requiring calcium administration.

X. Prognosis: Survival for 48 hours associated with full recovery.
XI. Disposition considerations: See anionic and nonionic detergents and soaps, above.

Bleach

I. Route of exposure: Oral, cutaneous, monocutaneous, ocular, inhalation.
II. Common generic and trade names:
  A. Liquid household bleaches usually contain from 3%–6% sodium hypochlorite. Concentration is higher in granular bleaches.
  B. Trade name: Clorox.
III. Uses: Household bleach (hypochlorite), commercial bleaches.
IV. Toxic mechanism:
  A. Irritating to all mucous membranes.
  B. Not associated with extensive tissue destruction or potential for stricture formation as with caustic alkaline corrosives. Exception: Commercial bleaches containing peroxides or perborates, which may be frankly caustic.
  C. Can produce intense eye irritation.
  D. Ingestion of hypochlorite in high concentrations can be sufficiently irritating to produce emesis and some gastric distress.
V. Range of toxicity:
  A. Toxic dose: Related to complications.
  B. Fatal dose: 30 ml in children if emesis does not occur.
VI. Clinical features:
  A. Nausea, vomiting, oropharyngeal irritation, intense eye irritation, coughing.
  B. May rarely see hyperchloremia and metabolic acidosis.

VII. Laboratory findings and evaluation:
    A. Electrolytes and renal function tests (BUN, creatinine).
    B. Arterial blood gases (if metabolic acidosis a consideration).
    C. Chest radiograph (if significant cough).
VIII. Treatment:
    A. Follow APTLS: See Chapter 8.
    B. Except for massive suicidal ingestions, do not induce emesis or lavage.
    C. Dilute by giving milk or water.
    D. Corrosive damage to GI tract is rare with household bleach ingestion, so unless there is clinical evidence of caustic ingestion (stridor, drooling, dysphagia), esophagoscopy not indicated.
    E. Industrial strength (greater than 5% concentration) bleach ingestions should be treated as caustic ingestion (see Chapter 73).
    F. Skin should be flushed with water.
    G. Eyes should be flushed immediately and irrigated for 15 minutes. If pain or irritation persists, consult ophthalmologist.
  IX. Prognosis: Prognosis excellent with early institution of therapy and good supportive care.
   X. Special considerations:
    A. Production of potentially lethal gases when other cleaning products are mixed with hypochlorite solutions contained in household bleaches.
      1. Addition of some bleaches to ammonia may cause liberation of chloramine gas.
      2. Addition of acid produces either hypochlorous acid or chlorine gas, depending on strength of acid.
      3. Addition of liquid dishwashing detergent may also cause formation of either hypochlorous acid or chlorine gas.
      4. Ammonia solutions can react with alkali to form large amounts of ammonia gas.
    B. Clinical presentation:
      1. Both ammonia and chloramine gas may produce some narcosis.
      2. Ammonia, chloramine, chlorine, hypochlorous acid gas produce severe pulmonary irritation, possibly pulmonary edema.
    C. Treatment:
      1. Systemic effects are treated supportively.
      2. Pulmonary effects can be treated with oxygen, positive-pressure assisted ventilation, and bronchodilators as needed.
  XI. Disposition considerations: See Anionic and nonionic detergents and soaps.

Strongly Acidic or Alkaline Products

   I. Route of exposure: Oral, cutaneous, mucocutaneous, ocular, inhalation.
  II. Common trade names:
    Electrasol
    Lysol Toilet Bowel Cleaner
    Liquid Plumber
    Easy Off Oven Cleaner

Top Job

Spic & Span

III. Action: See Chapter 73.

IV. Uses:

A. Electric dishwasher detergent, toilet bowl cleaner, drain cleaner, oven cleaner.

B. Selected household cleaners for walls and hard surfaces, selected laundry products containing high concentrations of sodium borates, carbonates, phosphates, silicates. Consult poison center (see Chapter 4 for listing) for specific product formulations.

V. Toxic mechanism:

A. Liquid products usually contain fairly concentrated hydrochloric acid.

B. Granular products contain sodium bisulfate.

C. Some toilet bowl cleaners contain hypochlorite in a fairly alkaline solution.

D. Concentrated ammonia products (oven cleaners, drain cleaners) are usually highly alkaline.

E. Also see Chapter 73.

VI. Range of toxicity: See Chapter 73.

VII. Clinical features: See Chapter 73.

VIII. Laboratory findings and evaluation: See Chapter 73.

IX. Treatment: See Chapter 73.

X. Prognosis: See Chapter 73.

XI. Special considerations: Certain alkaline ammonia products (oven, drain cleaners) are composed of solid granules coated with thin layer of paraffin to prevent immediate dissolution in water; this may delay corrosive effects. In this specific instance, emptying stomach may be safe and worthwhile if patient is seen within 30 minutes of ingestion and has no oropharyngeal burns and no pain to suggest esophageal or gastric burns.

XII. Disposition considerations: See Chapter 73.

Granular Soaps and Detergents

I. Route of exposure: Oral, cutaneous, mucocutaneous, ocular, inhalation.

II. Uses: Group includes household products intended for laundry, dishwashing (except automatic-dishwater detergents), cleaning of hard surfaces.

III. Toxic mechanism:

A. Low potential for systemic toxicity. Some laundry detergents and cleaners for hard surfaces are alkaline and have potential for causing esophageal burns, although these are usually minor and do not cause any mucosal injury.

B. Remaining products are expected at most to produce vomiting, diarrhea.

IV. Clinical features:

A. Nausea, vomiting, oropharyngeal irritation, intense eye irritation, coughing.

B. Rarely, hyperchloremia, metabolic acidosis.

V. Laboratory findings and evaluation:

A. Electrolytes, renal function tests (BUN, creatinine).

VI. Treatment:
    A. Follow APTLS: See Chapter 8.
    B. Except for massive suicidal ingestions, do not induce emesis or lavage.
    C. Dilute by giving milk or water.
    D. Skin should be flushed with water.
    E. Eyes should be flushed immediately and irrigated for 15 minutes. If pain or irritation persists, consult ophthalmologist.
    F. May require intravenous fluids if vomiting, diarrhea severe.
VII. Prognosis: Prognosis excellent with early therapy and good supportive care.
VIII. Special considerations:
    A. Some products contain enzymes or antiseptics, but these do not influence toxicity significantly.
    B. Liquid detergents:
        1. Similar composition to granular products, but toxicity even lower; however, liquid products likely to be ingested in larger quantities.
        2. Treatment remains the same.
        3. Liquid detergents may be part of mixture with weak alcohol solutions; however, concentration of alcohol is low, with little potential for systemic toxicity. Exception is very rare possibility of inducing hypoglycemia in pediatric age group.
IX. Disposition considerations: See anionic and nonionic detergents and soaps.

Liquid Hard Surface Cleaners

  I. Route of exposure: Oral, cutaneous, mucocutaneous, ocular, inhalation.
  II. Composition:
    A. Most contain either pine oil (mixture of turpene alcohols and turpene hydrocarbons or ethers along with borneol) or petroleum distillates.
    B. Amount of pine oil varies from trace amounts to impart pine odor up to 38%.
  III. Toxic mechanism:
    A. See Chapter 104.
    B. Pine oil has low aspiration potential because of low surface tension and addition of ingredients that cause some thickening.
    C. Some minor CNS narcotic effects unless ingestion large.
  IV. Clinical features:
    A. Pine oil causes irritation to eyes and mucous membranes.
    B. Hemorrhagic gastritis.
    C. Systemic effects may include weakness, CNS depression, hypothermia, respiratory failure.
  V. Laboratory findings and evaluation:
    A. Electrolytes, renal function tests (BUN, creatinine).
    B. Arterial blood gases (with respiratory distress)
    C. Blood glucose (check for hypoglycemia in presence of CNS depression, weakness).
    D. CBC and immediate spun hematocrit if signifiant GI bleeding.
    E. Stool hemoccult test.
    F. Chest radiograph (if significant respiratory symptoms).

VI. Treatment:
  A. Follow APTLS: See Chapter 8.
  B. It is important to determine exact pine oil content of product ingested.
  C. If large amount of a more potent preparation ingested, GI decontamination should proceed, with induction of emesis or lavage.
  D. If small amount ingested, dilution with milk probably sufficient.
  E. Treatment thereafter is supportive and symptomatic.
  F. Exposed skin should be flushed with water.
  G. Eyes should be irrigated with water for 15 minutes. If irritation or pain persists, consult an ophthalmologist.
VII. Prognosis: Prognosis good with appropriate treatment and supportive care.
VIII. Disposition considerations:
  A. Admission considerations:
    1. See General Admission Considerations (Chapters 17 and 18).
    2. All patients with the following symptoms should be admitted: Hemorrhagic gastritis; systemic effects such as weakness, CNS depression, hypothermia, respiratory failure.
    3. Suicide risk.
  B. Consultation considerations: See Anionic and nonionic detergents and soaps.
  C. Observation period: See Anionic and nonionic detergents and soaps.
  D. Discharge considerations: See Anionic and nonanionic detergents and soaps.

Bar Soaps

  I. Route of exposure: Oral, cutaneous, mucocutaneous, ocular, inhalation.
  II. Toxic mechanism: True soaps are salts of fatty acids; all have low toxicity.
  III. Clinical features: Some vomiting, diarrhea, other signs of mild GI irritation.
  IV. Laboratory findings and evaluation:
  A. Electrolytes and renal function tests (BUN, creatinine).
  V. Treatment:
  A. Follow APTLS: See Chapter 8.
  B. Except for massive suicidal ingestions, do not induce emesis or lavage. Attempts to perform lavage may be associated with sufficient sudsing to cause severe distension. Distention can be treated by administering weak alcohol solution.
  C. Dilute by giving milk or water. This will counter mild GI irritation.
  D. May require intravenous fluids if vomiting, diarrhea severe.
  VI. Prognosis: Excellent with early therapy and supportive care.
  VII. Special considerations: Deodorant soaps sometimes contain photosensitizing compounds, but presence of germicidal agents such as hexachlorophene has low potential for toxicity in concentrations used in commercial preparations.
  VIII. Disposition considerations:
  A. See Anionic and nonionic detergents and soaps.
  B. Patients generally do well and can be discharged home unless ingestion is associated with protracted vomiting, diarrhea, electrolyte imbalance.

Other Products

I. Fabric softeners:
   A. Generally nontoxic.
   B. Some preparations contain cationic surfactants, but concentration in liquid products is low and solid preparations do not lend themselves to massive ingestion.

II. Hand cleaners:
   A. Liquid hand cleaners:
      1. Most liquid hand cleaners are soaps, with few adverse effects. Potential for some toxicity from alcohol, essential oils that some contain.
   B. Powdered or cake hand cleaners:
      1. Powdered or cake hand cleaners are usually soaps containing only abrasive such as pumice and some sodium phosphate or carbonate. As a result, they have little toxicity excpet for some GI irritation.
      2. A few preparations contain high concentrations of boric acid. Symptoms may include hemorrhagic gastroenteritis, CNS depression, shock, kidney and hepatic injury. See also Chapters 73 and 119.
   C. Waterless hand cleaners:
      1. Waterless hand cleaners are usually soaps containing organic solvent such as naphtha in addition to anionic surfactant. Symptoms after large ingestions include CNS stimulation or narcosis, hemolysis, hepatic and renal injury. See also Anionic and Nonionic Detergents and Soaps, and Chapter 104.

III. Shampoos:
   A. Consist of synthetic ethanolamine nonionic surfactants, with only slightly greater toxicity than bar soaps.
   B. Toxic effects are similar to those of bar soaps, consisting mainly of GI irritation (vomiting and diarrhea), irritation of eyes.
   C. Some liquid soapless shampoos contain an anionic surfactant, which is somewhat more toxic; symptoms are the same.
   D. See Anionic and Nonionic Detergents and Soaps.

IV. Hair rinses:
   A. Hair rinses, including coloring products, have about same toxic potential as shampoos, except presence of silver nitrate and ammonia leads to greater toxicity.
   B. Hair lighteners with color are often quite alkaline and contain hydrogen peroxide, alcohol, propylene glycol.
   C. Conditioner rinses have even lower toxicity than shampoos.

V. Bath preparations:
   A. Bath salts or bubble bath often contain anionic surfactants or trisodium phosphate or both; may be moderately irritating, particularly with trisodium phosphate.
   B. Systemic toxicity rare except in borax-containing preparations, but requires very large quantities to be ingested.
   C. Bath oils often contain sulfated caster oil and fairly large amounts of perfumes (essential oils). Caster oil may cause diarrhea; essential oils may produce gastroenteritis (vomiting, diarrhea), CNS stimulation or depression, renal injury.

BIBLIOGRAPHY

Arena JM: Poisonings and other health hazards associated with use of detergents. *JAMA* 1964; 190:168–170.

Cann HM, Verhulst HL: Toxicity of household products and treatment of their ingestion. *AM J Dis Child* 1960; 100:157–160.

Done AK: The toxic emergency: Toxicology next to cleanliness. *Emerg Med* Aug 1981, pp 187–201.

Dreisbach RH, Robertson WO: *Handbook of Poisoning,* ed 12. Norwalk, Conn, Appleton-Century-Crofts, 1987.

Gosselin RE, Smith RP, Hodge HC: *Clinical Toxicology of Commercial Products,* ed 5. Baltimore, Williams & Wilkins Co, 1984.

Lawrence RA, Haggerty RJ: Household agents and their potential toxicity. *Modern Treatment* 1974; 8:511–527.

Litovitz T: The toxicity of household products. *Ear Nose Throat J* 1983; 62:7–18.

119

Antiseptics and Disinfectants

Robin M. Cuddy, M.D.

Although severe complications are generally uncommon, all antiseptics and disinfectants are capable of producing at least GI irritation with vomiting and possibly diarrhea, in addition to agitation, convulsions, and respiratory distress. Aside from dilution with milk or other demulcents and possibly gastric emptying, treatment is supportive and symptomatic.

Boric Acid

I. Route of exposure: Oral, transdermal, mucous membranes.
II. Common products containing borate:
    Boraxo Powdered Hand Soap
    Harris Famous Roach Tablets
    Murine Plus Eye Drops
    Flex-Care for Soft Contact Lenses
III. Pharmacokinetics:
    A. Onset of action: Rapidly absorbed; toxic symptoms may be delayed for several hours.
    B. Duration of action: About half excreted in urine in first 12 hours; remainder eliminated over 5–7 days.
    C. Elimination: Kidneys.
IV. Action:
    A. Boric acid produced by action of sulfuric acid on sodium borate.
    B. Only mildly bacteriostatic.
    C. Effective buffer against alkali.
    D. Causes powders to flow more freely.

V. Uses:
    A. Antiseptic.
    B. Buffer in talcum.
    C. Insecticides.
    D. Baby powder preparations.
    E. Eye washes.
VI. Toxic mechanism: Unknown. Toxic to all cells.
VII. Range of toxicity:
    A. Adults: Estimated fatal dose: 15–20 gm.
    B. Children: Estimated fatal dose: 5–6 gm.
    C. 2.9–4.4 gm boric acid in 1 tsp 100% boric acid.
VIII. Clinical features:
    A. GI: Abdominal pain, nausea, vomiting, bloody diarrhea.
    B. Skin: Erythroderma ("boiled lobster" appearance).
    C. CNS: Lethargy, seizures.
    D. Other: Cardiovascular collapse, renal failure.
IX. Laboratory findings and evaluation:
    A. Blood tests:
        1. Chemistry: Electrolytes (if vomiting and diarrhea severe); BUN and creatinine (if evidence of renal insufficiency).
        2. CBC and spun hematocrit.
        3. Type and screen.
        4. Blood glucose (rule out hypoglycemia in presence of lethargy or seizures).
    B. ECG (if impaired cardiovascular function).
    C. Urinalysis (if evidence of renal insufficiency).
X. General treatment:
    A. Follow APTLS: See Chapter 8.
    B. General management: Table 119–1 (see Chapter 12 for details).
XI. Specific management:
    A. Skin should be washed with soap and water. Exposed eyes should be irrigated with water for 15 minutes. If irritation or pain persists, consult ophthalmologist.

TABLE 119–1.

General Treatment

Treatment	Indicated	Of No Value	Contraindicated
O$_2$	±		
IV	+		
ECG monitor	±		
Forced diuresis		X	
Acidification			X
Alkalinization		X	
Emesis/lavage	+/+		
Charcoal	+		
Cathartic	+		

B. Monitor renal function, fluid and electrolyte balance carefully.

C. Seizures: See Chapter 22.

D. Dialysis:

    1. Consider **hemodialysis** in severely symptomatic adults.

    2. Consider **peritoneal dialysis** in infants.

XII. Prognosis:

  A. Expected response to treatment: In the past, more than 50% of infants with symptomatic boric acid poisoning died. This type of poisoning is now rare.

  B. Expected complications and long-term effects:

    1. Anuria.

    2. Skin infections.

XIII. Disposition considerations:

  A. Admission considerations:

    1. See General Admission Considerations (Chapters 17 and 18).

    2. All patients who are symptomatic or who have history of significant ingestion should be admitted.

    3. ICU: Hemodynamic instability.

  B. Consultation considerations:

    1. Nephrology consultation if dialysis indicated for renal impairment.

    2. Ophthalmologist for ocular exposure symptomatic after treatment.

  C. Observation period:

    1. Symptomatic patients should be admitted and not observed in emergency department.

    2. Since elimination may take several hours to days, asymptomatic patients with history of significant ingestion should be admitted and not observed expectantly in emergency department.

    3. Asymptomatic patients with insignificant ingestions who remain asymptomatic after 6–8 hours of observation may be discharged.

  D. Discharge considerations: See General Discharge considerations (Chapters 17 and 18).

Potassium Permanganate

  I. Route of exposure: Mucocutaneous.

  II. Pharmacokinetics:

    A. Immediate onset of irritant effects to esophageal and gastric surfaces.

    B. Systemic effects of minor importance because of poor absorption.

  III. Action: Oxidizing agent.

  IV. Uses: Disinfectant.

  V. Toxic mechanism:

    A. Alkaline caustic action on mucous membranes.

    B. Deaths have resulted from upper airway edema.

  VI. Range of toxicity:

    A. Fatal dose: Estimated at 10 gm in adults.

  VII. Clinical features:

    A. GI: Brown discoloration and edema of mucous membranes; abdominal pain.

      B. Pulmonary: Cough, laryngeal edema, stridor.

      C. Other: Cardiovascular collapse, renal failure.

VIII. Laboratory findings and evaluation:

      A. Blood tests:

          1. Chemistry: Electrolytes (if vomiting and diarrhea severe); BUN and creatinine (if evidence of renal insufficiency).

          2. CBC and spun hematocrit.

          3. Type and screen.

          4. Blood glucose (rule out hypoglycemia in presence of lethargy, seizures).

      B. ECG (if impaired cardiovascular function).

      C. Arterial blood gases, chest radiograph (if evidence of respiratory distress).

      D. Urinalysis (if evidence of renal insufficiency).

IX. General treatment:

      A. Follow APTLS: See Chapter 8.

      B. General management: Table 119–2 (see Chapter 12 for details).

  X. Specific management:

      A. Emergency cricothyroidotomy may be life-saving in presence of upper airway obstruction secondary to edema.

      B. Wash mucous membranes with water. Flush skin with water.

      C. Irrigate exposed eyes with water for 15 minutes; if pain or irritation persists, consult ophthalmologist.

      D. Dilute with milk, egg white, water.

      E. Esophagoscopy should be done within 24 hours to rule out esophageal injury.

      F. Monitor renal function, fluid and electrolyte balance. Dialysis may be required for severe renal impairment.

XI. Prognosis:

      A. Expected response to treatment:

          1. Death may occur up to 1 month after exposure (e.g., peritonitis).

      B. Expected complications and long-term effects:

          1. Anuria.

          2. Esophageal strictures.

TABLE 119–2.

General Treatment

Treatment	Indicated	Of No Value	Contraindicated
O$_2$	+		
IV	+		
ECG monitor	+		
Forced Diuresis		X	
Acidification			X
Alkalinization		X	
Emesis*/Lavage*			X/X
Charcoal*			X
Cathartic*			X

*Caustic ingestion.

XII. Disposition considerations:
    A. Admission considerations:
        1. See General admission considerations (Chapters 17 and 18).
        2. All patients who are symptomatic should be admitted.
        3. ICU: If hemodynamically unstable.
    B. Consultation considerations:
        1. Anesthesiology consultation for severe airway compromise.
        2. Nephrology consultation if dialysis indicated for renal impairment.
        3. Ophthalmologist for ocular exposure symptomatic after treatment.
        4. Gastroenterology consultation within 24 hours if endoscopy indicated.
    C. Observation period: Symptomatic patients should be admitted and not observed in emergency department.
    D. Discharge considerations: See General discharge considerations (Chapters 17 and 18).

Chlorate

    I. Route of exposure: Oral.
    II. Pharmacokinetics:
        A. Immediate onset of irritant effects to esophageal and gastric surfaces.
    III. Uses:
        A. Antiseptic.
        B. Mouthwash.
        C. Matches.
    IV. Toxic mechanism:
        A. Produces methemoglobinemia.
        B. Causes hemolysis.
        C. Toxic to proximal renal tubules (e.g., toxic nephritis).
        D. CNS depression.
    V. Range of toxicity:
        A. Fatal adult dose: Estimated at 15–30 gm.
        B. Fatal pediatric dose: Estimated at 2 gm.
    VI. Clinical features:
        A. GI: Gastritis, nausea, vomiting, abdominal pain.
        B. Pulmonary: Cyanosis resistant to oxygen therapy.
        C. CNS: Confusion, seizures.
        D. Hematology: Methemoglobinemia, hemolysis (see Chapter 102).
        E. Renal: Oliguria, anuria (e.g., toxic nephritis).
    VII. Laboratory findings and evaluation:
        A. Blood tests:
            1. Chemistry: Electrolytes (if vomiting and diarrhea severe); BUN and creatinine (if evidence of renal insufficiency).
            2. CBC and spun hematocrit.
            3. Type and screen.
            4. Blood glucose (rule out hypoglycemia in presence of mental status changes, depressed level of consciousness, seizures).
            5. Methemoglobin level (see Chapter 102).

B. ECG (if impaired cardiovascular function).

C. Arterial blood gases and chest radiograph (if evidence of respiratory distress).

D. Urinalysis (if evidence of renal insufficiency); check for hemoglobinuria.

VIII. General treatment:

A. Follow APTLS: See Chapter 8.

B. General management: Table 119–3 (see Chapter 12 for details).

IX. Specific management:

A. Wash mucous membranes with water. Flush skin with water.

B. Irrigate exposed eyes with water for 15 minutes; if pain or irritation persists, consult ophthalmologist.

C. Give 2–5 gm 1% sodium thiosulfate in 200 ml 5% sodium bicarbonate orally or intravenously. This inactivates chlorate and serves as specific antidote.

D. Assure adequate urine output and renal function. Consider alkaline diuresis if methemoglobinemia suspected. In preliminary animal studies, alkaline diuresis decreased renal necrosis and methemoglobinemia associated with chlorate poisoning.

E. Ascorbic acid and methylene blue have been used to combat formation of methemoglobin. Give 0.2 ml/kg methylene blue (IV over 5 minutes) and 500 mg–1 gm ascorbic acid (orally or by slow IV push) if patient is cyanotic or if methemoglobin level greater than 30% (see Controversies, below).

F. Monitor renal function, fluid and electrolyte balance.

G. For severe symptoms, consider exchange transfusions and hemodialysis for removal of chlorate.

X. Prognosis

A. Expected response to treatment:

1. Death may occur up to 1 week after poisoning, but if symptoms are mild or absent after first 12 hours, recovery expected.

TABLE 119–3.

General Treatment

Treatment	Indicated	Of No Value	Contraindicated
O$_2$ (100%)	+		
IV	+		
ECG monitor	+		
Forced diuresis†	?		
Acidification			X
Alkalinization†	?		
Emesis/lavage	+/+		
Charcoal	+		
Cathartic	+		
Dialysis*	±		

*Potential renal toxicity.
†Still experimental. Used effectively for treatment of methemoglobinemia in animal model (see below).

B. Expected complications:
 1. Anuria.
 2. Cardiopulmonary arrest.
 3. Seizures.
XI. Controversies:
 A. It is controversial as to whether methylene blue in high doses (cumulative dose >15 mg/kg) may actually increase level of methemoglobin by regenerating chlorate ion.
 B. Ascorbic acid has been used successfully for congenital forms of methemoglobinemia, but many believe it not useful in acquired (chemically induced) methemoglobinemia.
XII. Disposition considerations:
 A. Admission considerations:
 1. See General Admission Considerations (Chapters 17 and 18).
 2. All patients who are symptomatic should be admitted.
 3. See Chapter 102.
 4. ICU: If hemodynamically unstable.
 B. Consultation considerations:
 1. Nephrology consultation if dialysis indicated for renal impairment.
 2. Hematologist should be consulted for possible exchange transfusion in extremely symptomatic patients (especially neonates and children) in whom methemoglobinemia is unresponsive to methylene blue.
 3. Ophthalmologist for ocular exposure symptomatic after treatment.
 4. Inform public health authorities if poisoning secondary to environmental or occupational exposure.
 C. Observation period:
 1. Symptomatic patients should be admitted and not observed in emergency department.
 2. See Chapter 102.
 D. Discharge considerations:
 1. See General discharge considerations (Chapters 17 and 18).

Benzalkonium Chloride

I. Route of exposure: Oral, ocular, skin.
II. Common trade names:
 Roccal
 BTC
 Zephiran
III. Onset of action: Immediate corrosive effects on mucous membranes.
IV. Action: Cationic surfactant.
V. Uses: Germicide, sanitizer, disinfectant.
VI. Toxic mechanism:
 A. See Cationic detergents (Chapter 118).
 B. Interferes with many cellular functions. Nature of biochemical and pharmacologic effect responsible for systemic effects not known.
 C. Direct corrosive effects on GI tract.

VII. Range of toxicity:
  A. Toxic Dose: Estimated at 1–3 gm.
  B. Fatal dose: 100–700 mg/kg (laboratory mammals).
VIII. Clinical features:
  A. GI: Burning pain in mouth, throat, abdomen, accompanied by copious salivation, emesis. Severe cases may produce hemetemesis.
  B. Cardiovascular: Hypotension in severe poisoning.
  C. Neurological: Restlessness, confusion, weakness, CNS depression, seizures.
  D. Pulmonary: Dyspnea, cyanosis, respiratory paralysis.
 IX. Laboratory findings and evaluation:
  A. Blood tests:
    1. Chemistry: Electrolytes (If vomiting severe); BUN and creatinine (if evidence of renal insufficiency).
    2. CBC and spun hematocrit.
    3. Type and screen.
    4. Blood glucose (rule out hypoglycemia in presence of altered mental status, depressed level of consciousness, seizures).
  B. ECG (if impaired cardiovascular function).
  C. Arterial blood gases, chest radiograph (if evidence of respiratory distress).
  D. Urinalysis (if evidence of renal insufficiency).
  X. General treatment:
  A. Follow APTLS: See Chapter 8.
  B. General management: Table 119–4 (see Chapter 12 for details).
 XI. Specific management:
  A. Emergency cricothyroidotomy may be life-saving in presence of upper airway obstruction secondary to edema.
  B. Wash mucous membranes with water. Flush skin with water.
  C. Irrigate exposed eyes with water for 15 minutes; if pain or irritation persists, consult ophthalmologist.

TABLE 119–4.

General Treatment

Treatment	Indicated	Of No Value	Contraindicated
O₂	±		
IV	+		
ECG monitor	±		
Forced diuresis		X	
Acidification			X
Alkalinization		X	
Emesis*/lavage*			X/X
Charcoal†			X
Cathartic*			X

*If dilute solution (2% or less) has been ingested and little or no emesis has occurred spontaneously, gastric emptying by emesis or lavage may be attempted followed by cathartic.
†Charcoal contraindicated because may obscure mucosal damage during subsequent endoscopy.

D. Dilute with milk, egg white, water.
E. Hypotension: See Chapter 10.
F. Esophagoscopy should be done within 24 hours to rule out esophageal injury.
G. Monitor renal function, fluid and electrolyte balance. Dialysis may be required for severe renal impairment.
H. Seizures: See Chapter 22.
XII. Prognosis:
  A. Expected response to treatment:
    1. In fatal cases, death occurs rapidly, within 1–2 hours.
    2. If patient survives for 48 hours, recovery likely.
  B. Expected complications and long-term effects:
    1. Renal failure may develop secondary to prolonged hypotension.
XIII. Disposition considerations:
  A. Admission considerations:
    1. See General Admission Considerations (Chapters 17 and 18).
    2. All patients who are symptomatic should be admitted.
    3. ICU: If hemodynamically unstable.
  B. Consultation considerations:
    1. Anesthesiology consultation for severe airway compromise.
    2. Nephrology consultation if dialysis indicated for renal impairment.
    3. Ophthalmologist for ocular exposure symptomatic after treatment.
    4. Gastroenterology consultation within 24 hours if endoscopy indicated.
  C. Observation period:
    1. Symptomatic patients should be admitted and not observed in emergency department.
  D. Discharge considerations:
    1. See General Discharge Considerations (Chapters 17 and 18).

Phenol

I. See Chapter 75.

BIBLIOGRAPHY

Done AK: Disinfectant cleaners: Toxicology next to cleanliness. *Emerg Med* Aug 1981, pp 187–201.
Dreisbach RH, Robertson WO: Antiseptics, in *Handbook of Poisoning.* Norwalk, Conn, Appleton and Lange, 1987, pp 360–376.
Goldfrank LR, Flomenbaum NE, Lewin NA, et al: *Goldfrank's Toxicologic Emergencies,* ed 3. Norwalk, Conn, Appleton-Century-Crofts, 1986, pp 249–256.
Gosselin RE, Smith RR, Hodge HC: *Clinical Toxicology of Commercial Products,* ed 5. Baltimore, Williams & Wilkins Co, pp 109, 112, 118.
Lawrence RA, Haggerty RJ: Household products and their potential toxicity. *Modern Treatment* 1974; 8:511–527.
Litovitz T: The toxicity of household products. *Ear Nose Throat* 1983; 62:7–18.
Poisindex. Denver, Micromedex, Inc, 1986, 1987.

Miscellaneous

120

Salt (Sodium Chloride)

James J. Walter, M.D., F.A.C.E.P.

I. Route of exposure: Oral, rectal, intravenous.
II. Sources of salts involved in overdose:
    A. Severe salt intoxication:
        1. Ingestion of table salt or salt tablets by unattended infants, mentally retarded adults, or as intended overdose.
        2. Strong salt solution used as emetic or as gastric lavage solution, which was in practice until early 1970s.
        3. Use of salt water enemas.
        4. Inadvertent use of salt instead of sugar in preparation of infant formula.
        5. Excessive administration of skim milk to infants or inadequately diluted bouillion (home remedy for diarrhea).
        6. Excess salt intake and water deprivation as form of child abuse.
        7. Inadequately monitored intravenous infusion of saline solution (e.g., $NaHCO_3$, hypertonic saline solution).
III. Pharmacokinetics:
    A. Absorption: NaCl rapidly absorbed in any concentration and via any route of administration (orally, rectally, gastric lavage).
    B. Elimination: 90%–95% of intake excreted in urine.
IV. Action: Na^+ distributed in extracellular compartment; contributes to osmotic stability and preservation of normal muscle and nerve transmembrane potential. As NaCl and $NaHCO_3$, sodium salts play important role in regulating acid-base balance.
V. Uses:
    A. See Sources of salts involved in overdose.
    B. In United States, average adult consumes 10 gm salt per day (approximately 4 gm or 170 mEq Na^+/day).

VI. Toxic mechanism:
A. Hypernatremia occurs when proportion of Na⁺ to body water exceeds normal.
B. Increases in serum Na⁺ concentration cause shift of water from intracellular to extracellular space, resulting in cellular dessication.
C. CNS consequences are most serious. Combination of "brain shrinkage" and distention of intracranial blood vessels can result in subarachnoid, intraventricular, parenchymal hemorrhages.
D. Pulmonary congestion common if patient not simultaneously hypovolemic.
E. Renal damage consisting of vacuolization of renal tubular cells and acute tubular necrosis well documented and occurs often in severe hypernatremia.
F. Na⁺ can be quite toxic. One tablespoon salt (18 gm NaCl) absorbed and retained raises serum Na⁺ by 30 mEq/L in 3-year-old child. Since salt poisoning impairs ability of kidneys to excrete excess solute, significant acute ingestion can lead to striking hypernatremia, severe symptoms, and even death.

VII. Range of toxicity:
A. Toxic dose: It is estimated that ingestion of 0.5–1.0 gm/kg NaCl (8.5–17 mEq/kg Na⁺) is toxic in majority of patients.
B. Fatal dose: 3 gm/kg NaCl (50 mEq/kg Na⁺) likely fatal.
C. Dose conversions:
23 mg Na⁺ = 1 mEq Na⁺
59 mg NaCl contains 1 mEq Na⁺
1 gm NaCl contains 17 mEq Na⁺ (390 mg)
1 tsp NaCl = 6 gm NaCl, or 2,300 mg Na⁺, or 100 mEq Na⁺

VIII. Clinical features:
A. General: Fever occurs in majority of patients.
B. GI: Nausea, vomiting, diarrhea, abdominal cramping are usually earliest symptoms. Swollen tongue may be seen. Thirst often intense.
C. Neurologic: Weakness, irritability, headache, dizziness; progression to obtundation, convulsions, coma.
D. Cardiovascular: hypotension or hypertension may be seen; may depend on associated volume status.
E. Respiratory: Pulmonary congestion, respiratory distress common.

IX. Laboratory findings and evaluation:
A. Electrolyte panel:
1. Observe Na⁺ level closely (every 2–4 hours) initially as well as other electrolytes.
a. With Na⁺ levels 150–160 mEq/L, CNS symptoms are common, seizures can occur in 10% of patients.
b. With levels of 160–180 mEq/L, convulsions are more frequent, especially if treatment precipitates rapid fall in Na⁺ concentration (>1 mEq/L/hr).
2. Death frequent with serum Na⁺ levels 185 mEq/L.
B. Other tests dictated by clinical situation:
1. Arterial blood gases (with pulmonary edema).
2. Calculation of osmolarity.

X. General treatment:
   A. Follow APTLS: See Chapter 8.
   B. General management: Table 120–1 (see Chapter 12 for details).
XI. Specific treatment:
   A. Hypotension or shock: See Chapter 10.
   B. Hypernatremia:
      1. If serum sodium concentration <160 mEq/L, water may be given orally.
      2. If hypertonicity more marked, hypotonic saline solution should be given IV. Recommended hypotonic solution is D_5 0.45 NaCl or D_5 0.2 NaCl with 1 ampule sodium bicarbonate, supplemented with furosemide if needed in cases with associated volume excess.
      3. Infuse at two-thirds maintenance rate if patient not hypovolemic. Cerebral edema or seizures may occur if hypotonic saline solution administered too rapidly.
      4. If patient is hypovolemic, use normal saline solution.
      5. Goal is to lower Na^+ concentration no more than 10–15 mEq/L during first 24 hours and to restore osmolarity to normal over 36–72 hours. Check serum sodium every 2–4 hours during first 24 hours, then every 4–6 hours during the course of treatment.
      6. Once urine output established, add KCl 40 mEq/L.
   C. Peritoneal dialysis:
      1. Indications:
         a. Patient not responding to treatment.
         b. Na^+ >200 mEq/L.
         c. Renal impairment.
   D. Seizures:
      1. Consider mannitol 0.5–1.0 gm/kg to decrease intracranial pressure (controversial). This may be necessary if hypotonic saline solution has been administered too rapidly.
      2. See Chapter 22 for treatment recommendations.
XII. Prognosis:
   A. Expected response to treatment:
      1. Death frequent if serum levels >185 mEq/L.

TABLE 120–1.

General Treatment

Treatment	Indicated	Of No Value	Contraindicated
O_2	±		
IV	+		
ECG monitor	±		
Diuresis	+		
Acidification			X
Alkalinization		X	
Emesis*/lavage*		X/X	
Charcoal		X	
Cathartic		X	

*May be attempted if ingestion recent, especially with tablets.

2. Prognosis for full recovery good with appropriate supportive care, cautious administration of hypotonic intravenous fluid, rapid institution of dialysis if indicated.
   B. Expected complications and long-term effects: Intracerebral vascular injury from hyperosmolarity. Results in prolonged coma and seizures.
XIII. Disposition considerations:
   A. Admission considerations:
      1. See General Admission Considerations (Chapters 17 and 18).
      2. Ingestions >0.5–1.0 gm/kg have potential for serious toxicity.
      3. Signs and symptoms suggestive of toxic ingestion: fever, depressed level of consciousness, severe nausea, vomiting, abdominal pain.
      4. Serum sodium level >160 mEq/L regardless of symptoms.
      5. Suicide risk.
      6. ICU: If dialysis indicated.
   B. Consultation considerations: Nephrology or dialysis service.
   C. Observation period: Since salt is rapidly absorbed following ingestion, a few hours of observation with repeated serum Na^+ should suffice. Appropriate only for those patients initially asymptomatic with serum Na^+ <160 mEq/L and without underlying illness.
   D. Discharge considerations:
      1. General discharge considerations have been met (see Chapters 17 and 18).
      2. Significant ingestion (>0.5–1.0 gm/kg) has been ruled out.
      3. Attempts should not be made to lower Na^+ rapidly in the emergency department to allow for discharge, since precipitous falls in serum sodium may result in significant complications (e.g., cerebral edema, seizures).
      4. Suicide potential and psychiatric status have been appropriately evaluated.

BIBLIOGRAPHY

Barer J, Hill LL, Hill RM, et al: Fatal poisoning from salt used as an emetic. *Am J Dis Child* 1973; 125:889.

Finberg L, Guttrell C: Mass accidental salt poisoning in infancy. *JAMA* 1963; 184:187.

Johnston J, Robertson W, West J: Fatal ingestion of table salt by an adult. *West J Med* 1977; 126:141.

Levin T: What this patient didn't need: A dose of salts. *Hosp Prac* 1983; 18:95.

Saunders N, Balfe J, Laski B: Severe salt poisoning in an infant. *J Pediatr* 1976; 88:258.

Index